Prostate Cancer

Contemporary Cancer Research

Prostate Cancer

Biology, Genetics, and the New

Therapeutics

Edited by

Leland W. K. Chung, PhD

University of Virginia School of Medicine, Charlottesville, VA

William B. Isaacs, PhD

The Johns Hopkins University School of Medicine, Baltimore, MD

Jonathan W. Simons, MD

The Johns Hopkins Hospital, Baltimore, MD

Humana Press ✳ Totowa, New Jersey

© 2001 Humana Press Inc.
999 Riverview Drive, Suite 208
Totowa, New Jersey 07512

Due diligence has been taken by the publishers, editors, and authors of this book to assure the accuracy of the information published and to describe generally accepted practices. The contributors herein have carefully checked to ensure that the drug selections and dosages set forth in this text are accurate and in accord with the standards accepted at the time of publication. Notwithstanding, as new research, changes in government regulations, and knowledge from clinical experience relating to drug therapy and drug reactions constantly occurs, the reader is advised to check the product information provided by the manufacturer of each drug for any change in dosages or for additional warnings and contraindications. This is of utmost importance when the recommended drug herein is a new or infrequently used drug. It is the responsibility of the treating physician to determine dosages and treatment strategies for individual patients. Further it is the responsibility of the health care provider to ascertain the Food and Drug Administration status of each drug or device used in their clinical practice. The publisher, editors, and authors are not responsible for errors or omissions or for any consequences from the application of the information presented in this book and make no warranty, express or implied, with respect to the contents in this publication.

This publication is printed on acid-free paper. ∞
ANSI Z39.48-1984 (American Standards Institute) Permanence of Paper for Printed Library Materials.

Cover design by Patricia F. Cleary.
Cover artwork supplied by Dr. Leland W. K. Chung depicting Donald Coffey's Chinese brush painting (1994).

For additional copies, pricing for bulk purchases, and/or information about other Humana titles, contact Humana at the above address or at any of the following numbers: Tel: 973-256-1699; Fax: 973-256-8341; E-mail: humana@humanapr.com, or visit our Website: http://humanapress.com

Photocopy Authorization Policy:
Authorization to photocopy items for internal or personal use, or the internal or personal use of specific clients, is granted by Humana Press Inc., provided that the base fee of US $8.00 per copy, plus US $00.25 per page, is paid directly to the Copyright Clearance Center at 222 Rosewood Drive, Danvers, MA 01923. For those organizations that have been granted a photocopy license from the CCC, a separate system of payment has been arranged and is acceptable to Humana Press Inc. The fee code for users of the Transactional Reporting Service is: [0-89603-868-8/01 $10.00 + $00.25].

Printed in the United States of America. 10 9 8 7 6 5 4 3 2 1

Library of Congress Cataloging in Publication Data

Prostate cancer: biology, genetics and the new therapeutics/edited by Leland W.K. Chung, William B. Isaacs, Jonathan W. Simons.
        p. ; cm.—(Contemporary cancer research)
   Includes bibliographical references and index.
   ISBN 0-89603-868-8 (alk. paper)
      1. Prostate—Cancer. 2. Prostate—Cancer—Genetic aspects. 3.
   Prostate—Cancer—Treatment. I. Chung, Leland W. K. II. Isaacs. William Brewster. III.
   Simons, Jonathan W. IV. Series.
      [DNLM: 1. Prostatic Neoplasms—genetics. 2. Prostatic Neoplasms—pathology. 3.
   Prostatic Neoplasms—therapy. WJ 752 P96553 2001]
   RC280.P7 P7585 2001
   616.99'463—dc21
                                                                              00-040712

Contents

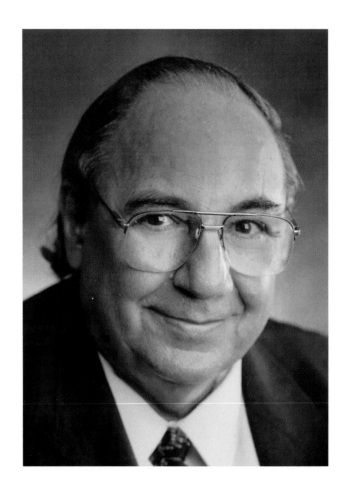

Donald S. Coffey, PhD.

Preface

This book embraces the wide field of prostate cancer genetics, biology, and therapy. It seems most appropriate to dedicate it to Donald S. Coffey, PhD, whose research vision is an inspiration to his colleagues and friends. Unraveling the secrets of prostate cancer is an intricate and sometimes frustrating process involving many researchers and many institutions. No one has seen through to the end of this road, and the list of researchers who have contributed to our understanding of the disease processes of prostate cancer is already a long one. But Donald Coffey stands out in his personal qualities as surely as in his roles as teacher and researcher. In the dedicatory article that begins this volume, Dr. Ward has spoken for all of us about Don Coffey's unique determination to build the road to defeat prostate cancer.

This book is divided into three sections: Cancer Genetics, Cancer Biology, and Cancer Therapeutics. These sections, like the skill and knowledge of the contributors, overlap in many dimensions. The divisions between sections are somewhat arbitrary and have been made expressly for the convenience of the reader. The reader will find chapters in each section that illuminate aspects of the genetics, biology, and therapy of prostate cancer. Nothing better illustrates the breadth of the research being conducted today by these distinguished groups, who truly understand and appreciate the power of multidisciplinary and translational approaches to deciphering the intricacy of the object of this research.

The first section of this book is devoted to Cancer Genetics. The effect that the progress in sequencing and characterizing the human genome has had on cancer genetics in general cannot be underestimated, both conceptually and methodologically. The section presented here on Cancer Genetics reflects this progress and provides a comprehensive review of our current understanding of the molecular genetic aspects of prostate cancer, as well as a roadmap for progress to come. In the initial chapter of this section, Drs. Isaacs, Walsh, and Xu provide an overview of the ongoing efforts to identify prostate cancer susceptibility genes through the study of hereditary prostate cancer (HPC) families. These extensive efforts by many laboratories have led to the realization that HPC is a highly heterogeneous disease, most likely due to a number of different HPC loci. Though four putative HPC loci have been localized through linkage studies, the cloning of the prostate equivalents of *BRCA1* and *BRCA2* has yet to be realized.

Dr. Bookstein provides an update on the status of our understanding of tumor suppressor genes inactivated in prostate cancer, including the recent exciting finding that the *PTEN* gene is frequently inactivated during prostate carcinogenesis, and how knowledge of such genes may be useful in diagnostics, prognostics, and therapeutics.

The reasons for renewed intense interest in androgen receptor (AR) and androgen metabolism are presented by the three chapters focused on this topic. By reviewing the evidence for frequent increases in AR gene copy number that accompany progression to hormone refractory disease, Dr. Visakorpi develops the interesting hypothesis that instead of being androgen independent, these tumors may be androgen *hyper*sensitive, owing to an overactivity of the AR pathway along with other molecular changes selected for during this process. Drs. Febbo and Kantoff summarize the fascinating data demonstrating the prostate cancer risk modifying properties attributable to polymorphic variants of the AR. Dr. Ross and colleagues extend this approach to include polymorphisms in other components of the androgen action pathway, as well as other prostate growth regulatory pathways as potentially important prostate cancer risk modifiers. These exciting and critically important areas and approaches of exploration will undoubtedly become more active as the extent of polymorphism in these and other critical prostate regulatory pathways are further defined and appreciated.

Although clinically localized prostate cancer is the research material that is most readily abundant and therefore most commonly studied, a full understanding of prostate carcinogenesis is impossible without examining the extremes of the disease progression spectrum, i.e., precursor lesions and lethal disease. Dr. Emmert-Buck and colleagues and Drs. Qian and Jenkins provide an exceptional overview of the genetic alterations found in PIN lesions using a wide variety of molecular techniques. An extensive study into the nature and extent of chromosome dosage changes that accompany prostate progression are described as well. Dr. Bova and colleagues have prepared an extensive historical review of several hundred prostate cancer autopsy studies, providing a conceptual framework to generate questions and approaches addressing the key mechanistic events underlying the lethal phenotype.

The lack of appropriate experimental models that accurately mimic the human disease has long been a problem for prostate cancer researchers. Drs. Sawyers and Reiter describe the series of recently developed prostate cancer xenograft models that they and others have developed and some of the elegant molecular biological insights that these models have already afforded.

One of the most active areas in the current molecular technology revolution is transcriptome profiling, coupled with proteomics or the ability to obtain a comprehensive view of gene expression patterns on a genome wide level. In addition to a discussion of this topic by Dr. Emmert-Buck and colleagues, Dr. Nelson describes his pioneering studies in this area, and provides an insightful outline of what the future holds for this promising approach.

The section on Cancer Biology includes a great deal of fresh and ongoing research, much of it suggesting some very welcome new possibilities for therapeutic intervention. Dr. Getzenberg describes the nuclear matrix and its role in regulating gene expression and alteration in cancer. The potential exists, after further refining the analytical techniques, for identifying new forms of nuclear matrix proteins and raising unique antibodies against them. This could provide badly needed new tools for prostate cancer diagnosis and therapeutic targeting. Dr. Hsieh describes another interesting cell structural component—cell adhesion molecules (CAMs)—and their role in regulating prostate development and carcinogenesis. The CAMs are a large family known to regulate key intercellular and intracellular communication pathways between and within cells. Dr. Hsieh summarizes recent advances in the study of CAMs in prostate biology and the potential application of CAMs to prostate cancer management.

Dr. Tindall and his colleague Dr. Mora carefully define the physiologic and pathophysiologic role of androgen receptor in prostate cancer cells. Their chapter clarifies the often confusing terminology of androgen-dependent and androgen-independent prostate cancer cells. They extensively describe ligand-dependent and -independent activation of androgen receptor in the context of normal and diseased tissues. Dr. Kung and his colleagues describe the roles of tyrosine kinases in prostate cancer cellular signaling. They have profiled tyrosine kinases in human prostate tumor models, and provide mechanistic insight into signal transduction pathways that may regulate the biology and behavior of prostate cancer cells at various stages of tumor progression.

Dr. Thompson and his colleagues introduce a new entity, Caveolin-1, as a metastasis-related gene in prostate cancer. This gene was discovered using a differential display PCR technique in an in vivo metastatic mouse prostate reconstitution model established in Dr. Thompson's laboratory. They propose that Caveolin-1 overexpression is associated with metastasis and androgen resistance. It is exciting to think about the potential role of Caveolin-1 as a survival factor, interacting with signal transduction cascades and serving to protect both natural and cytotoxic drug-mediated barriers to malignant progression.

Drs. Joseph and Isaacs review the process of angiogenesis in prostate cancer. Building on their own research expertise in this vital area, they explore the molecular and cellular basis of regulating angiogenesis in normal and pathologic conditions. Working through different targeting strategies to find a way to regulate angiogenesis is going to be a crucial step in defeating prostate cancer. Dr. Heston and his colleagues Drs. O'Keefe and Dr. Bacich describe an exciting potential new marker, prostate-specific membrane antigen (PSMA) for tumor-associated vasculature. PSMA is highly expressed in virtually all prostate tumors and metastases, and particularly in androgen refractory disease. They speculate that PSMA might be a highly valuable marker and treatment target not only for prostate cancer, but for several other solid tumors.

The basic biology and regulatory pathways controlling growth, progression to androgen independence, and resistance to chemotherapy are fundamental to the study of prostate cancer. Dr. Gleave and his colleagues, and Drs. Chung and Zhau provide new approaches and insights into targeting disease progression, based upon androgen withdrawal-induced apoptosis and stromal–epithelial interaction. Dr. Gleave and colleagues describe both human and mouse prostate cancer androgen-independent progression models, and begin to define potential therapeutic targets in these models using antisense strategy approaches. These approaches potentially could be applied either by themselves or in combination with other intervention strategies to block androgen-independent progression in clinical prostate cancers. Drs. Chung and Zhau summarize the basic concept of stromal–epithelial interaction in normal prostate growth and in malignant prostate cancer progression. By defining the potential mechanism and pathways between stromal and epithelial communication, they and their colleagues have moved the concept from the lab bench to the hospital bedside, using a gene therapy approach to deliver therapeutic genes to target cells, driven by tissue-specific promoters.

Overall, the section on Cancer Biology is devoted to the basic biology and regulatory mechanisms controlling prostate cancer growth and progression. These authors have unique experience and knowledge in their respective areas of expertise, and have indeed shone a new light on the future of prostate cancer diagnosis and treatment.

The section on Cancer Therapeutics is predicated on the view that the future of prostate cancer treatment will see incremental progress and improvements in patient survival in coming years, thanks to research in experimental therapeutics and pharmacology. Progress will be based on finding the intersections where discoveries on the level of basic science can be turned into medical opportunities. Historians will trace the improvement in prostate cancer survival in the 21st century to the foundations of scholarship laid, in large part, by Don Coffey and his many students in the fields of molecular pharmacology, cytotoxics, immunotherapy, antiprogression agents, nutrition, endocrinology, and gene therapy, to name only a few contributions.

In their chapter, Drs. Brooks and Dr. Nelson address the chemoprevention of prostate cancer, focusing on the identification of risk factors and particularly on the identification of a somatic molecular genetic lesion, in which cancers lose expression of the enzyme glutathione S-transferase-p (GSTP1).

Drs. Han and Partin discuss the current status of radical retropubic prostatectomy, finding that radical retropubic prostatectomy achieves excellent cancer control in men with clinically localized prostate cancer, even though there are some differences in tumor progression after surgery from different institutions. Drs. Ramakrishna and DeWeese similarly survey the current status of radiotherapy, and find that the skilled synthesis of current radiotherapy with the new molecular paradigms for therapy and risk stratification holds great promise for significant progress in the fight against prostate cancer.

Drs. Kamradt and Pienta review the status of chemotherapy in patients with hormone refractory prostate cancer. Currently, chemotherapy regimens are available that can reduce the burden of disease. Response rates are improving and patients are demonstrating clinical improvement. Also, the combination of chemotherapy with novel tumor growth suppressing agents offers a new paradigm for the management of hormone refractory prostate cancer in the next century. Dr. Nelson addresses the role of small bioactive peptides and cell surface peptidases in androgen independent prostate cancer. The propensity of prostate cancer to survive despite androgen withdrawal continues to haunt efforts to cure the disease. Recent advances have identified the roles of bioactive peptides, their receptors, and cell surface peptidases in this lethal phenotype of prostate cancer, and therapeutic intervention, based on this new understanding, is underway.

Drs. Tjoa and Murphy discuss progress in the development of a dendritic cell based vaccine for cancer of the prostate gland. Vaccine therapy may provide an alternative therapy for patients with hormone refractory metastatic prostate cancer. Administration of dendritic cells pulsed with PSMA peptides induced cellular immune responses against the tumor with virtually no adverse effects.

Hadley M. Wood and Dr. Carducci provide a brief overview of the current state of differentiation therapies. Recent new work in the field of antiproliferation agents, however, has been encouraging. Differentiation therapies, particularly in combination with each other, are demonstrating encouraging antitumor effects and lower negative side effects in advanced PCA. This area of research may develop drugs that will provide an effective, low toxicity first-line treatment for newly diagnosed patients with PCA.

Drs. Ferrer, Simons, and Rodriguez present a very thoughtful chapter on gene therapy, calling for research to be focused primarily on improved vector development for applications in urological disease—in particular, improved gene transfer *in situ*.

They argue that methods of augmenting current vector efficacy can be achieved by combination strategies. Efforts are being directed at radiosensitization, chemo-sensitization, and various combination strategies which may help optimize gene therapy efficacy.

In the final chapter of this section, Drs. Greenwald and Lieberman discuss chemo-prevention trials for prostate cancer. They consider that it will be important to convince the healthcare community and the general population of the practical value of a chemopreventive approach to carcinogenesis in its early stages before clinical symptoms are present. Developing methods that will enable clinicians to readily identify and stratify individuals at increased risk for prostate cancer is of critical importance to the optimization of the potential public health benefits of a chemopreventive approach.

As this book reveals, prostate cancer is a vast and multifaceted field of research. It may be that even the exact dimensions of this field are as yet imperfectly known and that the research done so far is only a beginning. Certainly the authors of this book are only a cross-section of the many research teams working across the nation and around the world. Unraveling the mysteries of prostate cancer will be a vast undertaking. But we have begun to do it, and when we reflect on the breadth and depth of the research that is attacking this problem, and on the inspiration provided by visionaries like Dr. Coffey, it begins to seem possible that some of the threads have come into our hands.

Leland W.K. Chung, PhD
William B. Isaacs, PhD
Jonathan W. Simons, MD

In Memoriam

We are indebted to the late Dr. Gerald Murphy for his contributions to this textbook and to prostate cancer research over his long and valuable career. He will be greatly missed by the research community.

Contributors

DEAN J. BACICH, PhD • *Department of Cancer Biology, The Lerner Research Institute, Cleveland Clinic Foundation, Cleveland, OH*

ROBERT BOOKSTEIN, MD • *Canji Inc., San Diego, CA*

G. STEVEN BOVA, MD • *Brady Urological Institute, The Johns Hopkins Hospital, Baltimore, MD*

JAMES D. BROOKS, MD • *Department of Urology, Stanford University Medical Center, Stanford, CA*

MICHAEL A. CARDUCCI, MD • *The Johns Hopkins Oncology Center, Baltimore, MD*

KIRK M. CHAN-TACK, MD • *Brady Urological Institute, The Johns Hopkins Hospital, Baltimore, MD*

LELAND W. K. CHUNG, PhD • *Molecular Urology and Therapeutics Program, The University of Virginia School of Medicine, Charlottesville, VA*

GERHARD A. COETZEE, PhD • *Departments of Preventive Medicine, Urology and Biochemistry, Keck School of Medicine at the University of Southern California, Norris Comprehensive Cancer Center, San Diego, CA*

KRISTINA A. COLE, MD, PhD • *Pathogenetics Unit, Laboratory of Pathology, National Cancer Institute, Bethesda, MD*

RALPH W. DEVERE WHITE, MD • *Department of Urology, UC Davis Cancer Center, UC Davis School of Medicine, Sacramento, CA*

THEODORE L. DEWEESE, MD • *Division of Radiation Oncology and the Brady Urological Institute, The Johns Hopkins Hospital, Baltimore, MD*

PAUL H. DURAY, MD • *Laboratory of Pathology, National Cancer Institute, Bethesda, MD*

MICHAEL R. EMMERT-BUCK, MD, PhD • *Pathogenics Unit, Laboratory of Pathology, National Cancer Institute, Bethesda, MD*

CHAD R. ENGLERT, MD • *Pathogenetics Unit, Laboratory of Pathology, National Cancer Institute, Bethesda, MD*

PHILLIP G. FEBBO, MD • *Lank Center for Genitourinary Oncology, Dana Farber Cancer Center, Harvard Medical School, Boston, MA*

FERNANDO FERRER, MD • *Brady Urological Institute, The Johns Hopkins Oncology Center, NIH, SPORE in Prostate Cancer, Baltimore, MD*

ROBERT H. GETZENBERG, PhD • *Prostate and Urological Cancer Center, The University of Pittsburgh Cancer Institute, Pittsburgh, PA*

JOHN W. GILLESPIE, MD • *Laboratory of Pathology, National Cancer Institute, Bethesda, MD*

MARTIN E. GLEAVE, MD • *Division of Urology, The University of British Columbia and the Prostate Center, Vancouver General Hospital, Vancouver, British Columbia, Canada*

ALEXEI GOLTSOV, PhD • *Department of Urology, Baylor College of Medicine, Houston, TX*

PETER GREENWALD, MD, DrPH • *Division of Cancer Prevention, National Cancer Institute, National Institutes of Health, Bethesda, MD*

MISOP HAN, MD • *Department of Urology, James Buchanan Brady Urological Institute, The John Hopkins University School of Medicine, Baltimore, MD*

WARREN D. W. HESTON, PhD • *Department of Cancer Biology and the Urology Institute, George M. O'Brien Urology Research Center/ The Lerner Research Institute, Cleveland Clinic Foundation, Cleveland, OH*

STEPHEN M. HEWITT, MD, PhD • *Laboratory of Pathology, National Cancer Institute, Bethesda, MD*

JER-TSONG HSIEH, PhD • *Department of Urology, University of Texas Southwestern Medical Center, Dallas, TX*

SUE ANN INGLES, PhD • *Departments of Preventive Medicine, Urology and Biochemistry, Keck School of Medicine at the University of Southern California, Norris Comprehensive Cancer Center, San Diego, CA*

JOHN T. ISAACS, PhD • *The Johns Hopkins Oncology Center, Baltimore, MD*

WILLIAM B. ISAACS, PhD • *Departments of Urology and Oncology, The Johns Hopkins University School of Medicine, Baltimore, MD*

ROBERT B. JENKINS, MD, PhD • *Laboratory of Medicine, Division of Laboratory Genetics, Mayo Clinic, Mayo Medical School, Rochestor, MN*

INGRID B. J. K. JOSEPH, DVM, PhD • *Johns Hopkins Oncology Center (currently with Abbott Laboratories), Baltimore, MD*

JEFFREY M. KAMRADT, MD • *University of Michigan Medical Center, Ann Arbor, MI*

PHILIP W. KANTOFF, MD • *Lank Center for Genitourinary Oncology, Dana Farber Cancer Center, Harvard Medical School, Boston, MA*

DAVID B. KRIZMAN, PhD • *Laboratory of Pathology, National Cancer Institute, Bethesda, MD*

HSING-JIEN KUNG, PhD • *Department of Biological Chemistry, UC Davis Cancer Center, UC Davis School of Medicine, Sacramento, CA*

WILLIAM W. LECATES, MD • *Brady Urological Institute, The Johns Hopkins Hospital, Baltimore, MD*

SIMON LEUNG, MB • *Division of Urology, University of British Columbia/Prostate Center, Vancouver General Hospital, Vancouver, British Columbia, Canada*

LIKUN LI, PhD • *Department of Urology, Baylor College of Medicine, Houston, TX*

RONALD LIEBERMAN, MD • *Division of Cancer Prevention, Prostate and Urologic Cancer Research Group, National Cancer Institute, National Institutes of Health, Bethesda, MD*

W. MARSTON LINEHAN, MD • *Urologic Oncology Branch, National Cancer Institute, Bethesda, MD*

HIDEAKI MIYAKE, MD, PhD • *Division of Urology, University of British Columbia and the Prostate Center, Vancouver General Hospital, Vancouver, British Columbia, Canada*

GLORIA R. MORA, PhD • *Departments of Biochemistry and Molecular Biology, Mayo Foundation, Rochester, MN*

GERALD P. MURPHY, MD, DSC • *Pacific Northwest Cancer Foundation, Seattle, WA*

COLLEEN NELSON, PhD • *Division of Urology, University of British Columbia and the Prostate Center, Vancouver General Hospital, Vancouver, British Columbia, Canada*

JOEL B. NELSON, MD • *Brady Urological Institute, The Johns Hopkins Medical Institution, (currently at the University of Pittsburgh, PA), Baltimore, MD*

PETER S. NELSON, MD • *Program in Genomics, Division of Human Biology, Fred Hutchinson Cancer Research Center, Seattle, WA*

WILLIAM G. NELSON, MD, PhD • *The Johns Hopkins Oncology Center, Baltimore, MD*

DENISE S. O'KEEFE, PhD • *Department of Cancer Biology, The Lerner Research Institute, Cleveland Clinic Foundation, Cleveland, OH*

DAVID K. ORNSTEIN, MD • *Urologic Oncology Branch, National Cancer Institute, Bethesda, MD*

ALAN W. PARTIN, MD, PhD • *Department of Urology, James Buchanan Brady Urological Institute, The John Hopkins University School of Medicine, Baltimore, MD*

EMANUEL F. PETRICOIN, PhD • *Center for Biologics and Research, Food and Drug Administration, Bethesda, MD*

KENNETH J. PIENTA, MD • *University of Michigan Medical Center, Ann Arbor, MI*

JUNQI QIAN, MD • *Department of Molecular Diagnostics, Bostwick Laboratories, Richmond, VA*

NAREN R. RAMAKRISHNA, MD, PhD • *Division of Radiation Oncology, The Johns Hopkins Hospital, Baltimore, MD*

JUERGEN K. V. REICHARDT, PhD • *Departments of Preventive Medicine, Urology and Biochemistry, Keck School of Medicine at the University of Southern California, Norris Comprehensive Cancer Center, San Diego, CA*

ROBERT E. REITER, MD • *Departments of Urology and Medicine, University of California, Los Angeles, CA*

CHENGZEN REN, MS • *Department of Urology, Baylor College of Medicine, Houston, TX*

PAUL RENNIE, PhD • *Division of Urology, University of British Columbia/Prostate Center, Vancouver General Hospital, Vancouver, British Columbia, Canada*

RONALD RODRIGUEZ, MD • *Brady Urological Institute, The Johns Hopkins Hospital, Baltimore, MD*

RONALD K. ROSS, MD • *Departments of Preventative Medicine, Urology and Biochemistry, Norris Comprehensive Cancer Center, Keck School of Medicine at the University of Southern California, San Diego, CA*

CHARLES L. SAWYERS, MD • *Departments of Urology and Medicine, University of California, Los Angeles, CA*

JONATHAN W. SIMONS, MD • *Brady Urological Institute, The Johns Hopkins Hospital, Baltimore, MD. (Currently at the Winship Cancer Institute, The Emory University School of Medicine, Atlanta, GA)*

SALAHALDIN TAHIR, PhD • *Department of Urology, Baylor College of Medicine, Houston, TX*

CLIFFORD G. TEPPER, PhD • *Department of Biological Chemistry, UC Davis Cancer Center, UC Davis School of Medicine, Sacramento, CA*

TIMOTHY C. THOMPSON, PhD • *Departments of Urology, Molecular and Cell Biology, and Radiology, Baylor College of Medicine, Houston, TX*

TERRY L. TIMME, PhD • *Department of Urology, Baylor College of Medicine, Houston, TX*

DONALD J. TINDALL, PhD • *Department of Urology, Mayo Foundation, Rochester, MN*

BENJAMIN A. TJOA, PhD • *Northwest Biotherapeutics Inc., Pacific Northwest Cancer Foundation, Seattle, WA*

TAPIO VISAKORPI, MD, PhD • *Laboratory of Cancer Genetics, Institute of Medical Technology, University of Tampere, Tampere, Finland*

CATHY D. VOCKE, PhD • *Urologic Oncology Branch, National Cancer Institute, Bethesda, MD*

PATRICK C. WALSH, MD • *Department of Urology, Johns Hopkins University School of Medicine/James Buchanan Brady Urological Institute, The Johns Hopkins Hospital, Baltimore, MD*

W. STEVEN WARD, PhD • *Institute for Biogenesis Research, Department of Anatomy and Reproductive Biology, University of Hawaii School of Medicine, Honolulu, HI*

HADLEY M. WOOD • *The John Hopkins University School of Medicine, Baltimore, MD*

JIANFENG XU, MD, DrPH • *Department of Public Health Sciences, Wake Forest University School of Medicine, Winston-Salem, NC*

GUANG YANG, MD, PhD • *Department of Urology, Baylor College of Medicine, Houston, TX*

HAIYEN E. ZHAU, PhD • *Molecular Urology and Therapeutics Program, University of Virginia School of Medicine, Charlottesville, VA*

PART I

INTRODUCTION

Building the Road to Defeat Prostate Cancer

A Dedication to Donald S. Coffey

W. Steven Ward, PhD

1. INTRODUCTION

Prostate Cancer: Biology, Genetics, and the New Therapeutics is dedicated to Donald S. Coffey, PhD. The fact that so many distinguished scientists readily agreed to contribute a substantial effort to this volume says more about the honor and respect this field has for Don Coffey than we could ever hope to convey in a short introduction. But part of the labor of love that went into this book dictates that we attempt to include a few words of a personal nature about the man we are honoring. Readers who do not know Don Coffey can assume that he is a leader in the field of prostate cancer research because a volume was dedicated to him on the subject. But why did the authors of these chapters choose *this* scientist to honor, and why was *this* title chosen to represent the work that would honor him?

Those of us who know him best will understand why we have chosen to begin with the story of a personal encounter. Years ago, when I left Don Coffey's lab to begin my own at another institution, he drew a diagram on a napkin to illustrate a point that his life embodies. It was essentially the one reproduced in Fig. 1, but without any of the words. He was telling me to examine any scientific problem from as many different angles as possible—that the worst mistake would be to limit myself to my favorite approach. During his 40 years at Johns Hopkins University, in which he focused primarily on prostate cancer, he taught many of the current leaders in the field by his example. The key to his art of penetrating focus was to approach one problem from several different viewpoints. This is how Don Coffey approaches everything in life, especially those things for which we honor him most—his scientific creativity, his unfaltering integrity, his brilliant and charismatic leadership, his passionate teaching, and his boundless humanity. With this introduction, we will address the two questions posed in the first paragraph in an effort to document at least a part of what he has given to the study of prostate cancer, and to the students he will eventually leave behind. Happily, this will be an incomplete task, since as of this writing, Don Coffey's laboratory is at its peak of activity, with no sign of slowing down.

From: *Prostate Cancer: Biology, Genetics, and the New Therapeutics*
Edited by: L. W. K. Chung, W. B. Isaacs, and J. W. Simons © Humana Press Inc., Totowa, NJ

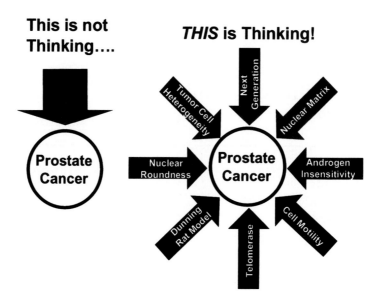

Fig. 1. This figure illustrates the penetrating creative focus that Don Coffey has applied to his lifelong goal of studying prostate cancer. The diagram is modified from one that he has used to illustrate how to think about any problem. One approaches the problem from as many different angles and viewpoints as possible. The individual arrows are labeled with the areas in which Don Coffey has made major contributions in the understanding of prostate cancer.

2. APPROACHING PROSTATE CANCER WITH AN OPEN MIND

Let us begin with Don Coffey's scientific contributions to our study of prostate cancer—the immediate subject of this book. It is important to note at the outset that he has made significant contributions in basic cell biology, to our understanding of the mechanisms of prostate cancer progression, and directly to clinical aspects of the disease, including the development of new treatments. Thus, his scientific accomplishments have spanned every aspect of the disease.

Don Coffey was a successful chemical engineer, beginning at North American Rayon in Tennessee when he made the decision to commit his life's work to the study of cancer. He moved on to another engineering job at Westinghouse in Baltimore, so that he could be closer to Johns Hopkins University, where he enrolled in graduate school in 1960. His dissertation focused on the role of sulfhydryl groups in D-amino-acid oxidase. Throughout his career, he would apply these experiences in engineering, chemistry, and biochemistry as major elements of his arsenal in solving difficult problems in prostate cancer in ways that no one else had considered. But it was mainly his ability to see the problem with an unbiased focus that would permit him to design these ground-breaking experiments. Don Coffey made multiple contributions to our knowledge of prostate cancer, as suggested in Fig. 1, but space permits us to describe only a few.

2.1. Androgen Insensitivity in Prostate Cancer

Don Coffey began his work on prostate cancer by studying the effects of androgens. When he began his work, the biggest problem was that of androgen insensitivity.

Charles Huggins had demonstrated that metastatic prostate cancer responded to androgen withdrawal, but it was quickly understood that this treatment only prolonged the life of the patients. The cancer nearly always progressed to a stage where it could grow independently of androgens. Coffey approached this problem by attempting to understand the basics of the normal prostate's dependency on androgens *(7–9)*. This subject would remain a major focus of his career. Together with John Isaacs, he first developed methods to experimentally identify androgen-insensitive tumors *(18)*, and then demonstrated that progression to androgen insensitivity was a clonal selection of a few cells rather than an induction of many *(20)*. This work has tremendous implications in the ongoing clinical debate on whether to treat patients with hormonal therapy early or late in the course of their disease, and Don Coffey has frequently been asked to comment on the results of clinical trials on major symposia panels because of this work.

2.2. The Dunning Rat Prostate Cancer Cell Lines

Early in his career, Coffey recognized the need for a good animal model to study prostate cancer. In 1977, he and two other groups reported that the Dunning R-3327 was an important model for prostate cancer *(30)*. Shortly thereafter, his laboratory developed androgen-independent lines from this original spontaneous tumor that would serve as important models for the development of androgen insensitivity and metastasis *(17–19)*. Today, this model continues to be one of the most important animal models for prostate cancer. Using this model, tumor metastasis genes have been isolated from human cancers, chemotherapy regimes have been designed, and the development of androgen insensitivity has been understood.

2.3. Genetic Instability and Tumor Cell Heterogeneity

Coffey's work on the development of androgen insensitivity led him directly into a new field in cancer research—which embraced the idea that an individual patient's tumor consists of a population of cells that are extremely heterogenous genetically, phenotypically, and behaviorally. This concept had already been suggested by the mechanism proposed by Coffey and Isaacs for the development of androgen insensitivity— clonal selection. Why were these androgen-insensitive cells present in the tumor in the first place? One possible answer is that heterogeneous cells are a hallmark of all cancers. Coffey approached this possibility first by developing some ideas on mechanisms of genetic instability and presenting them at a meeting he hosted at Johns Hopkins University on the subject of tumor cell heterogeneity *(1–3)*. He then took a more direct approach with a typically unique set of experiments. Together with a urologic oncology fellow named Mitchell Benson, he isolated the cells from the Dunning rat prostate cancer line and separated them by two different physical parameters *(1–3)*. Individual clones isolated from this separation were grown, the resulting cells were separated again, and the heterogeneity was repeated. These experiments demonstrated that the tumors contained phenotypically heterogeneous cells, and that each individual cell produced heterogeneous clones. This finding had tremendous implications for the development of drug resistance in all tumors, and for the progression of cancers over the long periods of time that they exist in patients.

2.4. The Nuclear Matrix and Prostate Cancer

Many researchers are familiar with Don Coffey because of his most important contribution to cell biology, seemingly unrelated to prostate cancer—the discovery of the nuclear matrix. However, even this important foray into the world of nuclear structure was directly related to his focus on prostate cancer. Drawing on his engineering background, Coffey focused on the structure of the cell. He reasoned that since pathologists routinely diagnosed cancer just by examining H&E stained cells, there must be an important structural aberration in the cancer cell that was distorted enough to be visible by light microscopy. He consulted a pathologist and learned that this aberration was usually a distorted nuclear shape. Coffey then hypothesized that a structural component of the nucleus must be responsible for its shape, and that one or more of these components was mutated or missing in cancer. Since the whole area of nuclear structure was in its infancy, he had to start at the beginning with the isolation and characterization of the normal structure. Together with a postdoctoral fellow, Ronald Berezney, he demonstrated that there was indeed such a structure, which they termed the nuclear matrix *(4,6)*. More importantly, Coffey's laboratory demonstrated that DNA synthesis occurred on the nuclear matrix *(5,24,31)*.

The discovery of the nuclear matrix launched an entire field of study in cell biology. Furthermore, Coffey eventually verified his original hypothesis that proteins of the nuclear matrix could be used to diagnose prostate cancer *(16,26,27)*. The principles of the nuclear matrix have also been used by one of Don Coffey's trainees to develop the most active chemotherapy protocols to date in the treatment of androgen-insensitive, metastatic prostate cancer *(23,28,29)*.

2.5. Nuclear Morphology and Cell Motility

The work on the nuclear matrix initiated with the study of the cancer-cell nucleus led to another fascinating and extremely important method of analyzing cancer specimens. Coffey was determined to answer a perplexing clinical question in prostate cancer—that of predicting which patients would fail surgery. A certain percentage of patients develop metastatic disease long after their surgery, even when the surgical margins are negative for disease and the lymph nodes are free of tumor cells. Because some of the patients' disease progressed even when the tumor appeared to be physically restricted to the prostate, Coffey reasoned that the difference between those tumors that eventually progressed after surgery and those that did not was an early event in the development of the tumor. Returning to his earlier lessons on the importance of nuclear structure to cell function, he hypothesized that the degree of distortion of the roundness of the nucleus could be quantified to predict the progression to metastatic disease. Together with David Diamond, a resident in the lab, he demonstrated that the degree of roundness could be used to predict which patients with organ-confined tumors would be most likely to develop metastatic prostate cancer *(13,14)*. This technique resulted in a surprising number of publications, and is to date the single best predictor of metastasis in this group of patients.

But Coffey was not yet satisfied that he fully understood the relationship between nuclear structure and cancer. After many discussions with fellow scientists, and much thinking about the problem, he finally concluded that the distortions in nuclear shape in the cancer cells on paraffin-embedded slides were really snapshots of very dynamically motile cells, and he began an intensive study on cell shape and motility. Coffey's approach was, once again, typically unique. Together with Allan Partin, and James Mohler, he first developed a visual grading system for motility using the Dunning cell lines *(22)*, and then a more sophisticated system using Fourier transform analysis of cell shape to quantitate motility *(25)*. An indication of the importance of this work, together with his analysis of nuclear shape, is that it earned Coffey the solicitation of several pathology departments across the country for chairmanship positions.

2.6. Other Contributions

Our discussion has covered only a few of Don Coffey's contributions to the study of prostate cancer. We do not have sufficient space to mention his ground-breaking work on telomerase in prostate cancer, his prolific contributions to the understanding of BPH, his work on genetic imprinting of the sex organs, and his contribution to the first gene-therapy trial for prostate cancer ever performed. What we have tried to emphasize is the creativity of his approach to studying the disease, and the wealth of discovery that has resulted from his multifaceted targeting of his goal of curing prostate cancer.

3. THE CHIEF OF PROSTATE CANCER

Don Coffey has also been a leader in the more traditional sense of the word. In 1982 he was featured in an issue of the *Hopkins Magazine*, in which the author remarked that everyone calls him " 'The Chief '. . . maybe because he addresses everyone as Chief " *(21)*. This appellation reveals far more than his familiar relationship with all those with whom he works. The Chief has taken on many leadership roles nationwide for the betterment of both the research itself and for the researchers. His ability to be a fair and compassionate leader as well as a highly successful one has required him to turn down far more leadership positions, both at Hopkins and nationwide, than it was possible for him to accept. Moreover, most of these roles were thrust upon him either by necessity or, more often, by popular demand. We will list only a few of these roles in an effort to document his leadership.

In 1971, Don Coffey began an 18-yr tenure on the NIH's National Prostatic Cancer Project, culminating in his chairmanship of the group from 1988 to 1989. This group was largely responsible for keeping prostate cancer at the forefront of the NIH's funding consideration, and Coffey was a constant advocate for the support of prostate-cancer research. He has served many leadership roles in the American Association for Cancer Research (AACR), including the Scientific Planning Committee and the Program Committee, and he was elected President in 1996 (he is still President-Elect). One of his most important leadership roles has been to break the boundary between clinical and basic researchers. He has been so successful at presenting basic scientific data to clinicians and presenting clinical data to basic scientists that basic research has become an integral part of the largely clinical meetings of the American Urological Association. Because of his leadership and example, basic scientists can now be members of this society.

In addition to these (and many other national committee roles), Don Coffey has always served as an ad-hoc advisor, traveling to Capitol Hill at a moment's notice to testify or to lobby privately with US Congressmen about the importance of prostate cancer research. He has been a constant and tireless champion of the importance of prostate cancer research funding in the United States, and many of the programs now available to researchers are a direct result of his efforts. He has also challenged us directly, through various editorials, to think a little more honestly about the way we approach our science *(12)*, about prostate cancer *(10)*, and about the way the nation funds cancer research *(11)*. His leadership roles usually fall into one of two categories— addressing a need that no one else recognized, or taking action when everyone else wanted him to lead the charge.

4. THE TEACHER

Finally, a word must be said about Don Coffey the teacher. Many of the authors in this volume, recognized leaders in the field of prostate cancer research, were trained in Don Coffey's laboratory. He has trained basic scientists to study prostate cancer, and he has trained physicians to study the clinical aspects of the disease. His trainees often become leaders in their fields, but they are not limited to prostate cancer, and this reveals something important about the man. In addition to his excellence in teaching science, Coffey's approach to working with young people is to focus on their dreams and talents, always putting their success ahead of his own. As Director of Urologic Research in the Department of Urology at Johns Hopkins University, he felt it was important to offer the broadest possible spectrum of research subjects to anyone who was in his laboratory. Although his immediate goal has always been to study cancer, he worked just as hard on projects relating to infertility or bladder infection if a student expressed a sincere desire to study such a topic that was outside his immediate research interests. All of his students could expect a lifetime of support from their mentor, and scientists who have never worked directly with him have benefitted from his dedication to serving others.

Don Coffey's lifelong dedication to selfless teaching has had a profound impact on the study of prostate cancer in this country. Through his teaching, he has produced two or three generations of researchers with the same dedication and standards of excellence he lives by. These researchers and their colleagues will undoubtedly contribute to the eventual cure of prostate cancer. Don Coffey has also earned the undying love and respect of all he has trained.

5. LOOKING AHEAD: THE TWENTY-FIRST CENTURY

This introduction to *Prostate Cancer: Biology, Genetics, and the New Therapeutics* is far too short to adequately describe all of the contributions Don Coffey has made to the study of prostate cancer and to its eventual cure. Our hope is to document enough to at least answer the two questions posed in the first paragraph. We have chosen to honor *this* scientist because he has made such unique and prolific contributions to the study of prostate cancer. We have chosen this title because it reflects the creativity and forward-thinking of the man this volume honors.

All that remains is to make a few comments on the book itself. The editors felt that the best way to honor Don Coffey was not to dwell on what has been accomplished, but to face forward and make an attempt to chart the path into the future. The major drawback of our effort is that we were unable to ask the one person who would be best suited for this task, since Don Coffey will not know of the existence of the volume until it is presented to him in its final form. Nevertheless, he has influenced the research of each one of those who were asked to participate in some way, and so he is participating in a way that is perhaps more real than any of the named authors. Many of his ideas, through lengthy discussions over many years, and much of his published research have been incorporated into each chapter. Each contributor has tried to formulate, to the best of their ability, a course for future research that is most likely to lead to finally curing this disease.

Thus, we have two hopes for this volume. First and foremost, it is a natural expression—and, therefore, a part of the immense legacy—that Don Coffey is still building for future generations of scientists. But we also hope that this effort will serve as a comprehensive guide to future researchers who are committed to the elimination of prostate cancer.

REFERENCES

1. Benson, M. C. and D. S. Coffey. 1983. Prostate cancer research: current concepts and controversies. *Sem. Urol.* **1**: 323–330.
2. Benson, M. C., D. C. McDougal, and D. S. Coffey. 1984. The application of perpendicular and forward light scatter to assess nuclear and cellular morphology. *Cytometry* **5**: 515–522.
3. Benson, M. C., D. C. McDougal, and D. S. Coffey. 1984. The use of multiparameter flow cytometry to assess tumor cell heterogeneity and grade prostate cancer. *Prostate* **5**: 27–45.
4. Berezney, R. and D. S. Coffey. 1974. Identification of a nuclear protein matrix. *Biochem. Biophys. Res. Commun.* **60**: 1410–1417.
5. Berezney, R. and D. S. Coffey. 1975. Nuclear protein matrix: association with newly synthesized DNA. *Science* **189**: 291–293.
6. Berezney, R. and D. S. Coffey. 1976. The nuclear protein matrix: isolation, structure, and functions. *Adv. Enzyme Regul.* **14**: 63–100.
7. Brasel, J. A., D. S. Coffey, and H. G. Williams-Ashman. 1968. Androgen-induced changes in the DNA polymerase activity of coagulating glands of castrated rats. *Med. Exp. Int. J. Exp. Med.* **18**: 321–326.
8. Chung, L. W. and D. S. Coffey. 1971. Biochemical characterization of prostatic nuclei. II. Relationship between DNA synthesis and protein synthesis. *Biochim. Biophys. Acta* **247**: 584–596.
9. Coffey, D. S., R. R. Ichinose, J. Shimazaki, and H. G. Williams-Ashman. 1968. Effects of testosterone on adenosine triphosphate and nicotinamide adenine dinucleotide levels, and on nicotinamide mononucleotide adenylytransferase activity, in the ventral prostate of castrated rats. *Mol. Pharmacol.* **4**: 580–590.
10. Coffey, D. S. 1993. Prostate cancer. An overview of an increasing dilemma. *Cancer* **71**: 880–886.
11. Coffey, D. S. 1996. Prostate cancer metastasis: talking the walk (news; comment). *Nat. Med.* **2**: 1305,1306.
12. Coffey, D. S. 1999. The real final exam. *Prostate* **39**: 323–325.
13. Diamond, D. A., S. J. Berry, H. J. Jewett, J. C. Eggleston, and D. S. Coffey. 1982. A new method to assess metastatic potential of human prostate cancer: relative nuclear roundness. *J. Urol.* **128**: 729–734.
14. Diamond, D. A., S. J. Berry, C. Umbricht, H. J. Jewett, and D. S. Coffey. 1982. Computerized image analysis of nuclear shape as a prognostic factor for prostatic cancer. *Prostate* **3**: 321–332.

15. Feinberg, A. P. and D. S. Coffey. 1982. The concept of DNA rearrangement in carcinogenesis and development of tumor cell heterogeneity, in *Tumor Cell Heterogeneity*, vol. 4 (Owens, A. H., D. S. Coffey, and S. B. Baylin, eds.), Academic Press, New York, pp. 469–488.

16. Getzenberg, R. H., K. J. Pienta, E. Y. Huang, and D. S. Coffey. 1991. Identification of nuclear matrix proteins in the cancer and normal rat prostate. *Cancer Res.* **51**: 6514–6520.

17. Isaacs, J. T., W. Heston, R. M. Weissman, and D. S. Coffey. 1978. Animal models of the hormone-sensitive and -insensitive prostatic adenocarcinomas, Dunning R-3327-H, R-3327-HI, and R-3327-AT. *Cancer Res.* **38**: 4353–4359.

18. Isaacs, J. T., W. B. Isaacs, and D. S. Coffey. 1979. Models for development of nonreceptor methods for distinguishing androgen-sensitive and -insensitive prostatic tumors. *Cancer Res.* **39**: 2652–2659.

19. Isaacs, J. T., G. W. Yu, and D. S. Coffey. 1981. The characterization of a newly identified, highly metastatic variety of Dunning R 3327 rat prostatic adenocarcinoma system: the MAT LyLu tumor. *Investig. Urol.* **19**: 20–23.

20. Isaacs, J. T., N. Wake, D. S. Coffey, and A. A. Sandberg. 1982. Genetic instability coupled to clonal selection as a mechanism for tumor progression in the Dunning R-3327 rat prostatic adenocarcinoma system. *Cancer Res.* **42**: 2353–2371.

21. Levine, J. 1985. The man who says YES. *Johns Hopkins Mag.* **36**: 34–44.

22. Mohler, J. L., A. W. Partin, and D. S. Coffey. 1987. Prediction of metastatic potential by a new grading system of cell motility: validation in the Dunning R-3327 prostatic adenocarcinoma model. *J. Urol.* **138**: 168–170.

23. Naik, H., J. E. Lehr, and K. J. Pienta. 1996. Inhibition of prostate cancer growth by 9-aminocamptothecin and estramustine. *Urology* **48**: 508–511.

24. Pardoll, D. M., B. Vogelstein, and D. S. Coffey. 1980. A fixed site of DNA replication in eucaryotic cells. *Cell* **19**: 527–536.

25. Partin, A. W., J. S. Schoeniger, J. L. Mohler, and D. S. Coffey. 1989. Fourier analysis of cell motility: correlation of motility with metastatic potential. *Proc. Natl. Acad. Sci. USA* **86**: 1254–1258.

26. Partin, A. W., R. H. Getzenberg, M. J. Carmichael, D. Vindivich, J. Yoo, D. S. Coffey, et al. 1993. Nuclear matrix protein patterns in human benign prostatic hyperplasia and prostate cancer. *Cancer Res.* **53**: 744–746.

27. Partin, A. W., J. V. Briggman, E. N. Subong, R. Szaro, A. Oreper, S. Wiesbrock, J. Meyer, D. S. Coffey, and J. I. Epstein. 1997. Preliminary immunohistochemical characterization of a monoclonal antibody (PRO:4-216) prepared from human prostate cancer nuclear matrix proteins. *Urology* **50**: 800–808.

28. Pienta, K. J., B. C. Murphy, W. B. Isaacs, J. T. Isaacs, and D. S. Coffey. 1992. Effect of pentosan, a novel cancer chemotherapeutic agent, on prostate cancer cell growth and motility. *Prostate* **20**: 233–241.

29. Pienta, K. J. and J. E. Lehr. 1993. Inhibition of prostate cancer growth by estramustine and etoposide: evidence for interaction at the nuclear matrix. *J. Urol.* **149**: 1622–1625.

30. Smolev, J. K., W. Heston, W. W. Scott, and D. S. Coffey. 1977. Characterization of the Dunning R3327H prostatic adenocarcinoma: an appropriate animal model for prostatic cancer. *Can. Treat. Rep.* **61**: 273–287.

31. Vogelstein, B., D. M. Pardoll, and D. S. Coffey. 1980. Supercoiled loops and eucaryotic DNA replicaton. *Cell* **22**: 79–85.

PART II

CANCER GENETICS

2

Hereditary Prostate Cancer

William B. Isaacs, PhD, Jianfeng Xu, MD, DrPH, and Patrick C. Walsh, MD

1. INTRODUCTION

One of the triumphs of molecular genetics during the past two decades has been the elucidation of the molecular mechanisms responsible for the inherited predisposition for a number of common human cancers. Genes such as *BRCA1*, *BRCA2*, *VHL*, *APC* and *hMSH2*—in which changes as small as single nucleotide substitutions result in greatly increased organ-specific cancer risk—have been identified through studies of familial breast, renal, and colorectal cancers. Major efforts are now underway world-wide to identify and characterize hereditary prostate cancer (HPC) genes through the study of prostate cancer families. Four separate loci suspected to harbor such genes have been identified to date, and efforts to clone the specific genes are in progress. A primary goal of these efforts is the development of genetic tests to determine which individuals carry high-risk prostate cancer alleles. This chapter provides an overview of the evidence supporting a hereditary form of prostate cancer, and summarizes the efforts to identify and characterize the genes responsible for hereditary prostate cancer (HPC).

2. FAMILIAL CLUSTERING OF PROSTATE CANCER

Evidence demonstrating a familial clustering of prostate cancer has been available as early as 1960 *(7)*, and multiple subsequent studies have confirmed this observation *(43,54,57,71,78)* (reviewed in ref. *30*). Two major studies are of particular interest in the determination of whether or not prostate cancer clusters in families. Cannon et al. *(7)* published a genetic epidemiological study on prostate cancer in the Utah Mormon population. Notably, prostate cancer exhibited the fourth strongest degree of familial clustering after lip, skin melanoma, and ovarian cancer. Prostate cancer had a higher familiality than either colon or breast carcinoma, two solid tumors which are well-recognized as having a genetic or familial component.

A case-controlled study of patients treated for prostate cancer at Johns Hopkins was carried out to assess the extent of familial aggregation in prostate cancer *(80)*. Extensive cancer pedigrees were obtained on 691 men with prostate cancer and 640 spouse controls. A positive family history of prostate cancer was the only consistent risk factor found in this study. Men with an affected father or brother were twice as likely to develop prostate cancer as men with no relatives affected. There was also a trend of

From: *Prostate Cancer: Biology, Genetics, and the New Therapeutics*
Edited by: L. W. K. Chung, W. B. Isaacs, and J. W. Simons © Humana Press Inc., Totowa, NJ

increasing risk with increasing number of affected family members, so that men with two or three first-degree relatives affected had a fivefold and 11-fold increased risk of developing prostate cancer. Cox proportional hazards analysis in the case relatives revealed that risk was particularly increased to relatives of younger probands (<55 yr).

These studies suggest a familial clustering in risk to prostate cancer, but do not directly address the underlying etiologic mechanism. Indeed, familial clustering can reflect either a shared environmental risk factor or a genetic mechanism. Two approaches which can be used to distinguish these possibilities are twin studies and complex segregation analysis.

3. TWIN STUDIES

The goal of twin studies is to compare the similarities (concordance rate) of a trait or disease in monozygotic (MZ) and dizygotic (DZ) twins to dissect the genetic and environmental components of a familial aggregation. Several twin studies of prostate cancer reported higher concordance rates in MZ twins compared to that of DZ twins, implicating a genetic contribution for familial aggregation of prostate cancer. Grönberg et al. *(26)* studied an unselected Swedish twin population. In 4840 male twin pairs, 458 prostate cancers were identified. Sixteen of the 1649 monozygotic twin pairs were concordant for prostate cancer (1.0%), compared with 6 of the 2983 dizygotic twin pair concordant for prostate cancer (0.2%). Using a cohort of 31,848 veteran twins born during the years 1917–1927, Page et al. *(63)* identified 1009 prostate cancer cases. There was a significantly higher concordance rate among monozygotic twin pairs (27.1%) than among dizygotic twin pairs (7.1%). Thus, both of these studies are consistent with a genetic basis for a least a portion of familial prostate cancer.

4. COMPLEX SEGREGATION ANALYSIS

By testing the fit of several models of inheritance (e.g., a major Mendelian gene model, an environmental model, and/or a polygene model) for the distribution of a disease in families, complex segregation analysis can identify the specific model that best describes the disease transmission in such families. Three complex segregation analyses of prostate cancer have been reported, and each is consistent with the hypothesis that one or more autosomal dominant susceptibility gene(s) exist *(8,27,70)*. Carter et al. *(8)* performed the first complex segregation analysis on 691 families, determined through prostate cancer probands undergoing radical prostatectomy for clinically localized prostate cancer at Johns Hopkins Hospital. This analysis indicated that the familial aggregation of prostate cancer could be best explained by autosomal dominant inheritance of a rare (disease gene frequency $q = 0.003$) high-risk allele leading to the early onset of prostate cancer. The estimated cumulative risk of prostate cancer by age 85 yr was 88% for carriers, vs 5% for noncarriers. Importantly, this inherited form of prostate cancer was estimated to account for a significant proportion of early-onset disease (43% of cases diagnosed under 55) and to be responsible for ~9% of all prostate cancer occurrences overall.

Grönberg et al. *(27)* carried out segregation analysis in an unselected population-based sample of 2857 nuclear families ascertained through an affected father diagnosed with prostate cancer in Sweden during 1959–1963. The results suggested that the observed familial aggregation of prostate cancer is best explained by a high-risk allele inherited in a dominant mode, with a high population frequency and a moderate lifetime penetrance (63%). The third complex segregation analysis by Schaid et al. *(70)* was performed to assess the genetic contribution to age at diagnosis and familial aggregation of prostate cancer in a sample of 5486 men who underwent a radical prostatectomy for clinically localized prostate cancer in the Mayo Clinic during the period from 1966 to 1995. The best-fitting model to explain the age at diagnosis and the familial aggregation proposed a rare autosomal dominant susceptibility gene, with the best fit observed when probands were diagnosed at <60 yr. The frequency of the rare allele was estimated to be 0.006 in the population, and the penetrances were 89% by age 85 yr for the carriers and 3% for the noncarriers. Thus, although the estimated parameters varied, each of these analyses provided support for the existence of high-risk alleles for prostate cancer, acting in a dominant Mendelian fashion. These results indicate that the genetics of prostate cancer are probably similar to those of colon and breast cancer, where a subset of the disease occurs in individuals who inherit defective copies of one of a series of critical, rate-limiting steps required for neoplastic transformation.

5. LINKAGE STUDIES

With strong evidence for a genetic component in the etiology of prostate cancer and evidence for a major susceptibility gene, mapping the gene(s) using linkage analysis is a natural next step. Indeed, as linkage studies in families with multiple members affected with these diseases were critical to the identification of colon cancer and breast cancer susceptibility genes, likewise, linkage analyses in prostate cancer families is an active area of study in multiple centers internationally.

Yet the linkage analysis of prostate cancer has proven to be a difficult undertaking for a number of reasons. First, as prostate cancer is, at least clinically, a late-onset disease, even in cases with early age at diagnosis, individuals in the parental generation of the probands are usually deceased, and individuals in the offspring generations are usually too young to manifest the phenotype. These features combine to make many prostate cancer pedigrees only marginally informative for linkage analysis. Second, segregation analyses notwithstanding, multiple modes of inheritance (dominant, recessive, and X-linked) with multiple genes are probably involved in prostate cancer susceptibility (i.e., genetic and allelic heterogeneity), largely decreasing the power of any single family collection to detect the effect of any single major gene. Third, with such a high prevalence of disease, and a potentially powerful environmental etiologic component, phenocopies (nongene carriers with disease) are likely to be prevalent. Finally, incomplete and age-dependent penetrance of prostate cancer genes generally decreases the power to detect linkage. Despite these difficulties, linkage studies of prostate cancer have been widely pursued, and as of 1999, four separate loci suspected of harboring hereditary prostate cancer genes have been reported (Table 1). Three of these loci are on chromosome 1, and the fourth is on X chromosome. The finding of multiple distinct loci, and the high likelihood that multiple additional loci will be identified, emphasizes the extensive and potentially complex genetic heterogeneity that characterizes hereditary prostate cancer, and no single gene is likely to explain the majority of familial clustering of this disease.

Table 1
Prostate Cancer Susceptibility Loci Identified by Linkage Studies

Locus	Chromosomal Location	Reference
HPC1	1q24-25	Smith et al. 1996 *(76)*
HPCX	Xq27-28	Xu et al. 1998 *(88)*
PCAP	1q42-43	Berthon et al. 1998 *(3)*
CAPB	1p36	Gibbs et al. 1999 *(24)*

6. GENOME-WIDE SCREEN FOR LINKAGE

As a systematic approach to identify prostate cancer susceptibility genes, the first genome-wide scan for linkage for was performed on 66 prostate cancer families at Johns Hopkins Hospital *(76)*. Each of these families met an operational definition of hereditary prostate cancer—i.e., having at least three cases of prostate cancer in first-degree relatives. The average age at diagnosis in these families was 65, which is more than 5 yr less than the average age of diagnosis in the United States. A total of 341 dinucleotide repeat markers, covering the genome with ~10 cM resolution, were genotyped and analyzed in these families. Two-point parametric linkage analysis identified seven regions with lod score (i.e., *l*ogarithm of the *od*ds ratio in favor of linkage vs no linkage) >1. The highest lod score observed was 2.75 at marker *D1S218*, which maps to the long arm of chromosome 1 (*1q24-25*). The other regions with lod >1.0 were *1q33-42, 4q26-27, 5p12-13, 7p21, 13q31-33*, and *Xq27-28*. Three other genome-wide screens for prostate cancer susceptibility gene were performed, but detailed results have not been published *(3,24,61)*.

7. *HPC1*

The *1q24-25* region identified in the genome-wide screen by Smith et al. *(76)* was further studied in 25 additional HPC families—13 at Johns Hopkins, and the remaining 12 families from Sweden. In the total 91 families, the overall two-point lod score was 3.65 at a recombination fraction (θ) of 0.18 with marker *D1S2883*. Multipoint analyses using different combinations of three consecutive markers were performed, and lod scores >4 were observed. Significant evidence for locus heterogeneity was obtained by an admixture test with an estimate of 34% of families linked to the region. The maximum multipoint lod score under the assumption of heterogeneity (i.e., assuming that only some of the families studied are linked to this locus) was 5.43, near *D1S202*. Importantly, these findings observed using a dominant linkage model were supported by nonparametric analyses, which make no assumptions about the mode of inheritance, gene frequency, or gene penetrance. These analyses provided highly significant results, with a peak multipoint NPL score of 4.71 (p = 1E-5) in the same interval. This locus was termed *HPC1* for hereditary prostate cancer gene 1.

In a preliminary attempt to understand the characteristics of prostate cancer caused by the action of the putative *HPC1* gene, Grönberg et al. *(28)* studied a subset of 74 hereditary prostate cancer families at Johns Hopkins. The 74 families were divided into 2 groups: either potentially linked (33 families) or unlinked (44 families), on the basis of haplotype analysis in the region of *HPC1*. The mean age of prostate cancer at diagnosis for men in potentially linked families was significantly lower than for men in potentially unlinked families (63.7 vs 65.9 yr; $p = 0.01$). Interestingly, higher-grade cancers (grade 3) were more common in potentially linked families, and advanced-stage diseases was found in 41% of the case patients in potentially linked families compared with 31% in potentially unlinked families. Whether these observations are the result of *HPC1* cancers being intrinsically more aggressive, or whether they have similar biologic potential for progression—but are observed to do so more often because they are initiated earlier—is still unclear. Larger studies focusing on the clinical aspects of HPC will be needed to address these issues.

To refine the location of *HPC1*, a set of markers with higher resolution in the *1q24-25* region were genotyped in a total sample of 121 North American hereditary prostate cancer families. The peak multipoint lod score assuming heterogeneity was 4.27, observed at *D1S2138*, but the curve was broad with lod >3 over 18 cM region. Nonparametric analysis provided similar results. Stratification analyses were performed in an attempt to identify the characteristics of the subset of hereditary prostate cancer families most likely to be linked to *HPC1*. Stratified analyses focused on several categories. The first category was based on basic family characteristics such as mean age at diagnosis and number of affected members. In breast cancer families, these characteristics have important effects on the likelihood of linkage to *BRCA1* e.g., evidence for linkage to *BRCA1* is mainly observed in families with early age at diagnosis and families with more than three cases of breast cancer *(17)*. The second category was based on the occurrence (or lack of) apparent male-to-male disease transmission, which could distinguish potential autosomal from X-linked inheritance. Results from these stratified analyses yielded several interesting findings:

1. Evidence for linkage at *HPC1* in the 121 families was mainly from 64 families, with mean age at diagnosis less than 65. The peak multipoint lod score assuming heterogeneity was 5.41 in this set of families with the proportion of families linked to this locus estimated as 35%, while lod scores approached zero in this region in the remaining 57 families with mean age at diagnosis 65 and above.
2. Evidence for linkage at *HPC1* was stronger in the 68 families with at least five affected family members than in families with three and four affected family members.
3. Stronger evidence for linkage at *HPC1* was observed in the 81 families with male-to-male disease transmission. The peak multipoint lod score (assuming heterogeneity) was 3.99 in these families, with the proportion of linked families estimated to be 25%.

While this subset analysis is helpful in determining the characteristics of families most likely to be linked to *HPC1*, little additional positional information is provided—the lod score curves for each of these subsets remain broad, complicating gene localization studies.

The results of the analyses of *1q24-25* linkage by other research groups have been varied. Three independent studies corroborated linkage to *HPC1*, and an equal number have found no clear evidence of linkage to *HPC1*. Cooney et al. *(12)* reported a linkage study of *1q24-25* in 59 prostate cancer families, each with two or more affected individuals. The peak NPL score was 1.58 at *D1S466* ($p = 0.057$) in the total 59 families, but was 1.72 ($p = 0.045$) in the subset of 20 families which met the criteria for hereditary prostate cancer families (three or more affected individuals within one nuclear family; affected individuals in three successive generations; and/or clustering of two or more individuals affected <55 yr). Hsieh et al. *(34)* reported further evidence to support *HPC1*. In 92 unrelated families having three or more affected individuals, the NPL score was 1.71 ($p = 0.046$). The evidence for linkage was stronger in the 46 families, with mean age at diagnosis <67. The NPL score was 2.04 ($p = 0.023$). The strongest confirmatory study of HPC1 linkage to date comes from a study of 44 large Utah pedigrees, described by Neuhausen et al. *(62)*. In this collection of families, each with an average of 10.7 affected individuals, an overall lod score of 2.06 ($p = 0.002$) was observed at for the interval *D1S196-D1S416*. Interestingly, most of the evidence for linkage came from the quartile of families with the youngest average age of diagnosis (lod score = 2.82, $p = 0.0003$ at *D1S215–D1S222*).

In contrast to these confirmatory studies, McIndoe et al. *(53)* reported no evidence for linkage to the *HPC1* region in 49 high-risk prostate cancer families, using either a parametric lod score approach assuming homogeneity or nonparametric analysis. There was also no evidence for linkage in the 18 families with early age at diagnosis (<65 yr). It is worthwhile to note that they observed positive lod scores for some markers in this region, a lod of 0.49 at *D1S422* in the total sample. Berthon et al. *(3)* reported results of a genome-wide screen and results from the *1q24-25* region in 47 French and German families. For the three markers in the *HPC1* region, they found negative two-point lod scores assuming a dominant model. No results were reported for the families with early age of diagnosis or a large number of affected individuals. Eeles et al. *(19)* reported a linkage study of *1q24-25* in 136 prostate cancer families ascertained in United Kingdom, Quebec, and Texas, 76 of which have three or more affected individuals. They found negative NPL scores in this region in the total sample, but positive NPL scores in a subset of 35 families with four or more affected members.

Multiple factors such as genetic locus heterogeneity, proportion of families with early mean age at diagnosis, with large number of affected family members, and with male-to-male disease transmission, may explain the difference among the different linkage studies. In light of the abovementioned difficulties of prostate cancer linkage analysis, the number of families from any single study population may provide only limited power to detect or confirm any linkage. To increase the power to test linkage, a collaborative effort was made to examine the *HPC1* locus in a worldwide study. A combined analysis for six markers in the *1q24-25* regions was performed in 772 hereditary prostate cancer families ascertained by members of the International Consortium for Prostate Cancer Genetics (ICPCG) from North America, Australia, Finland, Norway, Sweden, and the United Kingdom *(87)*. Overall, there was some evidence for linkage, with a peak parametric multipoint lod score assuming heterogeneity (hlod) of 1.40 ($p = 0.01$) at *D1S212*. The estimated proportion of families (α) linked to the locus was 0.06 (1-lod support interval from 0.01 to 0.12). Some evidence for linkage was also observed using a nonparametric approach. Further parametric analysis revealed a significant effect of the presence of male-to-male disease transmission within the families. In the subset of 491 such families, the peak hlod was 2.56 ($p = 0.0006$) and $\alpha = 0.11$ (1-lod support interval from 0.04 to 0.19), compared to hlods of 0 in the remaining 281 families. Within the male-to-male disease transmission families, the increased with early mean age of diagnosis (<65, $\alpha = 0.19$, with 1-lod support interval from 0.06 to 0.34) and number of affected family members (≥ 5, $\alpha = 0.15$, with 1-lod support interval from 0.04 to 0.28). The highest α was observed for the 48 families that met all three criteria (peak hlod = 2.25, p = 0.001, α = 0.29, with 1-lod support interval from 0.08 to 0.53). These results support the finding of a prostate cancer susceptibility gene linked to *1q24-25*, albeit in a defined subset of prostate cancer families. Whereas *HPC1* accounts for only a small proportion of all hereditary prostate cancer families, it appears to play a more prominent role in the subset of families with multiple members affected at an early age, and with male-to-male disease transmission. As with any HPC gene, determination of the true impact of *HPC1* on familial prostate cancer will not be possible until the gene is cloned and mutations are characterized (e.g., frequency and penetrance).

8. HPCX

Previous suggestions of possible X-linkage of prostate cancer came from several population based studies *(10,33,56,59,72,85)* which found greater risks for brothers of prostate cancer patients as compared to sons of patients. Interestingly, a region on chromosome X was implicated in the genome-wide scan for linkage described by Smith et al. *(76)*. In a follow-up study, this region was analyzed in a combined study population of 360 prostate cancer families collected at four different sites in North America, Finland, and Sweden. Evidence of linkage to *Xq27-28* was observed at the locus termed *HPCX (86)*. The peak two-point lod score was 4.6 at *DXS1113*, and the peak multipoint lod score was 3.85 between *DXS1120* and *DXS297*. Significant evidence for locus heterogeneity was observed, with 16% of the families in the combined study population estimated to be linked to *HPCX*, and a similar proportion in each separate family collection. Heterogeneity analysis of the Hopkins HPC family collection suggests that families linked to either *HPC1* or *HPCX* comprise two independent groups of families, with only families in which there is no evidence of male-to-male disease transmission showing evidence of linkage to the X chromosome.

9. PCaP

By the combination of genome-wide screen and fine mapping on a selection of 47 French and German families, Berthon et al. *(3)* reported a prostate cancer susceptibility locus at *1q42-43 (PCaP)*. The maximum two-point lod score was 2.7 with marker *D1S2785*. Multipoint parametric analysis yielded a lod score assuming heterogeneity of 2.2 and nonparametric analysis yielded NPL score of 3.1. They estimated that 50% of the 47 families were linked to the locus.

10. CaPB

Based on initial results of a genome-wide screen in 70 prostate cancer families and candidate-region mapping in 71 additional families, Gibbs et al. *(24)* reported linkage to *1p36*. Further evaluation of this data set revealed the exciting observation of an association between *1p36* linkage and the presence of brain cancer in a subset of the linked prostate cancer families. The overall two-point lod score was 3.22 at *D1S507* for 12 families with a history of prostate cancer and a blood relative with primary brain cancer. In the younger age group (mean age at diagnosis <66 yr), a maximum two-point lod of 3.65 at *D1S407* was observed. This linkage was rejected in both early and late age onset families with no history of brain cancer. Interestingly, tumors of the CNS were the only cancers found to be in excess in a study of other cancers in multiplex prostate cancer families reported by Isaacs et al. *(37)*.

11. ISSUES ASSOCIATED WITH HPC GENE CLONING FOLLOWING LINKAGE

While the finding of linkage in HPC families is a critical observation in the pathway to gene identification, the regions identified as the potential locations of prostate-cancer susceptibility genes by linkage studies are usually broad, which causes great difficulty for fine-mapping and cloning the relevant genes. The reasons for this inability of linkage analysis to provide more precise or more reliable mapping information in prostate cancer are similar to the problems associated with linkage analyses of this disease previously discussed and include:

1. Limited number of informative recombinants caused by the small number of meioses in available family data.
2. Locus heterogeneity decreases the relevant number of families useful for fine mapping.
3. The number of relevant families may be further decreased by the presence of phenocopies, resulting in negative evidence for linkage in truly linked families, and by incomplete penetrance of disease alleles.
4. With few exceptions, lod scores for individual families are not large enough to unambiguously indicate whether a family is linked to a specific locus.
5. Without a clear clinical discriminator of genetic versus nongenetic cases, there is uncertainty whether a key recombinant in a linked families is a true recombinant or a phenocopy.

To supplement fine mapping efforts in linkage studies, association studies can be taken as an alternative approach.

12. ASSOCIATION STUDIES

Association studies are generally case-controlled studies based on a comparison of the frequency of an allele in unrelated cases and normal controls. A significant difference in the allele frequency between cases and controls can be expected if the allele sequence itself is causal, or if the allele is in linkage disequilibrium (LD) with a disease-causing mutation. Since LD can only be observed when two markers are closely linked, a significant finding of LD can pinpoint the location of the disease gene. Association studies are commonly used for testing the relevance of candidate genes as disease susceptibility genes, and for testing LD of anonymous marker alleles in the regions implicated through linkage studies. This approach is becoming increasingly popular as more candidate genes are identified and denser maps of single nucleotide polymorphisms (SNPs) become available.

Although association studies for fine mapping have been performed successfully in many simple Mendelian diseases, this approach presents some difficulty in complex diseases, particularly in genetically heterogeneous populations. Association studies are susceptible to etiological heterogeneity (genetic or environmental), inheritance (dominant, recessive, or X-linked), and locus heterogeneity, as well as allelic (same gene but different mutations) and founder (same mutation exists in different genetic background) heterogeneity. Despite these difficulties, a large number of association studies have been reported.

13. *BRCA1* AND *BRCA2*

As a result of various epidemiological studies over the past four decades, a link between prostate and breast-cancer etiology has been suspected for many years *(20,52,83)*. Anderson and Badzioch *(1)* observed an increase in breast cancer risk as a function of family history of prostate cancer in families ascertained through male or female probands having breast cancer. However, as mentioned above, an examination of a large number of prostate cancer families for other cancers by Isaacs et al. *(37)* found only tumors of the central nervous system to be in significant excess; the number of breast cancer cases was not significantly elevated in this study. More recent studies have demonstrated an association between *BRCA1* and *BRCA2* mutations and increased risk of prostate cancer in carriers *(18,22,74,81)*. The most direct evidence for a role of these genes in prostate cancer susceptibility comes from an observation of Ashkenazi men known to harbor *BRCA1* or *-2* gene mutations. In this cohort, the rate of prostate cancer diagnosis by age 70 was 16%, compared to 3.8% for nonmutation carriers. Furthermore in an extensive study of other cancers in *BRCA2* carriers from the Breast Cancer Linkage Consortium *(6)*, a strong association with prostate cancer was found (estimated RR = 4.65, 95% CI = 3.48-6.22) for mutation carriers, particularly for men below 65 yr of age (RR = 7.33). Other studies examining a role for these genes in prostate cancer have been less supportive of a prominent effect, although these studies have been mainly restricted to the Ashkenazi Jewish population. Lehrer et al. *(47)* reported an absence of *BRCA1* and *-2* founder mutations in Ashkenazi prostate cancer cases, although only a limited number of these men reported a positive family history of the disease. Langston et al. *(46)* found a *BRCA1* 185delAG mutation in an affected member of a Jewish prostate cancer family, although no other family members were tested. A study of multiplex Ashkenazi Jewish prostate cancer families by Wilkens et al. *(84)* did not find elevated rates of common mutations in either *BRCA1* or *-2*. A similar finding was reported by Nastiuk et al. *(60)* who determined the rate of founder *BRCA1* and *-2* mutations in early-onset prostate cancer to be the same as the general Ashkenazi population. While it is clear that mutations in *BRCA1* and *BRCA2* increase the risk for prostate cancer, particularly in the case of *BRCA2* for early-onset disease, the contribution of germline mutations in these genes to familial clustering of prostate cancer remains to be more fully determined.

14. ANDROGEN ACTION PATHWAY

It is becoming more apparent that common polymorphisms that result in quantitative or qualitative functional differences in protein products involved in normal tissue physiology may play an important role in modifying disease risk. For prostate cancer, polymorphic variants in a number of genes have been correlated with disease risk, including the androgen receptor, the related 5 alpha reductase gene, the vitamin D receptor, and various members of the cytochrome P450 family *(21,58,66)*. Of these, most attention has focused upon genes involved in androgen action *(69)*, particularly androgen-receptor polymorphisms which result in variable androgen-receptor activity. Specifically, there are two polymorphic triplet repeats in of exon 1 which code for polyglutamine (CAG) and polyglycine (GGN) repeats of varying lengths of between

11–31 and 10–22 residues, respectively *(16,36,50,75)*. Although variations in the polyglycine repeat length are of unknown biological consequence, it has been demonstrated that the polyglutamine repeat length is inversely related to the ability of the androgen receptor to stimulate androgen-specific transcriptional activity *(11,40,77)*. This is of particular interest, since the population with the shortest average glutamine repeat length observed is the African-American population, which has the highest incidence and mortality rates reported for prostate cancer, whereas Asian individuals, who have a low risk for prostate cancer, tend to have longer repeat lengths *(16,36)*. Indeed, a number of studies have documented the correlation between shorter AR polyglutamine repeats and increased prostate cancer risk *(25,39,79)*. Stanford et al. *(79)* demonstrated an additional effect of shorter polyglutamine repeats, so that men with short repeat lengths for both polymorphisms (CAG <22 and GGN < or = 16) had a twofold increase in risk compared to men with two long repeats. Platz et al. also noted an effect of the GGN repeat *(51)*. Several studies have suggested that *AR* genes with shorter repeat lengths may increase the risk of developing more aggressive prostate cancer *(25,32)*. Polymorphisms in other genes involved in androgen metabolism have also been implicated in determining the risk for prostate cancer development (e.g., 5 alpha reductase, 3 beta hydroxysteroid dehydrogenase) *(14,51,67,69)*. Further study is needed to determine the overall role of these polymorphisms in determining or modifying prostate cancer risk.

15. VITAMIN D RECEPTOR

Although conflicting reports exist, a variety of epidemiologic data support the hypothesis that vitamin D deficiency is a risk factor for prostate cancer *(5,13,23,48,73)*, and the ability of this vitamin to suppress the growth of prostate cancer cells has been documented in experimental settings *(44,55,64)*. The finding of polymorphisms within the 3′ untranslated region of the vitamin D receptor gene (VDR) which potentially affected receptor expression, led to studies examining the frequency of VDR alleles in prostate cancer cases compared to controls. Two studies found that having either one or two copies of the VDR allele containing a BsmI restriction enzyme site (i.e., allele *b*, or the putative less active variant) was associated with an increased prostate cancer risk *(35,82)*, and possibly with more advanced disease *(35)*. However, this result was not observed in a study by Kibel et al. *(42)*, which examined VDR genotypes in a study of men who had died from prostate cancer. In this study, there was an interesting tendency for men with a strong family history to be homozygous for the less active allele. An extensive case-control study in the Physicians' Health Study in Boston *(49)* examined both serum vitamin D metabolite levels (1,25 dihydroxyvitamin D) and VDR polymorphisms in cases and controls. Although there was no increased risk associated with the allelic variants overall, in men with plasma levels of vitamin D which were below the median level, a significant risk reduction was observed for homozygous carriers of the *B* allele. The interpretation of these data has been complicated by recent reports indicating that the polymorphisms examined in these studies do not affect receptor function as originally thought, suggesting that the observed associations may reflect the influence of a different, adjacent gene *(15,31)*.

16. REGIONS OF LOSS OF HETEROZYGOSITY

By analogy to other common cancers, characterization of somatic alterations in genes and/or chromosomal segments in sporadic prostate cancers can be used to identify candidate prostate cancer susceptibility genes. Work from a large number of laboratories has identified a number of commonly occurring alterations in prostate cancer DNA (reviewed in Isaacs and Bova *[38]*). In terms of linkage analysis, no significant findings have been reported to date for genes known to undergo somatic alterations in sporadic prostate cancer, although only a handful have been analyzed (e.g., PTEN, Mxi1, GSTP1, AR).

17. CLINICAL AND PATHOLOGICAL CHARACTERIZATION OF HEREDITARY PROSTATE CANCER

To determine whether any differences might distinguish hereditary prostate cancer from its sporadic counterpart, a number of clinical features of prostate cancer were examined by Carter et al. in patients with clinically localized disease as a function of a family history of prostate cancer *(9)*. Clinical stage at presentation, preoperative PSA level, final pathological stage, and prostate weight were examined in a series of ~650 patients divided among three categories. For individuals classified as having hereditary disease, three or more relatives were affected in a single generation, or prostate cancer occurred in each of three successive generations on either the proband's paternal or maternal lineages, or that there were two relatives affected below the age of 55. For the other groups, either no other family members were affected (i.e., sporadic), or other family members were affected, but not to the extent found in families classified as hereditary. In summary, no unique clinical or pathological characteristic distinguished hereditary prostate cancer in this group of patients in this study.

This parallel between hereditary and sporadic prostate cancer extends to the incidence of multifocality found for each of these categories. Studies of individuals harboring other cancer-susceptibility alleles, in which multiple cancer foci are often observed in target organs, might lead to the prediction that prostate cancer would be more multifocal in patients with a hereditary form of the disease. In a study by Bastacky et al. *(2)*, this was not the case. As has been previously observed, prostate cancer is generally multifocal, and no difference was observed between sporadic and hereditary cases in this respect. A study by Keetch et al. *(41)* was similar to the Bastacky study in that it examined the pathological characteristics of prostate cancers from men undergoing radical prostatectomy for treatment of clinically localized disease, as a function of family history. The only difference observed was that familial cancers tended to have a slightly lower Gleason score (6.6 vs 7.6.).

Several studies have examined the effect of family history on outcome of prostate cancer after treatment. Bova et al. *(4)* found no differences in progression rates as measured by PSA elevation in a cohort of radical prostatectomy patients classified as having hereditary prostate cancer compared to men with sporadic disease. Kupelian et al. *(45)* did observe a significant tendency for men with a positive family history to progress more rapidly after either surgical or radiation treatment for clinically localized disease. Regardless of treatment, Rodriguez et al. *(68)* made the observation that men with a family history of prostate cancer are more likely to die from their disease, and that this risk increased with the number of affected relatives, particularly if diagnosed before age 65. In contrast, Grönberg et al. *(29)* found no significant differences in either overall or prostate cancer-specific survival in familial or sporadic cases in a cohort of Swedish prostate cancer patients.

As described above, Grönberg et al. *(28)* examined the characteristics of prostate cancers in families linked to the *HPC1* locus on chromosome 1. This study found that tumors in families linked to this locus were usually diagnosed earlier and were more aggressive than prostate cancers in unlinked families or in sporadic cases. Families linked to *HPC1* had more female breast and colon cancers, but these differences did not reach statistical significance. The finding by Gibbs et al. *(24)* that linkage of prostate cancer susceptibility to *1p36* is found in families that have both primary brain and prostate cancers is particularly intriguing, suggesting that such families, while rare, define a more genetically homogeneous subset of hereditary prostate cancer. Only when the genes themselves are cloned and characterized will their contributions to the pathogenesis of this disease become evident.

REFERENCES

1. Anderson, D. E. and M. D. Badzioch. 1992. Breast cancer risks in relatives of male breast cancer patients. *J. Natl. Cancer Inst.* **84:** 1114–1117.
2. Bastacky, S. I., K. J. Wojno, P. C. Walsh, M. J. Carmichael, and J. I. Epstein. 1995. Pathological features of hereditary prostate cancer. *J. Urol.* **153:** 987–992.
3. Berthon, P., A. Valeri, A. Cohen-Akenine, E. Drelon, T. Paiss, G. Wohr, et al. 1998. Predisposing gene for early-onset prostate cancer, localized on chromosome 1q42.2-43. *Am. J. Hum. Genet.* **62:** 1416–1424.
4. Bova, G. S., A. W. Partin, S. D. Isaacs, B. S. Carter, T. L. Beaty, W. B. Isaacs, et al. 1998. Biological aggressiveness of hereditary prostate cancer: long-term evaluation following radical prostatectomy. *J. Urol.* **160:** 660–663.
5. Braun, M. M., K. Helzlsouer, B. Hollis, and G. Comstock. 1995. Prostate cancer and prediagnostic levels of serum vitamin D metabolites (Maryland, United States). *Cancer Causes Control* **6:** 235–239.
6. Breast Cancer Linkage Consortium. 1999. Cancer risks in BRCA2 mutation carriers. *J. Natl. Cancer Inst.* **91:** 1310–1316.
7. Cannon, L., D. Bishop, M. Skolnick, S. Hunt, J. Lyon, and C. Smart. 1982. Genetic epidemiology of prostate cancer in the Utah Mormon genealogy. *Cancer Surv.* **1:** 47–69.
8. Carter, B. S., T. Beaty, G. Steinberg, B. Childs, and P. Walsh. 1992. Mendelian inheritance of familial prostate cancer. *Proc. Natl. Acad. Sci. USA* **89:** 3367–3371.
9. Carter, B. S., G. Bova, T. Beaty, G. Steinberg, B. Childs, W. B. Isaacs, et al. 1993. Hereditary prostate cancer: epidemiologic and clinical features (review). *J. Urol.* **150:** 797–802.
10. Cerhan, J. R., A. S. Parker, S. Putnam, B. Chiu, C. Lynch, M. Cohen, et al. 1999. Family history and prostate cancer risk in a population-based cohort of Iowa men. *Cancer Epidemiol. Biomark. Prev.* **8:** 53–60.
11. Chamberlain, N. L., E. Driver, and R. Miesfeld. 1994. The length and location of CAG trinucleotide repeats in the androgen receptor N-terminal domain affect transactivation function. *Nucleic Acids Res.* **22:** 3181–3186.
12. Cooney, K. A., J. McCarthy, E. Lange, L. Huang, S. Miesfeldt, J. Montie, et al. 1997. Prostate cancer susceptibility locus on chromosome 1q: a confirmatory study (see comments). *J. Natl. Cancer Inst.* **89:** 955–959.

13. Corder, E. H., H. Guess, B. Hulka, G. Friedman, M. Sadler, R. Vollmer, B. et al. 1993. Vitamin D and prostate cancer: a prediagnostic study with stored sera. *Cancer Epidemiol. Biomark. Prev.* **2:** 467–472.

14. Devgan, S. A., B. Henderson, M. Yu, C. Shi, M. Pike, R. Ross, et al. 1997. Genetic variation of 3 beta-hydroxysteroid dehydrogenase type II in three racial/ethnic groups: implications for prostate cancer risk. *Prostate* **33:** 9–12.

15. Durrin, L. K., R. Haile, S. Ingles, and G. Coetzee. 1999. Vitamin D receptor 3′-untranslated region polymorphisms: lack of effect on mRNA stability. *Biochim. Biophys. Acta* **1453:** 311–320.

16. Edwards, A., H. Hammond, L. Jin, C. Caskey, and R. Chakraborty. 1992. Genetic variation at five trimeric and tetrameric tandem repeat loci in four human population groups. *Genomics* **12:** 241–253.

17. Easton, D. F., S. Narod, D. Ford, and M. Steel. 1994. The genetic epidemiology of BRCA1. Breast Cancer Linkage Consortium (letter). *Lancet* **344:** 761.

18. Easton, D. F., L. Steele, P. Fields, W. Ormiston, D. Averill, P. Daly, et al. 1997. Cancer risks in two large breast cancer families linked to BRCA2 on chromosome 13q12-13. *Am. J. Hum. Genet.* **61:** 120–128.

19. Eeles, R. A., F. Durocher, S. Edwards, D. Teare, M. Badzioch, R. Hamoudi, et al. 1998. Linkage analysis of chromosome 1q markers in 136 prostate cancer families. The Cancer Research Campaign/British Prostate Group U.K. Familial Prostate Cancer Study Collaborators. *Am. J. Hum. Genet.* **62:** 653–658.

20. Ekman, P., Y. Pan, C. Li, and J. Dich. 1997. Environmental and genetic factors: a possible link with prostate cancer. *Br. J. Urol.* **79(Suppl 2):** 35–41.

21. Febbo, P. G., P. Kantoff, E. Giovannucci, M. Brown, G. Chang, C. Hennekens, et al. 1998. Debrisoquine hydroxylase (CYP2D6) and prostate cancer. *Cancer Epidemiol. Biomark. Prev.* **7:** 1075–1078.

22. Ford, D., D. Easton, D. Bishop, S. Narod, and D. Goldgar. 1994. Risks of cancer in BRCA1-mutation carriers. Breast Cancer Linkage Consortium. *Lancet* **343:** 692–695.

23. Gann, P. H., J. Ma, C. Hennekens, B. Hollis, J. Haddad, and M. Stampfer. 1996. Circulating vitamin D metabolites in relation to subsequent development of prostate cancer. *Cancer Epidemiol. Biomark. Prev.* **5:** 121–126.

24. Gibbs, M., J. Stanford, R. McIndoe, G. Jarvik, S. Kolb, E. Goode, et al. 1999. Evidence for a rare prostate cancer-susceptibility locus at chromosome 1p36. *Am. J. Hum. Genet.* **64:** 776–787.

25. Giovannucci, E., M. Stampfer, K. Krithivas, M. Brown, D. Dahl, A. Brufsky, et al. 1997. The CAG repeat within the androgen receptor gene and its relationship to prostate cancer *Proc. Natl. Acad. Sci. USA* **94:** 3320–3323 (published erratum appears in *Proc. Natl. Acad. Sci. USA* **94:** 8272, 1997).

26. Grönberg, H., L. Damber, and J. Damber. 1994. Studies of genetic factors in prostate cancer in a twin population. *J. Urol.* **152:** 1484–1489.

27. Grönberg, H., L. Damber, J. Damber, and L. Iselius. 1997. Segregation analysis of prostate cancer in Sweden: support for dominant inheritance. *Am. J. Epidemiol.* **146:** 552–557.

28. Grönberg, H., S. Isaacs, J. Smith, J. Carpten, G. Bova, D. Freije, et al. 1997. Characteristics of prostate cancer in families potentially linked to the hereditary prostate cancer 1 (HPC1) locus (see comments). *JAMA* **278:** 1251–1255.

29. Grönberg, H., L. Damber, B. Tavelin, and J. Damber. 1998. No difference in survival between sporadic, familial and hereditary prostate cancer (In Process Citation). *Br. J. Urol.* **82:** 564–567.

30. Grönberg, H., F. Wiklund, and J. Damber. 1999. Age specific risks of familial prostate carcinoma: a basis for screening recommendations in high risk populations. *Cancer* **86:** 477–483.

31. Gross, C., I. Musiol, T. Eccleshall, P. Malloy, and D. Feldman. 1998. Vitamin D receptor gene polymorphisms: analysis of ligand binding and hormone responsiveness in cultured skin fibroblasts. *Biochem. Biophys. Res. Commun.* **242:** 467–473.

32. Hakimi, J. M., R. Rondinelli, M. Schoenberg, and E. Barrack. 1996. Androgen-receptor gene structure and function in prostate cancer. *World J. Urol.* **14:** 329–337.

33. Hayes, R. B., J. Liff, L. Pottern, R. Greenberg, J. Schoenberg, A. Schwartz, et al. 1995. Prostate cancer risk in U.S. blacks and whites with a family history of cancer. *Int. J. Cancer* **60:** 361–364.

34. Hsieh, C. L., I. Oakley-Girvan, R. Gallagher, A. Wu, L. Kolonel, C. Teh, et al. 1997. Prostate cancer susceptibility locus on chromosome 1q: a confirmatory study (letter; comment). *J. Natl. Cancer Inst.* **89:** 1893,1894.

35. Ingles, S. A., R. Ross, M. Yu, R. Irvine, G. La Pera, R. Haile, et al. 1997. Association of prostate cancer risk with genetic polymorphisms in vitamin D receptor and androgen receptor (see comments). *J. Natl. Cancer Inst.* **89:** 166–170.

36. Irvine, R. A., M. Yu, R. Ross, and G. Coetzee. 1995. The CAG and GGC microsatellites of the androgen receptor gene are in linkage disequilibrium in men with prostate cancer. *Cancer Res.* **55:** 1937–1940.

37. Isaacs, S. D., L. Kiemeney, A. Baffoe-Bonnie, R. Beaty, and P. Walsh. 1995. Risk of cancer in relatives of prostate cancer probands. *J. Natl. Cancer Inst.* **87:** 991–996.

38. Isaacs, W. B. and G. Bova. 1998. Prostate cancer, in *The Genetic Basis of Human Cancer* (Vogelstein. B. and K. W. Kinzler eds.). New York: McGraw-Hill, pp. 653–660.

39. Kantoff, P., E. Giovannucci, and M. Brown. 1998. The androgen receptor CAG repeat polymorphism and its relationship to prostate cancer. *Biochim. Biophys. Acta* **1378:** C1–5.

40. Kazemi-Esfarjani, P., M. Trifiro, and L. Pinsky. 1995. Evidence for a repressive function of the long polyglutamine tract in the human androgen receptor: possible pathogenetic relevance for the (CAG)n-expanded neuronopathies. *Hum. Mol. Genet.* **4:** 523–527.

41. Keetch, D. W., P. Humphrey, D. Smith, D. Stahl, and W. Catalona. 1996. Clinical and pathological features of hereditary prostate cancer. *J. Urol.* **155:** 1841–1843.

42. Kibel, A. S., S. Isaacs, W. Isaacs, and G. Bova. 1998. Vitamin D receptor polymorphisms and lethal prostate cancer. *J. Urol.* **160:** 1405–1409.

43. Krain, L. S. 1974. Some epidemiologic variables in prostatic carcinoma in California. *Prev. Med.* **3:** 154–159.

44. Krill, D., J. Stoner, B. Konety, M. Becich, and R. Getzenberg. 1999. Differential effects of vitamin D on normal human prostate epithelial and stromal cells in primary culture (In Process Citation). *Urology* **54:** 171–177.

45. Kupelian, P. A., V. Kupelian, J. Witte, R. Macklis, and E. Klein. 1997. Family history of prostate cancer in patients with localized prostate cancer: an independent predictor of treatment outcome. *J. Clin. Oncol.* **15:** 1478–1480.

46. Langston, A. A., J. Stanford, K. Wicklund, J. Thompson, R. Blazej, and E. Ostrander. 1996. Germline BRCA1 mutations in selected men with prostate cancer (letter). *Am. J. Hum. Genet.* **58:** 881–884.

47. Lehrer, S., F. Fodor, R. Stock, N. Stone, C. Eng, H. Song, et al. 1998. Absence of 185delAG mutation of the BRCA1 gene and 6174delT mutation of the BRCA2 gene in Ashkenazi Jewish men with prostate cancer. *Br. J. Cancer* **78:** 771–773.

48. Lyles, K. W., W. Berry, M. Haussler, J. Harrelson, and M. Drezner. 1980. Hypophosphatemic osteomalacia: association with prostatic carcinoma. *Ann. Intern. Med.* **93:** 275–278.

49. Ma, J., M. Stampfer, P. Gann, H. Hough, E. Giovannucci, K. Kelsey, et al. 1998. Vitamin D receptor polymorphisms, circulating vitamin D metabolites, and risk of prostate cancer in United States physicians. *Cancer Epidemiol. Biomark. Prev.* **7:** 385–390.

50. Macke, J. P., N. Hu, S. Hu, M. Bailey, V. King, T. Brown, et al. 1993. Sequence variation in the androgen receptor gene is not a common determinant of male sexual orientation. *Am. J. Hum. Genet.* **53:** 844–852.

51. Makridakis, N., R. Ross, M. Pike, L. Chang, F. Stanczyk, L. Kolonel, et al. 1997. A prevalent missense substitution that modulates activity of prostatic steroid 5alpha-reductase. *Cancer Res.* **57:** 1020–1022.

52. McCahy, P. J., C. Harris, and D. Neal. 1996. Breast and prostate cancer in the relatives of men with prostate cancer. *Br. J. Urol.* **78:** 552–556.

53. McIndoe, R. A., J. Stanford, M. Gibbs, G. Jarvik, S. Brandzel, C. Neal, et al. 1997. Linkage analysis of 49 high-risk families does not support a common familial prostate cancer-susceptibility gene at 1q24-25. *Am. J. Hum. Genet.* **61:** 347–353.

54. Meikle, A. W., J. Smith, and D. West. 1985. Familial factors affecting prostatic cancer risk and plasma sex-steroid levels. *Prostate* **6:** 121–128.

55. Miller, G. J., G. Stapleton, T. Hedlund, and K. Moffat. 1995. Vitamin D receptor expression, 24-hydroxylase activity, and inhibition of growth by 1alpha,25-dihydroxyvitamin D3 in seven human prostatic carcinoma cell lines. *Clin. Cancer Res.* **1:** 997–1003.

56. Monroe, K. R., M. Yu, L. Kolonel, G. Coetzee, L. Wilkens, R. Ross, et al. 1995. Evidence of an X-linked or recessive genetic component to prostate cancer risk (see comments). *Nat. Med.* **1:** 827–829.

57. Morganti, G., L. Cianferrari, A. Cresseri, G. Arrigoni, and F. Lovati. 1956. Recherches clinico-statistiques et genetiques sur les neoplasies de la prostate. *Acat. Genet. Statis.* **6:** 304,305.

58. Murata, M., T. Shiraishi, K. Fukutome, M. Watanabe, M. Nagao, Y. Kubota, et al. 1998. Cytochrome P4501A1 and glutathione S-transferase M1 genotypes as risk factors for prostate cancer in Japan. *Jpn. J. Clin. Oncol.* **28:** 657–660.

59. Narod, S. A., A. Dupont, L. Cusan, P. Diamond, J. Gomez, R. Suburu, et al. 1995. The impact of family history on early detection of prostate cancer (letter). *Nat. Med.* **1:** 99–101.

60. Nastiuk, K. L., M. Mansukhani, M. Terry, P. Kularatne, M. Rubin, J. Melamed, et al. 1999. Common mutations in BRCA1 and BRCA2 do not contribute to early prostate cancer in Jewish men (In Process Citation). *Prostate* **40:** 172–177.

61. Neuhausen, S. L., M. Skolnick, and L. Cannon-Albright. 1997. Familial prostate cancer studies in Utah. *Br. J. Urol.* **79(Suppl. 1):** 15–20.

62. Neuhausen, S. L., J. Farnham, E. Kort, S. Tavtigian, M. Skolnick, and L. Cannon-Albright. 1999. Prostate cancer susceptibility locus HPC1 in Utah high-risk pedigrees (In Process Citation). *Hum. Mol. Genet.* **8:** 2437–2442.

63. Page, W. F., M. Braun, A. Partin, N. Caporaso, and P. Walsh. 1997. Heredity and prostate cancer: a study of World War II veteran twins. *Prostate* **33:** 240–245.

64. Peehl, D. M., R. Skowronski, G. Leung, S. Wong, T. Stamey, and D. Feldman. 1994. Antiproliferative effects of 1,25-dihydroxyvitamin D3 on primary cultures of human prostatic cells. *Cancer Res.* **54:** 805–810.

65. Platz, E. A., E. Giovannucci, D. Dahl, K. Krithivas, C. Hennekens, M. Brown, et al. 1998. The androgen receptor gene GGN microsatellite and prostate cancer risk. *Cancer Epidemiol. Biomark. Prev.* **7:** 379–384.

66. Rebbeck, T. R., J. Jaffe, A. Walker, A. Wein, and S. Malkowicz. 1998. Modification of clinical presentation of prostate tumors by a novel genetic variant in CYP3A4. *J. Natl. Cancer Inst.* **90:** 1225–1229.

67. Reichardt, J. K., N. Makridakis, B. Henderson, M. Yu, M. Pike, and R. Ross. 1995. Genetic variability of the human SRD5A2 gene: implications for prostate cancer risk. *Cancer Res.* **55:** 3973–3975.

68. Rodriguez, C., E. Calle, L. Tatham, P. Wingo, H. Miracle-McMahill, M. Thun, et al. 1998. Family history of breast cancer as a predictor for fatal prostate cancer. *Epidemiology* **9:** 525–529.

69. Ross, R. K., M. Pike, G. Coetzee, J. Reichardt, M. Yu, H. Feigelson, et al. 1998. Androgen metabolism and prostate cancer: establishing a model of genetic susceptibility. *Cancer Res.* **58:** 4497–4504.

70. Schaid, D. J., S. McDonnell, M. Blute, and S. Thibodeau. 1998. Evidence for autosomal dominant inheritance of prostate cancer. *Am. J. Hum. Genet.* **62:** 1425–1438.
71. Schuman, L. M., J. Mandel, C. Blackard, H. Bauer, J. Scarlett, and R. McHugh. 1971. Epidemiologic study of prostate cancer: preliminary report. *Cancer Treat. Rep.* **61:** 181–186.
72. Schuurman, A. G., M. Zeegers, R. Goldbohm, and P. van den Brandt. 1999. A case-cohort study on prostate cancer risk in relation to family history of prostate cancer. *Epidemiology* **10:** 192–195.
73. Schwartz, G. G., and B. Hulka. 1990. Is vitamin D deficiency a risk factor for prostate cancer? (Hypothesis) *Anticancer Res.* **10:** 1307–1311.
74. Sigurdsson, S., S. Thorlacius, J. Tomasson, L. Tryggvadottir, K. Benediktsdottir, J. Eyfjord, et al. 1997. BRCA2 mutation in Icelandic prostate cancer patients. *J. Mol. Med.* **75:** 758–761.
75. Sleddens, H. F., B. Oostra, A. Brinkmann, and J. Trapman. 1993. Trinucleotide (GGN) repeat polymorphism in the human androgen receptor (AR) gene. *Hum. Mol. Genet.* **2:** 493.
76. Smith, J. R., D. Freije, J. Carpten, H. Grönberg, J. Xu, S. Isaacs, et al. 1996. Major susceptibility locus for prostate cancer on chromosome 1 suggested by a genome-wide search (see comments). *Science* **274:** 1371–1374.
77. Sobue, G., M. Doyu, T. Morishima, E. Mukai, T. Yasuda, T. Kachi, et al. 1994. Aberrant androgen action and increased size of tandem CAG repeat in androgen receptor gene in X-linked recessive bulbospinal neuronopathy. *J. Neurol. Sci.* **121:** 167–171.
78. Spitz, M. R., R. Currier, J. Fueger, R. Babaian, and G. Newell. 1991. Familial patterns of prostate cancer: a case-control analysis. *J. Urol.* **146:** 1305–1307.
79. Stanford, J. L., J. Just, M. Gibbs, K. Wicklund, C. Neal, B. Blumenstein, et al. 1997. Polymorphic repeats in the androgen receptor gene: molecular markers of prostate cancer risk. *Cancer Res.* **57:** 1194–1198.
80. Steinberg, G. D., B. Carter, T. Beaty, B. Childs, and P. Walsh. 1990. Family history and the risk of prostate cancer. *Prostate* **17:** 337–347.
81. Struewing, J. P., P. Hartge, S. Wacholder, S. Baker, M. Berlin, M. McAdams, et al. 1997. The risk of cancer associated with specific mutations of BRCA1 and BRCA2 among Ashkenazi Jews (see comments). *N. Engl. J. Med.* **336:** 1401–1408.
82. Taylor, J. A., A. Hirvonen, M. Watson, G. Pittman, J. Mohler, D. Bell. 1996. Association of prostate cancer with vitamin D receptor gene polymorphism. *Cancer Res.* **56:** 4108–4110.
83. Thiessen, E. U. 1974. Concerning a familial association between breast cancer and both prostatic and uterine malignancies. *Cancer* **34:** 1102–1107.
84. Wilkens, E. P., D. Freije, J. Xu, D. Nusskern, H. Suzuki, S. Isaacs, et al. 1999. No evidence for a role of BRCA1 or BRCA2 mutations in Ashkenazi Jewish families with hereditary prostate cancer. *Prostate* **39:** 280–284.
85. Woolf, C. M. 1960. An investigation of familial aspects of carcinoma of the prostate. *Cancer* **13:** 739–744.
86. Xu, J., D. Meyers, D. Freije, S. Isaacs, K. Wiley, D. Nusskern, et al. 1998. Evidence for a prostate cancer susceptibility locus on the X chromosome. *Nat. Genet.* **20:** 175–179.
87. Xu, J., and International Consortium for Prostate Cancer Genetics. 2000. Combined analysis of hereditary prostate cancer linkage to *1q24-25*: results from 772 hereditary prostate cancer families from the International Consortium for Prostate Cancer Genetics. *Am. J. Hum. Genet.* **66:** 945–957.

3

AR Gene Alterations in Prostate Cancer Progression

Tapio Visakorpi, MD, PhD

1. INTRODUCTION

In the 1940s, Huggins and Hodges *(13)* showed that androgen withdrawal alleviates the symptoms of prostate cancer. Since then, hormonal therapy has remained the standard treatment of the advanced form of the disease. Despite the improved early diagnosis of prostate cancer, about one-third of patients are still diagnosed at a clinically advanced stage *(21)*. The majority of prostate cancer patients receive hormonal treatment at some point. Most initially respond to the therapy *(11)*. Eventually, however, the disease progresses despite ongoing androgen withdrawal. Since there is no effective treatment for hormone refractory prostate cancer, the prognosis after relapse is poor. The failure of endocrine therapy is one of the main problems in the management of prostate cancer *(10,37)*.

The mechanisms that lead to prostate cancer progression are not fully understood. Several hypotheses on the molecular mechanisms of tumor recurrence have been presented. Although it was once believed that recurrent prostate tumors are androgen independent, it has now become evident that androgen signaling pathways may still play a role in disease progression despite ongoing androgen withdrawal. For example, levels of prostate specific antigen (PSA), whose expression is regulated by androgens, are elevated rather than decreased during progression of the disease *(33)*. Patients seem to benefit from ongoing androgen withdrawal even after progression *(23)*. To identify the mechanisms of treatment failure, we and others have aimed at detection of chromosomal alterations present in hormone refractory prostate carcinomas. Mapping such aberrations can subsequently be used as a starting point for positional cloning of genes that may be important to progression of the disease.

2. CHROMOSOMAL ALTERATIONS IN HORMONE REFRACTORY PROSTATE CANCER

Comparative genomic hybridization (CGH) is a relatively new molecular cytogenic technique that can be used to detect DNA sequence-copy-number changes *(15)*. CGH maps chromosomal regions that may harbor amplified oncogenes or deleted tumor suppressor genes. We and others have used CGH to detect genetic alterations in both hormone naïve and hormone refractory prostate carcinomas *(2,3,14,28,29,36,41)*. In primary untreated prostate cancer, the average number of chromosomal alterations

From: *Prostate Cancer: Biology, Genetics, and the New Therapeutics*
Edited by: L. W. K. Chung, W. B. Isaacs, and J. W. Simons © Humana Press Inc., Totowa, NJ

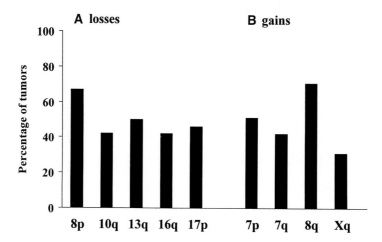

Fig. 1. A summary of the most commonly found DNA sequence copy number **(A)** losses, and **(B)** gains in hormone refractory prostate cancer by CGH (according to Nupponen et al. *[12]*, and Cher et al. *[15]*).

detectable by CGH is relatively low *(41)*. The loss of sequences predominates over gains, and high-level amplification of chromosomal regions is almost completely lacking in these tumors. This is a striking contrast to breast cancer, in which CGH often shows high-level amplification of many different regions *(16)*. On the other hand, hormone refractory prostate tumors contain almost three to four times more genetic changes than untreated tumors. In addition, gains and high-level amplification are often found *(29,41)*. These findings suggest that the underlying cause of the early development of prostate cancer may be inactivation of tumor suppressor genes, whereas late progression may involve amplification and activation of oncogenes. By comparing untreated primary and treated recurrent tumor pairs from the same patients, we have often found cases in which the tumor counterparts contain almost completely different chromosomal abnormalities *(29)*. Thus it seems that androgen ablation may act as a strong selection force in a similar fashion as the metastasis event.

Commonly found genetic alterations in hormone refractory prostate cancer include losses of 18p, 10q, 13q, 16q, and 17p, and gains of 7p, 7q, 8q, and Xq (Fig. 1). High-level amplification is especially prevalent in chromosomes 8q and Xq. The most common genetic alteration in hormone refractory tumors (found in 80–90% of cases) is the gain of 8q. It usually comprises the whole q-arm, although we have been able to identify two separate minimal commonly amplified regions (8q21 and 8q23-24), indicating that the gain has several target genes *(29)*. The well-known oncogene c-myc, located at 8q24, is a natural candidate target gene for the 8q gain. Other genes, such as eIF3-p40 *(30)* and PSCA *(35)* may also be involved in this amplification. The 8q gain is found in about 5% of untreated prostate carcinomas. Thus, it is not purely associated with the emergence of hormone refractory disease *(41)*.

In contrast, the gain of Xq has never been detected in hormonally untreated tumors *(29,41)*. When we analyzed the first prostate tumors by CGH, we found a case in which the hormone refractory tumor showed high-level amplification of Xp11-q13 region, while the untreated primary tumor from the same patient did not. This led us to believe

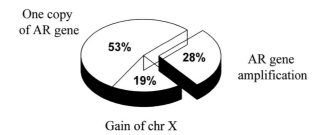

One copy of AR gene

53%

28%

AR gene amplification

19%

Gain of chr X

Fig. 2. The frequency of AR gene copy number alterations in locally recurrent hormone refractory prostate cancer.

that the amplification may be associated with the emergence of hormone refractory disease. We subsequently narrowed down the minimal regions of the amplification to Xcen-q13, which then suggested that the androgen receptor (*AR*) gene, located at Xq12, could be the target for amplification *(42)*.

3. AR

Androgen action is mediated to the target cells through a specific nuclear receptor (AR). AR belongs to a large steroid hormone receptor family, and it functions as a transcription factor. After binding to the ligand (androgens), the receptor is phosphorylated and homodimerized, and bound to the androgen responsive elements (AREs) located at the 5′ regions of the genes. Transcriptional activation by AR involves formation of a multiprotein complex, and the activity can be modulated by coactivators and corepressors. Although AREs have been recognized in the promoter regions of only a few genes, it is believed that the transcription of hundreds of genes is regulated by androgens and an AR-signaling pathway *(20)*.

4. *AR* GENE AMPLIFICATION

By fluorescence *in situ* hybridization (FISH), we have shown that the *AR* gene is truly amplified in about 30% of hormone refractory prostate carcinomas (Fig. 2). In addition, about 20% of hormone refractory tumors contain additional copies of chromosome X and the *AR* gene *(19,42)*. Hundreds of untreated prostate carcinomas have now been analyzed for *AR* gene-copy number, and none have shown high-level amplification of the gene *(1,19,42)*. It seems that the amplification occurs as the result of selection during androgen withdrawal. Similar examples of gene amplification leading to chemotherapy resistance have been reported. However, *AR* gene amplification is the first example of such a mechanism related to hormone therapy, suggesting that castration may act as an equally strong selection force as chemotherapy.

By mRNA *in situ* hybridization analyses, we have also shown that the amplification of the *AR* gene is associated with increased expression of the gene, as expected of the true target gene of amplification *(19)*. However, even the refractory tumors that do not contain *AR* gene amplification seem to strongly express *AR*, suggesting that the AR signaling pathway may also be active in the nonamplified cases. Consistent *AR* expression demonstrates a clear difference between breast and prostate cancer. Hormone refractory breast cancer typically loses the expression of the estrogen and progesterone receptor *(22)*.

There is little direct evidence that the amplified and overexpressed *AR* gene is functional in hormone refractory prostate tumors. The data that tumors which acquire *AR* gene amplification initially respond better to castration than tumors that do not acquire the amplification suggests that these tumors are sensitive to androgens *(19)*. In addition, the preliminary finding that patients with amplified *AR* gene responded better to second-line maximal androgen blockade (MAB) than patients without the amplification, indicates a functional AR signaling pathway *(31,32)*.

5. *AR* MUTATIONS

In addition to *AR* gene amplification, the gene can be altered by mutation. The role of such mutations in prostate cancer has been thoroughly studied. Still, the frequency of mutations is disputed. Several studies have screened untreated prostate tumors for *AR* gene mutations (reviewed in ref. *20*). Although two published articles *(9,40)* have suggested that a significant number of these tumors do contain mutations, most studies have concluded that such mutations are rare. Only a few studies *(6,7,19,38,39,40)* have analyzed hormone refractory tumors for *AR* gene mutations.

We have screened 31 locally-recurrent hormone refractory prostate carcinomas for mutations in all exons of the AR gene, and found only two mutations *(43)*. One of the mutations (Gly^{674}->Ala) was located at the hormone binding domain, but it did not alter the transactivational properties of the receptor molecule. The other was a CAG repeat-contraction mutation (CAG$_{20}$->CAG$_{18}$) in exon 1. The number of CAG repeats is believed to be associated with *AR* activity; the shorter the repeat, the higher the activity. Contraction of the CAG repeat could have some functional consequences. Although both these mutations occur in cases with *AR* gene amplification, the amplified *AR* genes generally represent the wild-type of the gene. These findings are consistent with studies suggesting that mutations are rare. Still, recent articles by Taplin and colleagues *(38,39)* have shown that *AR* mutations are common—found in about one-third of patients treated with the antiandrogen flutamide. These mutations cluster to codon 877, modulating the receptor molecule so that it can be paradoxically activated by flutamide. It seems that flutamide may select a cell clone which contains codon 877 mutation in the same way that castration selects the *AR* gene amplification.

6. MODULATION OF *AR* ACTIVATION

Recently, a number of coregulators of *AR* have been cloned. Such activators and repressors include Rb, ANPK(PKY), SNURF, ARIP3, ARA54, ARA55, and ARA70 *(8,12,18,25–27,44,45)*. These coregulators may modify the transcriptional activity of AR, and could theoretically play a role in the progression of prostate cancer. For example, an altered ARA70 expression level may lead to the agonist effect of antiandrogens such as flutamide *(24)*. However, studies of the coregulators have only been conducted with in vitro and animal models. Furthermore, it is not known whether they are altered in prostate cancer in vivo. It has also been shown in vitro that an AR signaling pathway could be activated by other growth factors, such as fibroblast and epidermal growth factors *(5)*. Like the coregulators, these mechanisms also require further study.

Two interesting studies on HER-2/neu (ERBB2) tyrosine kinase in prostate cancer were recently published. Using a xenograft model, Craft and a colleague *(4)* were able to show that androgen independent sublines of a xenograft expressed higher levels of HER-2/neu oncogene than the androgen dependent counterpart. The authors also found that by overexpressing HER-2/neu in a LNCaP cell line, the phenotype of the cells changed from an androgen dependent to an androgen independent one. Finally, they showed that overexpression of HER-2/neu increases the expression of PSA, especially at low androgen levels. Yeh and colleagues *(46)* also showed—by using DU145 and LNCaP cells—that HER-2/neu could induce PSA expression, possibly through a MAP kinase pathway. They suggested that HER-2 activates AR by promoting interaction between AR and AR coactivators, such as ARA70. These investigations clearly demonstrated a cross-communication between HER-2/neu tyrosine kinase and AR signaling pathways. It is possible that HER-2/neu and/or MAP kinase pathways may be involved in the recurrence of prostate cancer by activating AR in the presence of a low level of androgens (during castration) or in the absence of androgens. However, in vivo data on the role of these pathways in prostate cancer progression is still needed.

7. CONCLUSION

Studies on the emergence of hormone refractory prostate cancer during the last five years have emphasized the role of AR in treatment failure. The finding of *AR* gene amplification in many recurrent carcinomas suggests that these tumors may not be truly androgen independent; instead, they seem to be androgen hypersensitive. It is possible that cancer cells can overcome low androgen levels by overexpressing the *AR* gene. Yet in vitro and xenograft studies suggest that the AR pathway may be activated by other means than androgens. Thus, some hormone refractory prostate carcinomas may be almost androgen independent, but not necessarily independent of the AR signaling pathway (Fig. 3).

More studies are needed to understand how AR functions in the emergence of hormone refractory prostate cancer. One major shortcoming in prostate cancer research is the lack of good model systems. For example, there is no prostate cancer cell line or xenograft containing *AR* gene amplification. Such models would be crucial in studying questions such as how the amplified and overexpressed *AR* gene is activated, whether it needs a ligand, whether it could be autoactivated, or whether the activation could be turned off by antiandrogens or some other means.

The finding of *AR* gene amplification has many possible clinical implications. If the tumors with *AR* gene activation are truly androgen dependent and possibly androgen hypersensitive, one would expect that blocking the effects of residual androgens (by MAB) would be highly beneficial. And, our preliminary data suggest that this may well be the case *(31,32)*. To further study these questions, samples of recurrent tumors should routinely be obtained. Unfortunately, under current clinical practice it is difficult or impossible to obtain samples from metastatic sites of hormone refractory prostate cancer. One new possibility for obtaining recurrent samples is the collection of micrometastatic cells from the bone marrow of patients with disease progression *(34)*. Such samples could be extremely useful in the analyses of the AR signaling pathway and downstream genes. Further studies must be conducted to develop sample collection

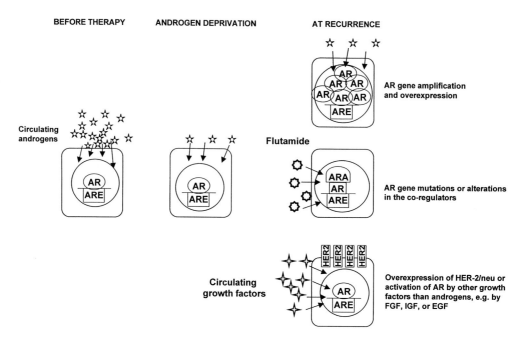

Fig. 3. Suggested mechanisms of disease progression during androgen withdrawal (AR=androgen receptor, ARE=androgen responsive element, ARA=androgen receptor-associated proteins).

procedures to ensure that enough recurrent cancer cells are retrieved for molecular analyses.

Finally, since it seems that the AR signaling pathway may be operational even during androgen withdrawal, the obvious question is whether new treatments, that are directed against the AR signaling pathway can be developed. It seems that traditional antiandrogens are not enough. New therapies could be directed against the AR itself, or against the alternative modes of AR activation.

REFERENCES

1. Bubendorf, L., J. Kononen, P. Koivisto, P. Schraml, H. Moch, T. C. Gasser, et al. 1999. Survey of gene amplifications during prostate cancer progression by high-throughput fluorescence in situ hybridization on tissue microarrays. *Cancer Res.* **59:** 803–806.
2. Cher, M. L., D. MacGrogan, R. Bookstein, J. A. Brown, R. B. Jenkins, and R. Jensen. 1994. Comparative genomic hybridization, allelic imbalances and fluorescence in situ hybridization on chromosome 8 in prostate cancer. *Genes Chromosomes Cancer* **11:** 153–162.
3. Cher, M. L., G. S. Bova, D. H. Small, P. R. Carroll, S. S. Pin, J. I. Epstein, et al. 1996. Genetic alterations in untreated metastases and androgen-independent prostate cancer detected by comparative genomic hybridization and allotyping. *Cancer Res.* **56:** 3091–3102.
4. Craft, N., Y. Shostak, M. Carey, and C. L. Sawyers. 1999. A mechanism for hormone-independent prostate cancer through modulation of androgen receptor signaling by the HER-2/neu tyrosine kinase. *Nat. Med.* **5:** 280–285.

5. Culig, Z., A. Hobisch, M. V. Cronauer, C. Radmayr, J. Trapman, A. Hittmair, et al. 1994. Androgen receptor activation in prostatic tumor cell lines by insulin-like growth factor-I, keratinocyte growth factor, and epidermal growth factor. *Cancer Res.* **54:** 5474–5478.
6. Elo, J. P., L. Kvist, K. Leionen, V. Isomaa, P. Henttu, O. Lukkarinen, et al. 1995. Mutated human androgen receptor gene detected in a prostatic cancer patient is also activated by estradiol. *J. Clin. Endocrinol. Metab.* **80:** 3494–3500.
7. Evans, B. A. J., M. E. Harper, C. E. Daniells, C. E. Watts, S. Matenhelia, J. Green, et al. 1996. Low incidence of androgen receptor gene mutations in human prostatic tumors using single strand conformation polymorphism analysis. *Prostate* **28:** 162–171.
8. Fujimoto, N., S. Yeh, H. Y. Kang, S. Inui, H. C. Chang, A. Mizokami, et al. 1999. Cloning and characterization of androgen receptor coactivator, ARA55, in human prostate. *J. Biol. Chem.* **274:** 8316–8321.
9. Gaddipati, J. P., D. G. McLeod, H. B. Heidenberg, I. A. Sesterhenn, M. J. Finger, J. W. Moul, et al. 1994. Frequent detection of codon 877 mutation in the androgen receptor gene in advanced prostate cancers. *Cancer Res.* **54:** 2861–2864.
10. Gittes, R. F. 1991. Carcinoma of the prostate. *N. Engl. J. Med.* **324:** 236–245.
11. Grayhack, J. T., T. C. Keeler, and J. M. Kozlowski. 1987. Carcinoma of the prostate. Hormonal therapy. *Cancer* **60(Suppl. 3):** 589–601.
12. Hsiao, P. W. and C. Chang. 1999. Isolation and characterization of ARA160 as the first androgen receptor N-terminal-associated coactivator in human prostate cells. *J. Biol. Chem.* **274:** 22,372–22,379.
13. Huggins, C. and C. V. Hodges. 1941. The effect of castration, of estrogens, and of androgen injection on serum phosphatase in metastatic carcinoma of prostate. *Cancer Res.* **1:** 293–297.
14. Joos, S., U. Bergerheim, Y. Pan, H. Matsuyama, M. Bentz, S. du Manoir, et al. 1995. Mapping of chromosomal gains and losses in prostate cancer by comparative genomic hybridization. *Genes Chromosomes Cancer* **14:** 267–276.
15. Kallioniemi, A., O. P. Kallioniemi, D. Sudar, D. Rutovitz, J. W. Gray, F. Waldman, et al. 1992. Comparative genomic hybridization for molecular cytogenetic analysis of solid tumors. *Science* **258:** 818–821.
16. Kallioniemi, A., O. P. Kallioniemi, J. Piper, M. Tanner, T. Stokke, L. Chen, et al. 1994. Detection and mapping of amplified DNA sequences in breast cancer by comparative genomic hybridization. *Proc. Natl. Acad. Sci. USA* **91:** 2156–2160.
17. Kallioniemi, O. P. and T. Visakorpi. 1996. Genetic basis and clonal evolution of human prostate cancer. *Adv. Cancer Res.* **68:** 225–255.
18. Kang, H. Y., S. Yeh, N. Fujimoto, and C. Chang. 1999. Cloning and characterization of human prostate coactivator ARA54, a novel protein that associates with the androgen receptor. *J. Biol. Chem.* **274:** 8570–8576.
19. Koivisto, P., J. Kononen, C. Palmberg, T. Tammela, E. Hyytinen, J. Isola, et al. 1997. Androgen receptor gene amplification: a possible molecular mechanism for failure of androgen deprivation therapy in prostate cancer. *Cancer Res.* **57:** 314–319.
20. Koivisto, P., M. Kolmer, T. Visakorpi, and O. P. Kallioniemi. 1998. Androgen receptor gene and hormonal therapy failure of prostate cancer. *Am. J. Pathol.* **152:** 1–9.
21. Kosary, C. L., L. A. G. Ries, B. A. Miller, B. F. Hankey, A. Harras, and B. K. Edwards. 1995. SEER Cancer Statistics Review, 1973–1992: Tables and Graphs. National Cancer Institute, NIH Pub. No. 96-2789, Bethesda, MD.
22. Kuukasjärvi, T., J. Kononen, H. Helin, K. Holli, and J. Isola. 1996. Loss of estrogen receptor in recurrent breast cancer is associated with poor response to endocrine therapy. *J. Clin. Oncol.* **14:** 2584–2589.
23. Labrie, F., A. Dupont, M. Giguere, J. P. Borsanyi, Y. Lacourciere, G. Monfette, et al. 1988. Benefits of combination therapy with flutamide in patients relapsing after castration. *Br. J. Urol.* **61:** 341–346.

24. Miyamoto, H., S. Yeh, G. Wilding, and C. Chang. 1998. Promotion of agonist activity of antiandrogens by the androgen receptor coactivator, ARA70, in human prostate cancer DU145 cells. *Proc. Natl. Acad. Sci. USA* **95:** 7379–7384.

25. Moilanen, A. M., U. Karvonen, H. Poukka, O. A. Jänne, and J. J. Palvimo. 1998. Activation of androgen receptor function by a novel nuclear protein kinase. *Mol. Biol. Cell* **9:** 2527–2543.

26. Moilanen, A. M., H. Poukka, U. Karvonen, M. Hakli, O. A. Jänne, and J. J. Palvimo. 1998. Identification of a novel RING finger protein as a coregulator in steroid receptor-mediated gene transcription. *Mol. Cell Biol.* **18:** 5128–5139.

27. Moilanen, A. M., U. Karvonen, H. Poukka, W. Yan., J. Toppari, O. A. Jänne, et al. 1999. A testis-specific androgen receptor coregulator that belongs to a novel family of nuclear proteins. *J. Biol. Chem.* **274:** 3700–3704.

28. Nupponen, N., E. Hyytinen, A. Kallioniemi, and T. Visakorpi. 1998. Genetic alterations is prostate cancer cell lines detected by comparative genomic hybridization. *Cancer Genet. Cytogenet.* **101:** 53–57.

29. Nupponen, N., L. Kakkola, P. Koivisto, and T. Visakorpi. 1998. Genetic alterations in hormone refractory recurrent prostate carcinomas. *Am. J. Pathol.* **153:** 141–148.

30. Nupponen, N., K. Porkka, L. Kakkola, M. Tanner, K. Persson, A. Borg, et al. 1999. Amplification and overexpression of p40 subunit of eukaryotic translation initiation factor 3 in breast and prostate cancer. *Am. J. Pathol.* **154:** 1777–1783.

31. Palmberg, C., P. Koivisto, E. Hyytinen, J. Isola, T. Visakorpi, O. P. Kallioniemi, et al. 1997. Androgen receptor gene amplification in a recurrent prostate cancer after monotherapy with nonsteroidal potent antiandrogen "Casodex" (bicalutamide) with a subsequent favorable response to maximal androgen blockade. *Eur. Urol.* **31:** 216–219.

32. Palmberg, C., P. Koivisto, L. Kakkola, T. L. J. Tammela, O. P. Kallioniemi, and T. Visakorpi. 2000. Androgen receptor gene amplification at the time of primary progression predicts response to combined androgen blockade as a second-line therapy in advanced prostate cancer. *J. Urol.* (in press).

33. Palmberg, C., P. Koivisto, T. Visakorpi, and T. L. J. Tammela. 1999. PSA decline is an independent prognostic marker in hormonally treated prostate cancer. *Eur. Urol.* **36:** 191–196.

34. Pantel, K., T. Enzmann, J. Kollermann, J. Caprano, G. Riethmuller, and M .W. Kollermann. 1997. Immunocytochemical monitoring of micrometastatic disease: reduction of prostate cancer cells in bone marrow by androgen deprivation. *Int. J. Cancer* **71:** 521–525.

35. Reiter, R. E., Z. Gu, T. Watanabe, G. Thomas, K. Szigeti, E. Davis, et al. 1998. Prostate stem cell antigen: a cell surface marker overexpressed in prostate cancer. *Proc. Natl. Acad. Sci. USA* **95:** 1735–1740.

36. Sattler, H. P., V. Rohde, H. Bonkhoff, T. Zwergel, and B. Wullich. 1999. Comparative genomic hybridization reveals DNA copy number gains to frequently occur in human prostate cancer. *Prostate* **39:** 79–86.

37. Stearns, M. E. and T. McGarvey. 1992. Biology of disease. Prostate cancer: therapeutic, diagnostic and basic studies. *Lab. Invest.* **67:** 540–552.

38. Taplin, M. E., G. J. Bubley, T. D. Shuster, M. E. Frantz, A. E. Spooner, G. K. Ogata, et al. 1995. Mutation of the androgen-receptor gene in metastatic androgen-independent prostate cancer. *N. Engl. J. Med.* **332:** 1393–1398.

39. Taplin, M. E., G. J. Bubley, Y. J. Ko, E. J. Small, M. Upton, B. Rajeshkumar, et al. 1999. Selection for androgen receptor mutations in prostate cancers treated with androgen antagonist. *Cancer Res.* **59:** 2511–2515.

40. Tilley, W. D., G. Buchanan, T. E. Hickey, and J. M. Bentel. 1996. Mutations in the androgen receptor gene are associated with progression of human prostate cancer to androgen independence. *Clin. Cancer Res.* **2:** 277–285.

41. Visakorpi, T., A. Kallioniemi, A.-C. Syvänen, E. Hyytinen, R. Karhu, T. Tammela, et al. 1995. Genetic changes in primary and recurrent prostate cancer by comparative genomic hybridization. *Cancer Res.* **55:** 342–347.

42. Visakorpi, T., E. Hyytinen, P. Koivisto, M. Tanner, R. Keinänen, C. Palmberg, et al. 1995. In vivo amplification of the androgen receptor gene and progression of human prostate cancer. *Nat. Genet.* **9:** 401–406.

43. Wallen, M. J., M. Linja, K. Kaartinen, J. Schleutker, and T. Visakorpi. 1999. Androgen receptor gene mutations in hormone refractory prostate cancer. *J. Pathol.* **189:** 559–563.

44. Yeh, S. and C. Chang. 1996. Cloning and characterization of a specific coactivator, ARA70, for the androgen receptor in human prostate cells. *Proc. Natl. Acad. Sci. USA* **93:** 5517–5521.

45. Yeh, S., H. Miyamoto, K. Nishimura, H. Kang, J. Ludlow, P. Hsiao, et al. 1998. Retinoblastoma, a tumor suppressor, is a coactivator for the androgen receptor in human prostate cancer DU145 cells. *Biochem. Biophys. Res. Commun.* **248:** 361–367.

46. Yeh, S., H. K. Lin, H. Y. Kang, T. H. Thin, M. F. Lin, and C. Chang. 1999. From HER2/Neu signal cascade to androgen receptor and its coactivators: a novel pathway by induction of androgen target genes through MAP kinase in prostate cancer cells. *Proc. Natl. Acad. Sci. USA* **96:** 5458–5463.

4

Lethal Metastatic Human Prostate Cancer
Autopsy Studies and Characteristics of Metastases

G. Steven Bova, MD, Kirk M. Chan-Tack, MD, and William W. LeCates, MD

1. INTRODUCTION

Death from prostate cancer is common in the United States, where an estimated 31,900 men will die from this disease in 2000 *(38)*. Prostate cancer is the second most prevalent cause of cancer death in males in the United States, and is even more prevalent in countries as geographically varied as Trinidad, Norway, Sweden, Cuba, Venezuela, Denmark, New Zealand, the Netherlands, Australia, Ireland, Hungary, and Finland (in decreasing order of reported death rate) *(38)*.

Prostate cancer mortality has a significant impact, even in nations that have relatively low prostate cancer death rates. In Japan, for example, where the prostate cancer death rate is one-third the US rate, approx 6400 men die each year from metastatic prostate cancer *(38)*.

Metastatic prostate cancer is presently incurable, and most men diagnosed with metastatic disease succumb over a period of months to years *(57)*. Recent advances in biology and chemistry have raised new hopes of finding effective therapy for metastatic prostate cancer. Specific anatomic and microscopic patterns of prostate cancer may reflect molecular changes, which can now be dissected to the DNA, RNA, carbohydrate, lipid, and protein level. The phenotypic review presented in this chapter reveals findings that reflect recent observations suggesting that prostate cancer is not a homogeneous disease at the molecular level *(22)*. A better understanding of the phenotypic spectrum of lethal prostate cancer may allow more a focused identification of new therapeutic molecular targets related to these various phenotypes.

We have recently initiated a "molecular" autopsy study of prostate cancer in an attempt to find meaningful patterns in the clinical, gross, microscopic, and molecular pathology of prostate cancer. Early results of this project suggest that the study of multiple metastatic lesions from multiple patients will allow a prioritization of molecular changes in this disease *(12)*.

Although the tendency of prostate cancer to spread to bone is well-known, a detailed discussion of clinical and pathologic patterns in lethal prostate cancer has been relatively rare in the literature. Between 1902 and 1992, autopsy studies of prostate cancer

From: *Prostate Cancer: Biology, Genetics, and the New Therapeutics*
Edited by: L. W. K. Chung, W. B. Isaacs, and J. W. Simons © Humana Press Inc., Totowa, NJ

from the United States, Japan, Germany, Sweden, England, and Australia have been reported in the literature.

We reviewed 271 autopsy studies of metastatic prostate cancer, identified by MEDLINE search to 1966 and manual search prior to 1966. Common clinical manifestations were clarified through a review of related case reports and experimental studies of metastasis.

Combining results from 19 studies that met specific criteria, the most common reported sites of metastasis were lymph nodes (74%), bone (69%), lung (40%), liver (28%), and adrenal (11%). Lymph node metastasis was most commonly found in the iliac and para-aortic regions, with para-aortic node involvement often occurring in the absence of iliac node involvement. Reported sites of bone metastasis appeared to be highly dependent on the extent of bone sampling at autopsy. Bone metastases were typically solely osteoblastic in individual patients, but were both osteolytic and osteoblastic in approx 20% of cases. Osteolytic metastases predominated in 15–30% of reported cases. Lung metastasis occurred with variable x-ray, pathologic, and clinical findings. Lung metastases usually showed diffuse lymphatic spread, and in some cases were associated with progressive dyspnea. Asymptomatic nodular lung metastases were also common. Adrenal metastasis was reported to occur in an average of 11% of patients who died of metastatic disease, but no cases of associated adrenal dysfunction were reported.

Meningeal metastasis was reported in 1–18% of cases in the five studies reporting such metastases, and parenchymal brain metastasis was reported in 2% of cases in the two studies reporting this finding. Breast metastasis has also been described, but only in patients treated with estrogen therapy.

The histology of metastases is rarely discussed in the literature. Urinary symptoms are the most common presenting manifestations of prostate cancer in men with proven metastatic disease at diagnosis. Back pain is also a common presenting symptom, and anemia, weakness, and weight loss are less common clinical signs upon diagnosis of metastatic disease. The immediate cause of death from metastatic prostate cancer is not discussed in most published autopsy studies.

Although bone metastasis has received significant attention in the literature, prostate cancer metastasis to lymph nodes, lung, and liver is also common. According to published data, 30% of men who die of prostate cancer have no demonstrated bone metastases. Patterns of prostate cancer involvement at common sites of metastasis such as bone and lung show surprising variability in pathologic and clinical features. Less common sites of involvement, such as adrenal and cranial dura and breast, should be considered during the clinical and pathologic evaluation of patients with metastatic prostate cancer. For improved knowledge of phenotypic variation in prostate cancer, future autopsy studies should clearly identify the specific anatomic sites and quantity of microscopic tissue analysis in each case. Although the isolated molecular analysis of prostate cancers has recently taken center stage in published studies, often ignoring patient-specific factors, observations which integrate phenotypic and molecular data may provide key insights for differentiation of putative prostate cancer clinical subtypes.

2. METHODS

Medline was accessed through the NCBI Pubmed Database (http://www.ncbi.nlm.nih.gov/entrez/) and searched for Medline-indexed titles and abstracts published between January 1966 and January 2000 obtained with the following Boolean search query: (((((((("prostatic diseases"[MeSH Terms] OR "prostate"[MeSH Terms]) OR prostate[Text Word]) OR prostatic[All Fields]) AND ((((("neoplasms"[MeSH Terms] OR cancer[Text Word]) OR ("carcinoma"[MeSH Terms] OR carcinoma[Text Word])) OR ("adenocarcinoma"[MeSH Terms] OR adenocarcinoma[Text Word])) OR ("neo-plasms"[MeSH Terms] OR neoplasm[Text Word])) OR ("neoplasms"[MeSH Terms] OR neoplasia[Text Word]))) AND ((((("autopsy"[MeSH Terms] OR autopsy[Text Word]) OR ("autopsy"[MeSH Terms] OR postmortem[Text Word])) OR ("autopsy" [MeSH Terms] OR necropsy[Text Word])) OR (("mortality"[MeSH Terms] OR "death"[MeSH Terms]) OR death[Text Word]))) AND ((("neoplasm metastasis" [MeSH Terms] OR metastasis[Text Word]) OR ("neoplasm metastasis"[MeSH Terms] OR metastases[Text Word])) OR ("secondary"[Subheading] OR metastatic[Text Word]))) AND notpubref[sb]) ["prostate" or "prostatic"] and ["cancer" or "carcinoma" or "adenocarcinoma" or "neoplasm" or "neoplasia"] and ["autopsy" or "postmortem" or "necropsy" or "death"] and ["metastasis" or "metastases" or "metastatic"]. References published prior to 1966 and some later references were obtained through citations which met the above criteria in reviewed papers. Non-English-language papers were initially reviewed by title only, and then through translation for selected papers.

References were initially selected if they reported autopsy findings of metastatic prostate cancer. Additional references were obtained by manual searching of the Science Citation Index for articles citing these primary references. References were excluded from the summarizing review if they imposed additional restrictions on patient selection—e.g., including only patients with lung metastasis *(80)*. References were also excluded if they failed to separate cases of nonmetastatic prostate cancer from cases of metastatic cancer, or failed to report the total number of patients with metastasis at a given site *(3,79,80)*. In some studies, authors did not specifically state whether cases with local extension also had distant metastasis. In other studies, the authors drew on a database where "metastatic" was defined to include local extension of the primary tumor *(63)*. In these studies, the total number of patients with metastasis may include some patients with local extension only. Thus, the results may understate the true incidence of site-specific cases among patients with metastasis *(17,26,30, 34,52,63,78,83)*. When possible, cases of local extension in the absence of observed metastasis were excluded. In cases where articles derived data solely from a subset of autopsy reports fully covered in another study, the former was excluded *(2,36)*. Studies which had partial overlap were retained *(68,82)*. Finally, studies using only clinical or radiographic means to diagnose metastatic disease were excluded *(16)*. Only non-excluded references were used in calculating summary data, but observations from excluded references may be cited in the discussion of results.

All averages were calculated by averaging the percentage of metastases found in each individual study. Averages were not weighted by the number of autopsies reviewed. This method was used to minimize error resulting from variations in autopsy technique and data quality over time and among centers, as some of the very large studies provide minimal information on tissue-sampling protocol and other variables. In order to minimize the error caused by small sample size that may be introduced by unweighted averaging, studies with less than 10 autopsies of metastatic prostate cancer were excluded *(21)*.

3. OVERVIEW OF SITES INVOLVED IN METASTASIS

In the 19 studies which met selection criteria (Table 1), the most common reported sites of metastatic involvement were lymph nodes (74%), bone (69%), lung (39%), liver (40%), and adrenal (11%). Lymph node metastasis was most commonly found in the iliac and para-aortic regions, with para-aortic involvement often occurring in the absence of iliac involvement. Thoracic, supraclavicular- and inguinal-node involvement was also well-described in the literature. Bone metastasis most commonly occurred in the vertebrae and pelvis, although involvement of sternum, ribs, femur, humerus, and skull was also common. Lesions were typically described as osteoblastic, but often showed osteolytic changes as well. Lung metastasis was reported to occur with variable X-ray and pathologic and clinical findings. Lung metastasis, which reportedly showed diffuse lymphatic spread, has been repeatedly associated with progressive dyspnea. Asymptomatic nodular lung metastases were also commonly described. Adrenal metastasis was reported to occur in an average of 11% of patients who died of metastatic disease. More recent studies reported a higher frequency of adrenal metastasis. Meningeal metastasis was reported to be more frequent than parenchymal brain metastasis, occurring in an average of 9% (range 1–18%) and 2% of cases, respectively. Several studies which reported no meningeal metastasis and did not state whether the meninges/brain were examined were excluded from these analyses. Breast metastasis has also been described, but only in patients treated with estrogen therapy.

4. HISTOLOGIC PATTERNS OF METASTATIC PROSTATE CANCER AT AUTOPSY

There are relatively few published studies on the histology of prostate cancer metastases. One study published by Brawn and Speights *(14)* found that in 200 consecutive staging lymphadenectomies with metastasis, 84% showed entirely gland-forming or greater than 50% gland-forming patterns—while in metastases from 100 autopsies of widely disseminated prostate cancer, 70% of metastases were entirely non-gland-forming. In five patients with staging lymphadenectomies who also were examined at autopsy, metastases at autopsy were found to be predominantly or completely non-gland-forming, while metastases at staging lymphadenectomy showed completely or predominantly gland-forming patterns. Takahashi, Muyuzumi, and Satoh *(75)* studied prostate cancer histopathology in 27 cases from biopsy and autopsy material. A change to a higher grade occurred from prostate biopsy to prostate at autopsy in 15% of cases. A higher grade was present in metastases at autopsy vs prostate at autopsy in 11% of cases.

5. CLINICAL PRESENTATION OF METASTATIC PROSTATE CANCER

Patients who die of metastatic prostate cancer are either diagnosed with metastatic disease at the time of presentation, or are initially believed to have disease confined to the prostate, receive local treatment, and later manifest signs of metastasis. Of those men who are known to have metastatic disease at the time of presentation, the most common presenting symptoms are urinary in nature. Of 79 patients presenting with metastasis, Bumpus *(16)* reported that 47 (60%) had urinary symptoms as the presenting symptom. Frequency was most common, occurring in 22 (28%), followed by hesitancy in 13 (17%), incontinence in 2 (3%), and urinary retention in 1 (1%). Barringer *(4)* described urinary symptoms in 115 of 145 cases (79%) presenting with distant metastasis or local extension. These symptoms included dribbling, dysuria, frequency, difficult urination, or nocturia. Eight of 145 (6%) presented with hematuria, and 25 (17%) showed hematuria as a secondary sign at presentation. Slack, Brady, and Murphy *(70)* described urinary frequency, obstruction, or both in 43% of 321 patients with metastatic prostate cancer at diagnosis.

Pain was the presenting symptom in 34% of patients with metastatic prostate cancer at presentation in the series of 79 patients reported by Bumpus *(16)*. The back, thigh, and chest were the most common sites of pain. Two of the cases that presented initially with pain in the chest and shoulders later progressed to paraplegia *(16)*. Barringer reported that only 7 of 145 patients (5%) with distant metastasis or local extension presented with pain as the first symptom. Sites of pain in these patients included the back, hip, heel, groin, buttocks, thigh, and leg. Slack, Brady, and Murphy *(70)* described pain as the presenting symptom in 26% in 321 patients with metastatic prostate cancer.

Additional presenting signs and symptoms in cases of metastatic prostate cancer include anemia, weakness, and weight loss. Slack, Brady, and Murphy *(70)* reported that one or more of these symptoms occurred in 17% of 321 patients with metastatic prostate cancer at diagnosis. Smith et al. *(71)* described five cases in which spinal cord compression was the initial manifestation of metastatic prostate cancer. Leg edema was reported as a presenting symptom in two of 79 cases from Bumpus *(16)* and one of 145 cases from Barringer *(4)*. Barringer also reported constipation, rectal bleeding, and unilateral testicular swelling as presenting symptoms in one case *(4)*.

6. CAUSE OF DEATH IN METASTATIC PROSTATE CANCER

Cause of death is rarely discussed explicitly in published autopsy studies of metastatic prostate cancer. In a study of 55 cases published in 1935, Graves and Militzer *(36)* described the immediate cause of death as pyelonephritis in 28%, pyelonephritis and pneumonia in 13%, pneumonia in 10%, and cachexia in 10%. The remaining cases were listed as "other" or "unknown." Schoonees et al. *(68)* described 61% of 324 patients in their 1972 series as dying of "prostate cancer," but no immediate cause of death was stated. Cardiovascular and respiratory conditions were reported as the cause of death in 33% of the cases.

7. LYMPH NODE METASTASIS

Lymph nodes are the most common reported site of metastasis in prostate cancer. At autopsy, an average of 74% of patients with metastasis have evidence of nodal involvement (Table 1). Of patients with nodal metastasis, para-aortic and iliac nodes are most commonly involved (Table 2). Nodes in the chest are involved in as many as 43% of patients with nodal metastasis *(8)*. Supraclavicular and inguinal nodes are often not examined in autopsy studies, but were shown to be commonly involved by some reports. For example, Berge and Lundberg found left and right supraclavicular-node involvement in 43% and 31% of patients respectively, and left and right inguinal nodes in 15% and 14% of patients respectively *(8)*. Other observed sites include mesenteric, cervical, and axillary lymph nodes (Table 2).

Table 1
Metastatic Prostate Cancer at Autopsy: Sites of Metastasis

	Autopsy dates	Site	Autopsy cases	Cases with metastasis	Bone	Lymph	Lung	Liver	Adrenal	Other
Kaufmann, E., 1902	1891–1900	Germany	22	20	16 (80%)	17 (85%)	a	a	a	a
Thomson Walker, J.W., 1905	1866–1904	Middlesex Hospital, London	10	10[b]	c	7 (70%)	3 (30%)	3 (30%)	0	Pancreas (1); kidney (1); testicle (1); peritoneum (1); colon (1)
Rau, W., 1922	1909–1919	Dresden, Germany	26	23	16 (70%)	17 (74%)	8 (35%)	4 (17%)	0	Kidney (1); ureter (1); pleura (1); skeletal muscle (1); mediastinum (1); peritoneum (1); 2.4 sites/pt
Caulk, J.R. and Boon-Itt, S.B., 1932	a 1932	Barnes Hospital, St. Louis	15	5	1 (20%)	a	0	1 (20%)	0	Urethra (1); ureter (1); kidney (1); myocardium (1); bladder (2); peritoneum (2); pleura (2);
Mintz, E.R. and Smith, G.G., 1934	a 1934	Massachusetts General, Boston City and Palmer Hospitals, Boston	100	87[b]	c	a	24 (28%)	20 (23%)	1 (1%)	Peritoneum (3); kidney (3); ureter (1); pancreas (1); gallbladder (1); pericardium (1); diaphragm (1); eye (1); penis (1); skin (1); esophagus (2); stomach (3); jejunum (1); cecum (1); large intestine (3)
Muir, E.G., 1934	a 1934	Middlesex Hospital, London	24	19	7 (37%)	18 (95%)	5 (26%)	4 (21%)	2 (11%)	Kidney (1); skin (1); dura (1); heart (1); ureter (1)
Graves, R.C. and Militzer, R.E., 1935	1928–1934	Pondville Hospital, Massachusetts	38	38	c a	33 (87%)	14 (37%)	9 (24%)	1 (3%)	Pleura (3); peritoneum (1); diaphragm (1); thyroid (1); pancreas (1)

Willis, R.A., 1952	1930–1933	Austin and Alfred Hospitals, Melbourne, Australia	15	11	3 (27%)	9 (81%)	6 (54%)	3 (27%)	1 (9%)	Dura (2); spleen (1)
Elkin, M. and Mueller, H.P., 1954	1928–1948	Pondville Hospital, Massachusetts	104	97 (mixed—some did but most did not receive hormonal therapy)[b]	68 (70%)	a	40 (41%)	23 (24%)	13 (13%)	Pleura (11); kidneys (4); spleen (3); thyroid (2); pancreas (2); gallbladder (1); diaphragm (1); heart (1); testicle (1)
Franks, L.M., 1956	a 1956	London	53	43 (41/43[b] received hormonal therapy)	37 (86%)	22 (51%)	7 (16%)	10 (23%)	3 (7%)	Kidney (1); spleen (1); peritoneum (2); skin (2); testis (1); breast (2)
Schoonees, R. et al., 1972	1950–1959	Buffalo, New York	56	39 (incl 12 local ext only; no hormonal therapy)[b]	22/27 (81%)	16/27 (59%)	13/27 (48%)	9/27 (33%)	8/27 (30%)	Pituitary (2); brain and spinal cord (4)
Viadana, E. et al., 1976	1956–1965	Buffalo, New York	56	56 (therapy)	43 (77%)	a	31 (55%)	24 (43%)	a	CNS (10); "endocrine" (15)
Berge, T. and Lundberg, S., 1977	1958–1969	Malmo, Sweden	1332	299 (no treatment information)	235 (79%)	261 (87%)	139 (47%)	83 (28%)	41 (14%)	Brain (7); meninges (18); trachea (1); pleura (55); oral cavity (1); small intest. (1); pancreas (4); peritoneum (15); myocardium (4); pericardium (4); spleen (18); pituitary (8); thyroid (6); kidney (5); ureter (1); bladder and urethra (1); testis (5); penis (1); breast (20 = 7%); skin (3); muscle (1)

(continued)

Table 1 (*continued*)

	Autopsy dates	Site	Autopsy cases	Cases with metastasis	Bone	Lymph	Lung	Liver	Adrenal	Other
Slack, Nelson H. et al., 1983	1970–1979	Buffalo, New York	113	113 (most rec hormonal therapy)	105 (93%)	70 (62%)	53 (47%)	47 (42%)	*a*	3.43 sites/pt (bone = 1 site); abdominal viscera (75)
Saitoh, H. et al., 1984	1958–1979	Annuals of Pathological Autopsy Cases, Japan	1885	1367 (no therapy information)[b]	913 (67%)	930 (68%)	671 (49%)	487 (36%)	237 (17%)	Bladder (536); kidneys (145); peritoneum (135); rectum (126); ureter (119); pleura (113); pancreas (68); intestines (60); spleen (57); seminal vesicles (53); heart (42); skin (36); brain (29); thyroid (29)
de la Monte, S.M. et al., 1986	1968–1984	Johns Hopkins Hospital	276	89 (48 estrogen ther; orchiec (no est); 33 no hormonal therapy)[b]	62 (70%)	62 (70%)	41 (46%)	27 (30%)	8 (20%)	8.7 sites/pt; seminal vesicles (57); bladder (23); soft tissues (36); serosal surfaces (33); ureters (19); large bowel (12); CNS (13)
Makarova, G.V. et al., 1987	*a* 1987	City Clinical Hospital No. 60, Moscow	227	227 on (no information therapy)	130 (57%)	161 (71%)	42 (19%)	52 (23%)	6 (3%)	Pleura (32)
Harada, M. et al., 1992	*a* 1992	Japan	137	127 (all with clinical diagnosis; no information on therapy)	111 (87%)	113 (89%)	64 (50%)	42 (33%)	25 (20%)	Kidney (7); spleen (4); pancreas (3); heart (3); breast (3); thyroid (2); testis (2); pituitary (1); meninges (1)
Average					**61%**	**81%**	**38%**	**28%**	**10%**	

[a]Not reported or cannot calculate incidence.
[b]Includes local extension.
[c]Bone not examined or authors describe bone examination as inadequate.

Table 2
Sites of Lymphatic Metastases in Patients with Lymphatic Metastases

	Cases with lymph metastases	Iliac	Para-aortic	Chest	Supraclavicular	Inguinal	Other
Kaufmann, E., 1902	17	8 (47%)	7 (41%)	Mediastinum 4 (24%); bronchial 4 (24%)	2 (12%)	a	Mesenteric 4 (24%); cervical 1 (6%)
Thomson Walker, J.W., 1905	7	3 (43%)	4 (57%)	a	a	a	Mesenteric 1 (14%); portal 1 (14%)
Muir, E.G., 1934	17	17 (100%)	10 (59%)	Thoracic 5 (29%)	5 (29%)	5 (29%)	
Berg, T. and Lundberg, S., 1977	261	119 (46%)	198 (76%)	Mediastinum 111 (43%)	Left 111 (43%); right 80 (31%)	Left 40 (15%); right 36 (14%)	Axillary, left 14 (5.3%); axillary, right 80 (31%)
Saitoh, H. et al., 1984	930	158 (17%)	Para-aortic 298 (32%); retroperitoneum 408 (44%)	Mediastinum 38 (4%) lung hilus 199 (21%)	a	149 (16%)	Axillary 33 (4%); neck and clavicle 249 (27%); para-tracheal 129 (14%); mesentery 90 (10%); liver hilus 61 (7%); stomach 42 (5%); pancreas 84 (9%)

[a] Not reported.

Sites of lymph node metastasis may provide information about the route by which prostate cancer spreads. In a series of 178 cancerous lymph nodes studied at autopsy, Arnheim *(3)* described para-aortic nodes as containing prostate cancer metastases more often than iliac nodes, noting that the drainage of lymph through iliac to para-aortic nodes suggests that iliac nodes should be more commonly involved. Since lymphatics follow the vascular supply to the prostate, and since multiple anastomoses exist throughout the lymphatic system, it is expected that some lymph fluid returning from the prostate bypasses the iliac nodes and is filtered first by the para-aortic nodes. If this fluid contains metastatic prostate cancer cells, the fact that para-aortic lymph node involvement occurs more commonly may simply reflect a greater number of para-aortic nodes, and thus a greater chance for these metastatic cells to implant and grow in these sites. Other autopsy studies support the finding that para-aortic nodes may be more common sites for metastasis than iliac nodes *(8,63,78)*. Saitoh et al. *(64)* examined 476 cases of lymph node metastasis at autopsy and proposed two types of lymphatic involvement. One group of patients showed involvement of pelvic and para-aortic nodes, while the second group showed involvement of para-aortic nodes without pelvic-node involvement. Liver and lung metastasis was more common in the second group, while local disease was more extensive in the first. According to the authors, these findings suggest that in some cases prostate cancer spreads to para-aortic nodes via a systemic hematogenous route or by the vertebral venous system, while in other cases prostate cancer spreads to para-aortic nodes via lymphatics. In summary, para-aortic lymph node metastases are more commonly detected than pelvic lymph node metastases at autopsy. Various explanations for this finding have been presented, but none have been proven.

8. BONE METASTASIS

Bone metastasis is a well-known feature of prostate cancer *(24,84)*. In the 15 autopsy studies reporting bone findings in our sample, the average incidence of bone marrow metastasis in patients with metastatic disease was 70%, ranging from 27–93% (Table 1). Exclusion of non-prostate cancer deaths revealed an even higher incidence of bone metastasis. Franks described bone metastasis in 86% of patients who died with metastatic disease and in 98% of patients who died of prostate cancer *(34)*. However, life-threatening lung and liver metastasis have been reported to occur in the absence of bone metastasis *(63)*.

The most common reported sites of metastatic lesions in bone are lumbar vertebrae, and the pelvis, ribs, and sternum (Table 3). Femoral metastasis is reported to occur in 8–37% of patients with bone metastasis, while humeral metastasis is less common, reported in 1–8%. Metastasis to the skull, clavicles, and scapulae is reported to occur in less than 5% of patients with bone metastasis *(34,36,40,50,56,63)*. In 111 patients with bone metastasis described by Harada et al., 38 cases (34%) showed metastasis to the vertebrae only and 2 (2%) to pelvic bones only. All other cases showed bone metastasis in two or more areas (e.g., vertebrae and pelvis). No cases showed metastasis to sternum, ribs, or femur without bone metastasis also present at other sites *(40)*. Other rare sites described in the literature include temporal bone, jaw, and bones of the orbit *(11,32,62)*. Even bone that appears normal grossly and by scintigraphy may contain

Table 3
Sites of Bone Metastases in Patients with Bone Metastases

	Cases with bone metastases	Vertebrae	Pelvis	Sternum	Ribs	Femur	Humerus	Skull	Other
Graves, R.C. and Militzer, R.E., 1935	76[b]	Lumbar 48 (63%); dorsal 19 (25%); cervical 3 (4%)	69 (92%)	a	18 (24%)	28 (37%)	4 (5%)	1 (1%)	Clavicle 2 (5%), scapula 2 (5%)
Walther, H.E., 1948	47	40 (85%)	18 (38%)	12 (25%)	19 (40%)	19 (40%)	a	11 (23%)	
Franks, L.M., 1956	37	33 (89%)	15 (41%)	6 (16%)	14 (38%)	5 (14%)	3 (8%)	a	
Saitoh, H. et al., 1984	913	Lumbar 201 (22%); thoracic 66 (7%); cervical 6 (1%); unknown 190 (21%)	Ilium 70 (8%); pubis 36 (4%); ischium 5 (1%); sacrum 21 (2%); unknown 39 (4%)	126 (14%)	156 (17%)	69 (8%)	12 (1%)	28 (3%)	Clavicle 11 (1%), scapula 6 (1%)
Makarova, G.V. et al., 1987	130	110 (85%)	62 (50%)	a	37 (30%)	a	a	a	
Harada, M. et al., 1992	111	106 (96%)	36 (32%)	38 (34%)	33 (30%)	16 (14%)	1 (1%)	2 (2%)	Clavicle 1 (1%), scapula 1 (1%)

[a]Not reported.
[b]Includes some patients studied only by roentgenogram.

tumor microemboli, as demonstrated by Wood et al. *(86)*. Of 43 prostate cancer patients with no evidence of metastatic disease, these authors found tumor microemboli by bone marrow aspiration in 19 (44%).

Many authors comment on the limitations of autopsy techniques in the detection of bone metastasis, attributing higher estimates of bone metastasis incidence to more careful searches *(10,29,34,52,78)*. Clinical bone scintigraphy studies suggest that the incidence of bone metastasis to various sites may be higher than that described in autopsy studies, especially at less accessible sites such as the skull, femur, and humerus *(54)*. Morgan et al. *(54)* described bone scintigraphy results showing 93% of 71 patients to have vertebral metastasis, 89% pelvic metastasis, 83% ribs or sternum, 63% skull, 49% femur, 34% humerus, 32% shoulder, 4% distal leg, and 1% distal arm.

Prostate cancer bone metastasis was first reported in the medical literature by Thompson in 1854 *(77)*. The existence of much earlier cases is suggested by anthropologists' findings in a 14th-century skeleton of a 45 to 55-yr-old male unearthed in Canterbury, England. This skeleton showed multiple areas of external new bone growth, involving thoracic and lumbar vertebrae, bilateral pelvis, proximal femora, bilateral ribs, sternum, right clavicle, occipital skull, and bilateral mandibular rami. Many other bones were unavailable for study, including most of the skull, scapulae, most ribs, and the proximal humeri. Radiographic study showed diffuse sclerotic changes with smaller areas of lytic changes. Considering the distribution and radiographic features of the lesions as well as the age and sex of the skeleton, metastatic prostate cancer was the leading diagnosis and was considered more likely than other causes of osteoblastic changes such as Paget disease of bone, based on radiographic findings. The authors cite reports of other medieval prostate cancer cases from Denmark, Switzerland, and Japan. Two of these cases describe skeletons of elderly men showing osteoblastic lesions in a distribution similar to but less extensive than the authors' Canterbury case. The third case, from 4th–7th-century Japan, showed osteoblastic lesions involving the entire skeleton *(1)*.

The method by which prostate cancer spreads to bone is controversial. Three paths have been proposed: lymphatic, local venous, and arterial. Based on autopsy case reports, Roberts *(61)* proposed that tumors spread via lymphatics associated with spinal ligaments. Also using autopsy material, Warren, Harris, and Graves *(84)* suggested perineural lymphatics as a probably route of dissemination. Lymph node involvement, however, does not seem to be a prerequisite for bone metastasis. In a series of 113 autopsies, Slack et al. *(70)* described an absence of lymph node involvement in 40% of patients with demonstrated bone metastasis. Bone is known to lack lymphatics, making this an unlikely route *(60)*.

Prostate cancer may spread to bone through local venous pathways. In 1940, Batson *(5)* proposed that spread occurs through the vertebral venous system. He demonstrated the connections of this system with prostatic venous drainage by injecting dye into the dorsal vein of the penis in cadavers. The dye was visualized in a pattern simulating the pattern of spread of prostate cancer in the vertebral column. Similar injection experiments in rhesus monkeys showed that with abdominal straining, the same distribution of dye was achieved. Franks repeated the cadaver injection experiments, reproducing Batson's results *(34)*. Further support for local venous dissemination came from Suzuki et al. *(74)*, who performed CT examination of vertebrae at autopsy and concluded that the pattern of metastasis within individual vertebrae follows venous rather than arterial distributions.

Alternative theories propose that spread to the vertebral column may be explained by the presence of red marrow, a "fertile soil" for cancer metastasis, rather than by the proximity of vertebrae to the prostate *(60)*. Dodds, Caride, and Lytton *(28)* searched for differences in the distribution of bone metastasis in prostate cancer vs nonprostatic cancers. By examining scintigrams of 73 patients with prostate cancer and 63 with nonprostatic cancers, they found no statistically significant differences in the distribution of bone metastasis. They proposed that these results support the widespread dissemination of tumor cells by passage through pulmonary capillaries and into the arterial circulation, rather than by local spread through Batson's plexus. Other authors have conducted similar studies, and found the pattern of dissemination of prostate cancer to differ from that of breast or lung cancer, supporting a role for Batson's plexus *(25,73)*.

Prostate cancer metastasis classically stimulates osteoblastic activity in the surrounding bone *(24,84)*. However, osteolytic changes are not uncommon. Elkin and Mueller *(30)* reported roentgenographic evidence from 61 patients with prostate-cancer bone metastasis. Of these, 39 (64%) showed blastic lesions, 10 (13%) lytic, and 14 (23%) mixed. Kaufmann described 14 of 16 cases of metastatic disease in bone as osteoblastic *(44)*. Suzuki et al. *(74)* found predominantly blastic lesions in 28 of 34 vertebrae examined at autopsy by computed tomography. Osteolytic lesions predominated in 6 of 34 vertebrae. Metastasis was usually observed to affect the peripheral part of the vertebral body, with an equal tendency to involve the anterior and posterior parts of the vertebrae. The spinous and transverse processes were never found to be involved without involvement of the vertebral body. In a series of clinical cases of metastatic prostate cancer, Plesnicar *(57)* noted 19 of 51 patients to have predominantly osteoblastic lesions initially, with osteolytic lesions developing only after disease progression following endocrine therapy. Simultaneously appearing osteoblastic and osteolytic lesions were noted in 25 of 51 patients. These patients were noted to have a greater number of metastases and a more limited response to endocrine therapy than the patients who initially had predominantly osteoblastic lesions. However, no difference was noted in the histologic degree of differentiation of the primary tumors between the two groups.

Pathologic fracture was described by Mintz and Smith as a rare feature of prostate cancer bone metastasis *(52)*. In a series of 87 autopsies on patients with metastatic disease, they described "a few" pathologic femur and rib fractures and one pathologic clavicle fracture. In addition, they cited reports of pathologic fracture of pubic rami from the literature, although none was observed in their series. In 75 cases of metastasis to bone, Graves and Militzer *(36)* observed pathologic fractures in five cases (7%): 2 femora, 1 clavicle, 1 pubis, and 1 lumbar vertebrae. In a 1909 review of 43 cases of prostate cancer bone metastasis, Blumer describes pathologic fracture in 5 of 43 (12%) cases, occurring most frequently in the femur, humerus, and clavicle *(10)*. Clain *(23)* reported on bone metastasis in 2001 cases of carcinoma from various primary sites, including 107 cases of prostate cancer. Pathologic fractures were reported in 8% of bone metastasis from all sources. None of the reports of pathologic fractures described the relationship between osteoblastic or osteolytic appearance or the tendency for pathologic fracture.

Paraplegia is one of the most severely debilitating consequences of prostate cancer vertebral metastasis. In the first reported case of bone metastasis, Thompson described paraplegia secondary to spinal cord compression by prostate cancer bone metastasis *(77)*. In 107 cases of prostate cancer metastatic to bone, Clain *(23)* described paraplegia in eight cases (8%). Blumer *(10)* reviewed 23 cases of bone metastasis reported in the literature prior to 1909. Eight of 23 cases (35%) developed paraplegia, four with loss of sphincter control and hyperreflexia. Mintz and Smith *(52)* mentioned paraplegia from spinal cord compression in metastatic prostate cancer as occurring in two of 200 clinical cases (1%) reviewed. Flynn and Shipley *(33)* reviewed the presentation and treatment of spinal cord compression caused by metastatic prostate cancer. The incidence of cord compression is described as related to the histologic grade of the primary tumor, occurring in 3% of patients with well-differentiated tumors, 4% of patients with moderately differentiated tumors, and 12% of patients with poorly differentiated tumors. Pain is described as the initial symptom of spinal cord compression, with weakness, sensory deficit and autonomic dysfunction following. The thoracic spine is reported to be the most commonly involved site of spinal cord compression, with involvement in 73% of 69 sites of spinal compression in 56 patients followed by Flynn and Shipley *(33)*. Smith et al. followed 26 patients with spinal cord compression caused by metastatic prostate cancer. Seven of the 26 (27%) patients experienced recurrent compression following treatment *(71)*.

9. LUNG METASTASIS

On average, lung metastasis is reported in 40% of patients with metastatic prostate cancer at autopsy, with reports ranging from 16–56% (Table 1). Pulmonary metastasis from prostate cancer is often difficult to distinguish clinically from primary lung cancers, and may take a variety of forms *(35)*. Elkin and Mueller described lung findings at autopsy in their 40 patients with lung metastasis as either consisting of multiple small nodules, diffuse lymphatic disease with hilar adenopathy, or grossly normal lungs with microscopic metastasis only *(30)*. Lome and John *(48)* reported four cases of undiagnosed prostate cancer presenting as progressive dyspnea secondary to pulmonary lymphangitic carcinomatosis. They described the typical clinical findings of prostate cancer metastatic to pulmonary lymphatics as dyspnea, cough, and subacute cor pulmonale, while nodular metastases were described as usually asymptomatic. Uncommon clinical presentations of prostate cancer lung metastasis includes superior vena cava syndrome *(35,53)* and malignant pleural effusion *(19,81)*. Lee et al. *(45)* reported a rare case of endobronchial metastasis of prostate cancer presenting with hemoptysis. The metastases showed a prominent mucinous component also present in the primary tumor. Four other cases of prostate cancer endobronchial metastasis were reviewed from the literature. Two of these cases also presented with hemoptysis, and none showed a mucinous component.

Autopsy studies suggest that the lymphangitic form of prostate cancer lung metastasis is more common than the nodular pattern. In an autopsy study of 15 cases of prostate cancer lung metastases, Legge, Good, and Ludwig *(46)* found diffuse lymphatic involvement in 12 cases (80%) and nodular metastases in three (20%) cases. Varkarakis et al. *(80)* studied X-ray and autopsy findings in 26 patients with prostate cancer lung metastasis. At autopsy, metastasis was present in lymphatics in only 15 of 26 cases; in lymphatics and parenchyma in four cases, and in lymphatics, parenchyma, and pleura in five cases. All but one of 26 cases of lung metastasis also showed bone metastasis. This is consistent with the findings of Saitoh et al. *(63)* who described metastasis to lung without other metastatic sites in only four of 1367 cases of metastatic disease. Bromberg et al. described a case of nodular pulmonary metastases without involvement of any other sites, and reported two similar cases from the literature *(15)*.

10. LIVER METASTASIS

Liver metastases are present in an average of 28% of patients who die of metastatic disease. The reported autopsy incidence of liver metastasis ranges from 14–43% (Table 1). Prostate cancer liver metastasis rarely occurs in the absence of metastasis to other sites. Saitoh et al. *(63)* described isolated metastasis to liver in only five of 1367 cases of metastatic disease. In 22 autopsy cases with liver metastasis, Mintz and Smith *(52)* described the gross appearance of the lesions as typically small, multiple, and firm, with only two cases of massive liver involvement by metastases. Jaundice was described in one of the 22 cases. Additional cases involving jaundice and death from hepatic failure have been reported *(9,51)*.

11. ADRENAL METASTASIS

Adrenal glands are the fifth most common reported site for metastasis in prostate cancer after lymph nodes, bone, lung, and liver. Approximately 11% of patients with metastatic prostate cancer will have adrenal metastasis, with reports ranging from 0–30% (Table 1). Studies published prior to the introduction of hormonal therapy in 1941 *(42)* tend to report a low incidence of adrenal metastasis, with an average of 3% *(36,52,56,58,78)*. Studies published after the introduction of hormonal therapy report an average incidence of adrenal metastasis of 16% *(8,17,26,30,34,40,50,63,68, 70,82,83,85)*. De la Monte et al. *(26)* compared the pattern of metastasis in patients who died of prostate cancer and received estrogen therapy with those who died of prostate cancer but did not receive estrogen therapy. They found a significantly increased incidence of metastasis to adrenal cortex (31 vs 7%), dura mater, and liver (48 vs 10%). The authors propose that the tendency for estrogen-treated tumor cells to metastasize to liver and adrenal may be the result of androgen concentration in these tissues caused by, for example, nonsuppressed adrenal androgen production and testosterone-estradiol-binding globulin in the liver. This potentially increased tendency for adrenal metastasis to occur after hormonal therapy is still in doubt, since one study reporting a 30% incidence of adrenal metastasis *(68)* included only patients whose initial diagnosis of prostate cancer occurred at autopsy. These patients presumably had not received estrogen or other androgen-ablation therapy.

12. BREAST METASTASIS

Breast metastasis was described in three of the studies in our sample: Franks *(34)* in two of 43 cases (5%), Berge and Lundberg *(8)* in 20 of 299 cases (7%), and Harada *(40)* in three of 127 cases (2%). Although only Franks confirmed that 95% of patients in the study were treated with hormonal therapy, all three studies were carried out after 1941, when hormonal therapy became widely used *(31)*. An autopsy study by Salyer and Salyer *(65)* examined 46 cases of estrogen-treated advanced prostate cancer where breast tissue was available and found clinically inapparent carcinoma in 11 (24%). These lesions were judged to be metastatic from the prostate based on the similarity in appearance to the known prostatic primary and its metastases, and based on the absence of any intraductal component in the breast lesions.

Prostate cancer metastatic to the breast was first reported in 1946 *(18,31)*. By 1951, 11 cases had been reported in the literature, all associated with estrogen therapy of total dose from 200 to 40,280 mg. Of the 11 cases, seven showed bilateral lesions *(18)*. Lo, Chomet, and Rubenstone *(47)* presented three cases of prostate cancer metastatic to the breast and reviewed 15 cases from the literature. All reported patients received estrogen therapy, 16 developed gynecomastia, and 15 had palpable lesions. The authors noted that Batson's cadaver injection experiments showed connection of the prostatic venous drainage to breast tissue via pelvic, vertebral, and intercostal veins. Benson *(7)* proposed that the increased vascularity of breast tissue secondary to estrogen therapy may be responsible for an increased likelihood of breast metastasis. Green and Klima *(37)* reported two cases from the literature of breast metastasis in estrogen-treated prostate cancer and reviewed 33 cases, noting that 67% were bilateral and that 70% had developed gynecomastia. Twelve out of 13 cases evaluated by immunohistochemistry stained positive for prostatic acid phosphatase or prostate-specific antigen (PSA). Green and Klima also reported 10 cases from the literature of primary breast cancer developing in estrogen-treated prostate cancer patients. Despite the apparent association between breast metastasis and estrogen therapy, some authors question the link, referring to the large number of patients treated with estrogen therapy and the relative rarity of breast metastasis *(69)*. Since the general abandonment of estrogen therapy in favor of various other antiandrogen treatments, there is no published data on the changing incidence of breast metastasis, and more modern autopsy studies are needed to examine this question.

13. BRAIN AND MENINGEAL METASTASIS

Metastasis of prostate cancer to brain parenchyma was reported to occur in 2% of cases by two studies in our sample. Meningeal metastasis was reported in 7% of cases by five studies. Additional studies reported only "CNS" metastasis, failing to clearly distinguish parenchymal from meningeal metastasis *(17,82)*. Some authors note that incomplete autopsies may contribute to an inaccurately low reported incidence of intracranial metastasis *(52)*.

Berge and Lundberg *(8)* reported parenchymal brain metastasis (2.3%) to be less common than meningeal metastasis (6.0%). Sarma and Godeau *(66)* reported parenchymal brain metastasis in three of 126 (2%) prostate cancer autopsy cases reviewed. One of these cases had only a single cerebral lesion, with disease otherwise confined to the prostate. The one patient diagnosed with an intracranial lesion premortem developed seizures. Smith, Kasdon, and Hardy *(72)* reported two clinical cases of intracranial disease, one without evidence of any other sites of metastasis. Catane et al. *(20)* found parenchymal brain metastasis in four of 91 (4.4%) autopsy cases reviewed. All of these cases had bone and lung metastasis. Brain lesions were asymptomatic, and were diagnosed at autopsy in three of the four cases. Taylor et al. *(76)* reviewed 126 complete autopsies in cases of prostate cancer, and found 14 (11%) with intracranial metastasis. Five patients had asymptomatic intracranial metastasis diagnosed at autopsy. Symptoms present in other patients included dysphagia, hoarseness, slurred speech, vertigo, deafness, vision changes, unilateral weakness, facial numbness, and headache. Four patients died as a result of the intracranial metastasis. The cause of death in these patients was subdural hematoma, aspiration as a result of cranial-nerve damage, respiratory arrest as a result of brain compression, and carcinomatous meningitis. Survival from time of prostate cancer diagnosis to death ranged from 1–14 yr. Twelve of the 14 patients had dural involvement, with subdural hemorrhage in eight. Four of the 12 patients with dural metastasis had local extension to parenchyma, cranial nerves, or pituitary. Of the two cases without dural metastasis, one case showed a cerebellar metastasis, and the other showed a pituitary metastasis. Lynes et al. *(49)* cited a series of studies of intracranial prostate cancer metastases showing that 67% involved meninges, 25% involved the cerebrum, and 8% involved the cerebellum.

14. OTHER SITES OF METASTASIS

Metastasis to the testes, penis, and ureter is rare in prostate cancer. Testicular metastasis was reported in five of the studies in our sample, showing an average incidence of 3% (Table 1). In 1951, Bradham *(13)* reported a case, and found only three other cases in the literature. Grignon, Shum, and Hayman *(39)* reviewed 1715 solid-tumor metastases in the testes and found prostate cancer to be the second most common source after lung cancer. Epididymal metastasis from prostate cancer has also been reported. Rizk et al. *(59)* presented a case and found 12 other cases described in the literature. Metastasis to the penis was reported by two studies in our sample, each as an isolated case. Mugharbil et al. *(55)* described a case of metastasis to the penis and presented 54 cases from the literature. Clinical presentation was variable and included priapism, painless penile mass, and less commonly, urinary retention *(67)*. Ureteral involvement may occur through local extension as well as through metastasis. True metastatic lesions of the ureters are rare. Benejam, Carroll, and Loening presented a case and described only 11 other cases reported in the literature *(6)*.

Splenic metastasis was noted in eight studies in our sample. According to those studies, the incidence of splenic metastasis ranges from 1–9% with an average of 4% (Table 1). Pancreatic metastasis was noted by nine studies with an average incidence of 3% ranging from 1–10%. Gastrointestinal metastasis was reported by four studies *(8,17,52,63)*. Saitoh et al. *(63)* reported intestinal metastasis in 4% of 1367 cases, and Berge and Lundberg *(8)* described metastasis to the small intestine in <1% of 299 cases. Mintz and Smith *(52)* described metastasis to the esophagus, stomach, and small and large intestine, with the incidence of each ranging from 1–3% *(52)*. De la Monte *(26)* et al. reported large intestine metastasis in 14% of 89 cases. Byar *(17)* described metastasis to colon or ileum occurring in 1–2% of cases. Peritoneal metastasis was reported by seven studies in our sample to occur in an average of 6% of patients who died of metastatic prostate cancer. Renal metastasis was reported by 10 studies to occur in an average of 5% of patients who died of metastatic prostate cancer. Thyroid metastasis occurred in an average of 2% of patients who died of metastatic prostate cancer, based on five studies in our sample reporting thyroid metastasis.

Prostate cancer metastasizes to other unusual sites. Myocardial metastasis was present in four of 299 cases (1%) of metastatic disease autopsied by Berge and Lundberg *(8)*. Caulk and Boon-Itt described myocardial metastasis in one of five autopsy cases *(21)*, and Walther *(83)* reported myocardial metastasis in one of 81 cases. Other studies report cardiac metastasis, but do not distinguish pericardial from myocardial metastasis *(30,40,63)*. Metastasis to skeletal muscle has also been reported *(58)*. Prostate cancer has been reported as an uncommon source of skin metastasis *(81)*. Katske, Waisman, and Lupu described two cases and reviewed 18 cases from the literature *(43)*. Affected sites included the groin, abdomen, chest, scalp, and face. Four of the 18 reviewed cases had no evidence of metastasis at other sites. Reports of unusual head and neck involvement include those of metastasis to the vocal cords *(39)* and parotid gland *(41)*. De Potter et al. reported seven cases of prostate cancer metastasis to the eye *(27)*.

15. CONCLUSION

Autopsy studies consistently describe prostate cancer metastasis involving the lymph nodes, bone, lungs, and liver. The traditional understanding that prostate cancer causes osteoblastic metastasis to the pelvis and spine holds true on average, but a review of autopsy studies shows great variability in the site and appearance of bone metastasis. None of the bones closely studied have been found to be spared the ravages of prostate cancer. Lymph nodes show equal variability in involvement by metastasis. In addition, less common sites of involvement, such as adrenal, dura and breast, should be considered during the clinical and pathologic evaluation of patients with metastatic prostate cancer.

The clinical manifestations of prostate cancer metastasis show variability as well. Bone pain and spinal cord compression are debilitating and well-known. Pathologic fracture is also a debilitating consequence of metastatic prostate cancer. Lung metastasis and dural metastasis are two additional sites of involvement that significantly contribute to the great morbidity and mortality of metastatic prostate cancer.

Autopsy is potentially the most powerful technique available for the study of metastatic disease. The addition of molecular analysis to standard anatomic and histologic examinations makes autopsy an even more broad and flexible means of studying metastatic disease. The limitations of autopsy in the past are apparent from the literature. Uniformity in procedures and full descriptions of the postmortem examination are essential for producing reliable data. To avoid the confusion of wide variation in the incidence of bone metastasis, for example, autopsy reports must explicitly state which bones were examined and what techniques were used. Histology at sites other than the primary tumor has been poorly described in most autopsy studies. Finally, clinical data are usually limited or absent, especially in more recent autopsy studies. Only rarely was the immediate cause of death reported. With improved documentation and technique, modern autopsy studies which combine a knowledge of tumor phenotype and molecular genotype are poised to make major contributions to the advancement of current understanding and treatment of metastatic prostate cancer.

REFERENCES

1. Anderson, T., J. Wakely, and A. Carter. 1992. Medieval example of metastatic carcinoma: a dry bone, radiological, and SEM study. *Am. J. Phys. Anthropol.* **89:** 309–323.
2. Araki, H., T. Mishina, K. Miyakoda, T. Fujiwara, and T. Kobayashi. 1980. An epidemiological survey of prostatic cancer from the Annual of the Pathological Autopsy Cases in Japan. *Tohoku J. Exp. Med.* **130:** 159–164.
3. Arnheim, F. K. 1948. Carcinoma of the prostate: a study of the post mortem findings in one hundred and seventy-six cases. *J. Urol.* **60:** 599–603.
4. Barringer, B. S. 1921. Carcinoma of prostate. *Surg. Gynecol. Obstet.* **34:** 168–176.
5. Batson, O. V. 1940. The function of the vertebral veins and their role in the spread of metastases. *Ann. Surg.* **112:** 138–149.
6. Benejam, R., T. J. Carroll, and S. Loening. 1987. Prostate carcinoma metastatic to ureter. *Urology* **29:** 325–327.
7. Benson, W. R. 1957. Carcinoma of the prostate with metastases to breasts and testis. *Cancer* **10:** 1235.
8. Berge, T. and S. Lundberg. 1977. Cancer in Malmo 1958–1969. An autopsy study. *Acta Pathol. Microbiol. Scand. Suppl.* 1–235.
9. Bleichner, J. C., B. Chun, and R. S. Klappenbach. 1986. Pure small-cell carcinoma of the prostate with fatal liver metastasis. *Arch. Pathol. Lab. Med.* **110:** 1041–1044.
10. Blumer, G. 1909. A report of two cases of osteoplastic carcinoma of the prostate with a review of the literature. *Johns Hopkins Hospital Bulletin* **20:** 200–204.
11. Boldt, H. C. and J. A. Nerad. 1998. Orbital metastases from prostate carcinoma. *Arch. Ophthalmol.* **106:** 1403–1408.
12. Bova, G. S., M. A. Eisenberger, M. Carducci, S. S. Pin, D. F. Jarrard, J. I. Epstein, et al. 1996. Molecular autopsy study of lethal prostate cancer. *J. Urol.* **155:** 529A.
13. Bradham, A. C. 1951. Prostatic carcinoma with metastasis to the testicle. *J. Urol.* **66:** 122.
14. Brawn, P. N. and V. O. Speights. 1989. The dedifferentiation of metastatic prostate carcinoma. *Br. J. Cancer* **59:** 85–88.
15. Bromberg, W. D., F. D. Gaylis, K. D. Bauer, and A. J. Schaeffer. 1989. Isolated pulmonary metastases from carcinoma of the prostate: a case report and deoxyribonucleic acid analysis using flow cytometry. *J. Urol.* **141:** 137–139.
16. Bumpus, H. C. 1921. Carcinoma of the prostate: a clinical study. *Surg. Gynecol. Obstet.* **32:** 31–43.
17. Byar, D. P. 1977. VACURG studies on prostatic cancer and its treatment, in *Urologic Pathology: The Prostate* (Tannenbaum, M., ed.), Lea & Febiger, Philadelphia, PA, 241–267.
18. Campbell, J. H., and S. D. Cummins. 1951. Metastases, simulating mammary cancer, in prostatic carcinoma under estrogenic therapy. *Cancer* **4:** 303–311.
19. Carrascosa, M., J. L. Perez-Castrillon, M. A. Mendez, L. Cillero, and R. Valle. 1994. Malignant pleural effusion from prostatic adenocarcinoma resolved with hormonal therapy. *Chest* **105:** 1577,1578.
20. Catane, R., J. Kaufman, C. West, C. Merrin, Y. Tsukada, and G. P. Murphy. 1976. Brain metastasis from prostatic carcinoma. *Cancer* **38:** 2583–2587.
21. Caulk, J. R. and S. B. Boon-Itt. 1932. Carcinoma of the prostate. *Am. J. Cancer* **16:** 1024–1052.
22. Cher, M. L., G. S. Bova, D. H. Moore, E. J. Small, P. R. Carroll, S. S. Pin, et al. 1996. Genetic alterations in untreated prostate cancer metastases and androgen independent pros-

tate cancer detected by comparative genomic hybridization and allelotyping. *Cancer Res.* **56:** 3091–3102.

23. Clain, A. 1964. Secondary malignant disease of bone. *Br. J. Cancer*, 15–29.
24. Cone, S. M. 1898. A case of carcinoma metastases in bone from a primary tumor of the prostate. *Johns Hopkins Hospital Bulletin* **9:** 114–118.
25. Cumming, J., N. Hacking, J. Fairhurst, D. Ackery, and J. D. Jenkins. 1990. Distribution of bony metastases in prostatic carcinoma. *Br. J. Urol.* **66:** 411–414.
26. de la Monte, S. M., G. W. Moore, and G. M. Hutchins. 1986. Metastatic behavior of prostate cancer. Cluster analysis of patterns with respect to estrogen treatment. *Cancer* **58:** 985–993.
27. De Potter, P., C. L. Shields, J. A. Shields, and D. J. Tardio. 1993. Uveal metastasis from prostate carcinoma. *Cancer* **71:** 2791–2796.
28. Dodds, P. R., V. J. Caride, and B. Lytton. 1981. The role of vertebral veins in the dissemination of prostatic carcinoma. *J. Urol.* **126:** 753–755.
29. Drury, R. A. B. 1964. Carcinomatous metastasis to the vertebral bodies. *J. Clin. Pathol.* **17:** 448–457.
30. Elkin, M. and H. P. Mueller. 1954. Metastases from cancer of the prostate: autopsy and roentgenological findings. *Cancer* **98:** 1246–1248.
31. Entz, F. H. 1948. Probable metastatic carcinoma of the male breast following stilbestrol therapy: case report. *J. Urol.* **59:** 1203–1207.
32. Flocks, R. H. and D. L. Boatman. 1973. Incidence of head and neck metastases from genitourinary neoplasms. *Laryngoscope* **83:** 1527–1539.
33. Flynn, D. F. and W. U. Shipley. 1991. Management of spinal cord compression secondary to metastatic prostatic carcinoma (review). *Urol. Clin. N. Am.* **18:** 145–152.
34. Franks, L. M. 1956. The spread of prostate cancer. *J. Path. Bact.* **72:** 603–611.
35. Gentile, P. S., H. W. Carloss, T. Y. Huang, L. T. Yam, and W. K. Lam. 1988. Disseminated prostatic carcinoma simulating primary lung cancer. Indications for immunodiagnostic studies. *Cancer* **62:** 711–715.
36. Graves, R. C. and R. E. Militzer. 1935. Carcinoma of the prostate with metastases. *J. Urol.* **33:** 235–251.
37. Green, L. K. and M. Klima. 1991. The use of immunohistochemistry in metastatic prostatic adenocarcinoma to the breast. *Hum. Pathol.* **22:** 242–246.
38. Greenlee, R. T., T. Murray, S. Bolden, and P. A. Wingo. 2000. Cancer Statistics, 2000. *Ca: Cancer J. Clin.* **50:** 7–33.
39. Grignon, D. J., J. Y. Ro, A. G. Ayala, and C. Chong. Carcinoma of prostate metastasizing to vocal cord (review). *Urology* **36:** 85–88.
40. Harada, M., M. Iida, M. Yamaguchi, and K. Shida. 1992. Analysis of bone metastasis of prostatic adenocarcinoma in 137 autopsy cases. *Adv. Exp. Med. Biol.* **324:** 173–182.
41. Hrebinko, R., S. R. Taylor, and R. R. Bahnson. 1993. Carcinoma of prostate metastatic to parotid gland. *Urology* **41:** 272, 273.
42. Huggins, C. and C. V. Hodges. 1941. The effect of castration, of estrogen and of androgen injection on serum phosphatases in metastatic carcinoma of the prostate. *Cancer Res.* **1:** 293–297.
43. Katske, F. A., J. Waisman, and A. Lupu. 1982. Cutaneous and subcutaneous metastases from carcinoma of prostate. *Urology* **19:** 373–376.
44. Kaufmann, E. 1902. Pathologische Anatomie der malignen Neoplasmen. *Deutsche Chirurgie* **53:** 381.
45. Lee, D. W., J. Y. Ro, A. A. Sahin, J. S. Lee, and A. G. Ayala. 1990. Mucinous adenocarcinoma of the prostate with endobronchial metastasis. *Am. J. Clin. Pathol.* **94:** 641–645.
46. Legge, D. A., C. A. Good, and J. Ludwig. 1971. Roentgenologic features of pulmonary carcinomatosis from carcinoma of the prostate. *Am. J. Roentgenol.* **111:** 360.

47. Lo, M. C., B. Chomet, and A. Rubenstone. 1978. Metastatic prostatic adenocarcinoma of male breast. *Urology* **11:** 641–646.

48. Lome, L. G. and T. John. 1973. Pulmonary manifestations of prostatic carcinoma. *J. Urol.* **109:** 680–685.

49. Lynes, W. L., D. G. Bostwick, F. S. Freiha, and T. A. Stamey. 1986. Parenchymal brain metastases from adenocarcinoma of prostate. *Urology* **28:** 280–287.

50. Makarova, G. V., L. M. Gorilovskii, and D. Okunev. 1987. Incidence and nature of metastases of prostatic cancer based on autopsy data (Russian). *Vopr. Onkol.* **33:** 78–83.

51. Mannion, R. A. and M. Johnson. 1993. Case report: accumulation of 99mTc-hydroxy-methylene diphosphonate by liver metastases of prostatic adenocarcinoma. *Clin. Radiol.* **47:** 209,210.

52. Mintz, E. R. and G. G. Smith. 1934. Autopsy findings in 100 cases of prostate cancer. *N. Engl. J. Med.* **211:** 479–487.

53. Montalban, C., M. A. Moreno, J. P. Molina, I. Hernanz, and C. Bellas. 1993. Metastatic carcinoma of the prostate presenting as a superior vena cava syndrome. *Chest* **104:** 1278–1280.

54. Morgan, J. W., K. A. Adcock, and R. Donohue. 1990. Distribution of skeletal metastases in prostatic and lung cancer. Mechanisms of skeletal metastases. *Urology* **36:** 31–34.

55. Mugharbil, Z. H., C. Childs, M. Tannenbaum, and H. Schapira. 1985. Carcinoma of prostate metastatic to penis. *Urology* **25:** 314,315.

56. Muir, E. G. 1934. Carcinoma of the prostate. *Lancet* **226:** 667–672.

57. Plesnicar, S. 1985. The course of metastatic disease originating from carcinoma of the prostate. *Clin. Exp. Metastasis* **3:** 103–110.

58. Rau, W. 1922. Eine vergleichende Statistik der 5 Kriegsjahren (1914–1919) und 5 Friedensjaren (1909–1914) sezierten Falle von Krebs und anderen malignen Tumoren am Pathologischen Institut des Stadtkrankenhauses Dresden-Friedrichstadt. *Z. Krebsforschung* **18:** 141.

59. Rizk, C. C., J. Scholes, S. K. Chen, J. Ward, and N. A. Romas. 1990. Epididymal metastasis from prostatic adenocarcinoma mimicking adenomatoid tumor. *Urology* **36:** 526–530.

60. Resnick, M. I. 1992. Hemodynamics of prostate cancer bone metastases. in *Prostate Cancer and Bone Metastasis*, vol. 324 (Karr, J. P. and Yamanaka, H., eds.), Plenum Press, New York, p. 77.

61. Roberts, O. W. 1927. Some notes on carcinoma of the prostate: including evidence of an intraspinous route of dissemination. *Br. J. Surg.* **15:** 652–660.

62. Sahin, A. A., J. Y. Ro, N. G. Ordonez, M. A. Luna, R. S. Weber, and A. G. Ayala. 1991. Temporal bone involvement by prostatic adenocarcinoma: report of two cases and review of the literature (review). *Head Neck* **13:** 349–354.

63. Saitoh, H., M. Hida, T. Shimbo, K. Nakamura, J. Yamagata, and T. Satoh. 1984. Metastatic patterns of prostatic cancer. Correlation between sites and number of organs involved. *Cancer* **54:** 3078–3084.

64. Saitoh, H., K. Yoshida, Y. Uchijima, N. Kobayashi, J. Suwata, and S. Kamata. 1990. Two different lymph node metastatic patterns of a prostatic cancer. *Cancer* **65:** 1843–1846.

65. Salyer, W. R. and D. C. Salyer. 1973. Metastases of prostate carcinoma to the breast. *J. Urol.* **109:** 671.

66. Sarma, D. P., and L. Godeau. 1983. Brain metastasis from prostatic cancer (review). *J. Surg. Oncol.* **23:** 173,174.

67. Savion, M., P. M. Livne, C. Mor, and C. Servadio. 1987. Mixed carcinoma of the prostate with penile metastases and priapism (review). *Eur. Urol.* **13:** 351,352.

68. Schoonees, R., L. D. Palma, J. F. Gaeta, R. H. Moore, and G. P. Murphy. 1972. Prostatic carcinoma treated at categorical center: clinical and pathologic observations. *NY State J. Med.* **72:** 1021–1027.

69. Scott, J., A. Robb-Smith, and I. Burns. 1974. Bilateral breast metastases from carcinoma of the prostate. *Br. J. Urol.* **46:** 209–214.

70. Slack, N. H., M. F. Brady, and G. P. Murphy. 1984. Prostatic carcinoma treated at a categorical center, 1970–1979. *NY State J. Med.* **83:** 699–705.
71. Smith, E. M., N. Hampel, R. Ruff, D. Bodner, and M. Resnick. 1993. Spinal cord compression secondary to prostate carcinoma: treatment and prognosis. *J. Urol.* **149:** 330–333.
72. Smith, V. C., D. Kasdon, and R. Hardy. 1980. Metastatic brain tumor from the prostate: two unusual cases. *Surg. Neurol.* **14:** 189–191.
73. Styles, C. 1989. The distribution of bone metastases as shown on isotope scanning: proposed modes of spread. *Australas. Radiol.* **33:** 226–228.
74. Suzuki, T., T. Shimizu, K. Kurokawa, H. Jimbo, J. Sato, and H. Yamanaka. 1994. Pattern of prostate cancer metastasis to the vertebral column. *Prostate* **25:** 141–146.
75. Takahashi, Y., T. Mayuzumi, and J. Satoh. 1986. Prostatic cancer: pathological analysis of autopsied cases (Japanese). *Hinyokika Kiyo.* **32:** 835–839.
76. Taylor, H. G., M. Lefkowitz, S. Skoog, B. Miles, D. McLeod, and J. Coggin. 1984. Intracranial metastases in prostate cancer. *Cancer* **53:** 2728–2730.
77. Thompson, H. 1854. *Tr. Path. Soc. Lond.* **5:** 204.
78. Thomson Walker, J. W. 1905. Malignant disease of the prostate: a statistical study based on the records of the Middlesex Hospital. *Arch. Middlesex Hosp.* **5:** 149.
79. Turner, J. W. 1940. Metastatic neoplasms: a clinical and roentgenological study of involvement of skeleton and lungs. *Am. J. Roentgenol.* **43:** 479–492.
80. Varkarakis, M. J., A. Winterberger, J. Gaeta, R. Moore, and G. Murphy. 1974. Lung metastases in prostatic carcinoma. Clinical significance. *Urology* **3:** 447–452.
81. Venable, D. D., D. Hastings, and R. Misra. 1983. Unusual metastatic patterns of prostate adenocarcinoma. *J. Urol.* **130:** 980–985.
82. Viadana, E., I. Bross, and J. Pickren. 1976. The metastatic spread of kidney and prostate cancers in man. *Neoplasma* **23:** 323–332.
83. Walther, H. E. 1948. *Die Voseherdruse. Krebsmetastasen*, Basel: Benno Schwabe & Co., pp. 436–444.
84. Warren, S., P. Harris, and R. Graves. 1936. Osseous metastasis of carcinoma of the prostate with special reference to the perineural lymphatics. *Arch. Pathol.* **22:** 139–160.
85. Willis, R. A. 1973. *The Spread of Tumors in the Human Body*, 3rd ed., Butterworth, London.
86. Wood, D. P., Jr., E. Banks, S. Humphreys, J. McRoberts, and V. Rangnekar. 1994. Identification of bone marrow micrometastases in patients with prostate cancer. *Cancer* **74:** 2533–2540.

5

Tumor Suppressor Genes in Prostate Cancer

Robert Bookstein, MD

1. DEFINITION AND GENERAL PROPERTIES OF TUMOR SUPPRESSOR GENES

The concept of tumor suppressor genes (TSGs) was originally proposed on the basis of cell-fusion studies between neoplastic and nonneoplastic cultured cells *(106,133).* These studies suggested the existence of chromosomal genetic elements in nonneoplastic cells that could suppress the malignant phenotype of fusion partners. Comings proposed that the process of neoplastic transformation involved the loss or inactivation of such suppressor elements, which in diploid organisms meant the alteration of both alleles of a given TSG locus *(47).* TSGs were thus viewed in counterpoise to the dominant oncogenes, for which proneoplastic activity was achieved via gain-of-function alterations (e.g., missense mutation, amplification, or overexpression) independent of the status of other alleles or loci *(15).* Both types of cancer genes have been integrated into general models of multistep carcinogenesis in which activated dominant oncogenes and inactivated TSGs contribute in a sequential or additive fashion to the process of cancer formation *(68).* Some workers have classified subgroups of TSGs that suppress only one aspect of the neoplastic phenotype, for example, "metastasis suppressors," such as nm23-H1, or "invasion suppressors," such as E-cadherin, but their genetic mechanism of loss or inactivation is analogous to that of all TSGs, and they are not otherwise distinguished here.

The term "tumor suppressor gene" may be misapplied to any genetic element that can be demonstrated experimentally to suppress growth in vitro or tumorigenicity in vivo upon transfer to cancerous recipient cells. This overlooks the corollary requirement for the inactivation of such genes during tumorigenesis by loss-of-function mutation, methylation-based gene silencing, transcriptional downregulation, or perhaps modification of the gene product *(103).* In other words, functional characterization of TSGs must be made in the context of identification based on altered gene structure or expression. Without this criterion, it is difficult to distinguish specific tumor suppression from nonspecific or toxic effects of heterologously (over) expressed transgenes. The best specificity control in this regard is the *lack* of suppressive function in recipient cells with wild-type function of the TSG in question. The induction of neoplastic properties in previously normal cells or tissues by TSG blockade, or the finding of

From: *Prostate Cancer: Biology, Genetics, and the New Therapeutics*
Edited by: L. W. K. Chung, W. B. Isaacs, and J. W. Simons © Humana Press Inc., Totowa, NJ

elevated cancer susceptibility in animals with germline TSG inactivation (e.g., knockout mice), are also useful indicators of TSG function.

The first paradigmatic TSG to be identified was *RB1*, which plays a critical role in the genesis of retinoblastoma, a rare intraocular cancer of early childhood *(18)*. Its distinct hereditary transmission pattern in some families, with affected members of both sexes in consecutive generations, was strongly suggestive of the involvement of an autosomal dominant genetic trait. In 1971, Knudson proposed the "two-hit" hypothesis, which offered a unifying genetic model for both familial and sporadic retinoblastoma based on biallelic mutation of a tumor suppressor-type locus, Rb *(136)*. Sporadic cases were predicted to result from somatic mutation of both Rb alleles in retinal precursor cells, whereas familial cases were thought to be caused by the germline inheritance of one mutant Rb allele followed by somatic mutation of the second allele. The susceptibility trait was localized to chromosome band 13q14 by linkage and cytogenetic studies in families *(73,253)*, and the responsible gene, *RB1*, was shown to suffer both germline and somatic inactivating mutations in retinoblastoma patients and tumors just as predicted *(60,74,79,149)*. Its biallelic inactivation in tumor cells supported the notion that wild-type *RB1* acted dominantly at the cellular level to prevent tumor formation.[*] The ability of a single TSG to suppress the neoplastic phenotype was first demonstrated by *RB1* gene transfer to established retinoblastoma tumor cells *(112)*. The *RB1* gene product, a phosphoprotein of 110 kDa apparent molecular wt (pRb), has been extensively characterized. Its best-understood function is as a component of the cell cycle machinery, in particular as a central negative regulator of the G_1/S transition *(86,302)*. Hypophosphorylated pRb binds to and inactivates E2F-1, a transcription factor that upregulates the expression of genes necessary for S-phase DNA synthesis *(35)*. pRb is phosphorylated by activated cyclin-dependent kinase (CDK) complexes, releasing active E2F-1 and thereby promoting S-phase progression. Indeed, a key negative regulator of CDK4, p16^{Ink4a} encoded by *CDKN2A*, is more frequently mutated than *RB1* in human cancers *(125)*. The two genes appear to be altered in a mutually exclusive fashion in several tumor types *(116,142,212,246)*. Although both genes are believed to act similarly in a single cell cycle-regulatory pathway, it remains unclear why certain cancers—e.g., retinoblastoma, osteosarcoma, and small-cell lung cancer— are associated with *RB1* mutation, whereas others such as melanoma and pancreatic cancers are particularly associated with *CDKN2A* mutation.

From these and many other studies, several general inferences about tumor suppressor genes have been made. First, mutant alleles of TSGs may be transmitted in the germline, and may cause unusual cancer susceptibilities in families. Second, any given TSG may be involved in multiple cancer types, but with widely varying frequencies of alteration. Mechanisms of alteration may also vary by cancer type. Third, the transfer of wild-type TSGs into tumor cells is capable of suppressing the neoplastic phenotype despite the presence of oncogenic mutations in multiple cancer loci *(88)*. The latter result, which has been widely supported using numerous TSGs, may be surprising in light of the multistep model of carcinogenesis if a given mutation were to act only at a certain cancer stage. It also suggested a potential therapeutic approach to cancer—

---

[*] The dominant inheritance pattern of mutant alleles in pedigrees is a result of the near-certainty of subsequent somatic mutation in at least one susceptible retinal precursor cell.

tumor suppressor gene therapy. Fourth, TSGs may have major roles in fundamental cellular processes such cell division, apoptosis, adhesion, or motility; and other genes in these pathways may also act as TSGs. The extrapolation of these general features of TSGs to prostate cancer genetics is explored in the remainder of this chapter.

2. POSITIONAL CLONING AND IDENTIFICATION OF PROSTATE TSGS

Because they were originally defined in the context of various chromosomal regions via linkage, karyotyping, and allelotypic analyses, many TSGs have been identified by positional cloning approaches in which genetic position and structural alteration are the primary identifying criteria. TSGs obtained in this way have included *RB1*, *APC*, *CDKN2A* (p16^{Ink4}), *Smad4*, *FHIT*, and *PTEN/MMAC1*. Positional and structural information also played a role in revising the perception of *TP53* as a TSG rather than an overexpressed 53 kDa oncoprotein as it was originally characterized. Most of these TSGs were not originally identified by their involvement in prostate cancers *per se*, and most are infrequently mutated in primary prostatic cancers (*see* Section 3). Therefore, there has been considerable interest in identifying TSGs with a principal role in primary prostate cancer or familial prostate cancer susceptibility based on linkage, karyotypic, or allelotypic changes particular to this cancer type.

The identification of genetic regions that confer hereditary prostate cancer predisposition has been a challenging area of intense focus for a number of research groups, and is reviewed separately in this volume. Studies of chromosomal number and structure in prostate cancer cells—including metaphase karyotyping, interphase (FISH) karyotyping, and comparative genomic hybridization (CGH)—have been reviewed elsewhere *(27,206)*. Primary prostate cancer offers special technical challenges for many of these methods because of their limited ability to be grown in culture and their extensive admixture of neoplastic and nonneoplastic cells. Furthermore, careful analysis of cancerous prostate glands has revealed frequent multifocality of disease with extensive genetic heterogeneity among tumor foci *(174,188)*. These features compromise methods that have proven successful in other cancer types.

Analysis of allelic loss ("LOH") is a molecular genetic translation of some of these chromosome-based methods with special utility in the search for TSGs. In the study of retinoblastoma and other cancers, the "second hit" to a TSG locus was often found to involve chromosomal loss (with or without reduplication) or regional conversion of the wild-type allele after mutational inactivation of other allele *(32)*. These changes may not be observed in chromosomal dosage-based methods. LOH analysis is also adept at detecting small, subkaryotypic heterozygous interstitial deletions. Yet normal-cell admixture and genetic heterogeneity remain compromising factors. These drawbacks may be partially surmounted by establishment of quantitative criteria for "allelic imbalance" *(171)* and by laser-capture microdissection to study microscopic islands of tumor cells *(64)*. Another issue for both karyotypic and allelotypic analyses is the interpretation of detected alterations, because aneuplodies and allelic imbalances may reflect the generalized instability of tumor cell genomes rather than the specific involvement of TSGs. The latter may be distinguished on the basis of higher rates of loss compared to "background," but this criterion is rather vague. Homozygous genetic deletions are generally less common and far smaller in size than allelic losses, but are more likely to be specific for TSG inactivation. The presence of overlapping homozygous deletions in a region of frequent allelic loss is optimal indirect evidence of somatic TSG involvement.

Despite all these caveats and limitations, karyotypic, allelotypic, and CGH analyses have suggested a number of common regions of genetic change in prostate cancers that support the existence of novel TSGs. Regional genetic losses on chromosome arms 2q, 5q, 6q, 7q, 8p, 10q, 13q, 16q, 17p, and 18q have been identified *(10,23,28,31,41,51,146, 155,167,265,290,311)*, which include known TSGs such as *RB1* on 13q14, *TP53* on 17p13, *CDH1* (E-cadherin) on 16q22, and *Smad4* (DPC4) on 18q21. Direct evidence for the involvement of these TSGs in prostate cancer is discussed in Section 3. A comprehensive review of studies of all of these genetic regions is beyond the scope of this chapter. Among the genetic regions without "known" TSGs, the 8p arm has received the greatest attention because of its high rate of allelic loss in prostate cancer and several other types of cancer *(22,51,76,129,297)*. Selected 8p loci are lost in up to 80% of primary and metastatic prostate cancers *(41)*, as well as in microdissected primary foci and PIN lesions *(65,294)*, suggesting a role in early prostatic oncogenesis. Attempts to refine the localization of TSGs by use of more polymorphic loci and more tumors have met with limited success on 8p, yielding up to three distinct consensus regions that may reflect either genetic or methodological complexity, or both *(75,174,221,305)*. These regions were not small or precise enough to support practical positional cloning.

In a study of 8p allelic loss, Bova et al. *(22)* detected a homozygous deletion of the macrophage scavenger receptor gene *(MSR,* located on 8p22) in one metastatic prostate cancer sample. Because this marker was within a consensus region of allelic loss, physical mapping of the single homozygous deletion was undertaken that defined a small critical region (730–970 kb) suitable for positional cloning *(24)*. By a combination of cDNA selection, exon trapping and genomic sequencing, only *MSR* and one additional novel gene, *N33*, was identified within this region *(16,172)*. Evaluation of *N33* yielded inconclusive evidence for its identification as a TSG in prostate as well as colorectal cancer. Methylation-based gene silencing was detected in most colorectal cell lines and tumors examined, whereas methylation and expression were unaltered in prostate cell lines and tumors. Although aberrant promoter hypermethylation is recognized as a mechanism of TSG inactivation (e.g., for *CDKN2A)*, cancer-associated hypermethylation is certainly not restricted to TSGs. DNA sequence alterations of *N33* were not found in either tumor type, and *N33* gene transfer in colorectal cancer cells showed no evidence of tumor suppression in vitro or in vivo *(170)*. Subsequently, Ahuja et al. *(2)* found that *N33* methylation was associated with both aging and neoplasia in human colonic epithelium. In a recent study of 47 tumor cell lines with 140 randomly spaced markers on chromosome 8p, Levy et al. *(153)* found a pancreatic cancer cell line with a homozygous deletion that overlapped the one mapped by Bova et al. *(24)*; *N33* is located within both of these deletions.[*]

Two other candidate TSGs have been identified in positional cloning efforts on chromosome 8p21.3-p22. One, known as *PRLTS* for "PDGF β receptor-like tumor suppressor," was located within a consensus region of allelic loss in hepatocellular, colorectal, and lung cancers *(77)*. Heterozygous genomic rearrangement of this gene was detected

---

[*] *N33* may also be within a small LOH region in non-small-cell lung cancer (NSCLC) *(152)*.

in one NSCLC tumor, and localized somatic mutations were observed in an additional 3 of 107 tumors. In a subsequent study of *PRLTS* in prostate cancer, one missense mutation was detected in 69 primary or metastatic specimens *(140)*. Functional characterization of *PRLTS* has not been reported. In another study, a gene called *FEZ1* was identified within a consensus region of allelic loss in primary esophageal squamous carcinomas located >2 Mb centromeric to *MSR* in 8p22. Somatic mutations were identified in two primary esophageal carcinomas and one prostate cell line from a total of 194 cancer samples or cell lines examined. A homozygous genomic DNA alteration was detected by Southern blotting in one of 18 tumor cell lines. Lack of expression, or expression of abnormally-spliced transcripts, were observed frequently among these samples or cell lines. Functional characterization of *FEZ1* has not been reported. These findings with *N33*, *PRLTS* and *FEZ1* suggest that definitive identification of TSGs in homozygous deletion and allelic loss regions may not always be straightforward.

A recent successful example of allelotyping and homozygous deletion mapping has emerged from studies of chromosome 10q in prostate, brain, and other cancers *(5,28,78,91,120,167,258)*, in which frequent abnormalities of a common 10q22-q25 region were noted. The gene encoding Mxi1, a functional antagonist of the proto-oncogene product c-Myc, was mapped into this genetic region and was therefore examined as a promising candidate TSG by Eagle et al. *(61)*. Between this and a follow-up study *(225)*, point mutations of this gene were detected in 12 of 20 primary prostate cancers, but affected only a minor subset of cells in each sample (1–19%, mean 5%); the significance of this mutational pattern is unclear. Other workers have not detected *MXI1* mutations, even with the use of microdissection *(127,144)*. These findings complicate the interpretation of TSG activity by *MXI1* gene transfer *(301)* and murine knockout *(240)*. In 1997, a gene called *PTEN* or *MMAC1* located at 10q23.3 was identified that was mutated in brain, prostate, and other cancer types *(158,259)*, and was also responsible for the inheritance of Cowden disease, a hamartomatous polyposis and cancer predisposition syndrome. This gene is further discussed in Section 3. Another candidate TSG in brain cancer, *DMBT1*, is located distally at 10q25.3-q26.1 *(189,258)*. Examination of this gene in prostate cancer has not been reported.

An alternative approach to the positional identification of novel TSGs involves testing for suppression activity of subchromosomal segments transferred to recipient tumor cells by microcell fusion. The chromosomal segments then define critical regions for positional cloning. For example, microcell-mediated transfer of human chromosome 11, or fragments thereof, into highly metastatic sublines of Dunning R-3327 rat prostatic cancer cells was shown to specifically suppress their metastatic phenotype but not their primary tumorigenicity *(114)*. Positional cloning within one small retained region yielded *KAI1*, a gene on human chromosome 11p11.2 that suppressed the metastasis of the AT6.1 subline *(58)*. *KAI1* was found to be downregulated in 70% of primary prostate cancers, but mutations have not been detected *(57)* and allelic losses are infrequent *(128)*. Although the mechanism of *KAI1* downregulation is unknown, its expression was shown to be directly activated by wild-type p53 *(181)*. *KAI1* was previously cloned as a leukocyte cell-surface antigen (CD82); its biochemical function and mechanism of metastasis suppression are unknown. Another cell-surface marker, CD44—encoded in chromosome 11p13—suppressed the metastatic properties of the

AT3.1 subline *(81)*. Other human chromosomes with metastasis-suppressing activity in R-3327 derivatives include chromosome 7q *(204)*, chromosome 8p *(115,203)*, chromosome 10q *(202)*, and chromosome 17 *(34,230)*. Potential issues in this approach include the genetic relevance of Dunning sublines to human disease. Chromosome 17q, which harbors a number of suppressor loci including *nm23-H1* and *BRCA1*, was shown to suppress the tumorigenicity of human prostate-cell line PPC-1 *(193)*, and the pter-q11 region of human chromosome 10 was found to suppress tumorigenicity and induce apoptosis of human prostate cell line PC-3 *(236)*. By similar methods, chromosome 8p was shown to suppress or reduce the tumorigenicity of two different colorectal cancer cell lines *(102,271)*. All chromosome transfer-based approaches are subject to the problem of assessing function of multiple transferred genes without knowledge of their structural alterations in host cells.

A number of methods have been developed for the identification of genes that are underexpressed in cancer cells compared to their normal counterparts, with the notion that some of these may be TSGs. Such methods include cDNA subtraction, representational difference analysis (RDA) on cDNA, differential display, comparative expressed sequence tag (EST) database analysis, and gene expression microarrays. Positional information is not used to select genes, although any genes obtained may be mapped after the fact. The application of such methods in prostate cancer has yielded a number of genes differentially expressed between tumor and normal tissue or among different tumors *(33,298)*, but structural or functional evidence for the identification of novel prostate TSGs by these means has not been forthcoming. Although comparative expression studies may have a number of uses, expression differences may be caused by variations in cellular composition (e.g., of stromal or inflammatory cells) between normal vs tumor tissue rather than changes in epithelial gene expression *per se.*

Several strategies for the functional cloning and identification of TSGs have also been proposed, including the use of "genetic suppressor elements" (retroviral expression constructs driving antisense cDNAs that may transform cells by blocking TSG function) *(97,159)*. Novel prostate TSGs using these methods have not been reported.*

3. TSG MUTATIONS OR EXPRESSION ABNORMALITIES IN PROSTATE CANCER

The genes reviewed in this section are well-established TSGs based on the existence of inactivating mutations in one or more human cancer types. Most of these genes also have demonstrable tumor suppressor activity in gene transfer experiments and/or induce a cancer susceptibility phenotype in mouse knockouts. A few genes are included that are downregulated rather than mutated in cancer, yet have compelling functional and mechanistic evidence for their role as TSGs. The preference for mutational vs expression evidence is threefold: first, mutations detected by standard methods are clonal and are likely to arise through a process of clonal selection. Second, altered gene expression, which may reflect global expression reprogramming controlled by other master regulators, is less likely than mutation to be a primary selectable change. Third, expres-

---

* A gene called *CATR1* has been defined functionally via an antisense approach in the tumorigenic conversion of a human squamous carcinoma cell line *(156)*. It was mapped to 7q31-32, near a small chromosomal region of allelic loss in prostate and breast cancer *(148,267,310,311)*.

sion data are potentially subject to confounding effects of variable tissue composition as described above. A rationale for examining the involvement of these TSGs in prostate cancer is the potential similarity of oncogenic mechanisms across cancer types. Genes excluded from this section include the androgen receptor gene (which appears to become oncogenic by activating mutations and/or amplification as discussed elsewhere), other dominant oncogenes and growth factors, potential hereditary predisposition genes (e.g., *BRCA1*),[†] DNA damage response or repair (mutator) genes[§] (e.g., *MLH1* and *MSH2*), detoxification genes (e.g., *GSTP1*), differentially expressed genes lacking mutational or functional characterization, and TSGs not yet characterized in prostate cancer.[¶] The focus here is on the evidence supporting a role for each gene in the genesis or progression of prostate cancer, which includes, at a minimum, rates of mutation or loss of expression (stratified by disease stage, if available). Measurement of allelic loss is insufficiently specific on its own, and is only considered in conjunction with mutational analysis.

3.1. APC *(chromosome 5q21)*

Mutant alleles of *APC* determine the (dominant) inheritance of familial adenomatous polyposis coli *(96)* and occur somatically as an early step in sporadic colorectal tumorigenesis (reviewed in ref. *132*). Truncating point mutations accompanied by allelic loss are typical, suggesting a classical two-hit (recessive) mechanism at the cellular level *(154)*. Tumor suppression by *APC* gene transfer has been demonstrated *(95)*, and the Min (multiple intestinal neoplasia) mouse strain is mutant for an allele of murine *APC (262)*. *APC* negatively regulates cellular levels of β-catenin (encoded by *CTNNB1*), a protein that mediates positive growth or survival signals via cadherins from the extracellular environment and that can be activated by mutation in colon, prostate, ovarian and other cancers *(118,213,234,254,296)*. Only one missense *APC* mutation was detected in 53 primary or metastatic prostate cancers examined *(263,300)*, suggesting the lack of involvement of this gene (but not the pathway) in prostatic oncogenesis.

3.2. CDH1 *(E-cadherin) (chromosome 16q22)*

The cadherins are a family of transmembrane glycoproteins that mediate cell-cell adhesion in a calcium dependent, homotypic manner in a wide variety of tissues *(216)*. E-cadherin is the major adhesion molecule of many epithelial layers, including prostatic glandular epithelium, and its role in the process of epithelial neoplasia has been intensively studied. *CDH1* encoding E-cadherin qualifies as a TSG because it is mutationally inactivated in about 50% of sporadic lobular breast carcinomas and diffuse gastric carcinomas in association with allelic loss *(12,13,208)*. Furthermore, heterozygous germline mutations were shown to predispose to hereditary diffuse gastric cancer in rare families *(98)*, and *CDH1* gene transfer suppressed tumor cell invasiveness *(292)*. Overt *CDH1* mutation is common in only these two cancer types, and is detected infre-

---

[†] Although *BRCA1* has been characterized as a TSG, somatic mutations are rare and its role in prostate cancer, if any, is more likely to be via prediposition rather than somatic alteration.

[§] Haber and Harlow *(103)* not unreasonably classified DNA mismatch repair genes as TSGs based on their genetic mechanism of biallelic inactivation. They are excluded here because of limited space.

[¶] E.g., *VHL*, involved in Von-Hippel Lindau syndrome and renal cell carcinoma, studies of which have not been reported in prostate cancer.

quently in other cancers *(231)*. Decreased expression of E-cadherin is commonly found in many epithelial neoplasms and is closely related to cancer invasiveness *(218)*, poor cellular differentiation/higher grade, and poor prognosis in colorectal, breast and prostate cancers, among others *(216)*. For example, in primary prostate cancer Umbas et al. showed that decreased or absent E-cadherin staining by immunohistochemistry (IHC) was strongly associated with higher Gleason grade (having near-perfect discrimination at the extremes of Gleason 4 vs 10) *(283)*, with advanced disease stage, and with shortened progression-free or overall survival after radical prostatectomy (RP) *(282)*. In multivariate analysis, E-cadherin staining was an independent predictor of high-stage disease at the time of RP *(180)*. Surprisingly, all 10 pelvic nodal metastases examined expressed E-cadherin despite its downregulation in primaries, suggesting selection for its reexpression in successfully established metastatic foci.

Mechanisms of *CDH1* downregulation in prostate cancer are not entirely clear *(216)*. Methylation-associated silencing of *CDH1* has been detected frequently in prostate and other tumor cell lines in culture as well as in breast cancer tissue *(90,309)*, but mutations and methylation are not usually found in primary prostate cancer specimens *(216)*. Decreased expression of E-cadherin, however, is associated with 16q allelic loss *(214)*. Normal expression and localization of E-cadherin is dependent on its proper association with α-catenin, which anchors it to the cytoskeleton and allows Wnt pathway signaling. Indeed, occasional mutation or deletion of *CTNNA1* encoding α-catenin has been found in colorectal or prostate cancer cell lines *(191,286)*, the invasiveness of which was suppressed by *CTNNA1* reexpression *(67)*. In IHC of primary prostate cancer, reduced α-catenin levels were associated with reduced levels of E-cadherin and with poor prognosis *(1,229)*. Therefore, *CTNNA1* also may be a TSG in its own right and a component of an adhesion and cell-signalling pathway that may be altered by mutations in any of *CDH1*, *CTNNA1* or *CTNNB1*.

3.3. CDKN1B $(p27^{Kip1})$ *(chromosome 12p13)*

Two families of proteins negatively regulate the cell cycle by binding to and inhibiting the cyclin dependent kinases (Cdks), which are a set of enzyme complexes required for cell cycle progression. The Cip/Kip proteins (p21, p27, and p57) inhibit most of these kinases, whereas inhibition by Ink4 proteins (p15, p16, p18, and p19) are restricted to Cdk4 or Cdk6. All CDK inhibitors (CDKIs) can inhibit cell cycle progression when overexpressed in most normal or tumor cells, and thus they have been considered good candidates for TSGs. However, extensive mutational screening has shown that only *CDKN2A* and *CDKN2B* encoding p16^{Ink4a} and p15^{Ink4b} are commonly mutated in the germline or in cancer cells; *CDKN1B* mutation is very rare *(126)*. p27^{Kip1} has been distinguished from other CDKIs as a potentially useful prognostic marker in many cancer types including colorectal, breast and prostate cancers, wherein decreased levels are unfavorable *(49,164,223,279)*. In prostate cancer, low p27 expression was associated with increased tumor grade and likelihood of recurrence, and with decreased survival time *(49)* and was an independent predictor of RP treatment failure in node-negative patients *(279)*. Multiple posttranscriptional mechanisms regulate p27 abundance and function, including translational efficiency, phosphorylation, ubiquitin-mediated degradation rate, and subcellular localization. The basis of cancer downregulation is variable or unclear *(45)*. Downregulation of p27 is also found in benign prostatic hyperplasia, but through a transcriptional mechanism *(48)*. One unusual feature of p27 cancer biology is that in heterozygous *CDKN1B* knockout mice, which are hypersensitive to radiation and carcinogen-induced neoplasia, tumors retain wild-type structure and expression of the second *CDKN1B* allele *(70)*. It is not clear whether p27 can also operate through this so-called haplo-insufficiency mechanism in human tumorigenesis.

3.4. CDKN2A (p16^{Ink4a}) (chromosome 9p21)

As introduced in Section 3.3., p16^{Ink4a} is a specific inhibitor of Cdk4 or Cdk6 complexes, and is commonly deleted or mutated in human cancers—especially in brain, bladder, esophageal, head and neck, and pancreatic cancers—in combination with 9p21 allelic loss *(30,123,125,161,163,243,245)*. Germline *CDKN2A* mutation confers familial melanoma in humans *(71)*. Because a primary function of Cdk4/cyclin D is the phosphorylation-mediated inactivation of pRb, growth suppression by *CDKN2A* gene transfer requires wild-type *RB1 (138,166)*. The reciprocal mutation of *CDKN2A* and *RB1* was noted in Section 1. Genetic analysis of *CDKN2* is complicated by the presence of a second upstream promoter and first exon (1β) that splices to common exons 2 and 3 employs an alternative reading frame (ARF) compared to p16 *(261)*. Hence, the sequence of the encoded protein (p14^{ARF} in humans) is completely dissimilar to that of p16 *(227)*. p14^{ARF} has been shown to have a specific function, unrelated to Cdk inhibition, in blocking the inhibitory activity of mdm2 on p53 *(273,313)*. Therefore, one 9p21 locus encodes gene products that critically support two major tumor suppression pathways—those of *RB1* and *TP53 (44)*. Most deletions (but not point mutations) *(226)* of *CDKN2* ablate both gene products and inactivate both pathways; this may explain why deletions in particular are so common in tumors. Another mechanism of *CDKN2* inactivation is p16^{Ink4a} promoter-specific methylation and silencing, which has been documented extensively in tumor cell lines and some primary tumor types *(85,110, 185)*. Methylation of the p14^{ARF}-specific promoter has not been reported.

Analyses of *CDKN2* inactivation in prostate cancer—usually performed without knowledge of the existence of p14^{ARF}—have shown that missense mutations of p16^{Ink4a} are rare *(37,43,122,139,215,268)*. To indirectly detect the presence of homozygous deletions (HZD) in tumor cells of clinical specimens containing contaminating normal cells, Cairns et al. used PCR of microsatellite polymorphisms to look for "retention of heterozygosity" at *CDKN2* within larger regions of allelic loss caused by the amplification solely of normal cell DNA *(30)*; HZD was thereby inferred in 3 (38%) of 8 prostate tumors. Allelic loss alone was commonly found *(30,122)*. p16^{Ink4a} promoter methylation was detected in three (13%) of 24 primary and one of 12 metastatic prostate cancers *(122)*. Quantitative RT-PCR was used to show decreased expression of p16^{Ink4a} mRNA in 26 (43%) of 60 primary tumors (mechanism not determined), but no correlation with either tumor stage or grade was found *(43)*. Although these findings suggest the potential involvement of *CDKN2* inactivation in prostate cancer, especially by homozygous deletion or methylation, additional studies with larger clinical sample sizes are needed. In prostate cancer cell lines, p16^{Ink4a} promoter methylation and gene silencing were detected in PC3, PPC-1 and TSU-Pr1 cells, which contain wild-type pRb, but not in DU145 and LNCaP cells—the former of which expresses a mutated pRb *(122)*. LNCaP cells expressed both wild-type p16 and pRb, but p16 expression was reported to be downregulated by androgens *(165)*.

3.5. FHIT *(chromosome 3p14)*

FHIT (fragile histidine triad) was positionally cloned in a region of allelic loss and cancer-related chromosome breakage. Partial or complete homozygous deletions of the gene have been observed in several tumor types, including cancers of the head and neck, gastrointestinal tract, and lung *(209,252,289)*. More common are abnormalities of FHIT mRNA detected by RT-PCR that manifest primarily as heterogeneous, aberrant splice products of unclear mechanism and significance *(82)*. As expected from its sequence, FHIT has dinucleoside $5',5'''$ -P^1,P^3-triphosphate hydrolase activity in vitro *(9)*; transfer of both wild-type and hydrolase-inactive FHIT alleles suppressed the tumorigenicity of FHIT-mutant tumor cells *(251)*. The single study of FHIT in prostate cancer found predominantly full-length FHIT mRNA expression in all samples, with aberrant splice products at equivalent low levels in both tumor and normal prostate samples *(147)*. Therefore, there is no evidence so far for *FHIT* involvement in prostate cancer.

3.6. Maspin *(chromosome* 18q21*) (239)*

Maspin was identified by subtractive hybridization and differential display methods as a cytoplasmic serine protease inhibitor (serpin)-like protein that was expressed in human mammary epithelial cells and downregulated in breast carcinoma cells *(217,314)*. Other members of the serpin family include plasminogen activator inhibitors PAI-1 and -2, which are also considered metastasis suppressors *(7)*; all share tissue plasminogen activator (tPA) as a target of their inhibitory activities *(248)*. Expression of exogenous maspin by gene transfection, or direct addition of recombinant protein in culture, suppressed the in vivo metastasis of breast cancer cells, or the in vitro invasiveness and motility of prostate cancer cells, respectively *(247,314)*. Maspin expression was low or absent in all prostate cancer cell lines and in 5 of 10 prostate-tumor specimens compared to epithelial cells *(284,312)*. Transcription of maspin mRNA was found to be repressed by the androgen receptor (AR) in a ligand independent fashion in both prostatic epithelial cells and in an androgen responsive prostate cancer cell line[*] *(312)*. One published mutational analysis detected only an apparent polymorphism *(284)*. A major role for maspin in prostate cancer progression remains speculative, pending study of additional tumor samples.

3.7. NME1 *(nm23-H1) (chromosome 17q22)*

This gene was among the first isolated on the basis of differential expression by comparative screening of murine cDNA libraries with labelled RNAs from metastatic vs nonmetastatic mouse melanoma cells *(260)*. Expression of the two human homologs, nm23-H1 and nm23-H2, is inversely correlated with the grade, metastatic potential, and prognosis of human breast cancer but not colorectal cancer, for example *(14,109,194)*. Transfer of this gene into metastatic tumor cells with low nm23 levels

---

[*] This does not explain the *differential* loss of maspin expression in prostate cancer cells.

reduced their ability to metastasize *(150,151)*. nm23 has nucleoside diphosphate kinase activity, as suggested by its sequence *(84)*, but its mechanism of metastasis suppression remains unclear *(169)*. In three IHC studies of nm23 expression in prostate cancer, one reported less nm23-H1 expression in metastases than in primary tumors *(141)*, whereas another detected high expression in prostate neoplasms of all stages, including metastases and PIN lesions *(196)*. Igawa et al. found the highest nm23 protein expression in stage D cancers and, based on their data that mRNA levels were elevated in cycling vs growth-arrested prostate cancer cells, proposed that nm23 expression was related to cell proliferative status *(117)*. The failure to generalize an inverse correlation of nm23 expression and metastasis in many cancer types leaves its potential role in prostatic oncogenesis uncertain.

3.8. RB1 *(chromosome 13q14)*

The general properties of *RB1* were reviewed in Section 1. Based on its fundamental role in human tumorigenesis and the cell cycle, *RB1* structure and expression was initially examined in a set of prostate cancer cell lines and tumor specimens *(20,21)*. In DU145 cells, point mutation-induced skipping of *RB1* exon 21 during mRNA processing resulted in readthrough of a mutant pRb lacking 35 amino acids. *RB1* gene transfer into DU145 cells had little effect on cell growth in culture, but markedly inhibited their tumorigenicity in nude mice. Reduced or absent pRb expression by Western blot and IHC was observed in two of six metastatic prostate cancer specimens, one of which contained a 103 bp deletion of the *RB1* promoter together with allelic loss *(20)*. Single-strand conformation polymorphism (SSCP) analysis of the entire coding region of *RB1* in 25 primary prostate cancers detected two missense mutations and two frameshift-inducing deletions in four cases (16%) *(143)*. In immunohistochemical studies, Phillips et al. reported that pRb was absent in 7 (16%) of 43 prostate cancers of various stages *(220)*, and Ittmann and Weiczorek showed reduced or absent pRb in 33% of primary stage B prostate cancers with 13q14 allelic loss (itself found in 35% of cases, for a ~12% overall rate of decreased pRb). Theodorescu et al. found that reduced pRb immunostaining was an independent predictor of decreased disease-specific survival *(276)*. On the other hand, pRb was present in 117 of 118 primary T1-2M0 prostate cancers in a Finnish study *(287)*, which also failed to detect any prognostic value even in modestly heterogeneous pRb expression (<90% of nuclei positive). Despite some inconsistencies, these studies suggest a role for *RB1* inactivation in the genesis and/or the progression of some prostate cancers. When combined with evidence of *CDKN2* inactivation, it can be surmised that the Rb pathway is an important target for selective alterations during prostatic oncogenesis.

3.9. PTEN *or* MMAC1 *(chromosome 10q23)*

PTEN / MMAC1 was positionally cloned based on loss of heterozygosity and HZDs in breast, brain, and prostate cancers *(158,259)*. Germline mutations of this gene appear to be responsible for the hamartomatous polyposis syndromes of Cowden and Bannayan-Zonana, as well as some cases of juvenile polyposis *(160,179,210)*; determinants of the different clinical manifestations in these diseases are unclear. Deletions or mutations have been identified primarily in Grade IV gliomas of brain (glioblastoma multiforme), *(54,59)*, endometrial carcinomas *(232,274)*, endometrioid ovarian carcinomas *(207)*, and prostate carcinomas *(121)*, with lower mutational frequencies in a number of other cancer types *(72, 275)*. *PTEN* gene transfer has been shown to reduce in vitro cellular proliferation, soft agar colony formation, and tumorigenicity of *PTEN*-mutant glioblastoma cancer cells *(38,80,190)*, and heterozygous *PTEN* knockout mice have a phenotype of multitissue hyperplasia/dysplasia and tumor formation *(50,222, 255)*. As suggested by its sequence, *PTEN* encodes a 55 kDa protein with phosphoserine/threonine/tyrosine phosphatase activity *(195)* and extensive homology to tensin, a protein that anchors focal adhesions to the cytoskeleton for purposes of extracellular adhesion and signal transduction. Tamura et al. have proposed that phosphorylated focal adhesion kinase (P-FAK), a component of the focal adhesion complex, is itself a physiological substrate for $p55^{PTEN}$ *(269,270)*. On the other hand, Maehama and Dixon have shown that recombinant $p55^{PTEN}$ is a phosphatidylinositol (PtdIns) 3-phosphatase that catalyzes the dephosphorylation of the lipid second messenger $PtdIns(3,4,5)P_3$ to $PdtIns(4,5)P_2$, thereby opposing the activity of PtdIns 3-kinase *(175)*. The latter function is supported by a dramatic inverse correlation between the expression of wild-type *PTEN* and the phosphorylation and activation status of protein kinase B (PKB or Akt) *(39,52,53,157,255,306)*, a downstream effector in the PtdIns 3-kinase pathway that mediates a number of cell growth, survival, and homeostatic signals in cancer and normal cells *(176)*.

Inactivating mutations of *PTEN/MMAC1* were present in three of five human prostate cancer cell lines (LNCaP, PC-3 and H660) *(158,259)* and in 7 (64%) of 11 prostate xenograft lines *(293)* (Table 1). In another set of 10 xenograft lines, only one had a *PTEN* deletion or mutation, but five of the remaining nine lines lacked *PTEN* mRNA and protein expression by Northern and Western blot, respectively *(303)*. Short-term culture of one line with the demethylating agent 5-azadeoxycytidine restored *PTEN* mRNA expression, suggesting a mechanism of methylation-associated gene silencing as with *CDKN2A*. Among more than a half dozen mutational analyses of stage B-D clinical prostate cancer samples, *PTEN* mutations were infrequent in early-stage primary disease (~7% *in toto*) but were found in about one-third of metastases (Table 1). Although these mutation rates are significant and approach those of *TP53*, they are generally much less than rates of chromosome 10q allelic loss. The basis of this discrepancy is uncertain.[*] In a follow-up study of other clinicopathological correlates by Giri et al. *(83)*, *PTEN*-mutant tumors were found to have increased microvessel density, which is associated with increased metastatic potential in prostate and other cancer types. These data depend on "retention of heterozygosity" analysis as a surrogate for homozygous deletion, and may also be biased by the greater technical challenge of detecting mutations in early-stage cancers. A recent immunohistochemical study of 109 paraffin-embedded radical prostatectomy specimens showed a lack of PTEN staining in tumor cells in about 20% of cases overall, associated with higher Gleason score and more advanced stage *(184)*. A role for *PTEN/MMAC1* in prostatic oncogenesis appears to be firmly established despite the relatively limited number of published studies at this time.

---

[*] Three possibilities may be considered: excess LOH targets other TSGs on chromosome 10q; excess LOH targets PTEN alleles with cryptic mutations or epigenetic silencing; or excess LOH reflects nonspecific genetic instability.

Table 1
**Meta-Analysis of 8 Mutation Screening Studies of *PTEN/MMAC1*
in Prostate Cancer (1997–1998)[a]**

Investigator	Total no.	1° PCa	1° PCa Stage B,C	Met. PCa	Comments
Cairns *(29)*	80		3/60 (5%)	7/20 (35%)	6 ROH + 4 Seq
Dong *(56)*	40		1/40 (3%)		1 Seq
Feilotter *(69)*	25		1/25 (4%)		1 Seq; preselected for LOH; HZD not examined
Gray *(92)*	37	5/37 (14%)			5 Seq, 4 in Stage D cases
Pesche *(219)*	6	1/6 (17%)			1 Seq, preselected for LOH
Teng *(275)*	6	0/6 (0%)			Preselected for LOH; HZD not examined
Suzuki *(264)*	19			6/19 (32%)	2 HZD + 4 Seq; heterogeneity among mult. tumors
Wang *(299)*	60		8/60 (13%)		8 ROH
TOTALS	273	6/49 (12%)	13/185 (7%)	13/39 (33%)	

[a] Primary prostate cancer specimens (1° PCa) were classified as stage B or C if the appropriate data were supplied; otherwise, primary cancers include disease stages B–D (or II–IV) *(241)*. Met. PCa: metastatic tumor specimens; ROH: "retention of heterozygosity" within larger regions of LOH, suggestive of homozygous deletion (HZD); Seq: sequence variants (somatic mutations).

3.10. Smad2, Smad4 *(DPC4) (chromosome 18q21) and* TGFβRII *(chromosome 3p22) (272)*

Transforming growth factor β (TGFβ) is a ubiquitous growth-inhibitory factor for epithelial cells, and decreased responsiveness to this factor is a common feature of epithelial cancers *(6)*. Molecular components of the TGFβ signalling pathway include the Type I and II TGFβ receptors (TGFβRI and TGFβRII), which are transmembrane serine/threonine kinases, and their intracellular substrates, which consist of hetero-oligomers of Smad4 with Smad2 or other Smad family members *(249)*. *Smad2, Smad4* and *TGFβRII* are targets for mutational inactivation in colorectal cancer *(66,178,277)*; *Smad4* (DPC4) mutations are especially frequent in pancreatic cancers *(104)*. *Smad2* and *Smad4* are both located in 18q21, a region of frequent allelic loss in many cancer types, including prostate *(281)*. However, between two studies of *Smad4* in prostate cancer, no deletions or mutations were found in four cell lines, eight primary tumor samples selected for 18q21 LOH, and 45 unselected tumor samples *(173,244)*. *Smad2* mutations are found in a small fraction (~7%) of colorectal and lung cancers *(66,280)*, and *TGFβRII* mutations are most common in colorectal and gastric cancers with microsatellite instability *(89,288)*; mutation screening of these genes in prostate cancer has not been reported. Decreased TGFβRII expression was found in primary prostate cancers compared to that in benign prostatic tissue, especially in those of higher histological grade *(130,304)*. LNCaP was examined as a TGFβ-resistant cell line in two studies, which came to opposing conclusions about the lack of Type I vs Type II receptors in this cell *(100,131)*. The molecular basis of TGFβ resistance in prostate cancer remains an area of active investigation.

3.11. **TP53** *(p53) (chromosome 17p13)*

p53, encoded by "the most frequently mutated gene in human cancer," was originally identified as a cellular protein stably associated with the large T antigen of SV40
and E1B gene product of adenovirus in transformed murine cells *(211)*. Although initially considered an oncogene, wild-type p53 can in fact suppress the neoplastic phenotype of *TP53*-mutated cancer cells *(36)*. *TP53* is mutated in over 50% of colon, lung,
breast, brain, and bladder cancers, usually in association with loss of the wild-type
allele *(93)*. Germline mutation of *TP53* results in the Li-Fraumeni syndrome, a cancer
predisposition syndrome of multiple, early-onset sarcomas, breast cancers, and brain
tumors *(177)*. p53 functions to induce either G1 cell cycle arrest or programmed cell
death in response to many types of cellular stress, including DNA damage, hypoxia,
heat shock, nucleotide depletion, and pH change *(224)*. The loss of this checkpoint
pathway in cancer cells is believed to promote genetic instability and the acquisition of
additional mutations *(145)*. At the biochemical level, p53 is a transcription factor that
controls the expression of other genes carry out its function. Three principal transcriptional targets for wild-type p53 are the proapoptotic protein Bax, the cyclin-dependent
kinase inhibitor CDKN1A (p21^{Cip1}), and the ubiquitin ligase mdm-2, which negatively
regulates p53 stability in an inhibitory feedback loop *(224)*.

Most cancer-derived *TP53* mutations are missense nucleotide changes leading to
amino acid substitutions in functionally conserved protein domains. Such mutant proteins lack biochemical, cellular, and tumor suppressor function, but (in an inversion of
the pattern expected for other mutated TSGs) invariably accumulate to high levels that
can be detected by IHC *(237)*. Although elevated levels of p53 with wild-type sequence
may also occur as a transient response to the cellular stimuli noted above, with appropriate criteria most IHC+ tumors are found to carry *TP53* mutations *(19,105)*. A meta-
analysis of 16 immunohistochemical studies of p53 in 1439 prostate cancer cases is
shown in Table 2. Positive nuclear immunostaining is least frequent in small, organ-
confined primary tumors (~3%), is present in ~14% of locally advanced (Stage III,
$T_3N_0M_0$) primary cancers, and is found most frequently in recurrent primary disease or
hormone-refractory bony metastases (~50%) *(198)*. The increasing fraction of IHC+
cases with disease stage suggests a role for *TP53* in prostate cancer progression and the
potential value of p53 IHC for prediction of clinical course. Positive immunostaining
in primary tumors has been associated with high histologic grade *(124,182)*, androgen
independence *(198)*, DNA aneuploidy, high cell proliferation rate, higher recurrence
rate *(308)*, and shorter survival after RP *(25,276,291)* or radiation therapy *(94,238)*,
although other studies have failed to find prognostic utility *(233,256,285)*. Molecular
genetic analysis of *TP53* has indicated a predominance of missense mutations, especially G:C->A:T transitions in "hot-spot" CpG dinucleotides *(19,197)*. In a problematic twist, these methods have amply demonstrated genetic heterogeneity among
multifocal primary tumors *(188,233)*, and have also suggested that *TP53*-mutated cells
are clonally selected during the process of metastasis *(197,257)*. Heterogeneity or technical differences may lead to the somewhat dissimilar results obtained by one group,
which has detected a higher frequency of missense mutations with unusual features in
primary prostate cancer as well as in benign prostatic hyperplasia *(42,99,186,187)*.

Table 2
Meta-Analysis of 16 IHC Studies of p53 in Prostate Cancer (1992–1997)[a]

Investigator	Total no.	Hormone sensitive					Hormone refractory	
		1° PCa Stage A–D $T_xN_xM_x$	1° PCa Stage A, B T0-2N0M0	1° PCa Stage C T3N0M0	1° PCa Stage D T_xN1-3 or M1	met. PCa Stage D T_xN1-3 or M1	1° PCa	met. PCa
Aprikian *(3)*	93	3/38 (8%)				4/35 (11%)	6/10 (60%)	6/10 (60%)
Berner *(11)*	84	6/34 (18%)					19/50 (38%)	
Bookstein *(19)*	143		3/74 (4%)	8/36 (22%)	8/33 (24%)			
Brooks *(26)*	80	2/38 (5%)				15/42 (36%)		
Eastham *(63)*	86		0/18 (0%)	2/21 (10%)		11/47 (23%)		
Heidenberg *(107)*	61	6/27 (22%)				4/8 (50%)	6/26 (62%)	
Henke *(108)*	73	7/73 (10%)						
Hughes *(113)*	67	10/36 (28%)				16/31 (52%)		
Kallakury *(124)*	107	15/107 (14%)						
McDonnell *(183)*	43							22/43 (51%)
Navone *(198)*	97	0/36 (0%)				0/8 (0%)	2/9 (22%)	21/44 (48%)
Salem *(235)*	96			10/96 (10%)				
Shurbaji *(250)*	109	23/109 (21%)						
Thomas *(278)*	68		0/10 (0%)	5/32 (16%)	4/26 (15%)			
Visakorpi *(291)*	137	23/137 (17%)						
Voeller *(295)*	95	4/85 (4%)				1/10 (10%)		
TOTALS	1439	98/720 (14%)	3/102 (3%)	25/185 (14%)	12/59 (20%)	51/181 (28%)	43/95 (45%)	49/97 (51%)

[a] Included studies contained more than 50 cases (except for McDonnell et al., who studied only bone-marrow biopsies) and were screened for rough comparability of case selection, staging, and staining methods and criteria. Results were stratified by consensus disease stage where possible *(241)*. "Hormone sensitive" group includes "hormone untreated" and "unknown," whereas "hormone refractory" indicates relapse or progression after hormone therapy. Stage A–D, $T_xN_xM_x$ group consists of untreated primary tumors for which IHC data were not explicitly stratified by stage.

The role of *TP53* in prostate cancer has also been addressed functionally by gene transfer into TSU-Pr1 and PC-3 prostate tumor cell lines, both lacking endogenous wild-type p53 protein *(119)*. Wild-type p53 expression inhibited colony formation compared to mutant p53 in these assays. The use of *TP53* for in vivo gene therapy of prostate cancer is discussed in Section 4. below.

4. APPLICATION OF TSGS IN PROSTATE CANCER DIAGNOSIS, PROGNOSIS, AND THERAPY

Aside from the self-evident benefits of increased mechanistic understanding of the cancer process, what utility can be assigned to the class of tumor suppressor genes in particular? For the pursuit of new therapeutic agents, the dominant oncogenes would appear to be more appropriate targets for traditional small-molecule drug design, with its emphasis on inhibition of function. In the areas of diagnostic classification, prognostication, and selection of therapies, TSGs should offer some value as fundamental determinants of neoplasia. The most promising application to emerge to date is immunohistochemistry of p53 (especially in combination with that of antiapoptosis protein bcl-2), which may predict recurrence after RP *(25,192)* and response to external-beam radiotherapy *(40,228,238)* or drug therapies *(55)*. As reviewed here, only a few other TSGs have shown prognostic utility so far, and superiority over standard clinicopathological indices is not yet established. Predictive genetic risk assessment awaits characterization of one or more prostate cancer predisposition loci, which may or may not turn out to be TSGs. Mouse germline knockouts of TSGs have not yet yielded new animal models for human prostate cancer, although the initial findings of prostatic hyperplasia/dysplasia with both the *PTEN/MMAC1* and *Mxi1* knockouts are promising. One leading area for rapid utility of TSGs is in cancer-gene therapy, in which replacement of missing gene functions has great theoretical appeal. At the same time, major technical challenges—especially in the efficiency of gene delivery and the management of immune response—must be overcome. Gene therapy is fully covered elsewhere; thus, its review here is brief and selective.

4.1 p53 Gene Therapy

TP53 is attractive as a transgene for cancer gene therapy because of its potential to induce apoptosis in p53-mutant cancer cells, especially in combination with chemotherapeutic agents or irradiation. Adenovirus is the most efficient gene delivery vector in common use *(17)*. Recombinant adenoviruses expressing wild-type p53 (rAd-p53) are currently in clinical trials for several cancer indications including lung *(242,266)*, head and neck, liver-metastatic colorectal, ovarian *(8)*, and prostate cancers (e.g., NIH/ ORDA Gene Therapy Protocols 9706-192 and 9710-217); the results of prostate trials are not yet published. A number of preclinical studies in nude mouse models have shown reduced tumor growth with rAd-p53 delivered by intratumoral or intraperitoneal (ip) injection into sc or ip tumors formed from p53-mutant human prostate cancer cell lines DU145, PC-3 and TSU-Pr1 *(4,87,200,307)*, as well as p53-wild-type C4-2, a subline of LNCaP *(137)*. Nielsen and colleagues have shown improved efficacy of rAd-p53 combined with paclitaxel (Taxol) and other chemotherapeutic agents in several cancer models including prostate *(101,201)*. Using an orthotopic PC-3 xenograft model with spontaneous metastatic progression, Eastham et al. *(62)* have shown reduced primary tumor growth and reduced frequency of progression following single orthotopic injections of rAd-p53. Insofar as metastatic progression in clinical prostate cancer is associated with selection of p53-mutant populations in primary tumors, this therapeutic approach may have direct clinical relevance.

CDKN1A (p21^{Cip1}) and *CDKN2A* (p16^{Ink4a}) have also been used as transgenes in similar vectors and prostate cancer models as *TP53*. In one comparative study, Ad-p53 proved to be more efficacious than vectors with either cell cycle regulator *(87)*.

4.2. CD66a / BGP / C-CAM Gene Therapy

Human CD66a—also known as biliary glycoprotein (BGP)—and its rat homolog C-CAM, are adhesive cell surface glycoproteins with homotypic binding properties. Decreased expression of this cell surface molecule has been demonstrated in rodent cancers, in human colon and prostate carcinomas, and in preneoplastic lesions of these tissues *(134,199,205)*. C-CAM1 gene transfer into prostate cancer cell line PC-3 reduced their anchorage-dependent and independent growth rates in vitro and their tumorigenicity in vivo, whereas transfection of an antisense C-CAM vector increased the tumorigenicity of a formerly nontumorigenic prostatic epithelial cell line *(111)*. These studies were used to justify the development of adenovirus-mediated C-CAM1 or CD66a gene therapy for prostate cancer *(135,168)*. In two preclinical studies, intratumoral administration of rAd-C-CAM1 or -CD66a into sc PC-3 or DU145 xenografts, respectively, inhibited tumor growth in a dose and schedule dependent manner *(162,168)*. In a recent twist in the understanding of C-CAM1 biology, Comegys et al. *(46)* found that C-CAM1-overexpressing PC-3 clones regained their tumorigenic phenotype and increased their in vivo growth rates compared to parental clones while maintaining high levels of C-CAM1 expression and a growth retarded phenotype in vitro. The "revertant" clones also showed evidence of decreased rather than increased cellular differentiation. The implication of these results for CD66a gene therapy remains to be determined.

REFERENCES

1. Aaltomaa, S., P. Lipponen, M. Ala-Opas, M. Eskelinen, and V. M. Kosma. 1999. Alpha-catenin expression has prognostic value in local and locally advanced prostate cancer. *Br. J. Cancer* **80:** 477–482.
2. Ahuja, N., Q. Li, A. L. Mohan, S. B. Baylin, and J.-P. J. Issa. 1998. Aging and DNA methylation in colorectal mucosa and cancer. *Cancer Res.* **58:** 5489–5494.
3. Aprikian, A. G., A. S. Sarkis, W. R. Fair, Z. F. Zhang, Z. Fuks, and C. Cordon-Cardo. 1994. Immunohistochemical determination of p53 protein nuclear accumulation in prostatic adenocarcinoma. *J. Urol.* **151:** 1276–1280.
4. Asgari, K., I. A. Sesterhenn, D. G. McLeod, K. Cowan, J. W. Moul, P. Seth, et al. 1997. Inhibition of the growth of pre-established subcutaneous tumor nodules of human prostate cancer cells by single injection of the recombinant adenovirus p53 expression vector. *Int. J. Cancer* **71:** 377–382.
5. Atkin, N. B. and M. C. Baker. 1985. Chromosome study of five cancers of the prostate. *Hum. Genet.* **70:** 359–364.
6. Attisano, L., J. L. Wrana, F. Lopez-Casillas, and J. Massague. 1994. TGF-beta receptors and actions. *Biochim. Biophys. Acta* **1222:** 71–80.

7. Bajou, K., A. Noel, R. D. Gerard, V. Masson, N. Brunner, C. Holst-Hansen, et al. 1998. Absence of host plasminogen activator inhibitor 1 prevents cancer invasion and vascularization. *Nat. Med.* **4:** 923–928.

8. Barinaga, M. 1997. From bench top to bedside. *Science* **278:** 1036–1039.

9. Barnes, L. D., P. N. Garrison, Z. Siprashvili, T. Druck, and C. M. Croce. 1997. Fhit, a putative tumor suppressor in humans, is a dinucleoside $5',5'''$-P^1,P^3-triphosphate hydrolase. *Biochemistry* **35:** 11,529–11,535.

10. Bergerheim, U. S. R., K. Kunimi, V. P. Collins, and P. Ekman. 1991. Deletion mapping of chromosomes 8, 10, and 16 in human prostate carcinoma. *Genes Chromosomes Cancer* **3:** 215–220.

11. Berner, A., G. Geitvik, F. Karlsen, S. D. Fossa, J. M. Nesland, and A. L. Borresen. 1995. TP53 mutations in prostatic cancer. Analysis of pre- and post-treatment archival formalin-fixed tumour tissue. *J. Pathol.* **176:** 299–308.

12. Berx, G., A.-M. Cleton-Jansen, K. Strumane, W. J. F. de Leeuw, F. Nollet, F. v. Roy, et al. 1996. E-cadherin is inactivated in a majority of invasive human lobular breast cancers by truncation mutations throughout its extracellular domain. *Oncogene* **13:** 1919–1925.

13. Berx, G., F. Nollet, and F. van Roy. 1998. Dysregulation of the E-cadherin/catenin complex by irreversible mutations in human carcinomas. *Cell Adhes. Commun.* **6:** 171–184.

14. Bevilacqua, G., M. E. Sobel, L. A. Liotta, and P. S. Steeg. 1989. Association of low nm23 RNA levels in human primary infiltrating ductal breast carcinomas with lymph node involvement and other histopathological indicators of high metastatic potential. *Cancer Res.* **49:** 5185–5190.

15. Bishop, J. 1987. The molecular genetics of cancer. *Science* **235:** 305–311.

16. Bookstein, R., G. S. Bova, D. MacGrogan, A. Levy, and W. B. Isaacs. 1997. Tumour-suppressor genes in prostatic oncogenesis: a positional approach. *Br. J. Urol.* **79 (Suppl. 1):** 28–36.

17. Bookstein, R., W. Demers, R. Gregory, D. Maneval, J. Park, and K. Wills. 1996. p53 gene therapy in vivo of hepatocellular and liver metastatic colorectal cancer. *Sem. Oncol.* **23:** 66–77.

18. Bookstein, R. and W.-H. Lee. 1991. Molecular genetics of the retinoblastoma suppressor gene, in *Critical Reviews in Oncogenesis* (Perucho, M. and E. Pimentel, eds.), CRC, Orlando, FL, pp. 211–227.

19. Bookstein, R., D. MacGrogan, S. G. Hilsenbeck, F. Sharkey, and D. C. Allred. 1993. p53 is mutated in a subset of advanced-stage prostate cancers. *Cancer Res.* **53:** 3369–3373.

20. Bookstein, R., P. Rio, S. Madreperla, F. Hong, C. Allred, W. E. Grizzle, et al. 1990. Promoter deletion and loss of retinoblastoma gene expression in human prostate carcinoma. *Proc. Natl. Acad. Sci. USA* **87:** 7762–7766.

21. Bookstein, R., J.-Y. Shew, P.-L. Chen, P. Scully, and W.-H. Lee. 1990. Suppression of tumorigenicity of human prostate carcinoma cells by replacing a mutated *RB* gene. *Science* **247:** 712–715.

22. Bova, G. S., B. S. Carter, M. J. G. Bussemakers, M. Emi, Y. Fujiwara, N. Kyprianou, et al. 1993. Homozygous deletion and frequent allelic loss of chromosome 8p22 loci in human prostate cancer. *Cancer Res.* **53:** 3869–3873.

23. Bova, G. S. and W. B. Isaacs. 1996. Review of allelic loss and gain in prostate cancer. *World J. Urol.* **14:** 338–346.

24. Bova, G. S., D. MacGrogan, A. Levy, S. S. Pin, R. Bookstein, and W. B. Isaacs. 1996. Physical mapping of chromosome 8p22 markers and their homozygous deletion in a metastatic prostate cancer. *Genomics* **35:** 46–54.

25. Brewster, S. F., J. D. Oxley, M. Trivella, C. D. Abbott, and D. A. Gillatt. 1999. Preoperative p53, bcl-2, CD44 and E-cadherin immunohistochemistry as predictors of biochemical relapse after radical prostatectomy. *J. Urol.* **161:** 1238–1243.

26. Brooks, J. D., G. S. Bova, C. M. Ewing, S. Piantadosi, B. S. Carter, J. C. Robinson, et al. 1996. An uncertain role for p53 gene alterations in human prostate cancers. *Cancer Res.* **56:** 3814–3822.

27. Brothman, A. R., T. M. Maxwell, J. Cui, D. A. Deubler, and X. L. Zhu. 1999. Chromosomal clues to the development of prostate tumors. *Prostate* **38:** 303–312.

28. Brothman, A. R., D. M. Peehl, A. M. Patel, and J. E. McNeal. 1990. Frequency and pattern of karyotypic abnormalities in human prostate cancer. *Cancer Res.* **50:** 3795–3803.

29. Cairns, P., K. Okami, S. Halachmi, N. Halachmi, M. Esteller, J. G. Herman, et al. 1997. Frequent inactivation of PTEN/MMAC1 in primary prostate cancer. *Cancer Res.* **57:** 4997–5000.

30. Cairns, P., T. J. Polascik, Y. Eby, K. Tokino, J. Califano, A. Merlo, et al. 1995. Frequency of homozygous deletion at p16/CDKN2 in primary human tumours. *Nat. Genet.* **11:** 210–212.

31. Carter, B. S., C. M. Ewing, W. S. Ward, B. F. Treiger, T. W. Aalders, J. A. Schalken, et al. 1990. Allelic loss of chromosomes 16q and 10q in human prostate cancer. *Proc. Natl. Acad. Sci. USA* **87:** 8751–8755.

32. Cavenee, W. K., T. P. Dryja, R. A. Phillips, W. F. Benedict, R. Godbout, B. L. Gallie, et al. 1983. Expression of recessive alleles by chromosomal mechanisms in retinoblastoma. *Nature* **305:** 779–784.

33. Chang, G. T. G., L. J. Blok, M. Steenbeek, J. Veldscholte, W. M. van Weerden, G. J. van Steenbrugge, et al. 1997. Differentially expressed genes in androgen-dependent and -independent prostate carcinomas. *Cancer Res.* **57:** 4075–4081.

34. Chekmareva, M. A., C. M. Hollowell, R. C. Smith, E. M. Davis, M. M. LeBeau, and C. W. Rinker-Schaeffer. 1997. Localization of prostate cancer metastasis-suppressor activity on human chromosome 17. *Prostate* **33:** 271–280.

35. Chellappan, S. P., S. Hiebert, M. Mudryj, J. M. Horowitz, and J. R. Nevins. 1991. The E2F transcription factor is a cellular target for the RB protein. *Cell* **65:** 1053–1061.

36. Chen, P.-L., Y. Chen, R. Bookstein, and W.-H. Lee. 1990. Genetic mechanisms of tumor suppression by the human p53 gene. *Science* **250:** 1576–1580.

37. Chen, W., C. M. Weghorst, C. L. K. Sabourin, Y. Wang, D. Wang, D. G. Bostwick, et al. 1996. Absence of p16/MTS1 gene mutations in human prostate cancer. *Carcinogenesis* **17:** 2603–2607.

38. Cheney, I. W., D. E. Johnson, M.-T. Vaillancourt, J. Avanzini, A. Morimoto, G. W. Demers, et al. 1998. Suppression of tumorigenicity of glioblastoma cells by adenovirus-mediated MMAC1/PTEN gene transfer. *Cancer Res.* **58:** 2331–2334.

39. Cheney, I. W., S. T. C. Neuteboom, M.-T. Vaillancourt, M. Ramachandra, and R. Bookstein. 1999. Adenovirus-mediated gene transfer of MMAC1/PTEN to glioblastoma cells inhibits S phase entry by the recruitment of p27Kip1 into cyclin E/CDK2 complexes. *Cancer Res.* **59:** 2318–2323.

40. Cheng, L., T. J. Sebo, J. C. Cheville, T. M. Pisansky, J. Slezak, E. J. Bergstralh, et al. 1999. p53 protein overexpression is associated with increased cell proliferation in patients with locally recurrent prostate carcinoma after radiation therapy. *Cancer* **85:** 1293–1299.

41. Cher, M. L., G. S. Bova, D. H. Moore, E. J. Small, P. R. Carroll, S. S. Pin, et al. 1996. Genetic alterations in untreated prostate cancer metastases and androgen independent prostate cancer detected by comparative genomic hybridization and allelotyping. *Cancer Res.* **56:** 3091–3102.

42. Chi, S.-G., R. W. D. White, F. J. Meyers, D. B. Siders, F. Lee, and P. H. Gumerlock. 1994. p53 in prostate cancer: frequent expressed transition mutations. *J. Natl. Cancer Inst.* **86:** 926–933.

43. Chi, S.-G., R. W. D. White, J. T. Muenzer, and P. H. Gumberlock. 1997. Frequent alteration of CDKN2 (p16^{INK4A}/MTS1) expression in human primary prostate carcinomas. *Clinical Cancer Res.* **3:** 1889–1897.

44. Chin, L., J. Pomerantz, and R. A. DePinho. 1998. The Ink4a/ARF tumor suppressor: one gene—two products—two pathways. *Trends Biol. Sci.* **23:** 291–296.

45. Clurman, B. E. and P. Porter. 1998. New insights into the tumor suppressor function of p27Kip1. *Proc. Natl. Acad. Sci. USA* **95:** 15,158–15,160.

46. Comegys, M. M., M. P. Carriero, J. F. Brown, A. Mazzacua, D. L. Flanagan, A. Makarovskiy, et al. 1999. C-CAM1 expression: differential effects on morphology, differentiation state and suppression of human PC-3 prostate carcinoma cells. *Oncogene* **18:** 3261–3276.

47. Comings, D. E. 1973. A general theory of carcinogenesis. *Proc. Natl. Acad. Sci. USA* **70:** 3324–3328.

48. Cordon-Cardo, C., A. Koff, M. Drobnjak, P. Capodieci, I. Osman, S. S. Millard, et al. 1998. Distinct altered patterns of p27Kip1 gene expression in benign prostatic hyperplasia and prostatic carcinoma. *J. Natl. Cancer Inst.* **90:** 1284–1291.

49. Cote, R. J., Y. Shi, S. Groshen, A. C. Feng, C. Cordon-Cardo, D. Skinner, et al. 1998. Association of p27Kip1 levels with recurrence and survival in patients with stage C prostate carcinoma. *J. Natl. Cancer Inst.* **90:** 916–920.

50. Cristofano, A. D., B. Pesce, C. Cordon-Cardo, and P. P. Pandolfi. 1998. Pten is essential for embryonic development and tumour suppression. *Nat. Genet.* **19:** 348–355.

51. Cunningham, J. M., A. Shan, M. J. Wick, S. K. McDonnell, D. J. Schaid, D. J. Tester, et al. 1996. Allelic imbalance and microsatellite instability in prostatic adenocarcinoma. *Cancer Res.* **56:** 4475–4482.

52. Davies, M. A., D. Koul, H. Dhesi, R. Berman, T. J. McDonnell, D. McConkey, et al. 1999. Regulation of Akt/PKB activity, cellular growth, and apoptosis in prostate carcinoma cells by MMAC/PTEN. *Cancer Res.* **59:** 2551–2556.

53. Davies, M. A., Y. Lu, T. Sano, X. Fang, X., P. Tang, R. LaPushin, et al. 1998. Adenoviral transgene expression of MMAC/PTEN in human glioma cells inhibits Akt activation and induces anoikis. *Cancer Res.* **58:** 5285–5290.

54. Davies, M. P., F. E. Gibbs, H. Halliwell, K. A. Joyce, M. M. Roebuck, M. L. Rossi, et al. 1999. Mutation in the PTEN/MMAC1 gene in archival low grade and high grade gliomas. *Br. J. Cancer* **79:**, 1542–1548.

55. DiPaola, R. S. and J. Aisner. 1999. Overcoming bcl-2- and p53-mediated resistance in prostate cancer. *Semin. Oncol.* **26 (Suppl. 2):** 112–116.

56. Dong, J.-T., T. W. Sipe, E.-R. Hyytinen, C.-L. Li, C. Heise, D. E. McClintock, et al. 1998. PTEN/MMAC1 is infrequently mutated in pT2 and pT3 carcinomas of the prostate. *Oncogene* **17:** 1979–1982.

57. Dong, J.-T., H. Suzuki, S. S. Pin, G. S. Bova, J. A. Schalken, W. B. Isaacs, et al. 1996. Down-regulation of the KAI1 metastasis suppressor gene during the progression of human prostatic cancer infrequently involves gene mutation or allelic loss. *Cancer Res.* **56:** 4387–4390.

58. Dong, J. T., P. W. Lamb, C. W. Rinker-Schaeffer, J. Vukanovic, T. Ichikawa, J. T. Isaacs, et al. 1995. KAI1, a metastasis suppressor gene for prostate cancer on human chromosome 11p11.2. *Science* **268:** 884–886.

59. Duerr, E. M., B. Rollbrocker, Y. Hayashi, N. Peters, B. Meyer-Puttlitz, D. N. Louis, et al. 1998. PTEN mutations in gliomas and glioneuronal tumors. *Oncogene* **16:** 2259–2264.

60. Dunn, J. M., R. A. Phillips, A. J. Becker, and B. L. Gallie. 1988. Identification of germline and somatic mutations affecting the retinoblastoma gene. *Science* **241:** 1797–1800.

61. Eagle, L. R., X. Yin, A. R. Brothman, B. J. Williams, N. B. Atkin, and E. V. Prochownik. 1995. Mutation of the MXI1 gene in prostate cancer. *Nat. Genet.* **9:** 249–255.

62. Eastham, J. A., W. Grafton, C. M. Martin, and B. J. Williams. 2000. Suppression of primary tumor growth and the progression to metastasis with p53 adenovirus in human prostate cancer. *J. Urol.* **164:** 814–819.

63. Eastham, J. A., A. M. F. Stapleton, A. E. Gousse, T. L. Timme, G. Yang, K. M. Slawin, et al. 1995. Association of p53 mutations with metastatic prostate cancer. *Clin. Cancer Res.* **1:** 1111–1118.

64. Emmert-Buck, M. R., R. F. Bonner, P. D. Smith, R. F. Chuaqui, Z. Zhuang, S. R. Goldstein, et al. 1996. Laser capture microdissection. *Science* **274:** 998–1001.

65. Emmert-Buck, M. R., C. D. Vocke, R. O. Pozzatti, P. H. Duray, S. B. Jennings, C. Florence, et al. 1995. Allelic loss on chromosome 8p12-21 in microdissected prostatic intraepithelial neoplasia. *Cancer Res.* **55:** 2959–2962.

66. Eppert, K., S. W. Scherer, H. Ozcelik, R. Pirone, P. Hoodless, H. Kim, et al. 1996. MADR2 maps to 18q21 and encodes a TGFβ-regulated MAD-related protein that is functionally mutated in colorectal carcinoma. *Cell* **86:** 543–552.

67. Ewing, C. M., N. Ru, R. A. Morton, J. C. Robinson, M. J. Wheelock, K. R. Johnson, et al. 1995. Chromosome 5 suppresses tumorigenicity of PC3 prostate cancer cells: correlation with re-expression of α-catenin and restoration of E-cadherin function. *Cancer Res.* **55:** 4813–4817.

68. Fearon, E. R. and B. Vogelstein. 1990. A genetic model for colorectal tumorigenesis. *Cell* **61:** 759–767.

69. Feilotter, H. E., M. A. Nagai, A. H. Boag, C. Eng, and L. M. Mulligan. 1998. Analysis of PTEN and the 10q23 region in primary prostate carcinomas. *Oncogene* **16:** 1743–1748.

70. Fero, M. L., E. Randel, K. E. Gurley, J. M. Roberts, and C. J. Kemp. 1998. The murine gene p27Kip1 is haplo-insufficient for tumour suppression. *Nature* **396:** 177–180.

71. Fitzgerald, M. G., D. P. Harkin, D. P., S. Silva-Arrieta, D. J. MacDonald, L. C. Lucchina, H. Unsal, et al. 1996. Prevalence of germ-line mutations in p16, p19ARF, and CDK4 in familial melanoma: analysis of a clinic-based population. *Proc. Natl. Acad. Sci. USA* **93:** 8541–8545.

72. Forgacs, E., E. J. Biesterveld, Y. Sekido, K. Fong, S. Muneer, I. I. Wistuba, et al. 1998. Mutation analysis of the PTEN/MMAC1 gene in lung cancer. *Oncogene* **17:** 1557–1565.

73. Francke, U. 1976. Retinoblastoma and chromosome 13. *Birth Defects* **12:** 131–137.

74. Friend, S. H., R. Bernards, S. Rogelj, R. A. Weinberg, J. M. Rapaport, D. M. Albert, et al. 1986. A human DNA segment with properties of the gene that predisposes to retinoblastoma and osteosarcoma. *Nature* **323:** 643–646.

75. Fujiwara, Y., M. Emi, H. Ohata, Y. Kato, T. Nakajima, T. Mori, et al. 1993. Evidence for the presence of two tumor suppressor genes on chromosome 8p for colorectal carcinoma. *Cancer Res.* **53:** 1172–1174.

76. Fujiwara, Y., H. Ohata, M. Emi, K. Okui, K. Koyama, E. Tsuchiya, et al. 1994. A 3-Mb physical map of the chromosome region 8p21.3-p22, including a 600-kb region commonly deleted in human hepatocellular carcinoma, colorectal cancer, and non-small cell lung cancer. *Genes Chromosomes Cancer* **10:** 7–14.

77. Fujiwara, Y., H. Ohata, T. Kuroki, K. Koyama, E. Tsuchiya, M. Monden, et al. 1995. Isolation of a candidate tumor suppressor gene on chromosome 8p21.3-p22 that is homologous to an extracellular domain of the PDGF receptor beta gene. *Oncogene* **10:** 891–895.

78. Fults, D., C. A. Pedone, G. A. Thomas, and R. White. 1990. Allelotype of human malignant astrocytoma. *Cancer Res.* **50:** 5784–5789.

79. Fung, Y. K. T., A. L. Murphree, A. T'Ang, J. Qian, S. H. Hinrichs, and W. F. Benedict. 1987. Structural evidence for the authenticity of the human retinoblastoma gene. *Science* **236:** 1657–1661.

80. Furnari, F. B., H. Lin, H.-J. S. Huang, and W. K. Cavenee. 1997. Growth suppression of glioma cells by PTEN requires a functional phosphatase catalytic domain. *Proc. Natl. Acad. Sci. USA* **94:** 12,479–12,484.

81. Gao, A. C., W. Lou, J. T. Dong, and J. T. Isaacs. 1997. CD44 is a metastasis suppressor gene for prostatic cancer located on human chromosome 11p13. *Cancer Res.* **57:** 846–849.

82. Gayther, S. A., P. Barski, S. J. Batley, L. Li, K. A. Foy, S. N. Cohen, et al. 1997. Aberrant splicing of the TSG101 and FHIT genes occurs frequently in multiple malignancies and in normal tissues and mimics alterations previously described in tumours. *Oncogene* **15:** 2119–2126.

83. Giri, D. and J. Ittman. 1999. Inactivation of the PTEN tumor suppressor gene is associated with increased angiogenesis in clinically localized prostate carcinoma. *Hum. Pathol.* **30:** 419–424.

84. Golden, A., M. Benedict, A. Shearn, N. Kimura, A. Leone, and L. A. Liotta. 1992. Nucleoside diphosphate kinases, nm23, and tumor metastasis: possible biochemical mechanisms. *Cancer Treat. Res.* **63:** 345–358.

85. Gonzalez-Zulueta, M., C. M. Bender, A. S. Yang, T. Nguyen, R. W. Beart, J. M. Tornout, et al. 1995. Methylation of the 5′ CpG island of the p16/CDKN2 tumor suppressor gene in normal and transformed human tissues correlates with gene silencing. *Cancer Res.* **55:** 4531–4535.

86. Goodrich, D. W., N. P. Wang, Y.-W. Qian, E. Y.-H. P. Lee, and W.-H. Lee. 1991. The retinoblastoma gene product regulates progression through the G1 phase of the cell cycle. *Cell* **67:** 293–302.

87. Gotoh, A., C. Kao, S.-C. Ko, K. Hamada, T.-J. Liu, and L. W. K. Chung. 1997. Cytotoxic effects of recombinant adenovirus p53 and cell cycle regulator genes (p21WAF1/CIP1 and p16CDKN2) in human prostate cancers. *J. Urol.* **158:** 636–641.

88. Goyette, M. C., K. Cho, C. L. Fasching, D. B. Levy, K. W. Kinzler, C. Paraskeva, et al. 1992. Progression of colorectal cancer is associated with multiple tumor supressor gene defects but inhibition of tumorigenicity is accomplished by correction of any single defect via chromosome transfer. *Mol. Cell. Biol.* **12:** 1387–1395.

89. Grady, W. M., L. L. Myeroff, S. E. Swinler, A. Rajput, S. Thiagalingam, J. D. Lutterbaugh, et al. 1999. Mutational inactivation of transforming growth β receptor type II in microsatellite stable colon cancers. *Cancer Res.* **59:** 320–324.

90. Graff, J. R., J. G. Herman, R. G. Lapidus, H. Chopra, R. Xu, D. F. Jarrard, et al. 1995. E-cadherin expression is silenced by DNA hypermethylation in human breast and prostate carcinomas. *Cancer Res.* **55:** 5195–5199.

91. Gray, I. C., S. M. Phillips, S. J. Lee, J. P. Neoptolemos, J. Weissenbach, and N. K. Spurr. 1995. Loss of the chromosomal region 10q23-25 in prostate cancer. *Cancer Res.* **55:** 4800–4803.

92. Gray, I. C., L. M. D. Stewart, S. M. A. Phillips, J. A. Hamilton, N. E. Gray, G. J. Wa tson, et al. 1998. Mutation and expression analysis of the putative prostate tumour-suppressor gene PTEN. *Br. J. Cancer* **78:** 1296–1300.

93. Greenblatt, M. S., W. P. Bennett, M. Hollstein, and C. C. Harris. 1994. Mutations in the p53 tumor suppressor gene: clues to cancer etiology and molecular pathogenesis. *Cancer Res.* **54:** 4855–4878.

94. Grignon, D. J., R. Caplan, F. H. Sarkar, C. A. Lawton, E. H. Hammond, M. V. Pilepich, et al. 1997. p53 status and prognosis of locally advanced prostatic adenocarcinoma: a study based on RTOG 8610. *J. Natl. Cancer Inst.* **89:** 158–165.

95. Groden, J., G. Joslyn, W. Samowitz, D. Jones, N. Bhattacharyya, L. Spirio, et al. 1995. Response of colon cancer cell lines to the introduction of APC, a colon-specific tumor suppressor gene. *Cancer Res.* **55:** 1531–1539.

96. Groden, J., A. Thliveris, W. Samowitz, M. Carlson, L. Gelbert, H. Albertsen, et al. 1991. Identification and characterization of the familial adenomatous polyposis coli gene. *Cell* **66:** 589–600.

97. Gudkov, A. V., A. R. Kazarov, R. Thimmapaya, S. A. Axenovich, I. A. Mazo, and I. B. Roninson. 1994. Isolation of genetic suppressor elements from a retroviral normalized cDNA library: identification of a kinesin associated with drug sensitivity and senescence. *Proc. Natl. Acad. Sci. USA* **91:** 3744–3748.

98. Guilford, P., J. Hopkins, J. Harraway, M. McLeod, N. McLeod, P. Harawira, et al. 1998. E-cadherin germline mutations in familial gastric cancer. *Nature* **392:** 402–405.

99. Gumerlock, P. H., S.-G. Chi, X.-B. Shi, H. J. Voeller, J. W. Jacobson, E. P. Gelmann, et al. 1997. p53 abnormalities in primary prostate cancer: single-strand conformation polymorphism analysis of complementary DNA in comparison with genomic DNA. *J. Natl. Cancer Inst.* **89:** 66–71.

100. Guo, Y. and N. Kyprianou. 1998. Overexpression of transforming growth factor (TGF) beta1 type II receptor restores TGF-beta1 sensitivity and signaling in human prostate cancer cells. *Cell Growth Differ.* **9:** 185–193.

101. Gurnani, M., P. Lipari, J. Dell, B. Shi, and L. L. Nielsen. 1999. Adenovirus-mediated p53 gene therapy has greater efficacy when combined with chemotherapy against human head and neck, ovarian, prostate, and breast cancer. *Cancer Chemother. Pharmacol.* **44:** 143–151.

102. Gustafson, C. E., P. J. Wilson, R. Lukeis, E. Woollatt, L. Annab, L. Hawke, et al. 1996. Functional evidence for a colorectal cancer tumor suppressor gene at chromosome 8p22-23 by monochromosome transfer. *Cancer Res.* **56:** 5238–5245.

103. Haber, D. and E. Harlow. 1997. Tumour-suppressor genes: evolving definitions in the genomic age. *Nat. Genet.* **16:** 320–322.

104. Hahn, S. A., M. Schutte, A. T. M. S. Hoque, C. A. Moskaluk, L. T. da Costa, E. Rosenblum, et al. 1996. DPC4, a candidate tumor suppressor gene at human chromosome 18q21.1. *Science* **271:** 350–353.

105. Hall, P. A. and D. P. Lane. 1994. p53 in tumour pathology: can we trust immunohistochemistry?—revisited! *J. Pathol.* **172:** 1–4.

106. Harris, H., O. J. Miller, G. Klein, P. Worst, and T. Tachibana. 1969. Suppression of malignancy by cell fusion. *Nature* **223:** 363–368.

107. Heidenberg, H. B., I. A. Sesterhenn, J. P. Gaddipati, C. M. Weghorst, G. S. Buzard, J. W. Moul, et al. 1995. Alteration of the tumor suppressor gene p53 in a high fraction of hormone refractory prostate cancer. *J. Urol.* **154:** 414–421.

108. Henke, R.-P., E. Kruger, H. Ayhan, D. Hubner, P. Hammerer, and H. Huland. 1994. Immunohistochemical detection of p53 protein in human prostatic cancer. *J. Urol.* **152:** 1297–1301.

109. Hennessy, C., J. A. Henry, F. E. B. May, B. R. Westley, B. Angus, and T. W. J. Lennard. 1991. Expression of the antimetastatic gene nm23 in human breast cancer: an association with good prognosis. *J. Natl. Cancer Inst.* **83:** 281–285.

110. Herman, J. G., A. Merlo, L. Mao, R. G. Lapidus, J.-P. J. Issa, N. E. Davidson, et al. 1995. Inactivation of the CDKN2/p16/MTS1 gene is frequently associated with aberrant DNA methylation in all common human cancers. *Cancer Res.* **55:** 4525–4530.

111. Hsieh, J. T., W. Luo, W. Song, Y. Wang, D. Kleinerman, N. T. Van, et al. 1995. Tumor suppressive role of an androgen-regulated epithelial cell adhesion molecule (C-CAM) in prostate carcinoma cell revealed by sense and antisense approaches. *Cancer Res.* **55:** 190–197.

112. Huang, H.-J. S., J.-K. Yee, J.-Y. Shew, P.-L. Chen, R. Bookstein, T. Friedmann, et al. 1988. Suppression of the neoplastic phenotype by replacement of the retinoblastoma gene product in human cancer cells. *Science* **242:** 1563–1566.

113. Hughes, J. H., M. B. Cohen, and R. A. Robinson. 1995. p53 immunoreactivity in primary and metastatic prostatic adenocarcinoma. *Mod. Pathol.* **8:** 462–466.

114. Ichikawa, T., Y. Ichikawa, J. Dong, A. L. Hawkins, C. A. Griffin, W. B. Isaacs, et al. 1992. Localization of metastasis suppressor gene(s) for prostatic cancer to the short arm of human chromosome 11. *Cancer Res.* **52:** 3486–3490.

115. Ichikawa, T., N. Nihei, H. Suzuki, M. Oshimura, M. Emi, Y. Nakamura, et al. 1994. Suppression of metastasis of rat prostatic cancer by introducing human chromosome 8. *Cancer Res.* **54:** 2299–2302.

116. Ichimura, K., E. E. Schmidt, H. M. Goike, and V. P. Collins. 1996. Human glioblastomas with no alterations of the CDKN2A (p16Ink4a, MTS1) and CDK4 genes have frequent mutations of the retinoblastoma gene. *Oncogene* **13:** 1065–1072.

117. Igawa, M., D. B. Rukstalis, T. Tanabe, and G. W. Chodak. 1994. High levels of nm23 expression are related to cell proliferation in human prostate cancer. *Cancer Res.* **54:** 1313–1318.

118. Ilyas, M., I. P. M. Tomlinson, A. Rowan, M. Pignatelli, and W. E. Bodmer. 1997. β-Catenin mutations in cell lines established from human colorectal cancers. *Proc. Natl. Acad. Sci. USA* **94:** 10,330–10,334.

119. Isaacs, W. B., B. S. Carter, and C. M. Ewing. 1991. Wild-type p53 suppresses growth of human prostate carcinoma cancer cells containing mutant p53 alleles. *Cancer Res.* **51:** 4716–4720.

120. Ittman, M. 1996. Allelic loss on chromosome 10 in prostate adenocarcinoma. *Cancer Res.* **56:** 2143–2147.

121. Ittman, M. 1998. Chromosome 10 alterations in prostate adenocarcinoma (review). *Oncol. Rep.* **5:** 1329–1335.

122. Jarrard, D. F., G. S. Bova, C. M. Ewing, S. S. Pin, S. H. Nguyen, S. B. Baylin, et al. 1997. Deletional, mutational, and methylation analyses of CDKN2 (p16/MTS1) in primary and metastatic prostate cancer. *Genes Chromosomes Cancer* **19:** 90–96.

123. Jen, J., W. Harper, S. H. Bigner, D. D. Bigner, N. Papadopoulos, S. Markowitz, et al. 1994. Deletion of p16 and p15 genes in brain tumors. *Cancer Res.* **54:** 6353–6358.

124. Kallakury, B. V. S., J. Figge, J. S. Ross, H. A. G. Fisher, H. L. Figge, and T. A. Jennings. 1994. Association of p53 immunoreactivity with high Gleason tumor grade in prostatic adenocarcinoma. *Hum. Pathol.* **25:** 92–97.

125. Kamb, A., N. A. Gruis, J. Weaver-Feldhaus, Q. Liu, K. Harshman, S. V. Tavitian, et al. 1994. A cell cycle regulator potentially involved in the genesis of many tumor types. *Science* **264:** 436–440.

126. Kawamata, N., R. Morosetti, C. Miller, D. Park, K. S. Spirin, T. Nakamaki, et al. 1995. Molecular analysis of the cyclin-dependent kinase inhibitor gene p27Kip1 in human malignancies. *Cancer Res.* **55:** 2266–2269.

127. Kawamata, N., D. Park, S. Wilczynski, J. Yokota, and H. P. Hoeffler. 1996. Point mutations of the MXI1 gene are rare in prostate cancers. *Prostate* **29:** 191–193.

128. Kawana, Y., A. Komiya, T. Ueda, N. Nihei, H. Kurmochi, H. Suzuki, et al. 1997. Location of KAI1 on the short arm of human chromosome 11 and frequency of allelic loss in advanced human prostate cancer. *Prostate* **32:** 205–213.

129. Kerangueven, F., L. Essioux, A. Dib, T. Noguchi, F. Allione, J. Geneix, et al. 1995. Loss of heterozygosity and linkage analysis in breast carcinoma: indication for a putative third susceptibility gene on the short arm of chromosome 8. *Oncogene* **10:** 1023–1026.

130. Kim, I. Y., H. J. Ahn, D. J. Zelner, J. W. Shaw, S. Lang, M. Kato, et al. 1996. Loss of expression of transforming growth factor beta type I and type II receptors correlates with tumor grade in human prostate cancer tissues. *Clin. Cancer Res.* **2:** 1255–1261.

131. Kim, I. Y., H. J. Ahn, D. J. Zelner, J. W. Shaw, J. A. Sensibar, J. H. Kim, et al. 1996. Genetic change in transforming growth factor beta (TGF-beta) receptor type I gene correlates with insensitivity to TGF-beta 1 in human prostate cancer cells. *Cancer Res.* **56:** 44–48.

132. Kinzler, K. and B. Vogelstein. 1996. Lessons from hereditary colorectal cancer. *Cell* **87:** 159–170.

133. Klein, G., U. Bregula, F. Wiener, and H. Harris. 1971. The analysis of malignancy by cell fusion. I. Hybrids between tumour cells and L cell derivatives. *J. Cell Sci.* **8:** 659–672.

134. Kleinerman, D., P. Troncoso, T. Brooks, A. Eschenbach, S.-H. Lin, and J. T. Hsieh. 1995. The expression of epithelial cell adhesion molecule (C-CAM) in human prostate development and in prostate carcinoma: implication as a tumor suppressor. *Cancer Res.* **55:** 1215–1220.

135. Kleinerman, D. I., W. W. Zhang, S. H. Lin, T. V. Nguyen, A. Eschenbach, and J. T. Hsieh. 1995. Application of a tumor suppressor (C-CAM1)-expressing recombinant

adenovirus in androgen-independent human prostate cancer therapy: a preclinical study. *Cancer Res.* **55:** 2831–2836.

136. Knudson, A. G. 1971. Mutation and cancer: statistical study of retinoblastoma. *Proc. Natl. Acad. Sci. USA* **68:** 820–823.

137. Ko, S. C., A. Gotoh, G. N. Thalmann, H. E. Zhau, D. A. Johnston, W. W. Zhang, et al. 1996. Molecular therapy with recombinant p53 adenovirus in an androgen-independent, metastatic human prostate cancer model. *Hum. Gene Ther.* **7:** 1683–1691.

138. Koh, J., G. H. Enders, B. D. Dynlacht, and E. Harlow. 1995. Tumor-derived p16 alleles encoding proteins defective in cell-cycle inhibition. *Nature* **375:** 506–510.

139. Komiya, A., H. Suzuki, S. Aida, R. Yatani, and J. Shimazaki. 1995. Mutational analysis of CDKN2 (CDK4I/MTS1) gene in tissues and cell lines of human prostate cancer. *Jpn. J. Cancer Res.* **86:** 622–625.

140. Komiya, A., H. Suzuki, T. Ueda, S. Aida, N. Ito, T. Shiraishi, et al. 1997. PRLTS gene alterations in human prostate cancer. *Jpn. J. Cancer Res.* **88:** 389–393.

141. Konishi, N., S. Nakaoka, T. Tsuzuki, K. Matsumoto, Y. Kitahori, Y. Hiasa, et al. 1993. Expression of nm23-H1 and nm23-H2 proteins in prostate carcinoma. *Jpn. J. Cancer Res.* **84:** 1050–1054.

142. Kratzke, R. A., T. M. Greatens, J. B. Rubins, M. A. Maddaus, D. E. Niewoehner, G. A. Niehans, et al. 1996. Rb and p16Ink4a expression in resected non-small cell lung tumors. *Cancer Res.* **56:** 3415–3420.

143. Kubota, Y., K. Fujinami, H. Uemura, Y. Dobashi, H. Miyamoto, Y. Iwasaki, et al. 1995. Retinoblastoma gene mutations in primary human prostate cancer. *Prostate* **27:** 314–320.

144. Kuczyk, M. A., J. Serth, C. Bokemeyer, J. Schwede, R. Herrmann, S. Machtens, et al. 1998. The MXI1 tumor suppressor gene is not mutated in primary prostate cancer. *Oncol. Rep.* **5:** 213–216.

145. Lane, D. P. 1992. p53, guardian of the genome. *Nature* **358:** 15,16.

146. Latil, A., J. C. Baron, O. Cussenot, G. Fournier, T. Soussi, L. Boccon-Gibod, et al. 1994. Genetic alterations in localized prostate cancer: identification of a common region of deletion on chromosome arm 18q. *Genes Chromosomes Cancer* **11:** 119–125.

147. Latil, A., I. Bieche, G. Fournier, O. Cussenot, S. Pesche, and R. Lidereau. 1998. Molecular analysis of the FHIT gene in human prostate cancer. *Oncogene* **16:** 1863–1868.

148. Latil, A., O. Cussenot, G. Fournier, J.-C. Baron, and R. Lidereau. 1995. Loss of heterozygosity at 7q31 is a frequent and early event in prostate cancer. *Clin. Cancer Res.* **1:** 1385–1389.

149. Lee, W.-H., R. Bookstein, F. Hong, L.-J. Young, J.-Y. Shew, and E. Y.-H. P. Lee. 1987. Human retinoblastoma susceptibility gene: cloning, identification, and sequence. *Science* **235:** 1394–1399.

150. Leone, A., U. Flatow, J. V. Houtte, and P. S. Steeg. 1993. Transfection of human nm23-H1 into the human MDA-MB-435 breast carcinoma cell line: effects on tumor metastatic potential, colonization and enzymatic activity. *Oncogene* **8:** 2325–2333.

151. Leone, A., U. Flatow, C. R. King, M. A. Sandeen, I. M. K. Margulies, L. A. Liotta, et al. 1991. Reduced tumor incidence, metastatic potential, and cytokine responsiveness of nm23-transfected melanoma cells. *Cell* **65:** 25–35.

152. Lerebours, F., S. Olschwang, B. Thuille, A. Schmitz, P. Fouchet, B. Buecher, et al. 1999. Fine deletion mapping of chromosome 8p in non-small-cell lung carcinoma. *Int. J. Cancer* **81:** 854–858.

153. Levy, A., U.-C. Dang, and R. Bookstein. 1999. High-density screen of human tumor cell lines for homozygous deletions of loci on chromosome arm 8p. *Genes Chromosomes Cancer* **24:** 42–47.

154. Levy, D. B., K. J. Smith, Y. Beazer-Barclay, S. R. Hamilton, B. Vogelstein, and K. W. Kinzler. 1994. Inactivation of both APC alleles in human and mouse tumors. *Cancer Res.* **54:** 5953–5958.

155. Li, C., C. Larsson, A. Futreal, J. Lancaster, C. Phelan, U. Aspenblad, et al. 1998. Identification of two distinct deleted regions on chromosome 13 in prostate cancer. *Oncogene* **16:** 481–487.

156. Li, D., H. Yan, J. Chen, B. C. Casto, K. S. Theil, and G. E. Milo. 1996. Malignant conversion of human cells by antisense cDNA to a putative tumor suppressor gene. *Carcinogenesis* **17:** 1751–1755.

157. Li, J., L. Simpson, M. Takahashi, C. Miliaresis, M. P. Myers, N. Tonks, et al. 1998. The PTEN/MMAC1 tumor suppressor induces cell death that is rescued by the AKT/protein kinase B oncogene. *Cancer Res.* **58:** 5667–5672.

158. Li, J., C. Yen, D. Liaw, K. Podsypanina, S. Bose, S. I. Wang, et al. 1997. PTEN, a putative protein tyrosine phosphatase gene mutated in human brain, breast and prostate cancer. *Science* **275:** 1943–1947.

159. Li, L., and S. N. Cohen, S. N. 1996. tsg101: a novel tumor susceptibility gene isolated by controlled homozygous functional knockout of allelic loci in mammalian cells. *Cell* **85:** 319–329.

160. Liaw, D., D. J. Marsh, J. Li, P. L. M. Dahia, S. I. Wang, Z. Zheng, et al. 1997. Germline mutations of the PTEN gene in Cowden disease, an inherited breast and thyroid cancer syndrome. *Nat. Genet.* **16:** 64–67.

161. Liggett, W. H. and D. Sidransky. 1998. Role of the p16 tumor suppressor gene in cancer. *J. Clin. Oncol.* **16:** 1197–1206.

162. Lin, S. H., Y. S. Pu, W. Luo, Y. Wang, and C. J. Logothetis. 1999. Schedule-dependence of C-CAM1 adenovirus gene therapy in a prostate cancer model. *Anticancer Res.* **19:** 337–340.

163. Liu, Q., S. Neuhausen, M. McClure, C. Frye, J. Weaver-Feldhaus, N. A. Gruis, et al. 1995. CDKN2 (MTS1) tumor suppressor gene mutations in human tumor cell lines. *Oncogene* **10:** 1061–1067.

164. Loda, M., B. Cukor, S. W. Tam, P. Lavin, M. Fiorentino, G. F. Draetta, et al. 1997. Increased proteasome-dependent degradation of the cyclin-dependent kinase inhibitor p27 in aggressive colorectal carcinomas. *Nat. Med.* **3:** 231–234.

165. Lu, S., S. Y. Tsai, and M. J. Tsai. 1997. Regulation of androgen-dependent prostatic cancer cell growth: androgen regulation of CDK2, CDK4, and CKI p16 genes. *Cancer Res.* **57:** 4511–4516.

166. Lukas, J., D. Parry, L. Aagaard, D. J. Mann, J. Bartkova, M. Strauss, et al. 1995. Retinoblastoma protein-dependent cell-cycle inhibition by the tumour suppressor p16. *Nature* **375:** 503–506.

167. Lundgren, R., N. Mandahl, S. Heim, J. Limon, H. Henrikson, and F. Mitelman. 1992. Cytogenetic analysis of 57 primary prostatic adenocarcinomas. *Genes Chromosomes Cancer* **4:** 16–24.

168. Luo, W., M. Tapolsky, K. Earley, C. G. Wood, D. R. Wilson, C. J. Logothetis, et al. 1999. Tumor-suppressive activity of CD66a in prostate cancer. *Cancer Gene Ther.* **6:** 313–321.

169. MacDonald, N. J., A. D. L. Rosa, M. A. Benedict, J. M. Freije, H. Krutsch, and P. S. Steeg. 1994. A serine phosphorylation of Nm23, but not its nucleoside diphosphate kinase activity, correlates with suppression of tumor metastatic potential. *J. Biol. Chem.* **268:** 25,780–25,789.

170. MacGrogan, D. and R. Bookstein. 1997. Tumour suppressor genes in prostate cancer. *Sem. Cancer Biol.* **8:** 11–19.

171. MacGrogan, D., A. Levy, D. Bostwick, M. Wagner, D. Wells, and R. Bookstein. 1994. Loss of chromosome arm 8p loci in prostate cancer: mapping by quantitative allelic imbalance. *Genes Chromosomes Cancer* **10:** 151–159.

172. MacGrogan, D., A. Levy, G. S. Bova, W. B. Isaacs, and R. Bookstein. 1996. Structure and methylation-associated silencing of a gene within a homozygously deleted region of human chromosome band 8p22. *Genomics* **35:** 55–65.

173. MacGrogan, D., M. Pegram, D. Slamon, and R. Bookstein. 1997. Comparative mutational analysis of DPC4 (Smad4) in prostatic and colorectal carcinomas. *Oncogene* **15:** 1111–1114.

174. Macintosh, C. A., M. Stower, N. Reid, and N. J. Maitland. 1998. Precise microdissection of human prostate cancers reveals genotypic heterogeneity. *Cancer Res.* **58:** 23–28.

175. Maehama, T. and J. E. Dixon. 1998. The tumor suppressor, PTEN/MMAC1, dephosphorylates the lipid second messenger, phosphatidylinositol 3,4,5,-triphosphate. *J. Biol. Chem.* **273:** 13,375–13,378.

176. Maehama, T. and J. E. Dixon. 1999. PTEN: a tumour suppressor that functions as a phospholipid phosphatase. *Trends Cell Biol.* **9:** 125–128.

177. Malkin, D., F. P. Li, L. C. Strong, J. Fraumeni, C. E. Nelson, D. H. Kim, et al. 1990. Germ line p53 mutations in a familial syndrome of breast cancer, sarcomas, and other neoplasms. *Science* **250:** 1233–1238.

178. Markowitz, S., J. Wang, L. Myeroff, R. Parsons, L. Sun, J. Lutterbaugh, et al. 1995. Inactivation of the type II TGFβ receptor in colon cancer cells with microsatellite instability. *Science* **268:** 1336–1338.

179. Marsh, D. J., P. L. M. Dahia, Z. Zheng, D. Liaw, R. Parsons, R. J. Gorlin, et al. 1997. Germline mutations in PTEN are present in Bannayan-Zonana syndrome. *Nat. Genet.* **16:** 333–334.

180. Marzo, A. M. de, B. Knudsen, K. Chan-Tack, and J. I. Epstein. 1999. E-cadherin expression as a marker of tumor aggressiveness in routinely processed radical prostatectomy specimens. *Urology* **53:** 707–713.

181. Mashimo, T., M. Watabe, S. Hirota, S. Hosobe, K. Miura, P. J. Tegtmeyer, et al. 1998. The expression of the KAI1 gene, a tumor metastasis suppressor, is directly activated by p53. *Proc. Natl. Acad. Sci. USA* **95:** 11,307–11,311.

182. Matsushima, H., T. Kitamura, T. Goto, Y. Hosaka, Y. Homma, and K. Kawabe. 1997. Combined analysis with Bcl-2 and p53 immunostaining predicts poorer prognosis in prostatic carcinoma. *J. Urol.* **158:** 2278–2283.

183. McDonnell, T. J., N. M. Navone, P. Troncoso, L. L. Pisters, C. Conti, A. Eschenbach, et al. 1997. Expression of bcl-2 oncoprotein and p53 protein accumulation in bone marrow metastases of androgen independent prostate cancer. *J. Urol.* **157:** 569–574.

184. McMenamin, M. E., P. Soung, S. Perera, I. Kaplan, M. Loda, and W. R. Sellars. 1999. Loss of PTEN expression in paraffin-embedded primary prostate cancer correlates with high Gleason score and advanced stage. *Cancer Res.* **59:** 4291–4296.

185. Merlo, A., J. G. Herman, L. Mao, D. J. Lee, E. Gabrielson, P. C. Burger, et al. 1995. 5′ CpG island methylation is associated with transcriptional silencing of the tumor suppressor p16/CDKN2/MTS1 in human cancers. *Nat. Med.* **1:** 686–692.

186. Meyers, F. J., S.-G. Chi, J. R. Fishman, R. White, and P. H. Gumerlock. 1993. p53 mutations in benign prostatic hyperplasia. *J. Natl. Cancer Inst.* **85:** 1856–1858.

187. Meyers, F. J., P. H. Gumerlock, S. G. Chi, H. Borchers, A. D. Deitch, and R. White. 1998. Very frequent p53 mutations in metastatic prostate carcinoma and in matched primary tumors. *Cancer* **83:** 2534–2539.

188. Mirchandani, D., J. Zheng, G. J. Miller, A. K. Ghosh, D. K. Shibata, R. J. Cote, et al. 1995. Heterogeneity in intratumor distribution of p53 mutations in human prostate cancer. *Am. J. Pathol.* **147:** 92–101.

189. Mollenhauer, J., S. Wiemann, W. Scheurlen, B. Korn, Y. Hayashi, K. K. Wilgenbus, et al. 1997. DMBT1, a new member of the SRCR superfamily, on chromosome 10q25.3-26.1 is deleted in malignant brain tumours. *Nat. Genet.* **17:** 32–39.

190. Morimoto, A. M., A. E. Berson, G. H. Fujii, D. Teng, S. V. Tavtigian, R. Bookstein, et al. 1999. Phenotypic analysis of human glioma cells expressing the MMAC1 tumor suppressor phosphatase. *Oncogene* **18:** 1261–1266.

191. Morton, R. A., C. M. Ewing, A. Nagafuchi, S. Tsukita, and W. B. Isaacs. 1993. Reduction of E-cadherin levels and deletion of the α-catenin gene in human prostate cancer cells. *Cancer Res.* **53:** 3585–3590.

192. Moul, J. W. 1999. Angiogenesis, p53, bcl-2 and Ki-67 in the progression of prostate cancer after radical prostatectomy. *Eur. Urol.* **35:** 399–407.

193. Murakami, Y. S., A. R. Brothman, R. J. Leach, and R. L. White. 1995. Suppression of malignant phenotype in a human prostate cancer cell line by fragments of normal chromosomal region 17q. *Cancer Res.* **55:** 3389–3394.

194. Myeroff, L. L. and S. D. Markowitz. 1993. Increased nm23-H1 and nm23-H2 messenger RNA expression and absence of mutations in colon carcinomas of low and high metastatic potential. *J. Natl. Cancer Inst.* **85:** 147–152.

195. Myers, M. P., J. P. Stolarov, C. Eng, J. Li, S. I. Wang, M. H. Wigler, et al. 1997. P-TEN, the tumor suppressor from human chromosome 10q23, is a dual-specificity phosphatase. *Proc. Natl. Acad. Sci. USA* **94:** 9052–9057.

196. Myers, R. B., S. Srivastava, D. K. Oelschlager, D. Brown, and W. E. Grizzle. 1996. Expression of nm23-H1 in prostatic intraepithelial neoplasia and adenocarcinoma. *Hum. Pathol.* **27:** 1021–1024.

197. Navone, N. M., M. E. Labate, P. Troncoso, L. Pisters, C. J. Conti, A. Eschenbach, et al. 1999. p53 mutations in prostate cancer bone metastases suggest that selected p53 mutants in the primary site define foci with metastatic potential. *J. Urol.* **161:** 304–308.

198. Navone, N. M., P. Troncoso, L. L. Pisters, T. L. Goodrow, J. L. Palmer, W. W. Nichols, et al. 1993. p53 protein accumulation and gene mutation in the progression of human prostate carcinoma. *J. Natl. Cancer Inst.* **85:** 1657–1669.

199. Neumaier, M., S. Paululat, A. Chan, P. Matthaes, and C. Wagener. 1993. Biliary glycoprotein, a potential human cell adhesion molecule, is down-regulated in colorectal carcinomas. *Proc. Natl. Acad. Sci. USA* **90:** 10,744–10,748.

200. Nielsen, L. L., M. Gurnani, J. Syed, J. Dell, B. Hartman, M. Cartwright, et al. 1998. Recombinant E1-deleted adenovirus-mediated gene therapy for cancer: efficacy studies with p53 tumor suppressor gene and liver histology in tumor xenograft models. *Hum. Gene Ther.* **9:** 681–694.

201. Nielsen, L. L., P. Lipari, J. Dell, M. Gurnani, and G. Hajian. 1998. Adenovirus-mediated p53 gene therapy and paclitaxel have synergistic efficacy in models of human head and neck, ovarian, prostate, and breast cancer. *Clin. Cancer Res.* **4:** 835–846.

202. Nihei, N., T. Ichikawa, Y. Kawana, H. Kuramochi, H. Kugo, M. Oshimura, et al. 1995. Localization of metastasis suppressor gene(s) for rat prostatic cancer to the long arm of human chromosome 10. *Genes Chromosomes Cancer* **14:** 112–119.

203. Nihei, N., T. Ichikawa, Y. Kawana, H. Kuramochi, H. Kugoh, M. Oshimura, et al. 1996. Mapping of metastasis suppressor gene(s) for rat prostate cancer on the short arm of human chromosome 8 by irradiated microcell-mediated chromosome transfer. *Genes Chromosomes Cancer* **17:** 260–268.

204. Nihei, N., S. Ohta, H. Kuramochi, H. Kugoh, M. Oshimura, J. C. Barrett, et al. 1999. Metastasis suppressor gene(s) for rat prostate cancer on the long arm of human chromosome 7. *Genes Chromosomes Cancer* **24:** 1–8.

205. Nollau, P., H. Scheller, M. Kona-Horstmann, S. Rohde, F. Hagenmuller, C. Wagener, et al. 1997. Expression of CD66a (human C-CAM) and other members of the carcinoembryonic antigen gene family of adhesion molecules in human colorectal adenomas. *Cancer Res.* **57:** 2354–2357.

206. Nupponen, N. and T. Visakorpi. 1999. Molecular biology of progression of prostate cancer. *Eur. Urol.* **35:** 351–354.

207. Obata, K., S. J. Morland, R. H. Watson, A. Hitchcock, G. Chenevix-Trench, E. J. Thomas, et al. 1998. Frequent PTEN/MMAC mutations in endometrioid but not serous or mucinous epithelial ovarian tumors. *Cancer Res.* **58:** 2095–2097.

208. Oda, T., Y. Kanai, T. Oyama, K. Yoshiura, Y. Shimoyama, W. Birchmeier, et al. 1994. E-cadherin gene mutations in human gastric carcinoma cell lines. *Proc. Natl. Acad. Sci. USA* **91:** 1858–1862.

209. Ohta, M., H. Inoue, M. G. Cotticelli, K. Kastury, R. Baffa, J. Palazzo, et al. 1996. The FHIT gene, spanning the chromosome 3p14.2 fragile site and renal carcinoma-associated t(3;8) breakpoint, is abnormal in digestive tract cancers. *Cell* **84:** 587–597.

210. Olschwang, S., O. M. Serova-Sinilnikova, G. M. Lenoir, and G. Thomas. 1998. PTEN germ-line mutations in juvenile polyposis coli. *Nat. Genet.* **18:** 12–14.

211. Oren, M. and V. Rotter. 1999. Introduction: p53—the first twenty years. *Cell Mol. Life Sci.* **55:** 9–11.

212. Otterson, G. A., R. A. Kratzke, A. Coxon, Y. W. Kim, and F. J. Faye. 1994. Absence of p16^{Ink4a} protein is restricted to the subset of lung cancer lines that retains wildtype RB. *Oncogene* **9:** 3375–3378.

213. Palacios, J. and C. Gamallo. 1998. Mutations in the beta-catenin gene (CTNNB1) in endometrioid ovarian carcinomas. *Cancer Res.* **58:** 1344–1347.

214. Pan, Y., H. Matsuyama, N. Wang, S. Yoshihiro, L. Haggarth, C. Li, et al. 1998. Chromosome 16q24 deletion and decreased E-cadherin expression: possible association with metastatic potential in prostate cancer. *Prostate* **36:** 31–38.

215. Park, D. J., S. P. Wilczynski, E. Y. Pham, C. W. Miller, and H. P. Koeffler. 1997. Molecular analysis of the INK4 family of genes in prostate carcinomas. *J. Urol.* **157:** 1995–1999.

216. Paul, R., C. M. Ewing, D. F. Jarrard, and W. B. Isaacs. 1997. The cadherin cell-cell adhesion pathway in prostate cancer progression. *Br. J. Urol.* **79 (Suppl. 1):** 37–43.

217. Pemberton, P. A., A. R. Tipton, N. Pavloff, J. Smith, J. R. Erickson, Z. M. Mouchabeck, et al. 1997. Maspin is an intracellular serpin that partitions into secretory vesicles and is present at the cell surface. *J. Histochem. Cytochem.* **45:** 1697–1706.

218. Perl, A.-K., P. Wilgenbus, U. Dahl, H. Semb, and G. Christofori. 1998. A causal role for E-cadherin in the transition from adenoma to carcinoma. *Nature* **392:** 190–193.

219. Pesche, S., A. Latil, F. Muzeau, O. Cussenot, G. Fournier, M. Longy, et al. 1998. PTEN/ MMAC1/TEP1 involvement in primary prostate cancers. *Oncogene* **16:** 2879–2883.

220. Phillips, S. M. A., C. M. Barton, S. J. Lee, D. G. Morton, D. M.A. Wallace, N. R. Lemoine, et al. 1994. Loss of the retinoblastoma susceptibility gene (RB1) is a frequent and early event in prostatic tumorigenesis. *Br. J. Cancer* **70:** 1252–1257.

221. Pineau, P., H. Nagai, S. Prigent, Y. Wei, G. Gyapay, J. Weissenbach, et al. 1998. Identification of three distinct regions of allelic deletions on the short arm of chromosome 8 in hepatocellular carcinoma. *Oncogene* **18:** 3127–3134.

222. Podsypanina, K., L. H. Ellenson, A. Nemes, J. Gu, M. Tamura, K. M. Yamada, et al. 1999. Mutation of Pten/Mmac1 in mice causes neoplasia in multiple organ systems. *Proc. Natl. Acad. Sci. USA* **96:** 1563–1568.

223. Porter, P. L., K. E. Malone, P. J. Heagerty, G. M. Alexander, L. A. Gatti, E. J. Firpo, et al. 1997. Expression of cell-cycle regulators p27Kip1 and cyclin E, alone and in combination, correlate with survival in young breast cancer patients. *Nat. Med.* **3:** 222–225.

224. Prives, C. and P. A. Hall. 1999. The p53 pathway. *J. Pathol.* **187:** 112–126.

225. Prochownik, E. V., G. L. Eagle, D. Deubler, X. L. Zhu, R. A. Stephenson, L. R. Rohr, et al. 1998. Commonly occuring loss and mutation of the MXI1 gene in prostate cancer. *Genes Chromosomes Cancer* **22:** 295–304.

226. Quelle, D. E., M. Cheng, R. A. Ashmun, and C. J. Scherr. 1997. Cancer-associated mutations at the INK4a locus cancel cell cycle arrest by p16INK4a but not by the alternative reading frame protein p19ARF. *Proc. Natl. Acad. Sci. USA* **94:** 669–673.

227. Quelle, D. E., F. Zindy, R. A. Ashmun, and C. J. Scherr. 1995. Alternative reading frames of the INK4a tumor suppressor gene encode two unrelated proteins capable of inducing cell cycle arrest. *Cell* **83:** 993–1000.

228. Rakozy, C., D. J. Grignon, Y. Li, E. Gheiler, B. Gururajanna, J. E. Pontes, et al. 1999. p53 gene alterations in prostate cancer after radiation failure and their association with clinical outcome: a molecular and immunohistochemical analysis. *Pathol. Res. Pract.* **195:** 129–135.

229. Richmond, P. J. M., A. J. Karayiannakis, A. Nagafuchi, A. V. Kaisary, and M. Pignatelli. 1997. Aberrant E-cadherin and α-catenin expression in prostate cancer: correlation with patient survival. *Cancer Res.* **57:** 3189–3193.

230. Rinker-Schaeffer, C. W., A. L. Hawkins, N. Ru, J. Dong, G. Stoica, C. A. Griffin, et al. 1994. Differential suppression of mammary and prostate cancer metastasis by human chromosomes 17 and 11. *Cancer Res.* **54:** 6249–6256.

231. Risinger, J. I., A. Berchuck, M. F. Kohler, and J. Boyd. 1994. Mutations of the E-cadherin gene in human gynecologic cancers. *Nat. Genet.* **7:** 98–102.

232. Risinger, J. I., A. K. Hayes, A. Berchuck, and J. C. Barrett. 1997. PTEN/MMAC1 mutations in endometrial cancers. *Cancer Res.* **57:** 4736–4738.

233. Roy-Burman, P., J. Zheng, and G. J. Miller. 1997. Molecular heterogeneity in prostate cancer: can TP53 mutation unravel tumorigenesis? *Mol. Med. Today* **3:** 476–482.

234. Rubinfeld, B., P. Robbins, M. El-Gamil, I. Albert, E. Porfiri, and P. Polakis. 1997. Stabilization of beta-catenin by genetic defects in melanoma cell lines. *Science* **275:** 1790–1792.

235. Salem, C. E., N. A. Tomasic, D. A. Elmajian, D. Esrig, P. W. Nichols, C. R. Taylor, et al. 1997. p53 protein and gene alterations in pathological stage C prostate carcinoma. *J. Urol.* **158:** 510–514.

236. Sanchez, Y., M. Lovell, M. C. Marin, P. E. Wong, M. E. Wolf-Ledbetter, T. J. McDonnell, et al. 1996. Tumor suppression and apoptosis of human prostate carcinoma mediated by a genetic locus within human chromosome 10pter-q11. *Proc. Natl. Acad. Sci. USA* **93:** 2551–2556.

237. Save, V., K. Nylander, and P. A. Hall. 1998. Why is p53 protein stabilized in neoplasia? Some answers but many more questions! *J. Pathol.* **184:** 348–350.

238. Scherr, D. S., J. Wei, M. Chung, D. Felsen, R. Allbright, and B. S. Knudsen. 1999. BCL-2 and p53 expression in clinically localized prostate cancer predicts response to external beam radiotherapy. *J. Urol.* **162:** 12–16.

239. Schneider, S. S., C. Schick, K. E. Fish, E. Miller, J. C. Pena, S. D. Treter, et al. 1995. A serine proteinase inhibitor locus at 18q21.3 contains a tandem duplication of the human squamous cell carcinoma antigen gene. *Proc. Natl. Acad. Sci. USA* **92:** 3147–3151.

240. Schreiber-Agus, N., Y. Meng, T. Hoang, H. Hou, K. Chen, R. Greenberg, et al. 1998. Role of Mxi1 in ageing organ systems and the regulation of normal and neoplastic growth. *Nature* **393:** 483–487.

241. Schroder, F. H., P. Hermanek, L. Denis, W. R. Fair, M. K. Gospodarowicz, and M. Pavone-Macaluso. 1992. The TNM classification of prostate cancer. *Prostate* **(Suppl. 4):** 129–138.

242. Schuler, M., C. Rochlitz, J. A. Horowitz, J. Schlegel, A. P. Perruchoud, F. Kommoss, et al. 1998. A phase I study of adenovirus-mediated wild-type p53 gene transfer in patients with advanced non-small cell lung cancer. *Hum. Gene Ther.* **9:** 2075–2082.

243. Schutte, M., R. H. Hruban, J. Geradts, R. Maynard, W. Hilgers, S. K. Rabindran, et al. 1997. Abrogation of the Rb/p16 tumor-suppressive pathway in virtually all pancreatic carcinomas. *Cancer Res.* **57:** 3126–3130.

244. Schutte, M., R. H. Hruban, L. Hedrick, K. R. Cho, G. M. Nadasdy, C. L. Weinstein, et al. 1996. DPC4 gene in various tumor types. *Cancer Res.* **56:** 2527–2530.

245. Serrano, M. 1997. The tumor suppressor protein p16Ink4a. *Exper. Cell Res.* **237:** 7–13.

246. Shapiro, G. I., C. D. Edwards, L. Kobzik, J. Godleski, W. Richards, D. J. Sugarbaker, et al. 1995. Reciprocal Rb inactivation and p16Ink4 expression in primary lung cancers and cell lines. *Cancer Res.* **55:** 505–509.

247. Sheng, S., J. Carey, E. Seftor, L. Dias, M. J. C. Hendrix, and R. Sager. 1996. Maspin acts at the cell membrane to inhibit invasion and motility of mammary and prostatic cancer cells. *Proc. Natl. Acad. Sci. USA* **93:** 11,669–11,674.

248. Sheng, S., B. Truong, D. Fredrickson, R. Wu, A. B. Pardee, and R. Sager. 1998. Tissue-type plasminogen activator is a target of the tumor suppressor gene maspin. *Proc. Natl. Acad. Sci. USA* **95:** 499–504.

249. Shi, Y., A. Hata, R. S. Lo, J. Massague, and N. P. Pavletich. 1997. A structural basis for mutational inactivation of the tumour suppressor Smad4. *Nature* **388:** 87–93.

250. Shurbaji, M. S., J. H. Kalbfleisch, and T. S. Thurmond. 1995. Immunohistochemical detection of p53 protein as a prognostic indicator in prostate cancer. *Hum. Pathol.* **26:** 106–109.

251. Siprashvili, A., G. Sozzi, L. D. Barnes, P. McCue, A. K. Robinson, V. Eryomin, et al. 1997. Replacement of Fhit in cancer cells suppresses tumorigenicity. *Proc. Natl. Acad. Sci. USA* **94:** 13,771–13,776.

252. Sozzi, G., M. L. Veronese, M. Negrini, R. Baffa, M. G. Cotticelli, H. Inoue, et al. 1996. The FHIT gene at 3p14.2 is abnormal in lung cancer. *Cell* **85:** 17–26.

253. Sparkes, R. S., A. L. Murphree, R. Lingua, M. C. Sparkes, L. L. Field, S. J. Funderburk, et al. 1983. Gene for hereditary retinoblastoma assigned to human chromosome 13 by linkage to esterase D. *Science* **219:** 971–973.

254. Sparks, A. B., P. J. Morin, B. Vogelstein, and K. W. Kinzler. 1998. Mutational analysis of the APC/beta-catenin/Tcf pathway in colorectal cancer. *Cancer Res.* **58:** 1130–1134.

255. Stambolic, V., A. Suzuki, J. L. Pompa, G. M. Brothers, C. Mirtsos, T. Sasaki, et al. 1998. Negative regulation of PKB/Akt-dependent cell survival by the tumor suppressor PTEN. *Cell* **95:** 29–39.

256. Stapleton, A. M., P. Zbell, K. M. Kattan, G. Yang, T. M. Wheeler, P. T. Scardino, et al. 1998. Assessment of the biologic markers p53, Ki-67, and apoptotic index and predictive indicators of prostate carcinoma recurrence after surgery. *Cancer* **82:** 168–175.

257. Stapleton, A. M. F., T. L. Timme, A. E. Gousse, Q.-F. Li, A. A. Tobon, M. W. Kattan, et al. 1997. Primary human prostate cancer cells harboring p53 mutations are clonally expanded in metastases. *Clin. Cancer Res.* **3:** 1389–1397.

258. Steck, P. A., H. Lin, L. A. Langford, S. A. Jasser, D. Koul, W. K. Yung, et al. 1999. Functional and molecular analyses of 10q deletions in human gliomas. *Genes Chromosomes Cancer* **24:** 135–143.

259. Steck, P. A., M. A. Pershouse, S. A. Jassar, W. K. A. Yung, H. Lin, A. H. Ligon, et al. 1997. Identification of a candidate tumour suppressor gene, MMAC1, at chromosome 10q23.3 that is mutated in multiple advanced cancers. *Nat. Genet.* **15:** 356–362.

260. Steeg, P. S., G. Bivalacqua, L. Kopper, U. P. Thorgiersson, J. E. Talmadge, L. A. Liotta, et al. 1988. Evidence for a novel gene associated with low tumor metastatic potential. *J. Natl. Cancer Inst.* **80:** 200–204.

261. Stone, S., P. Jiang, P. Dayananth, S. V. Tavtigian, H. Katcher, D. Parry, et al. 1995. Complex structure and regulation of the p16 (MTS1) locus. *Cancer Res.* **55:** 2988–2994.

262. Su, L.-K., K. W. Kinzler, B. Vogelstein, A. C. Preisinger, A. R. Moser, C. Luongo, et al. 1992. Multiple intestinal neoplasia caused by a mutation in the murine homolog of the APC gene. *Science* **256:** 668–670.

263. Suzuki, H., S. Aida, S. Akimoto, T. Igarashi, R. Yatani, and J. Shimazaki. 1994. State of adenomatous polyposis coli gene and ras oncogenes in Japanese prostate cancer. *Jpn. J. Cancer Res.* **85:** 847–852.

264. Suzuki, H., D. Freije, D. R. Nusskern, K. Okami, P. Cairns, D. Sidransky, et al. 1998. Interfocal heterogeneity of PTEN/MMAC1 gene alterations in multiple metastatic prostate cancer tissues. *Cancer Res.* **58:** 204–209.

265. Suzuki, H., A. Komiya, M. Emi, H. Kuramochi, T. Shiraishi, R. Yatani, et al. 1996. Three distinct commonly deleted regions of chromosome arm 16q in human primary and metastatic prostate cancers. *Genes Chromosomes Cancer* **17:** 225–233.

266. Swisher, S. G., J. A. Roth, J. Nemunaitis, D. D. Lawrence, B. L. Kemp, C. H. Carrasco, et al. 1999. Adenovirus-mediated p53 gene transfer in advanced non-small-cell lung cancer. *J. Natl. Cancer Inst.* **91:** 763–771.

267. Takahashi, S., A. L. Shan, S. R. Ritland, K. A. Delacey, D. G. Bostwick, M. M. Lieber, et al. 1995. Frequent loss of heterozygosity at 7q31.1 in primary prostate cancer is associated with tumor aggressiveness and progression. *Cancer Res.* **55:** 4114–4119.

268. Tamimi, Y., P. P. Bringuier, F. Smit, V. Bokhoven, F. M. J. Debruyne, and J. A. Schalken. 1996. p16 mutations/deletions are not frequent events in prostate cancer. *Br. J. Cancer* **74:** 120–122.

269. Tamura, M., J. Gu, K. Matsumoto, S.-I. Aota, R. Parsons, and K. M. Yamada. 1998. Inhibition of cell migration, spreading, and focal adhesion by tumor suppressor PTEN. *Science* **280:** 1614–1617.

270. Tamura, M., J. Gu, T. Takino, and K. M. Yamada. 1999. Tumor suppressor PTEN inhibition of cell invasion, migration, and growth: differential involvement of focal adhesion kinase and p130Cas. *Cancer Res.* **59:** 442–449.

271. Tanaka, K., R. Kikuchi-Yanoshita, M. Muraoka, M. Konishi, M. Oshimura, and M. Miyaki. 1996. Suppression of tumorigenicity and invasiveness of colon carcinoma cells by introduction of normal chromosome 8p12-pter. *Oncogene* **12:** 405–410.

272. Tani, M., S. Takenoshita, T. Kohno, K. Hagiwara, Y. Nagamachi, C. C. Harris, et al. 1997. Infrequent mutations of the transforming growth factor beta-type II receptor gene at chromosome 3p22 in human lung cancers with chromosome 3p deletions. *Carcinogenesis* 1119–1921.

273. Tao, W. and A. J. Levine. 1999. p19(ARF) stabilizes p53 by blocking nucleo-cytoplasmic shuttling of Mdm2. *Proc. Natl. Acad. Sci. USA* **96:** 6937–6941.

274. Tashiro, H., M. S. Blazes, R. Wu, K. R. Cho, S. Bose, S. I. Wang, et al. 1997. Mutations in PTEN are frequent in endometrial carcinoma but rare in other common gynecological malignancies. *Cancer Res.* **57:** 3935–3940.

275. Teng, D. H.-F., R. Hu, H. Lin, T. Davis, D. Iliev, C. Frye, et al. 1997. MMAC1/PTEN mutations in primary tumor specimens and tumor cell lines. *Cancer Res.* **57:** 5221–5225.

276. Theodorescu, D., S. R. Broder, J. C. Boyd, S. E. Mills, and H. F. Frierson. 1997. p53, bcl-2 and retinoblastoma proteins as long-term prognostic markers in localized carcinoma of the prostate. *J. Urol.* **158:** 131–137.

277. Thiagalingam, S., C. Lengauer, F. S. Leach, M. Schutte, S. A. Hahn, J. Overhauser, et al. 1996. Evaluation of candidate tumour suppressor genes on chromosome 18 in colorectal cancers. *Nat. Genet.* **13:** 343–346.

278. Thomas, D. J., M. Robinson, P. King, T. Hasan, R. Charlton, J. Martin, et al. 1993. p53 expression and clinical outcome in prostate cancer. *Br. J. Urol.* **72:** 778–781.

279. Tsihlias, J., L. R. Kapusta, G. DeBoer, I. Morava-Protzner, I. Zbieranowski, N. Bhattacharya, et al. 1998. Loss of cyclin-dependent kinase inhibitor p27Kip1 is a novel prognostic factor in localized human prostate adenocarcinoma. *Cancer Res.* **58:** 524–528.

280. Uchida, K., M. Nagatake, H. Osada, Y. Tatabe, M. Kondo, T. Mitsudomi, et al. 1996. Somatic in vivo alterations of the JV18-1 gene at 18q21 in human lung cancers. *Cancer Res.* **56:** 5583–5585.

281. Ueda, T., A. Komiya, M. Emi, H. Suzuki, T. Shiraishi, R. Yatani, et al. 1997. Allelic losses on 18q21 are associated with progression and metastasis in human prostate cancer. *Genes Chromosomes Cancer* **20:** 140–147.

282. Umbas, R., W. B. Isaacs, P. P. Bringuier, H. E. Schaafsma, F. M. Karthaus, G. O. Oosterhof, et al. 1994. Decreased E-cadherin expression is associated with poor prognosis in patients with prostate cancer. *Cancer Res.* **54:** 3929–3933.

283. Umbas, R., J. A. Schalken, T. W. Aalders, B. S. Carter, H. F. M. Karthaus, H. E. Schaafsma, et al. 1992. Expression of the cellular adhesion molecule E-cadherin is reduced or absent in high-grade prostate cancer. *Cancer Res.* **52:** 5104–5109.

284. Umekita, Y., R. A. Hiipakka, and S. Liao. 1997. Rat and human maspins: structures, metastatic suppressor activity and mutation in prostate cancer cells. *Cancer Lett.* **113:** 87–93.

285. Uzoaru, I., M. Rubenstein, Y. Mirochnik, L. Slobodskoy, M. Shaw, and P. Guinan. 1998. An evaluation of the markers p53 and Ki-67 for their predictive value in prostate cancer. *J. Surg. Oncol.* **67:** 33–37.

286. Vermeulen, S. J., F. Nollet, E. Teugels, K. M. Vennekens, F. Malfait, J. Philippe, et al. 1999. The α-catenin gene (CTNNA1) acts as an invasion-suppressor gene in human colon cancer cells. *Oncogene* **18:** 905–915.

287. Vesalainen, S. and P. Lipponen. 1995. Expression of retinblastoma gene (Rb) protein in T12M0 prostatic adenocarcinoma. *J. Cancer Res. Clin. Oncol.* **121:** 429–433.

288. Vincent, F., M. Nagashima, S. Takenoshita, M. A. Khan, A. Gemma, K. Hagiwara, et al. 1997. Mutation analysis of the transforming growth factor-β type II receptor in human cell lines resistant to growth inhibition by transformin growth factor-β. *Oncogene* **15:** 117–122.

289. Virgilio, L., M. Shuster, S. M. Gollin, M. L. Veronese, M. Ohta, K. Huebner, et al. 1996. FHIT gene alterations in head and neck squamous cell carcinomas. *Proc. Natl. Acad. Sci. USA* **93:** 9770–9775.

290. Visakorpi, T., A. H. Kallioniemi, A.-C. Syvanen, E. R. Hyytinen, R. Karhu, T. Tammela, et al. 1995. Genetic changes in primary and recurrent prostate cancer by comparative genomic hybridization. *Cancer Res.* **55:** 342–347.

291. Visakorpi, T., O.-P. Kallioniemi, A. Heikkinen, T. Koivula, and J. Isola. 1992. Small subgroup of aggressive, highly proliferative prostatic carcinomas defined by p53 accumulation. *J. Natl. Cancer Inst.* **84:** 883–887.

292. Vleminckx, K., J. Vakaet, M. Mareel, W. Fiers, and F. van Roy. 1991. Genetic manipulation of E-cadherin expression by epithelial tumor cells reveals an invasion suppressor role. *Cell* **66:** 107–119.

293. Vlietstra, R. J., D. C. J, G. van Alewijk, K. G. L. Hermans, G. J. v. Steenbrugge, and J. Trapman. 1998. Frequent inactivation of PTEN in prostate cancer cell lines and xenografts. *Cancer Res.* **58:** 2720–2723.

294. Vocke, C. D., R. O. Pozzatti, D. G. Bostwick, C. D. Florence, S. B. Jennings, S. E. Strup, et al. 1996. Analysis of 99 microdissected prostate carcinomas reveals a high frequency of allelic loss on chromosome 8p12-21. *Cancer Res.* **56:** 2411–2416.

295. Voeller, H. J., L. Y. Sugars, T. Pretlow, and E. P. Gelmann. 1994. p53 oncogene mutations in human prostate cancer specimens. *J. Urol.* **151:** 492–495.

296. Voeller, H. J., C. I. Truica, and E. P. Gelmann. 1998. Beta-catenin mutations in human prostate cancer. *Cancer Res.* **58:** 2520–2523.

297. Vogelstein, B., E. R. Fearon, S. E. Kern, S. R. Hamilton, A. C. Preisinger, Y. Nakamura, et al. 1989. Allelotype of colorectal carcinomas. *Science* **244:** 207–211.

298. Wang, F.-L., Y. Wang, W.-K. Wong, Y. Liu, F. J. Addivinola, P. Liang, et al. 1996. Two differentially expressed genes in normal human prostate tissue and in carcinoma. *Cancer Res.* **56:** 3634–3637.

299. Wang, S. I., R. Parsons, and M. Ittman. 1998. Homozygous deletion of the PTEN tumor suppressor gene in a subset of prostate adenocarcinomas. *Clin. Cancer Res.* **4:** 811–815.

300. Watanabe, M., H. Kakuichi, H. Kato, T. Shiraishi, R. Yatani, T. Sugimura, et al. 1996. APC gene mutations in human prostate cancer. *Jpn. J. Clin. Oncol.* **26:** 77–81.

301. Wechsler, D. S., C. A. Shelly, C. A. Petroff, and C. V. Dang. 1997. MXI1, a putative tumor suppressor gene, suppresses growth of human glioblastoma cells. *Cancer Res.* **57:** 4905–4912.

302. Weinberg, R. A. 1995. The retinoblastoma protein and cell cycle control. *Cell* **81:** 323–330.

303. Whang, Y. E., X. Wu, H. Suzuki, R. E. Reiter, C. Tran, R. L. Vessella, et al. 1998. Inactivation of the tumor suppressor PTEN/MMAC1 in advanced human prostate cancer through loss of expression. *Proc. Natl. Acad. Sci. USA* **95:** 5246–5250.

304. Williams, R. H., A. M. Stapleton, G. Yang, L. D. Truong, E. Rogers, T. L. Timme, et al. 1996. Reduced levels of transforming growth factor beta receptor type II in human prostate cancer: an immunohistochemical study. *Clin. Cancer Res.* **2:** 635–640.

305. Wright, K., P. J. Wilson, J. Kerr, K. Do, T. Hurst, S.-K. Khoo, et al. 1998. Frequent loss of heterozygosity and three critical regions on the short arm of chromosome 8 in ovarian adenocarcinoma. *Oncogene* **17:** 1185–1188.

306. Wu, X., K. Senechal, M. S. Neshat, Y. E. Whang, and C. L. Sawyers. 1998. The PTEN/MMAC1 tumor suppressor phosphatase functions as a negative regulator of the phosphoinositide 3-kinase/Akt pathway. *Proc. Natl. Acad. Sci. USA* **95:** 15,587–15,591.

307. Yang, C., C. Cirielli, M. C. Capogrossi, and A. Passaniti. 1995. Adenovirus-mediated wild-type p53 expression induces apoptosis and suppresses tumorigenesis of prostatic tumor cells. *Cancer Res.* **55:** 4210–4213.

308. Yang, G., A. M. F. Stapleton, T. M. Wheeler, L. D. Truong, T. L. Timme, et al. 1996. Clustered p53 immunostaining: a novel pattern associated with prostate cancer progression. *Clin. Cancer Res.* **2:** 399–401.

309. Yoshiura, K., Y. Kanai, A. Ochiai, Y. Shimoyama, T. Sugimura, and S. Hirohashi. 1995. Silencing of the E-cadherin invasion-suppressor gene by CpG methylation in human carcinomas. *Proc. Natl. Acad. Sci. USA* **92:** 7416–7419.

310. Zenklusen, J. C., I. Bieche, R. Lidereau, and C. J. Conti. 1994. (C-A)$_n$ microsatellite repeat D7S522 is the most commonly deleted region in human primary breast cancer. *Proc. Natl. Acad. Sci. USA* **91:** 12,155–12,158.

311. Zenklusen, J. C., J. C. Thompson, P. Troncoso, J. Kagan, and C. J. Conti. 1994. Loss of heterozygosity in human primary prostate carcinomas: a possible tumor suppressor gene at 7q31.1. *Cancer Res.* **54:** 6370–6373.

312. Zhang, M., D. Magit, and R. Sager. 1997. Expression of maspin in prostate cells is regulated by a positive Ets element and a negative hormonal responsive element site recognized by androgen receptor. *Proc. Natl. Acad. Sci. USA* **94:** 5673–5678.

313. Zhang, Y., Y. Xiong, and W. G. Yarbrough. 1998. ARF promotes MDM2 degradation and stabilizes p53: ARF-INK4a locus deletion impairs both the Rb and p53 tumor suppression pathways. *Cell* **92:** 725–734.

314. Zou, Z., A. Anisowicz, M. J. C. Hendrix, A. Thor, M. Neveu, S. Sheng, et al. 1994. Maspin, a serpin with tumor-suppressing activity in human mammary epithelial cells. *Science* **263:** 526–529.

6

Androgen Receptor Polymorphisms and Prostate Cancer Risk

Phillip G. Febbo, MD and Philip W. Kantoff, MD

1. INTRODUCTION

Prostate cancer (CaP) has long been recognized as an androgen dependent tumor. In the 1940s, Huggins and Hodges demonstrated that patients experienced decreased CaP related bone pain after orchiectomy *(38)*. Subsequent clinical trials have shown decreased CaP-specific mortality in patients treated with orchiectomy or its equivalent *(21)*. Such observations have engendered great interest in the role that androgens play in the development of the prostate and prostate cancer (CaP).

Androgen signaling is mediated through the androgen receptor (AR), a member of the superfamily of nuclear receptors that are ligand dependent transcription factors. Inactivating mutations within the AR gene cause androgen insensitivity syndromes (AIS), supporting its critical role in androgen signaling. Along with these rare but highly penetrant mutations, the AR has frequent variations in its gene sequence, knownas polymorphisms. Most of these variations have an imperceptible or modest affect on AR function and consequently less obvious phenotypes.

The AR gene does not act as a dominant, tumor-causing gene linked with familial CaP. Although a locus on the X chromosome is in linkage disequilibrium with familial CaP, the particular region is distant from the AR gene *(83)*. However, the central role of AR in the development and growth of the prostate suggests that more subtle variations in AR function may alter the risk for CaP over time.

Over the past decade, there has been increasing interest in the functional characterization of polymorphisms within the AR gene. The extreme phenotypic effects caused by pathologic elongation of the AR polyglutamine tract, (i.e., Kennedy's syndrome or spinal and bulbar muscular atrophy (SBMA), stimulated further functional analysis of AR variants in vitro and increased investigation of the effects of normal variation on androgen dependent phenotypes such as CaP.

This chapter reviews the major functional domains of the AR, briefly discusses the polymorphisms and mutations identified within each domain of the AR, and reviews the literature examining the association between genetic polymorphisms within the AR and CaP.

From: *Prostate Cancer: Biology, Genetics, and the New Therapeutics*
Edited by: L. W. K. Chung, W. B. Isaacs, and J. W. Simons © Humana Press Inc., Totowa, NJ

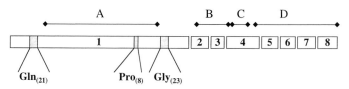

A = Transactivational domain (aa 141 - 338)
B = DNA Binding domain (aa 556 - 623)
C = Hinge Region/Nuclear Localization signal (aa 628 - 657)
D = Ligand Binding Domain (aa 666-918)

Fig. 1. Androgen receptor gene, exon structure (Exons 1–8), major functional domains (**A, B, C, D**), and location of polymorphic glutamine (Gln), proline (Pro), and Glycine (Gly) repeats *(11,13)*.

2. ANDROGEN RECEPTOR: GENE STRUCTURE, PROTEIN FUNCTION, AND LOCATION OF MUTATIONS AND POLYMORPHISMS

The discovery of uterine cells preferentially retaining radiolabeled estrogen over other steroid molecules *(41,70)* introduced the concept of intracellular steroid-specific binding proteins or receptors. Soon after, other binding proteins for steroid ligands were sought and found, including those for glucocorticoids, progesterones, and androgens *(4,5,20)*.

The *AR* was cloned in 1988 by several independent groups *(15,50,69)*. The cloning of the gene and identification of its open reading frame identified the AR as part of the nuclear receptor superfamily *(34)*. The AR is comprised of approx 918 amino acids, and shares the three major functional domains of this superfamily: 1) a transactivational domain; 2) a DNA binding domain; and 3) a ligand binding domain (Fig. 1) *(45,73)*. Chromosomal mapping experiments placed the AR on the X chromosome (Xq11-12) *(13,72)*.

AR acts as a transcription factor to control cell growth and differentiation. Unbound AR resides within both the cytoplasm and nucleus *(7,9,55,68,86)*. Androgens bind to the carboxy-terminus of the AR, most likely with a 1:1 stoichiometry (similar to the estrogen receptor *[26,63]*). After ligand binding, ARs dimerize and translocate to the nucleus *(7,55)*. The DNA binding domains of AR-dimers recognize specific sequences known as androgen response elements (AREs) adjacent to target genes *(37)*. Once bound to DNA, the AR initiates transcription through its association with the transcription initiation complex and a growing number of transcriptional coregulators *(30,31,84)*.

The DNA binding domain and the ligand binding domain of the *AR* are the most highly conserved regions across species and members of the nuclear receptor family *(34)*. The high level of conservation suggests a certain inflexibility regarding a fully functional AR tolerating amino acid substitutions within these regions. The multiple examples of AIS caused by single amino acid substitutions within the DNA or ligand binding domains support such a rigidity. The transactivational domain on the amino terminus is less conserved and less involved in single amino acid substitutions causing AIS. Within this region, three polymorphisms have been identified within the *AR*. The specific structure of these domains and the mutations or polymorphisms identified within each are discussed in Section 2.1.

2.1. DNA Binding Domain

The 66 amino acid DNA binding domain is rich in cystine, lysine, and arginine, and was predicted to associate with DNA based on its similarity to regions within known DNA binding proteins (e.g., TFIIIa) *(80,81)*. The amino acid sequence encodes two DNA binding "zinc fingers" *(29)*. The amino-terminus zinc finger is involved in DNA binding, and the second zinc finger is more likely involved in receptor dimerization and/or interaction with nuclear receptor coactivators. X-ray crystallography has confirmed and expanded the understanding of nuclear-receptor DNA binding *(62)*.

Within this region no common polymorphisms have been identified. This can probably be attributed to the profound effect that alterations may have on AR function, and thereby on resultant phenotype. Single amino acid substitutions within this region are sufficient to abrogate receptor function, and this region is commonly mutated in individuals with androgen insufficiency syndromes *(10)*. An amino acid substitution in this region (Arg608Lys) has been implicated in both androgen insufficiency and male breast cancer, suggesting that decreased AR function—although protective of CaP—may predispose individuals to breast cancer *(49)*. In all likelihood, any mutation resulting in androgen insensitivity would decrease sperm production and decrease the likelihood that such a mutation would be passed on contain enough frequency to be considered a polymorphism.

2.2. Carboxy Terminus (Ligand Binding Domain)

The carboxy terminus of each nuclear receptor contains the ligand binding domain, and has been implicated in many receptor functions including nuclear localization *(35)*, transcriptional regulation *(79)*, and receptor dimerization *(53)*. Like the DNA binding domain, mutations in the ligand binding domain frequently result in complete and partial AIS with a single amino acid substitution often sufficient to severely diminish AR function *(3,6,56)*. Again, even modest genetic variation within this region may result in decreased AR function and compromise propagation of any mutation.

Crystal structure analyses of nuclear-receptor family members (specifically the thyroid receptor) have revealed that the hydrophobic residues form a cavity, and in this region ligand binds *(77)*. A comparison between the X-ray structures of ligand-free Retinoid X receptor alpha, ligand bound Retinoid A receptor gamma and thyroid receptor alpha1 reveals a common tertiary structure called an antiparallel alpha-helical sandwich with 12 helices *(8)*. Based on the similarities in specific regions of the LBD, it was predicted that all members of the steroid receptor superfamily, including the AR, would have a similar structure *(82)*.

Although this region of the *AR* has been found to be frequently mutated in advanced CaP *(67)* and an androgen sensitive cell line (LNCaP) *(75)*, no common polymorphisms have been described. The single amino acid substitution seen in the LNCaP AR decreases ligand specificity and may confer a growth advantage upon these androgen dependent cells, since it renders the AR more promiscuous with regard to ligand specificity *(71,75)*. To date, no germline polymorphisms have been identified which correspond to this mutation.

2.3. Transactivational Domain (Amino terminus)

The amino terminus contains the transactivational domain of the AR required for transcriptional regulation *(43)*. Of the three major domains shared by nuclear receptors, this region exhibits the greatest variation between members of the superfamily *(34)*. Truncation mutations have demonstrated that this region, together with the DNA binding domain, is sufficient for transcriptional activation *(42,43)* and has constitutive activity approaching that of the intact, ligand bound receptor *(32)*. However, no single amino acid substitutions have been identified which result in AIS, although recently a frameshift mutation resulting in premature truncation (at 79 amino acids) and complete AIS has been identified *(85)*.

This segment of the AR contains mono-acidic repeats *(16)*. The AR is unique among the nuclear receptor superfamily with each of a polyglutamine tract, a polyglycine repeat, and a polyproline tract *(50)*. A similar polyglutamine repeat is also present in the glucocorticoid receptor and is found in the rat AR *(16)*.

The functional significance of the glutamine, glycine, and proline repeats remains an active area of investigation. Interestingly, these repeats—particularly the glutamine repeat—are highly polymorphic. Variations exist in the number of glutamine, glycine, and proline residues within and across racial/ethnic populations. The association between AR and these polymorphisms, AR function, and the risk of CaP is the focus of this chapter.

3. POLYMORPHISMS IDENTIFIED WITHIN THE AR

The *AR* was known to have regions of genetic variability, or polymorphisms, from its first identification *(50)*. The first polymorphism was a trinucleotide (CAG) repeat identified in the first exon resulting in a polyglutamine tract in the protein. This region was found to be highly polymorphic, but of uncertain significance *(64)*. Other polymorphisms were identified within the first exon, and subsequent investigations focused on the description of these polymorphisms and their effect on AR function and androgen-dependent phenotypes such as secondary sexual characteristics and CaP.

3.1. The CAG Repeat Polymorphism

The CAG repeat exists within exon 1 and begins at amino acid number 58 *(47)*. There are variable numbers of CAG repeats ranging from 13 to 32 in normal populations *(64)*. The CAG repeat is preserved across species and is found in the amino terminus of the rat and mouse, suggesting some functional importance *(14,17)*.

Pathologic elongation of the CAG repeat in the *AR* (>42 repeats) causes Kennedy's syndrome *(47)*. Kennedy's disease, or spinal and bulbar muscular atrophy (SBMA), was known to be X-linked with affected individuals exhibiting adult onset, progressive muscle weakness and atrophy and signs of androgen insensitivity *(2)*. A comparison of the *AR* sequence between affected and unaffected individuals demonstrated absolute association with an expanded CAG repeat and the disease (lod score 13.2 at 0 centimorgans) *(47)*. Progressive lengthening of CAG repeats above the threshold length causing SBMA, in a similar way as the CAG repeat expansions associated with Huntington's disease *(1)*, myotonic dystrophy *(11)*, and fragile X syndrome *(76)*, results in increasing severity of the muscular atrophy *(22)*.

The pathogenesis behind elongation of the CAG repeat remains unclear. AR with an expanded polyglutamine tract have normal ligand binding kinetics and intracellular localization compared to wild-type AR *(12)*. In vitro assays have demonstrated decreased transcriptional transactivation by AR with CAG repeat expansion, which probably accounts for the partial androgen insufficiency observed in individuals with SBMA *(52)*. However, this alone is not sufficient to account for the neurodegenerative process involved in SBMA, and some gain is likely to result in function of the AR, with pathologic elongation of the CAG repeat.

Recent data suggests that involvement of cellular caspases may contribute to the neurodegenerative phenotype of diseases caused by pathologic expansion of CAG repeats *(24)*. In the AR, cleavage at Asp146 by caspase-3, with release of the polyglutamine tract, has recently been shown to be necessary for AR-induced apoptosis and the formation of perinuclear aggregates in CAG-expanded AR (the pathologic finding in SBMA) *(25)*. In addition to this in vitro observation, the Huntington protein with an expanded CAG repeat was associated with caspase I activation in the CNS of affected individuals and mice *(54)*. Treatment of the transgenic mouse model for Huntington's disease with a dominant-negative Caspase I construct increased survival and decreased severity of the pathologic lesions associated with this disease.

While SBMA represents a phenotype caused by abnormal lengthening of the *AR* CAG repeat and a possible gain of function, three clinical observations suggest more subtle androgen-insufficient phenotypes are associated with normal variation of the CAG repeat. The first is the previously noted androgen insufficiency observed in individuals with SBMA who can exhibit gynecomastia and reduced fertility *(2)*. The second is an association between increased hirsutism (as measured by a Ferriman Gallwey score) and decreased CAG repeat length in a group of Hispanic women with normal testosterone levels seen at an infertility clinic ($p = 0.014$) *(48)*. Finally, sperm production in exquisitely androgen-sensitive men with CAG lengths greater than 28 repeats had a fourfold increase (95% CI 3.2–4.9) in their risk for abnormal sperm production *(74)*.

These observations and the severe phenotype of SBMA prompted in vitro functional analyses of *AR* with different CAG repeat lengths. Three studies have suggested that longer CAG repeat lengths were associated with decreased AR transactivation *(14,44,52)*. In the first two reports, *AR* constructs with 40 CAG repeats or greater were less able to transactivate a reporter gene than wild-type *AR (14,52)*. Subsequent reports have focused on the effect of CAG repeat-length variation within a normal range, and have demonstrated that such variation (e.g., 12 CAG repeats vs 20 CAG repeats) also had similar, although smaller, effects on AR transactivation or the phenotype of other AR mutations *(44,46,74)*. Thus, a functional consequence of this polymorphism has been well documented in vivo with Kennedy's disease and clinical observations suggesting partial androgen insufficiency as well as in vitro with decreased AR transactivational ability with increasing CAG length.

Although pathologic elongation of the CAG repeat is a rare event, the locus is highly variable within a normal range of CAG repeats *(64)*. Such variation is found within racial/ethnic populations, where significant differences exist. African-American individuals have, on average, a significantly shorter number of CAG repeats than Caucasian individuals, who in turn have a shorter average number of repeats than Asian

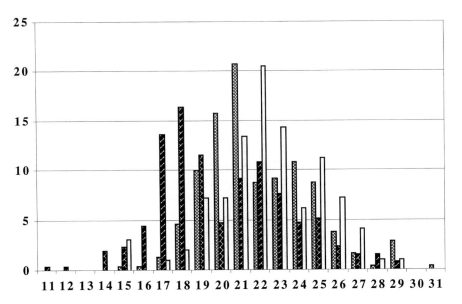

Fig. 2. AR CAG repeat polymorphism allele frequencies in three populations. Three racial/ethnic populations were genotyped for the length of the CAG repeat *(69)*.

individuals (Fig. 2) *(23)*. As a specific example from this study, 39.7 % of those partici-pants identified as African-American had CAG lengths <19 compared with 6.7%, 9.4%, and 6.2% of Caucasian, Mexican American, and Asian participants, respectively. This difference between African-American and Caucasian men was confirmed by a smaller study of men revealing a mean CAG length of 19.0 +/–3 ($n = 65$) vs 21.0 +/–3 ($n = 130$), respectively *(60)*.

The observed ethnic/racial differences in mean CAG length within the *AR* had a trend that paralleled racial/ethnic differences in CaP frequency. It was suggested that such genetic variation of the CAG polymorphism may contribute to the observed racial difference *(18)*. Because of this epidemiological observation and the growing in vitro data suggesting a modulatory affect of the CAG repeat on AR function, many independent groups have investigated the association between CAG length and risk of CaP in case-control series. Three major studies in this area are presented in Table 1 *(33,39,40,66)*.

This first report of a possible association between CAG and risk of CaP came from a small case-control study of men from Los Angeles county, California *(40)*. Within the Caucasian participants (57 cases, 39 controls), there was a slight excess of CaP in those men with CAG repeat length greater than 22 (OR = 1.25) *(40)*. The number of controls was subsequently expanded to 169 individuals (non-Hispanic Caucasian) and an Odds Ratio of 2.0 (95% CI 1.07–3.75) for men with a CAG repeat length of less than 20 compared to those in whom CAG >20 was observed *(39)*. This later study also looked a the subpopulation of men with advanced disease and found an increased OR of 2.36 (95% CI 1.02–5.49) for men with CAG length less than 20, although the num-bers within this subgroup were small (cases $n = 12$, controls $n = 14$) and the CI came very close to 1.00 (1.02) *(39)*.

Two larger studies subsequently established a link between CAG length and CaP risk. The largest study to date is a nested case-control study involving men enrolled in

Table 1
Summary of CAG Repeat and CaP Association Studies[a]

Author	*n* cases/ controls	CAG range	Analysis	OR(CI) all CaP	OR(CI) local low-grade	OR(CI) advanced/ high-grade
Ingles et al., (1997)	57/169	NA	CAG < 20 vs CAG ≥ 20	2.10[b] (1.11–3.99)	1.74 (0.78–3.87) *n* = 31	2.36[b] (1.02–5.49) *n* = 26
Giovannucci et al., (1997)	587/588	6–39	CAG$_x$ vs CAG$_{x-6}$[c]	1.28[b] (1.01–2.50)	1.02 (0.77–1.37) *n* = 309	1.75[b] (1.23–2.50) *n* = 269
Stanford et al., (1997)	301/277	11–32	CAG <22 vs CAG ≥ 222	1.23 (0.88–1.73)	1.26 (0.84–1.84) *n* = 152	1.20 (0.79–1.84) *n* = 129

[a]Three major case-control analyses of the association between AR CAG repeat polymorphism length and risk of CaP. (*n* = number, NA = not available, OR = odds ratio, CI = 95% confidence interval, local/ low-grade = clinical stage A or B, Gleason score ≤ 6, advanced/high-grade = clinical stage C or D, Gleason score ≥ 7).

[b]$p < 0.05$.

[c]OR calculated for individuals with 6 fewer CAG repeats compared to a reference individual.

the Physician's Health Study who had a confirmed diagnosis of CaP and matched controls *(33)*. In this study, shorter CAG length was associated with risk of higher-grade and higher-stage CaP (Table 2). For analysis, men were divided into quartiles of CAG length. When the lowest quartile was compared to the highest, men in the lowest quartile of CAG length had a 64% increase in their risk of aggressive CaP (defined as Gleason score ≥ 7 and/or Stage C or D).

Remarkably, CaP-specific mortality was associated with shorter CAG length within this study. In this analysis, the risk of CaP, aggressive CaP, and fatal CaP was compared between men whose CAG length differed by 6 repeats *(33)*. Compared to a reference individual (a man with 21 CAG repeats), the odds ratio for a man with six fewer CAG repeats (15) to die of CaP was 2.08 (95% CI 1.05-4.00) or double.

Another larger study also suggested that CAG length was associated with an increased risk of CaP, but the associations did not reach statistical significance *(66)*. This study included 301 cases and 277 controls, and suggested that a 3% decrement in the risk of CaP was associated with each additional CAG repeat *(66)*. This observation, although not statistically significant, was observed for both aggressive CaP and low-grade, less aggressive CaP.

All studies suggesting an association between CAG repeat length and CaP were performed in the United States. A recent case-control study examining a French and German cohort (105 controls, 132 sporadic CaP, and 131 members from families with a history of CaP (85 affected, 46 unaffected) found no association between CAG length and risk of CaP (OR 1.007, 95% CI 0.97 – 1.1, $p = 0.87$), or Gleason Score *(19)*. Such a negative finding may suggest that significant differences exist between specific populations with regard to the importance of the CAG repeat and CaP pathogenesis.

Table 2
Risk of CaP Associated with CAG Repeat Polymorphism Length in the AR[a]

Prostate cancer	Cases	Odds Ratio	95% CI	p value
Total	587	1.28	1.01–1.61	0.04
High-grade/stage	269	1.64	1.22–2.22	0.001
Low-grade/stage	309	1.02	0.77–1.37	0.86
High-grade	210	1.59	1.14–2.22	0.007
Advanced-stage	180	1.75	1.23–2.50	0.002
Metastatic (distant)	56	2.44	1.32–4.55	0.004
Fatal	43	2.08	1.05–4.00	0.04

[a]Participants in the Physician's Health Study diagnosed with CaP and matched controls were genotyped for CAG repeat length and the odds ratio for all CaP and CaP subgroups was derived for a CAG repeat decrement of 6 repeats. High-grade was defined as poorly differentiated and/or Gleason ≥ 7, High-stage and Advanced stage were defined as CaP of clinical stage C or D *(74)*.

The identification of an association between CAG length and risk of CaP resulted in subsequent investigation of the use of CAG length as a diagnostic marker. Studies of the contribution of CAG length to prediction of CaP surgical grade, systemic involvement, or disease specific mortality have been largely negative. One report suggested an 83% occurrence of lymph node positive disease for a small ($n = 59$) cohort of men with clinical prostate cancer and CAG length of 16 or 17, despite a lack of clinical evidence suggesting metastatic spread *(36)*.

A larger cohort of men ($n = 472$) who had undergone a radical prostatectomy at the Mayo Clinic was genotyped for CAG length, and no association was detected between CAG length and surgical stage, maximum Gleason score, or CaP recurrence (as determined by PSA failure or positive bone scan and/or CT scan) *(28)*. The mode CAG length within this population of 472 men was 21, similar to other Caucasian cohorts, and means according to pathological stage were as follows: A ($n = 80$) 21.5 ± 3.3, B (168) 21.9 ± 3.0, C (185) 21.6 ± 3.2, and D1 (39) 21.9 ± 2.0. There was no association between CAG length and Gleason grade ($p = 0.53$), no trend for shorter repeat length with increasing clinical stage ($p = 0.63$), and no significant correlation between pathological stage and CAG length was observed, although a trend for individuals with pathological stage C and D to have a higher proportion of CAG repeats <20 approached statistical significance ($p = 0.084$) *(28)*. The negative results of this study may have resulted from an inherent bias of a surgical cohort favoring low-stage, low-grade tumors for which the case-control studies have demonstrated a weaker association (null in Giovannucci et al.) as compared with high-grade, high-stage CaP. However, in a study of sequential patients with CaP at the Dana Farber Cancer Institute, no significant association between clinical stage, Gleason grade, and PSA was observed *(27)*.

Several groups have expanded our understanding of the importance of the CAG repeat within the AR in CaP by investigating alterations associated with CaP development or progression. In an initial study, 40 human CaP specimens were genotyped for CAG length and compared to genomic DNA *(61)*. Of the 40 tumors, only one contained a population of cells with a contracted CAG repeat from the germline length of 24 to a shorter length of 18 CAG repeats. CAG repeat alterations were also found in three out of 36 CaP tumors from Japanese men *(78)*. However, these differences were contractions or expansions of only a single CAG repeat, and two occurred in individuals with significant microsatellite instability, casting doubt on the importance of the observation in CaP development or progression. A final study found no significant alteration in CAG length in 18 hormone refractory CaP specimens or nine local CaP tumors *(59)*. Thus, given the infrequency of CAG repeat-length alterations in CaP, CAG contraction is probably not important in the pathogenesis of CaP.

Further questions regarding the CAG repeat in the AR include the association of this polymorphisms with CaP in racial/ethnic groups other than Caucasian (African-American and Asian), the effect of this polymorphism on protein structure and function, and the potential to use the CAG polymorphism in the setting of a model incorporating multiple polymorphisms along the androgen pathway in CaP. By itself, the magnitude of the biologic effect of variation in the CAG repeat does not appear large enough to be used as a marker of disease behavior for an individual. However, the risk attributable to variations of CAG length on the population is substantial and, in conjunction with other polymorphisms, may eventually play a role in a model predicting disease behavior *(58)*.

3.2. GGN Polymorphism

A second trinucleotide polymorphism which has been identified within exon 1 encodes a polyglycine tract of variable length *(65)*. Although referred to as a GGN polymorphism, the actual sequence is comprised of $(GGT)_{3}GGG(GGT)_{2}(GGC)_{4-25}$ with occasional variation of the internal $(GGT)2$ tract *(51)*. The most common number of GGN repeats in a Caucasian population is 23 (53.5%) and 24 (34%), and the maximum observed range is 10–31 *(51,57)*. Unlike the CAG repeat polymorphism, there is known syndrome attributed to pathologic elongation of this locus. The specific effects of this polymorphism on AR function have not yet been described, and this repeat is not conserved across species. However, given its variability, the association of GGN with CaP has been investigated *(57)*.

The CaP cohort from the Physician's Health Study was used to identify an association between the GGN polymorphism and CaP risk. In this preliminary study, increased distance from the mean number of GGN repeats (i.e., 23) was associated with a decreased risk of CaP *(57)*. The specific association found was with each repeat (either additional repeats or missing repeats) away from the mean, and there was an 8% decrement in risk for CaP ($p = 0.04$). An association between GGN repeat length and CaP risk was not supported in a French and German group, although the number of affected individuals was smaller, introducing an increased potential for a beta error *(19)*.

If the association between increased CaP risk and GGN length of 23 is valid, it may be suggested that AR transactivation is optimal, with 23 GGN repeats. Variation away from 23 repeats could potentially result in protein conformations that are less active and subsequently result in decreased androgen-stimulated transcription. Alternative explanations include decreased mRNA stability, decreased translation efficiency, or decreased protein stability, to name a few. As there are no functional studies addressing this question to date, any explanation remains speculative.

The GGN has also been tested for its association with CaP together with the CAG repeat polymorphism. There is no correlation between GGN allele length and the number of CAG repeats *(51)*. When investigated together, however, there is an increase in the strength of association between the two polymorphisms and CaP. The first published study of a combined effect on CaP reported that individuals with less than 16 CAG repeats and the mean number of GGN repeats (22 in that study) were at the highest risk for CaP *(66)*. Analysis of the Physician's Health Study CaP cohort confirms a trend toward both alleles contributing to CaP risk, with individuals showing the lowest number of CAG repeats (bottom quartile) and the mean number of GGN repeats (i.e., 23) having the highest risk of CaP (E. Giovannucci, unpublished results).

The associations between GGN repeat length and CaP risk remain few and without functional explanation. The preliminary studies so far justify further characterization of the functional effects of the GGN on the AR protein.

3.3. Other Polymorphisms

There are also short poly-proline tracts within the first exon of the AR, although these appear to be less variable and no associative study has yet addressed their role in the function of the AR or in CaP risk.

4. CONCLUSIONS AND FUTURE DIRECTIONS

The AR plays a central role in prostate development and probably CaP. The importance of the AR combined with the lifetime exposure to ligand probably account for the observed associations between modest variations in protein function and androgen dependent phenotypes.

The in vitro work presented here demonstrates a reproducible, yet modest, effect on AR function with progressive lengthening of the CAG repeat. The role of the GGN polymorphism remains unclear. Such variability of the AR is probably insufficient to have a major role in the progression of CaP, as indicated by the lack of somatic changes of the CAG repeat. However, even a very small variation of AR function over a lifetime—including very early developmental events—may alter the propensity for the prostate to undergo neoplastic transformation in the presence of androgens.

The modest effect for an individual can also translate into a significant effect for a population. It remains to be seen how the CAG repeat within the AR affects CaP incidence and behavior within African-American men who have increased rates of CaP and shorter CAG repeat lengths. The CAG repeat probably accounts for some of the racial/ethnic differences in CaP incidence and behavior, yet this link remains untested.

The examination of individual polymorphisms and their association with a phenotype such as CaP is an important first step, but will underestimate their potential influence. The AR is one part of a pathway including polypeptide regulatory proteins, membrane-bound receptors, and metabolic enzymes that comprise the androgen signaling pathway. Genetic variation within each component potentially influences the development of the prostate and CaP. Many groups are parsing out the independent effects of polymorphisms within each component of the androgen signaling pathway, and eventually we will be able to use combinatorial approaches to associate patterns of polymorphisms with CaP behavior. Thus, with a better understanding of the complex pattern of polymorphisms within the androgen signaling pathway, we hope to provide a more accurate prediction of the incidence and behavior of CaP for an individual.

With just under 200,000 men diagnosed with CaP each year, such predictive tools for CaP behavior are vital.

REFERENCES

1. Arbizu, T. 1983. A family with adult spinal and bulbar muscular atrophy, X-linked inheritance and associated testicular failure. *J. Neurol. Sci.* **59**: 371–382.

2. Batch, J. A., D. M. Williams, H. R. Davies, B. D. Brown, B. A. Evans, I. A. Hughes, et al. 1992. Androgen receptor gene mutations identified by SSCP in fourteen subjects with androgen insensitivity syndrome. *Hum. Mol. Genet.* **1**: 497–503.

3. Bauulieu, E. E., I. Jung, J. Blondea, and P. Robel. 1971. Androgen receptors in rat ventral prostate. *Adv. Biosci.* **7**: 179–191.

4. Baxter, J. and G. Tomkins. 1971. Specific cytoplasmic glucocorticoid hormone receptors in hepatoma tissue culture cells. *Proc. Natl. Acad. Sci. USA* **68**: 932–937.

5. Belsham, D. D., F. Pereira, C. R. Greenberg, S. Liao, and K. Wrogemann. 1995. Leu-676-Pro mutation of the androgen receptor causes complete androgen insensitivity syndrome in a large Hutterite kindred. *Hum. Mutat.* **5**: 28–33.

6. Blondeau, J. P., E. E. Baulieu, and P. Robel. 1982. Androgen-dependent regulation of androgen nuclear receptor in the rat ventral prostate. *Endocrinology* **110**: 1926–1932.

7. Bourguet, W., M. Ruff, P. Chambon, H. Gronemeyer, and D. Moras. 1995. Crystal structure of the ligand binding domain of the human nuclear receptor RXR-alpha. *Nature* **375**: 377–382.

8. Brinkmann, A. O., L. M. Lindh, D. I. Breedveld, E. Mulder, and H. J. van Der Molen. 1983. Cyproterone acetate prevents translocation of the androgen receptor in the rat prostate. *Mol. Cell Endocrinol.* **32**: 117–129.

9. Brinkmann, A. O. and J. Trapman. 1992. Androgen receptor mutants that affect normal growth and development. *Cancer Surv.* **14**: 95–111.

10. Brook, J. D., M. E. McCurrach, H. G. Harley, A. J. Buckler, D. Church, H. Aburatani, et al. 1992. Molecular basis of myotonic dystrophy: expansion of a trinucleotide (CTG) repeat at the 3′ end of a transcript encoding a protein kinase family member (published erratum appears in *Cell* 1992 Apr 17;69(2):385). *Cell* **68**: 799–808.

11. Brooks, B. P., H. L. Paulson, D. E. Merry, E. F. Salazar-Grueso, A. O. Brinkmann, E. M. Wilson, et al. 1997. Characterization of an expanded glutamine repeat androgen receptor in a neuronal cell culture system. *Neurobiol. Dis.* **3**: 313–323.

12. Brown, C. J., S. J. Goss, D. B. Lubahn, D. R. Joseph, E. M. Wilson, F. S. French, et al. 1989. Androgen receptor locus on the human X chromosome: regional localization to Xq11-12 and description of a DNA polymorphism. *Am. J. Hum. Genet.* **44**: 264–269.

13. Chamberlain, N. L., E. D. Driver, and R. L. Miesfeld. 1994. The length and location of CAG trinucleotide repeats in the androgen receptor N-terminal domain affect transactivation function. *Nucleic Acids Res.* **22**: 3181–3186.

14. Chang, C., G. Chodak, E. Sarac, H. Takeda, and S. Liao. 1989. Prostate androgen receptor: immunohistological localization and mRNA characterization. *J. Steroid Biochem.* **34**: 311–313.

15. Chang, C., J. Kokontis, and S. Liao. 1988. Structural analysis of complementary DNA and amino acid sequences of human and rat androgen receptors. *Proc. Natl. Acad. Sci. USA* **85**: 7211–7215.

16. Choong, C. S., J. A. Kemppainen, and E. M. Wilson. 1998. Evolution of the primate androgen receptor: a structural basis for disease. *J. Mol. Evol.* **47**: 334–342.

17. Coetzee, G. A. and R. K. Ross. 1994. Re: Prostate cancer and the androgen receptor (letter). *J. Natl. Cancer Inst.* **86**: 872,873.

18. Correa-Cerro, L., G. Wohr, J. Haussler, P. Berthon, E. Drelon, P. Mangin, et al. 1999. (CAG)nCAA and GGN repeats in the human androgen receptor gene are not associated with prostate cancer in a French-German population. *Eur. J. Hum. Genet.* **7:** 357–362.

19. Corvol, P., R. Falk, M. Freifeld, and C. Bardin. 1972. In vitro studies of progesterone binding protein in guinea pig uterus. *Endocrinology* **90:** 1464–1469.

20. Crawford, E., M. Eisenberger, D. McLeod, J. Spaulding, R. Benson, F. Orr, et al. 1989. A controlled trial of leuprolide with and without flutamide in prostatic carcinoma. *N. Engl. J. Med.* **321:** 419–424.

21. Doyu, M., G. Sobue, E. Mukai, T. Kachi, T. Yasuda, T. Mitsuma, et al. 1992. Severity of X-linked recessive bulbospinal neuronopathy correlates with size of the tandem CAG repeat in androgen receptor gene. *Ann. Neurol.* **32:** 707–710.

22. Edwards, A., H. A. Hammond, L. Jin, C. T. Caskey, and R. Chakraborty. 1992. Genetic variation at five trimeric and tetrameric tandem repeat loci in four human population groups. *Genomics* **12:** 241–253.

23. Ellerby, L. M., R. L. Andrusiak, C. L. Wellington, A. S. Hackam, S. S. Propp, J. D. Wood, et al. 1999. Cleavage of atrophin-1 at caspase site aspartic acid 109 modulates cytotoxicity. *J. Biol. Chem.* **274:** 8730–8736.

24. Ellerby, L. M., A. S. Hackam, S. S. Propp, H. M. Ellerby, S. Rabizadeh, N. R. Cashman, et al. 1999. Kennedy's disease: caspase cleavage of the androgen receptor is a crucial event in cytotoxicity. *J. Neurochem.* **72:** 185–195.

25. Estes, P., E. Suba, J. Lawler-Heavner, D. Elashry-Stowers, L. Wie, D. Toft, et al. 1987. Immunologic analysis of human breast cancer progesterone receptors. 1. Immunoaffinity purification of transformed receptors and production of monoclonal antibodies. *Biochemistry* **26:** 6250–6262.

26. Febbo, P., J. Manola, K. Krithivas, D. Casey, D. Farmer, and P. Kantoff. 1998. The CAG repeat in the human androgen receptor (hAR) gene and its association with clinical and pathological parameters of prostate cancer (CaP): a retrospective, single institution study (abstract). Proceedings AACR Special Conference on "New Research Approaches in the Prevention and Cure of Prostate Cancer."

27. Febbo, P., S. Ramakumar, K. Krithivas, D. Farmer, A. Chan, C. Wilcox, et al. 1998. The relationship between the cag repeat polymorphism in the human androgen receptor (ar) gene and pathologic stage (ps) in patients undergoing radical prostatectomy (rp) for prostate cancer (cap). ASCO Annual Meeting Proceedings, 17.

28. Freedman, L., B. Luisi, Z. Korszun, R. Basavapp, P. Sigler, and K. Yamamoto. 1988. The function and structure of the metal coordination sites within the glucocorticoid receptor DNA binding domain. *Nature* **334:** 543–546.

29. Froesch, B. A., S. Takayama, and J. C. Reed. 1998. BAG-1L protein enhances androgen receptor function. *J. Biol. Chem.* **273:** 11,660–11,666.

30. Fronsdal, K., N. Engedal, T. Slagsvold, and F. Saatcioglu. 1998. CREB binding protein is a coactivator for the androgen receptor and mediates cross-talk with AP-1. *J. Biol. Chem.* **273:** 31,853–31,859.

31. Gao, T., M. Marcelli, and M. J. McPhaul. 1996. Transcriptional activation and transient expression of the human androgen receptor. *J. Steroid Biochem. Mol. Biol.* **59:** 9–20.

32. Giovannucci, E., M. J. Stampfer, K. Krithivas, M. Brown, D. Dahl, A. Brufsky, et al. 1997. The CAG repeat within the androgen receptor gene and its relationship to prostate cancer (published erratum appears in *Proc. Natl. Acad. Sci. USA* 1997 Jul 22;94(15):8272). *Proc. Natl. Acad. Sci. USA* **94:** 3320–3323.

33. Green, S. and P. Chambon. 1986. A superfamily of potentially oncogenic hormone receptors. *Nature* **324:** 615–617.

34. Guiochon-Mantel, A., H. Loosfelt, P. Lescop, S. Sar, M. Atger, M. Perrot-Applant, et al. 1989. Mechanisms of nuclear localization of the progesterone receptor: evidence for interaction between monomers. *Cell* **57:** 1147–1154.

35. Hakimi, J. M., M. P. Schoenberg, R. H. Rondinelli, S. Piantadosi, and E. R. Barrack. 1997. Androgen receptor variants with short glutamine or glycine repeats may identify unique subpopulations of men with prostate cancer. *Clin. Cancer Res.* **3:** 1599–1608.

36. Ham, J., A. Thompson, M. Needham, P. Webb, and M. Parker. 1988. Characterization of reponse elements for androgens, glucocorticoids and progestins in mouse mammary tumor virus. *Nucl. Acids Res.* **16:** 5263–5276.

37. Huggins, C., R. Stevens, and C. Hodges. 1941. Studies in prostate cancer II, the effects of castration on advanced carcinoma of the prostate gland. *Arch. Surg.* **43:** 209.

38. Huntington's Disease Collaborative Research Group. 1993. A novel gene containing a trinucleotide repeat that is expanded and unstable on Huntington's disease chromosomes. *Cell* **72:** 971–983.

39. Ingles, S. A., R. K. Ross, M. C. Yu, R. A. Irvine, G. La Pera, R. W. Haile, et al. 1997. Association of prostate cancer risk with genetic polymorphisms in vitamin D receptor and androgen receptor (see comments). *J. Natl. Cancer Inst.* **89:** 166–170.

40. Irvine, R. A., M. C. Yu, R. K. Ross, and G. A. Coetzee. 1995. The CAG and GGC microsatellites of the androgen receptor gene are in linkage disequilibrium in men with prostate cancer. *Cancer Res.* **55:** 1937–1940.

41. Jensen, E., T. Sujuki, T. Kawashima, W. Stumpf, P. Jungblut, and E. DeSombre. 1968. A two-step mechanism for the interaction of estradiol with rat uterus. *Proc. Natl. Acad. Sci. USA* **59:** 632–638.

42. Jenster, G., H. A. van der Korput, C. van Vroonhoven, T. H. van der Kwast, J. Trapman, and O. Brinkmann. 1991. Domains of the human androgen receptor involved in steroid binding, transcriptional activation, and subcellular localization. *Mol. Endocrinol.* **5:** 1396–1404.

43. Jenster, G., H. A. van der Korput, J. Trapman, and A. O. Brinkmann. 1992. Functional domains of the human androgen receptor. *J. Steroid Biochem. Mol. Biol.* **41:** 671–675.

44. Kazemi-Esfarjani, P., M. A. Trifiro, and L. Pinsky. 1995. Evidence for a repressive function of the long polyglutamine tract in the human androgen receptor: possible pathogenetic relevance for the (CAG)n-expanded neuronopathies. *Human Molecular Genetics* **4:** 523–527.

45. Keller, E., W. Ershler, and C. Chang. 1996. The androgen receptor: a mediator of diverse responses. *Frontiers in Bioscience* **1:** d59–71.

46. Knoke, I., A. Allera, and P. Wieacker. 1999. Significance of the CAG repeat length in the androgen receptor gene (AR) for the transactivation function of an M780I mutant AR. *Hum. Genet.* **104:** 257–261.

47. LaSpada, A. R., E. M. Wilson, D. B. Lubahn, A. Harding and K. H. Fishbeck. 1991. Androgen receptor gene mutations in x-linked spinal and bulbar muscular atrophy. *Nature* **352:** 77–79.

48. Legro, R. S., B. Shahbahrami, R. A. Lobo, and B. W. Kovacs. 1994. Size polymorphisms of the androgen receptor among female Hispanics and correlation with androgenic characteristics. *Obstet. Gynecol.* **83:** 701–706.

49. Lobaccaro, J. M., et al. 1993. Androgen receptor gene mutation in male breast cancer. *Hum. Mol. Genet.* **2:** 1799–1802.

50. Lubahn, D. B., D. R. Joseph, M. Sar, J. Tan, H. N. Higgs, R. E. Larson, et al. 1988. The human androgen receptor: complementary deoxyribonucleic acid cloning, sequence analysis and gene expression in prostate. *Mol. Endocrinology* **2(12):** 1265–1271.

51. Lumbroso, R., L. K. Beitel, D. M. Vasiliou, M. A. Trifiro, and L. Pinsky. 1997. Codon-usage variants in the polymorphic (GGN)n trinucleotide repeat of the human androgen receptor gene. *Hum. Genet.* **101:** 43–46.

52. Mhatre, A., M. Trifiro, M. Kaufman, P. Kazemi-Esfarjani, D. Figlewicz, G. Rouleau, et al. 1993. Reduced transcriptional regulatory competence of the androgen receptor in X-linked spinal and bulbar muscular atrophy. *Nat. Genet.* **5:** 184–188.

53. O'Malley, B. 1990. The steroid receptor superfamily: more excitement predicted for the future. *Mol. Endocrinol.* **4:** 363–369.

54. Ona, V. O., M. Li, J. P. Vonsattel, L. J. Andrews, S. Q. Khan, W. M. Chung, et al. 1999. Inhibition of caspase-1 slows disease progression in a mouse model of Huntington's disease (see comments). *Nature* **399:** 263–267.

55. Paris, F., G. F. Weinbauer, V. Blum, and E. Nieschlag. 1994. The effect of androgens and antiandrogens on the immunohistochemical localization of the androgen receptor in accessory reproductive organs of male rats. *J. Steroid Biochem. Mol. Biol.* **48:** 129–137.

56. Peters, I., W. Weidemann, G. Romalo, D. Knorr, H. U. Schweikert, and K. D. Spindler. 1999. An androgen receptor mutation in the direct vicinity of the proposed C-terminal alpha-helix of the ligand binding domain containing the AF-2 transcriptional activating function core is associated with complete androgen insensitivity. *Mol. Cell Endocrinol.* **148:** 47–53.

57. Platz, E. A., E. Giovanucci, D. M. Dahl, K. Krithivas, C. H. Hennekens, M. Brown, et al. 1998. The androgen receptor gene GGN microsatellite and prostate cancer risk. *Cancer Epidemiol. Biomark. Prev.* **7:** 379–384.

58. Ross, R., M. Pike, G. Coetzee, J. Reichardt, M. Yu, H. Feigleson, et al. 1998. Androgen metabolism and prostate cancer: establishing a model of genetic susceptibility. *Cancer Res.* **58:** 4497–4504.

59. Ruizeveld de Winter, J. A., P. J. Janssen, H. M. Sleddens, M. C. Verleun-Mooijman, J. Trapman, A. O. Brinkmann, et al. 1994. Androgen receptor status in localized and locally progressive hormone refractory human prostate cancer. *Am. J. Pathol.* **144:** 735–746.

60. Sartor, O., Q. Zheng, and J. A. Eastham. 1999. Androgen receptor gene CAG repeat length varies in a race-specific fashion in men without prostate cancer. *Urology* **53:** 378–380.

61. Schoenberg, M. P., J. M. Hakimi, S. Wang, G. S. Bova, J. I. Epstein, K. H. Fischbeck, et al. 1994. Microsatellite mutation (CAG24→18) in the androgen receptor gene in human prostate cancer. *Biochem. Biophys. Res. Commun.* **198:** 74–80.

62. Schwabe, J. W., L. Chapman, J. T. Finch, and D. Rhodes. 1993. The crystal structure of the estrogen receptor DNA binding domain bound to DNA: how receptors discriminate between their response elements. *Cell* **75:** 567–578.

63. Seielstad, D., K. Carlson, J. Katzenellenbogen, P. Kushner, and G. Greene. 1995. Molecular characterization by mass spectrometry of the human estrogen receptor ligand binding domain expressed in Escherichia coli. *Mol. Endo.* **9:** 647–658.

64. Sleddens, H. F., B. A. Oostra, A. O. Brinkmann, and J. Trapman. 1992. Trinucleotide repeat polymorphism in the androgen receptor gene (AR). *Nucleic Acids Res.* **20:** 1427.

65. Sleddens, H. F., B. A. Oostra, A. O. Brinkmann, and J. Trapman. 1993. Trinucleotide (GGN) repeat polymorphism in the human androgen receptor (AR) gene. *Hum. Mol. Genet.* **2:** 493.

66. Stanford, J. L., J. J. Just, M. Gibbs, K. G. Wicklund, C. L. Neal, B. A. Blumenstein, et al. 1997. Polymorphic repeats in the androgen receptor gene: molecular markers of prostate cancer risk. *Cancer Res.* **57:** 1194–1198.

67. Taplin, M. E., G. J. Bubley, T. D. Shuster, M. E. Frantz, A. E. Spooner, G. K. Ogata, et al. 1995. Mutation of the androgen-receptor gene in metastatic androgen-independent prostate cancer (see comments). *N. Engl. J. Med.* **332:** 1393–1398.

68. Thompson, T. C. and L. W. Chung. 1984. Extraction of nuclear androgen receptors by sodium molybdate from normal rat prostates and prostatic tumors. *Cancer Res.* **44:** 1019–1026.

69. Tilley, W. D., M. Marcelli, J. D. Wilson, and M. J. McPhaul. 1989. Characterization and expression of a xDNA encoding the human androgen receptor. *Proc. Natl. Acad. Sci. USA* **86:** 327–331.

70. Toft, D. and J. Gorsky. 1966. A receptor molecule for estrogens: isolation from the rat uterus and preliminary characterization. *Proc. Natl. Acad. Sci. USA* **5:** 1574–1581.

71. Trapman, J. and A. O. Brinkmann. 1996. The androgen receptor in prostate cancer. *Pathol. Res. Pract.* **192:** 752–760.

72. Trapman, J., P. Klaassen, G. G. Kuiper, J. A. van der Korput, P. W. Faber, H. C. van Rooij, et al. 1988. Cloning, structure and expression of a cDNA encoding the human androgen receptor. *Biochem. Biophys. Res. Commun.* **153:** 241–248.

73. Tsai, S., M. Tsai, and B. O'Malley. 1991. The steroid receptor superfamily: transactivators of gene expression, in *Nuclear Hormone Receptors: Molecular Mechanisms, Cellular Functions, Clinical Abnormalities* (Parker, M. ed.), Academic Press, London, pp. 103–124.

74. Tut, T. G., F. J. Ghadessy, M. A. Trifiro, L. Pinsky, and E. L. Young. 1997. Long polyglutamine tracts in the androgen receptor are associated with reduced trans-activation, impaired sperm production, and male infertility. *J. Clin. Endocrinol. Metab.* **82:** 3777–3782.

75. Veldscholte, J., C. A. Berrevoets, C. Ris-Stalpers, G. G. Kuiper, G. Jenster, J. Trapman, et al. 1992. The androgen receptor in LNCaP cells contains a mutation in the ligand binding domain which affects steroid binding characteristics and response to antiandrogens. *J. Steroid Biochem. Mol. Biol.* **41:** 665–669.

76. Verkerk, A., M. Pieretti, J. Sutcliffe, Y. Fu, D. Kuhl, A. Pizzuti, et al. 1991. Identification of a gene (FMR-1) containing a CGG repeat coincident with a breakpoint cluster region exhibiting length variation in fragile X syndrome. *Cell* **65:** 905–914.

77. Wagner, R. L., J. W. Apriletti, M. E. McGrath, B. L. West, J. D. Baxter, and R. J. Fletterick. 1995. A structural role for hormone in the thyroid hormone receptor. *Nature* **378:** 690–697.

78. Watanabe, M., T. Uhijima, T. Shiraishi, R. Yatani, J. Shimazaki, T. Kotake, et al. 1997. Genetic alterations of androgen receptor gene in Japanese human prostate cancer. *Jpn. J. Clin. Oncol.* **27:** 389–393.

79. Waterman, M., S. Adler, C. Nelson, G. Greene, R. Evans, and M. Rosenfeld. 1988. A single domain of the estrogen receptor confers deozyribonucleic acid binding and transcriptional activation of the rat prolactin gene. *Mol. Endocrinol.* **2:** 14–21.

80. Weinberger, C., S. Hollenberg, E. Ong, J. Harmon, S. Brower, J. Cidlowski, et al. 1985. Identification of human glucocorticoid receptor complementary DNA clones by epitope selection. *Science* **228:** 740–742.

81. Weinberger, C., S. Hollenberg, M. Rosenfeld, and R. Evans. 1985. Domain structure of human glucocorticoid receptor and its relationship to the v-erbA oncogene product. *Nature* **318:** 670–672.

82. Wurtz, J.-M., W. Bourguet, J.-P. Renaud, V. Vivat, P. Chambon, D. Moras, et al. 1996. A canonical structure for the ligand binding domain of nuclear receptors. *Nature Structural Biol.* **3:** 87–94.

83. Xu, J., D. Meyers, D. Freije, S. Isaacs, K. Wiley, D. Nusskern, et al. 1998. Evidence for a prostate cancer susceptibility locus on the X chromosome. *Nat. Genet.* **20:** 175–179.

84. Yeh, S. and C. Chang. 1996. Cloning and characterization of a specific coactivator, ARA70, for the androgen receptor in human prostate cells. *Proc. Natl. Acad. Sci. USA* **93:** 5517–5521.

85. Zhu, Y. S., L. Q. Cai, J. J. Cordero, W. J. Canovatchel, M. D. Katz, and J. Imperato-McGinley. 1999. A novel mutation in the CAG triplet region of exon 1 of androgen receptor gene causes complete androgen insensitivity syndrome in a large kindred. *J. Clin. Endocrinol. Metab.* **84:** 1590–1594.

86. Zhuang, Y. H., M. Blauer, A. Pekki, and P. Tuohimaa. 1992. Subcellular location of androgen receptor in rat prostate, seminal vesicle and human osteosarcoma MG-63 cells. *J. Steroid Biochem. Mol. Biol.* **41:** 693–696.

7

The Genetic Epidemiology of Prostate Cancer

Closing in on a Complex Disease

Ronald K. Ross, MD, Juergen K.V. Reichardt, PhD, Sue Ann Ingles, PhD, and Gerhard A. Coetzee, PhD

1. INTRODUCTION

A full understanding of the etiology of prostate cancer is a goal we have yet to attain. Until recently, epidemiologists have focused mainly on possible environmental risk factors. After several decades of studies, no clear, single strong environmental risk factor has emerged, and this work has not led to a clear pathogenic pathway involving environmental influences *(39)*. The opportunities created by evolving molecular technology in recent years have led to an increasing emphasis on determining the possible genetic influences on risk. As prostate cancer is a highly familial disease, recent studies have attempted to exploit this powerful risk factor by conducting genetic linkage studies in large multiplex prostate cancer families searching for one or several single locus, high-penetrance susceptibility genes. Although this work has revealed several suggestive loci on several chromosomes *(41,49)*, confirmatory work for each of these to date has been largely inconclusive. Cloning of such a susceptibility gene for prostate cancer, a gene comparable in penetrance to the BRCA1 and BRCA2 loci for breast and ovarian cancer, remains elusive and is not likely to occur in the very near future. The alternative molecular epidemiologic focus in prostate cancer etiology has been on low-penetrance candidate genes, which are significant not only to familial prostate cancer, but even more so to the sporadic forms of the disease—because the products of these genes serve functions along plausible biologic pathways of prostate carcinogenesis.

2. ENVIRONMENTAL INFLUENCES

The demographic epidemiology of prostate cancer suggests that "environment" in the strictest sense has little or no importance in prostate cancer development—i.e., for a role of environmental chemical exposures that might be encountered in industrial urban living. For example, prostate cancer is not a disease that, at least historically, is strongly influenced by socioeconomic indicators. It is not a disease for which risk is strongly linked to urbanization or living in highly industrialized countries *(39)*. For example, Japan—one of the world's most industrialized nations—has one of the lowest prostate cancer rates in the world. Although a few occupational hazards, most

From: *Prostate Cancer: Biology, Genetics, and the New Therapeutics*
Edited by: L. W. K. Chung, W. B. Isaacs, and J. W. Simons © Humana Press Inc., Totowa, NJ

notably those linked to cadmium exposure, have been suggested to increase prostate cancer risk *(25)*, these can explain at most only a very tiny fraction of all prostate cancer occurrences.

Studies of environmental influences on prostate cancer risk have considered environment in a broader sense, by focusing particularly on the role of dietary influences. There are a number of promising leads regarding causative or protective dietary influences on prostate cancer development. These include dietary fat (increased risk), or some component of fat like the fatty acid α-linoleic acid *(15)*; the antioxidant carotenoid lycopene (found primarily in tomato and tomato products) for which there is both prospective epidemiologic dietary data *(14)* and serologic biomarker data *(12)* in support of a protective role for this micronutrient; calcium (increased risk), most likely through its interaction with vitamin D metabolic pathways *(16)*; vitamin E, another antioxidant vitamin that was almost inadvertently found to be associated with reduced risk of prostate cancer during analysis of a randomized clinical trial designed specifically to lower lung cancer risk in heavy cigarette smokers *(20)*; and selenium, a soil-based mineral with both antioxidant and proapoptotic properties, which like vitamin E was found to reduce prostate cancer risk as a secondary effect of a trial designed to reduce skin-cancer recurrences *(5)*. Other dietary factors, such as soybean-based foods (protective factors) and other plant-based estrogens (phytoestrogens), and dietary fiber (protective factors) have not been well-studied epidemiologically, but are of etiologic interest (phytoestrogens as a competitive inhibitor of androgens in prostate epithelium and as a possible explanation for part of the low risk of prostate cancer in Asians, and fiber as a mechanism to enhance fecal excretion and reduce enterohepatic recirculation of androgens) *(39)*.

The focus of this chapter is the nonenvironmental component of prostate cancer epidemiology, and several possible molecular or molecular genetic pathways are reviewed. Dietary hypotheses which clearly intersect with such molecular or molecular genetic pathways regarding prostate cancer etiology are examined.

3. MOLECULAR AND MOLECULAR GENETIC PATHWAYS

Other than age, the most important epidemiologic demographic risk factor for prostate cancer is race-ethnicity or the international variation in incidence *(39)*. African-American men have the highest rates of prostate cancer in the world by far, whereas Asian populations (native Japanese, Chinese, and Korean men) have the lowest. Early migrant studies suggested that rates of prostate cancer shift upon migration from low- to high-risk areas (an observation which stimulated interest in environmental influences on prostate cancer development). It is now clear that this shift is relatively small in comparison to the underlying differences in incidence across populations *(39)*. Therefore, attention has shifted to the possible contribution of genetic factors, and these observed racial-ethnic differences in incidence have driven much of the work on molecular genetic pathways of prostate carcinogenesis.

3.1. Androgen Metabolism Pathways

Of the etiologic pathways most commonly discussed in the study of prostate cancer, the one involving androgens and androgen metabolism clearly receives the most attention *(38)*. The prostate is an androgen-regulated organ which requires androgen influences for development and growth. It is generally agreed that androgens are the major stimulus for cell division in the prostate *(7)*. As cell proliferation and malignant transformation are inextricably tied *(32)*, the activity of androgens alone is sufficient to generate intense interest in androgens in prostate carcinogenesis. Other lines of evidence supporting the role of androgens in prostate cancer development have been previously reviewed *(38)*. These include the prominent requirement for androgens in experimental prostate carcinogenesis *(30)*; the absence of prostate cancer in men with underdeveloped prostates resulting from androgen deficiency—including eunuchs and men with constitutional 5-alpha reductase deficiency *(38)*; the uniform requirement for androgens in the growth and spread of prostate malignancies *(46)*; the rather strong relationship between circulating levels of testosterone and prostate cancer risk in the one adequate prospective serologic study conducted to date *(11)*; and the substantial differences in hormonal patterns among racial-ethnic groups at the extremes and in the middle of prostate cancer risk, which have demonstrated that high-risk populations (African-Americans) have increased androgen biosynthesis *(35)* whereas low-risk populations (Asians) have a reduced ability to bioactivate androgens *(36)*.

The genetic control of androgen biosynthesis, transport, and metabolism is a complex process which directly or indirectly involves hundreds of genes. Ross and colleagues, in proposing a polygenic model of prostate cancer etiology based around the androgen metabolic pathway, suggested criteria to use for justifying inclusion of certain genes in such a model and for initiating studies of particular genes *(38)*: The products of the genes under investigation must play critical roles in androgen stimulation of prostatic epithelium; polymorphic genetic markers must be known, and there must be evidence that various polymorphic alleles have functional consequences (or are linked to loci with functional relevance). Ross and colleagues suggested that since race-ethnicity is such a powerful factor in prostate cancer, allelic variation of the polymorphic markers across racial-ethnic groups at substantially different underlying risk of prostate cancer should occur in a manner predicted by the functional studies of the polymorphisms. In proposing such models, this group also suggested that there may be multiple functional polymorphisms in the same gene, so that a particular individual might carry both high-risk and low-risk markers and have an overall risk level from a particular gene that is no different from the population as a whole *(38)*.

The evaluation of the contribution of androgen metabolism genes to prostate cancer etiology is still in its earliest stages, but there have been preliminary evaluations of genes involved in androgen biosynthesis (CYP17, HSD3B2), androgen degradation (CYP3A4, HSD3, HSD3B2), androgen bioactivation (SRD5A2), androgen transport/transactivation (AR), and even "downstream" genes transactivated by the androgen receptor (PSA) *(50)*. However, the most extensive work to date has been on SRD5A2 and AR—the products of which both play major roles in androgen stimulation within prostate epithelial cells.

SRD5A2, the 5-alpha reductase type II gene, encodes the enzyme responsible for testosterone reduction in prostate epithelium to its more biologically active form (in terms of androgen receptor binding), dihydrotestosterone *(48)*. There are two 5-alpha reductase isozymes, and the type II enzyme is more active in prostate tissue. When the

SRD5A2 gene was originally cloned, a dinucleotide $(TA)_n$ repeat polymorphism was concurrently described in the 3' untranslated region (UTR) *(45)*. Although unique alleles of this polymorphism were eventually described for both African-Americans and Asians—and preliminary evidence suggested that for the former group at least, these alleles might be associated with an increased risk of prostate cancer *(37)*—more definitive studies have not shown any conclusive relationship between this marker and prostate cancer risk *(38)*. Complete sequencing of the coding region of 50 men with high and low levels of androstanediol glucuronide, a circulating biochemical correlate of 5-alpha reductase activity, revealed seven missense substitution mutations *(27)*—i.e., mutations resulting in an amino acid change. One of these, a valine to leucine substitution at codon 89 (V89L), has been shown to correlate with androstanediol levels (VV homozygotes showing the highest levels, LL homozygotes the lowest levels, and VL heterozygotes showing intermediate levels) across racial-ethnic groups *(27)*. Asian-Americans, a low-risk population for prostate cancer, have the highest proportion of LL homozygotes, the putative low-risk genotype, whereas African-Americans—the high-risk population—have the highest proportion of VV homozygotes. However, studies have not shown that this polymorphism is directly related to prostate cancer risk. A second missense substitution, an alanine to threonine substitution at codon 49 (A49T), has been preliminarily investigated to determine its relationship to prostate cancer. Variant alleles at this locus (TT or AT genotypes) are very rare in healthy men among all racial-ethnic groups investigated to date. However, presence of a T allele is strongly related to prostate cancer, especially advanced prostate cancer in both African-Americans and Latinos (RRs = 3.2 and 7.1 for prostate cancer overall and for advanced disease in African-Americans, $p = 0.04$ and 0.001, respectively; and RRs = 2.5 and 3.6 for prostate cancer overall and advanced disease in Latinos, $p = 0.08$ and 0.04, respectively) *(33)*. However, preliminary studies have not demonstrated A49T variant alleles to be associated with prostate cancer risk in Asian or non-Latino white populations. Reichardt and colleagues have conducted in vitro transfection assays which have demonstrated that the A49T mutation increases enzymatic activity, whereas the V89L mutation reduces kinetic properties of the enzyme compared to wild-type enzyme—findings which are generally compatible with projections from the epidemiologic data published to date *(33)*. The other five missense mutations have not yet been investigated in terms of their relationship to prostate cancer risk.

The *AR* gene is located on the X chromosome. Two polymorphic trinucleotide repeat sequences (a $[CAG]_n$ and a $[GGC]_n$) have been described in exon 1, the transcription modulatory domain of the gene. The *AR* transactivates genes with androgen-response elements in their promoter region, including those that control cell division in the prostate.

The $(CAG)_n$ has been the focus of particular attention *(6)*. An expansion of this repeat is the cause of an X-linked adult-onset motor neuron disease, spinal and bulbar muscular atrophy (Kennedy's disease) *(24)*. Whereas the range of CAG repeats in healthy men is between approx 6 and 39, men with Kennedy's disease have a minimum of 42 repeats. Coetzee and Ross, recognizing that men with Kennedy's disease also have evidence of reduced androgen activity—including low virilization, low fertility, and gynecomastia *(1)*—proposed that the length of this CAG may modify androgen transactivation activity and, thereby, modify prostate cancer risk *(6)*. This hypothesis was supported by transfection assays in which AR genes with Kennedy's disease-size CAGs were shown to have substantially reduced transactivation activity relative to genes with CAGs in the normal range *(47)*. The specific hypothesis proposed by Coetzee and Ross was that shorter CAGs would result in greater transactivation than longer CAGs, and that men with short CAG repeats would therefore have higher prostate cancer risk. This hypothesis received further support from these same types of in vitro transfection assay results, when it was demonstrated that CAG length corresponded in a linear inverse fashion with transactivation activity within the normal range of repeats (longer CAG, reduced transactivation) *(3)*. Indirect support for the hypothesis also came from studies of healthy men from different racial-ethnic groups which demonstrated that African-American men, as predicted, have shorter CAGs on average, and Asian men have longer CAGs on average compared to whites *(6)*. Subsequently, this investigative team showed that CAG length was related to prostate cancer in whites, so that men with fewer than 20 repeats (the median length in the healthy control men) had twice the risk of prostate cancer compared to men with 20 or more. Risk was greater for advanced disease at presentation than for men presenting with localized or occult disease *(21)*. This finding was verified in two other large studies in whites, both showing that shorter CAG repeats are associated with increased prostate cancer risk *(17,42)*. Two other studies have suggested that CAG repeat length can identify phenotypic subtypes among prostate cancer patients *(18,19)*.

One important biological issue is to understand the molecular basis for reduced transactivation activity with expanded CAG repeat lengths. In recent years, the importance of coactivator proteins in transcriptional activation has become increasingly apparent. Irvine and colleagues have recently shown that one family of such proteins, the p160 coactivator family, interacts with the AR subdomain that contains the polymorphic polyglutamine (polyQ) tract encoded by the CAG repeat in the AR gene. These investigators have demonstrated that with increasing polyQ length, p160-mediated coactivation is increasingly inhibited *(23)*.

Preliminary studies of the other trinucleotide repeat—a $(GGC)_n$ polymorphism also in exon 1—and its relationship to prostate cancer have produced provocative but inconclusive results *(22,42)*. The majority of healthy men of all racial-ethnic groups have a GGC_{16} allele. Two studies have suggested that non-GGC_{16} individuals may be at increased risk of prostate cancer *(22,42)*. The molecular basis for this effect is unknown.

Substantial epidemiologic evidence indicates that men with prostate cancer-affected brothers have substantially higher prostate cancer risk than those with prostate cancer-affected fathers (although the latter group still has substantially higher risk than the population as a whole) *(28)*. This generation "skip pattern" of familial risk is compatible with an X-linked inherited disorder, although other inheritance models are also plausible. As an X-linked disorder, the *AR* gene becomes a strong candidate gene for prostate cancer. Yet linkage studies of familial prostate cancer in multiplex families have not found any strong evidence of AR-linked inheritance *(43)*. Nonetheless, a third polymorphic marker in the *AR* gene, a StuI restriction fragment-length polymorphism (RFLP) located between the two trinucleotide repeat microsatellites, has been preliminarily reported to be associated with prostate cancer risk. An excess proportion of the

S1 allele (cut by the restriction enzyme) was found among prostate cancer patients with an affected brother (12 of 14, or 86%) compared to men with no such family history (118 of 204, or 58%) *(38)*.

A major goal of the polygenic etiologic model is to combine the effects of multiple genes in a particular metabolic pathway to create high (and/or low) risk genetic profiles for individuals or populations *(38)*. A category of candidate genes that remain largely unstudied in terms of prostate cancer development are the "downstream" genes which are transactivated by the *AR*. One such gene is the prostate-specific antigen (*PSA*) gene, encoding a tissue-specific protease produced by prostate epithelium, which has become a standard assay for monitoring prostate cancer progression. A major function of *PSA* is to cleave the major insulin-like growth-factor (IGF) binding protein, IGFBP-3, resulting in elevated levels of IGF-1. IGF signaling pathways have been proposed as a common etiologic pathway for multiple cancer sites, including the prostate. By regulating the IGF axis, PSA activity may alter prostate cancer risk. Ingles et al. recently studied a G/A substitution polymorphism in the promoter region of the PSA gene in conjunction with the polymorphic CAG repeat in exon 1 of the AR. Subjects with both a short CAG repeat and PSA genotype GG had a five-fold increase in prostate cancer risk overall and, based on small numbers, a more than 10-fold increase in advanced disease *(50)*.

3.2. Insulin-Like Growth Factor (IGF) Signaling Pathways

IGF-1 stimulates cell proliferation and reduces apoptosis in vitro in normal as well as malignant prostate epithelium *(8,9)*. Recently, a prospective study of 15,000 physicians (the Physician's Health Study) found that among 152 prostate cancer patients and 152 age-matched controls, men in the second, third, and fourth quartiles of IGF-1 at baseline had 1.9, 2.8, and 4.3 times the risk of subsequently developing prostate cancer compared to men in the lowest quartile *(4)*. Regulation of IGF-1 levels is complex and not fully understood, but includes both genetic and environmental influences and occurs systemically as well as at a local, tissue-specific level. Polymorphisms have been identified in the IGFBP-3 and IGF-1 genes. Although the functional significance of the former is unknown, the latter a dinucleotide (CA) repeat in the structural region of the IGF-1 gene has been shown to correlate with circulating IGF-1 levels *(34)*.

IGF signaling pathways, because of their importance in cell proliferation, are important in their own right as a potential etiologic pathway for prostate cancer. As noted here, the IGF pathway also clearly interfaces with androgen-transactivation pathways. Moreover, dietary restriction, which alters serum concentrations of IGF-1, reduces cancer incidence in rodents, whereas excess calories increases IGF-1 levels. Based on these observations, Burroughs et al. *(2)* have suggested that perhaps one of the apparent links between diet and prostate cancer might be mediated through IGF pathways.

3.3. Vitamin D Metabolism Pathways

A third etiologic pathway of current interest in prostate cancer development is the vitamin D metabolic pathway. Vitamin D or, more accurately, 1,25-dihydroxyvitamin D, the bioactive vitamin D metabolite is a potent antiproliferation agent in the prostate as well as a prodifferentiation agent for prostate cells in vitro *(31)*. As prostate cells themselves metabolize vitamin D compounds to 1,25-dihydroxyvitamin D, vitamin D stimulation of the prostate is—like IGF—under both local and systemic control.

The first prospective study of the relationship between circulating 1,25-dihydroxyvitamin D levels and subsequent risk of prostate cancer was highly provocative and stimulated additional interest in this field *(10)*. This study found that men who developed prostate cancer had substantially and significantly lower levels of 1,25-dihydroxyvitamin D levels than men who did not develop prostate cancer, regardless of the circulating level of 25-hydroxyvitamin D, the parent compound. Subsequent prospective studies have been less convincing *(13)*. The Physician's Health Study, for example, found no overall relationship between 1,25-dihydroxyvitamin D levels and prostate cancer risk. However, in a subsequent report from that study, a positive association was observed between estimated dietary intake of calcium and prostate cancer risk, which the authors suggested might be caused by a suppressive effect of calcium on conversion of 25-hydroxyvitamin D to 1,25-dihydroxyvitamin D *(16)*. In addition to its anticancer-like effects on cell lines, vitamin D has inhibitory effects on prostate growth in animal models *(40)*.

Vitamin D activity is mediated by the vitamin D receptor (VDR) encoded by the VDR gene. A number of polymorphisms with common allele variants have been identified in the VDR gene. Some of these have been shown to have biological correlates, such as associations with indices of bone mineral density (Vitamin D plays an important role in bone mineral metabolism) *(29)*. A few of these polymorphic markers have been preliminarily studied in relationship to prostate cancer risk. Ingles et al., for example, found that a bimodal polyA microsatellite in the 3′ UTR of the VDR gene was strongly related to prostate cancer risk in whites *(3)*. In this study, men with at least one "long" A allele had a 4.6-fold increase in prostate cancer risk compared to men homozygous for "short" polyA alleles. Moreover, of the 26 patients tested who presented with advanced disease, all had at least one long A allele, vs only 36/169 healthy control men of similar age *(3)*. Taylor and colleagues, reporting results of another case-control study of whites, found an association between prostate cancer risk and a second polymorphic marker, a TaqI RFLP. Individuals who had a TaqI T allele had a threefold higher prostate cancer risk than men who were tt homozygotes *(44)*.

Ingles et al. have also begun exploring the relationship between polymorphic markers of the VDR gene and prostate cancer risk in African-Americans *(21)*. There is, at most, a very weak linkage disequilibrium in the 3′ UTR area of the VDR gene in African-Americans. Therefore, these investigators devised a haplotype assay to directly examine two relevant polymorphic markers in combination (a *Bsm*I RFLP in intron 8 that is in linkage disequilibrium with the polyA microsatellite in whites and a marker that has been extensively studied in relationship to bone mineral density; and the polyA microsatellite itself). They found that the BsmIB/long polyA haplotype was associated with a twofold increase in the risk of advanced prostate cancer compared to individuals with no B/long A haplotypes, as predicted from the results of their study in whites *(21)*.

Only one other study to date has been published on VDR genotype and prostate cancer risk. That study had the advantage of available data on circulating vitamin D levels. The BsmI genotype in this study was associated with an increase in prostate cancer risk only among those men with low circulating levels of 25-hydroxyvitamin D *(26)*.

4. THE FUTURE OF MOLECULAR GENETIC STUDIES
OF PROSTATE CANCER

The rapidity of further advances in the field of molecular genetic epidemiology will be technology-driven, with opportunities developing for testing multiple polymorphic loci simultaneously on a single sample—thereby greatly enhancing efficiency in the study of gene-gene or gene-environment interactions in the context of polygenic etiologic models. The rate-limiting step in further development of such models will likely be the availability of DNA samples in epidemiologically, well-characterized populations of greatest interest in terms of prostate cancer risk (i.e., the elderly, African-Americans, and Asians, those with detailed baseline dietary histories, multiplex prostate cancer families, or those with baseline serologic or other biological samples for further molecular epidemiologic analyses). Nonetheless, it is virtually certain that the focus of epidemiologic research on prostate cancer in the next decade will be on the development and testing of such models, with the goal of gaining a detailed understanding of the complex molecular pathways leading to prostate carcinogenesis.

A major advantage to having mechanisms in place for securing and storing DNA samples in large epidemiologic studies of prostate cancer is that as new genes are discovered in a particular molecular pathway or new polymorphic loci are identified in genes already known to be involved in that pathway, these can readily be added onto the existing model to determine whether they contribute in a meaningful way in distinguishing between high and low-risk populations. Moreover, such banks of DNA samples will allow investigations into whether or in what ways one molecular genetic pathway (e.g., the androgen metabolism pathway) might interact with other pathways (e.g., IGF signaling and vitamin D metabolism pathways).

Well-characterized epidemiologic cohorts followed prospectively for prostate-cancer development have the additional advantage when used for building molecular genetic etiologic models of allowing the easy incorporation of environmental—for example, dietary—risk factors into the model, to determine whether these environmental factors might modify the effect of individual genes in the model or modify the entire molecular genetic pathway.

The long-term goal of such model building is to be able to use multiple genetic markers to define subgroups of the population at very high or very low risk of developing prostate cancer, and to use these to explain some of the important demographic aspects of prostate cancer epidemiology, especially the remarkable racial-ethnic variation in incidence. In addition to the obvious contributions such molecular genetic models will make to our basic understanding of prostate cancer pathogenesis, these models should provide a basis for better targeting populations for screening interventions and for developing primary prevention strategies aimed at the multigene products or at the genes themselves.

ACKNOWLEDGMENT

We are honored to participate in this volume, which pays tribute to the remarkable accomplishments of Donald Coffey. Don has led the crusade in the past several decades to give prostate cancer research national and international visibility and importance, at a time when prostate cancer has become the most commonly diagnosed cancer in the United States. He has done this with creative thinking about the prostate gland and how it functions, as well as with his own unique flair and humor. He has a special ability to bring scientists from diverse disciplines together for interdisciplinary meetings to establish research agendas to accomplish our common goals—to reduce morbidity and mortality from prostate cancer. Largely because of Don, achievement of these goals is on the horizon, and that horizon looks closer every day. We are all extremely grateful.

REFERENCES

1. Arbizu, T., J. Santamaria, J. M. Gomex, A. Quilez, and J. P. Serra. 1983. A family with adult spinal and bulbar muscular atrophy X-linked inheritance and associated with testicular failure. *J. Neurol. Sci.* **59:** 371–382.
2. Burroughs, K. D., S. E. Dunn, J. C. Barrett, and J. A. Taylor. 1999. Insulin-like growth factor-I: a key regulator of human cancer risk. *J. Natl. Cancer Inst.* **91:** 579–581.
3. Chamberlain, N. L., E. D. Driver, and R. L. Miesfeld. 1994. The length and location of CAG trinucleotide repeats in the androgen receptor N-terminal domain affect transactivation function. *Nucleic Acids Res.* **22:** 3181–3186.
4. Chan, J. M., M. J. Stampfer, E. Giovannucci, P. H. Gann, J. Ma, P. Wilkinson, et al. 1998. Plasma insulin-like growth factor-I and prostate cancer risk: a prospective study. *Science* **279:** 563–566.
5. Clark, L. C., B. Dalkin, A. Krongrad, G. Combs, B. W. Turnbull, E. H. Slate, et al. 1998. Decreased incidence of prostate cancer with selenium supplementation: results of a double-blind cancer prevention trial. *Br. J. Urol.* **81:** 730–734.
6. Coetzee, G. A. and R. K. Ross. 1994. Prostate cancer and the androgen receptor. *J. Natl. Cancer Inst.* **86:** 872,873.
7. Coffey, D. S. 1979. Physiological control of prostatic growth: an overview, in *Prostate Cancer*, Geneva, UICC Technical Report Series. International Union Against Cancer.
8. Cohen, P., D. M. Peehl, G. Lamson, and R. G. Rosenfeld. 1991. Insulin-like growth factors (IGFs), IGF receptors, and IGF-binding proteins in primary cultures of prostate epithelial cells. *J. Clin. Endocrinol. Metab.* **73:** 401–407.
9. Cohen, P., D. M. Peehl, and R. G. Rosenfeld. 1994. The IGF axis in the prostate. *Hormone Metab. Res.* **26:** 81–84.
10. Corder, E. H., G. D. Friedman, J. H. Vogelman, and N. Orentreich. 1995. Seasonal variation in vitamin D, vitamin D-binding protein, and dehydroepiandrosterone: risk of prostate cancer in black and white men. *Cancer Epidemiol. Biomark. Prev.* **4:** 655–659.
11. Gann, P. H., C. H. Hennekens, J. Ma, C. Longcope, and M. J. Stampfer. 1996. Prospective study of sex hormone levels and risk of prostate cancer. *J. Natl. Cancer Inst.* **88:** 1118–1126.
12. Gann, P. H., J. Ma, E. Giovannucci, W. Willett, F. Sacks, C. H. Hennekens, et al. 1999. Lower prostate cancer risk in men with elevated plasma lycopene levels: results of a prospective analysis. *Cancer Res.* **59:** 1225–1230.
13. Gann, P. H., J. Ma, C. H. Hennekens, B. W. Hollis, J. G. Haddad, and M. J. Stampfer. 1996. Circulating vitamin D metabolites in relation to subsequent development of prostate cancer. *Cancer Epidemiol. Biomark. Prev.* **5:** 121–126.
14. Giovannucci, E., A. Ascherio, E. B. Rimm, M. J. Stampfer, G. A. Colditz, and W. C. Willett. 1995. Intake of carotenoids and retinol in relation to risk of prostate cancer. *J. Natl. Cancer Inst.* **87:** 1767–1776.
15. Giovannucci, E., E. B. Rimm, G. A. Colditz, M. J. Stampfer, A. Ascherio, C. C. Chute, et al. 1993. A prospective study of dietary fat and risk of prostate cancer. *J. Natl. Cancer Inst.* **85:** 1571–1579.

16. Giovannucci, E., E. B. Rimm, A. Wolk, M. J. Ascherio, M. J. Stampfer, G. A. Colditz, et al. 1998. Calcium and fructose intake in relation to risk of prostate cancer. *Cancer Res.* **58:** 442–447.

17. Giovannucci, E., M. J. Stampfer, K. Krithivas, M. Brown, A. Brufsky, J. Talcott, et al. 1997. The CAG repeat within the androgen receptor gene and its relationship to prostate cancer. *Proc. Natl. Acad. Sci. USA* **94:** 3320–3323.

18. Hakimi, J. M., M. P. Schoenberg, R. H. Rondinelli, S. Piantadosi, and E. R. Barrack. 1997. Androgen receptor variants with short glutamine or glycine repeats may identify unique subpopulations of men with prostate cancer. *Clin. Cancer Res.* **3:** 1599–1608.

19. Hardy, D. O., H. I. Scher, T. Bogenreider, P. Sabbatini, Z. Zhang, D. M. Nanus, et al. 1996. Androgen receptor CAG repeat lengths in prostate cancer: correlation with age of onset. *J. Clin. Endocrinol. Metab.* **81:** 4400–4405.

20. Heinonen, O. P., D. Albanes, J. Virtamo, P. R. Taylor, J. K. Huttunen, A. M. Hartman, et al. 1998. Prostate cancer and supplementation with alpha-tocopherol and beta-carotene: incidence and mortality in a controlled trial. *J. Natl. Cancer Inst.* **90:** 440–446.

21. Ingles, S. A., G. A. Coetzee, R. K. Ross, B. E. Henderson, L. N. Kolonel, L. Crocitto, et al. 1998. Association of prostate cancer with vitamin D receptor haplotypes in African-Americans. *Cancer Res.* **58:** 1620–1623.

22. Ingles, S. A., R. K. Ross, M. C. Yu, R. A. Irvine, G. La Pera, R. W. Haile, et al. 1997. Association of prostate cancer risk with genetic polymorphisms in vitamin D receptor and androgen receptor. *J. Natl. Cancer Inst.* **89:** 166–170.

23. Irvine, R. A., H. Ma, M. Yu, R. K. Ross, M. R. Stallcup, and G. A. Coetzee. 1999. Inhibition of p160-mediated coactivation with increasing androgen receptor polyglutamine length. *Hum. Mol. Genet.* (submitted).

24. La Spada, A. R., E. M. Wilson, D. B. Lubahn, A. E. Harding, and K. H. Fischback. 1991. Androgen receptor gene mutations in X-linked spinal and bulbar muscular atrophy. *Nature* **352:** 77–79.

25. Lemen, R. A., J. S. Lee, J. K. Wagoner, and H. P. Blejer. 1976. Cancer mortality among cadmium production workers. *Ann. NY Acad. Sci.* **271:** 273–279.

26. Ma, J., M. J. Stampfer, P. H. Gann, H. L. Hough, E. Giovannucci, K. T. Kelsey, et al. 1998. Vitamin D receptor polymorphisms, circulating vitamin D metabolites, and risk of prostate cancer in United States physicians. *Cancer Epidemiol. Biomark. Prev.* **7:** 385–390.

27. Makridakis, N., R. K. Ross, M. C. Pike, L. Chang, F. Z. Stanczyk, L. N. Kolonel, et al. 1997. A prevalent missense substitution that modulates activity of prostatic steroid 5α-reductase. *Cancer Res.* **57:** 1020–1022.

28. Monroe, K. R., M. C. Yu, L. N. Kolonel, G. A. Coetzee, L. R. Wilkens, R. K. Ross, et al. 1995. Evidence of an X-linked genetic component to prostate cancer risk. *Nat. Med.* **1:** 827–829.

29. Morrison, N. A., R. Yeoman, P. J. Kelly, and J. A. Eisman. 1992. Contribution of trans-acting factor alleles to normal physiological variability: vitamin D receptor gene polymorphism and circulating osteocalcin. *Proc. Natl. Acad. Sci. USA* **89:** 6665–6669.

30. Noble, R. L. 1977. The development of prostatic adenocarcinoma in Nb rats following prolonged sex hormone administration. *Cancer Res.* **37:** 1929–1933.

31. Peehl, D. M., R. J. Skowronski, G. K. Leung, S. T. Wong, T. A. Stamey, and D. Feldman. 1994. Antiproliferative effects of 1,25-dihydroxyvitamin D3 on primary cultures of human prostatic cells. *Cancer Res.* **54:** 805–810.

32. Preston-Martin, S., M. C. Pike, R. K. Ross, P. A. Jones, and B. E. Henderson. 1990. Increased cell division as a cause of human cancer. *Cancer Res.* **50:** 7415–7421.

33. Makridakis, N. M., R. K. Ross, M. C. Pike, L. E. Crocitto, et al. 1999. Association of missense substitution in SRD5A2 gene with prostate cancer in African-American and Hispanic men in Los Angeles, USA. *Lancet* **354:** 975–978.

34. Rosen, C. J., E. S. Kurland, D. Vereault, R. A. Adler, P. J. Rackoff, W. Y. Craig, et al. 1998. Association between serum insulin growth factor-I (IGF-I) and a simple sequence repeat in IGF-I gene: implications for genetic studies of bone mineral density. *J. Clin. Endocrinol. Metab.* **83:** 2286–2290.

35. Ross, R. K., L. Bernstein, H. Judd, R. Hanisch, M. C. Pike, and B. E. Henderson. 1986. Serum testosterone levels in healthy young black and white men. *J. Natl. Cancer Inst.* **76:** 45–48.

36. Ross, R. K., L. Bernstein, R. A. Lobo, H. Shimizu, F. Z. Stanczyk, M. C. Pike, et al. 1992. 5-Alpha reductase activity and risk of prostate cancer among Japanese and US white and black males. *Lancet* **339:** 887–889.

37. Ross, R. K., G. A. Coetzee, J. Reichardt, E. Skinner, and B. E. Henderson. 1995. Does the racial-ethnic variation in prostate cancer risk have a hormonal basis? *Cancer* **75:** 1778–1782.

38. Ross, R. K., M. C. Pike, G. A. Coetzee, J. K. V. Reichardt, M. C. Yu, H. Feigelson, et al. 1998. Androgen metabolism and prostate cancer: establishing a model of genetic susceptibility. *Cancer Res.* **58:** 4497–4504.

39. Ross, R. K. and D. Schottenfeld. 1996. Prostate cancer, in *Cancer Epidemiology and Prevention, 2nd Ed.* (Schottenfeld, D. and J. F. Fraumeni, eds.), Oxford University Press, New York, pp. 1180–1206.

40. Schwartz, G. G., C. C. Hill, T. A. Oeler, M. J. Becich, and R. R. Bahnson. 1995. 1,25-dihydroxy-16-ene-23-yne-vitamin D3 and prostate cancer cell proliferation *in vivo*. *Urology* **46:** 365–369.

41. Smith, J. R., D. Freije, J. D. Carpten, H. Gronberg, J. Xu, S. D. Isaacs, et al. 1996. Major susceptibility locus for prostate cancer on chromosome 1 suggested by a genome-wide search. *Science* **274:** 1371–1374.

42. Stanford, J. L., J. J. Just, M. Gibbs, K. G. Wicklund, C. L. Neal, B. A. Blumenstein, et al. 1997. Polymorphic repeats in the androgen receptor gene: molecular markers of prostate cancer risk. *Cancer Res.* **57:** 1194–1198.

43. Sun, S., S. A. Narod, A. Aprikian, P. Ghadirian, and F. Labrie. 1995. Androgen receptor and familial prostate cancer. *Nat. Med.* **1:** 848,849.

44. Taylor, J. A., A. Hirvonen, M. Watson, G. Pittman, J. L. Mohler, and D. A. Bell. 1996. Association of prostate cancer with vitamin D receptor gene polymorphism. *Cancer Res.* **56:** 4108–4110.

45. Thigpen, A. E., D. L. Davis, T. Gautier, J. Imperato-McGinley, and W. Russell. 1992. The molecular basis of steroid 5-alpha-reductase deficiency in a large Dominican kindren. *N. Engl. J. Med.* **327:** 1216–1219.

46. Trump, D. L. and C. N. Robertson. 1993. Neoplasms of the prostate, in *Cancer Medicine* (Holland, J. F., E. Frei, III, and R. C. Bast, Jr., eds.), Lea and Febiger, Philadelphia, pp. 1562–1586.

47. Tut, T., F. J. Ghadessy, M. A. Trifiro, L. Pinsky, and E. L. Yong. 1997. Long polyglutamine tracts in the androgen receptor are associated with reduced trans-activation, impaired sperm production, and male infertility. *J. Clin. Endocrinol. Metab.* **82:** 3777–3782.

48. Wilson, J. D., J. E. Griffin, and D. W. Russell. 1993. Steroid 5 α-reductase 2 deficiency. *Br. J. Cancer* **14:** 577–593.

49. Xu, J., D. Meyers, D. Freije, S. Isaacs, K. Wiley, D. Nusskern, et al. 1998. Evidence for a prostate cancer susceptibility locus on the X chromosome. *Nat. Genet.* **20:** 175–179.

50. Xue, W., R. A. Irvine, M. C. Yu, R. K. Ross, G. A. Coetzee, S. A. Ingles. 2000. Susceptibility to prostate cancer: interaction between genotypes at the androgen receptor (AR) and prostate-specific antigen (PSA) loci. *Cancer Res.* **60:** 839–841.

8

Determination of Gene and Chromosome Dosage in Prostatic Intraepithelial Neoplasia and Prostatic Carcinoma by Molecular Cytogenetic Techniques

Junqi Qian, MD and Robert B. Jenkins, MD, PhD

1. INTRODUCTION

Prostate adenocarcinoma accounts for nearly one-third of all invasive cancers in American men, and has marked clinical variability *(48)*. Some cases metastasize early and result in patient death within a few years, while others are relatively indolent and the patient dies of other causes *(46,76)*. Within any selected group of men with clinically evident and localized prostate adenocarcinoma, treated by any modality, a small but finite proportion will suffer local progression and/or metastatic relapse within 5–10 yr *(5)*. This is partly the result of incomplete staging of those men treated by watchful waiting or radiotherapy *(18)*. The challenge for urologists and oncologists is to identify the tumors that will progress, and perhaps to treat them more aggressively. One of the highest priorities in prostate cancer research is to identify new laboratory tests, especially genetic markers which can more accurately predict the rate of tumor progression and how the tumor might respond to appropriate therapy *(37,63)*. To search for genetic markers, an understanding of the genetic mechanism for prostate cancer initiation and progression is critical. Progress in the genetic study of prostate cancer has been aided by recent technical and conceptual advances in molecular biology. An important approach for the study of prostate cancer is the determination of gene and chromosome dosage *(7,11,40)*.

High-grade prostatic intraepithelial neoplasia (PIN) represents the most likely precursor of prostatic adenocarcinoma *(26,28,58,59,68)*. It harbors substantial genetic changes, and these changes are similar to those in primary and metastatic carcinoma *(2,21,32,43,55,64,70,78)*. Despite attempts at early detection, prostate cancer is often diagnosed at an advanced state: approx 28% of patients have extraprostatic extension, and 25% have bone metastases which are incurable by current modalities. An understanding of the genetic events which accompany the progression of PIN to prostatic adenocarcinoma and the subsequent development of metastases is extremely useful for prevention, early detection, and treatment.

Fluorescence *in situ* hybridization (FISH), polymerase chain reaction (PCR), and comparative genomic hybridization (CGH) are commonly used techniques for detect-

From: *Prostate Cancer: Biology, Genetics, and the New Therapeutics*
Edited by: L. W. K. Chung, W. B. Isaacs, and J. W. Simons © Humana Press Inc., Totowa, NJ

ing gene and chromosome dosage in human specimens. The recently developed microarray techniques are also powerful tools for the study of tumor genomes. In this chapter, we discuss the utility of FISH, PCR, CGH, and microarrays in the determination of gene and chromosome dosage in cancer specimens. We also discuss the genetic anomalies associated with PIN and adenocarcinoma as detected by these techniques.

2. THE UTILITY OF VARIOUS INTERPHASE FISH TECHNIQUES

FISH is a useful method for the detection of gene and chromosome anomalies in cell lines (3), touch preparations from fresh tissue (78), isolated nuclei from formalin-fixed, paraffin-embedded tissue (1,80), and routine histologic sections from paraffin blocks (2,43,44,64). Analysis of interphase nuclei from archival blocks eliminates the need for fresh tissue. It also allows for a comparison of chromosome anomalies with other prognostic factors in prostate cancer (1,80). However, the various methods of FISH analysis of archival tissue in paraffin blocks have advantages and disadvantages (1,64,80). The selection of an appropriate method depends on the clinical or scientific hypothesis to be addressed.

In tissue sections, FISH allows precise histopathologic correlation of multiple foci of normal epithelium, premalignant lesions, and carcinoma within a single specimen, including the study of intratumoral heterogeneity (2,64,65). This is a useful approach for understanding carcinogenesis, especially for the study of clonal origin of multifocal prostate cancer (2,64,65). For example, analysis of chromosomal anomalies in PIN, atypical adenomatous hyperplasia, and prostatic carcinoma in whole-mount prostates have revealed similar genetic changes in carcinoma and PIN, but not in atypical adenomatous hyperplasia (2,64,65). FISH can easily distinguish chromosomal centromere gain and loss (1–3,43,44,64,65,78,80). With appropriate probes, the copy number of specific chromosomal regions can also be determined (43,44). However, accurate quantitative analyses of chromosome and gene copy number in tissue sections is not possible, because many nuclei are sliced or overlapped. Our data show that a significant proportion of signal loss with fluorescent-labeled centromere probes in tissue sections (mean, 23.7 to 31.2% in benign tissue and 21 to 26% in tumors) results from the artifact of nuclear truncation, causing artificial monosomy. This problem is partially overcome by using conservative abnormal criteria based on a statistical analysis of the FISH signals observed in normal epithelium and inspection of the distribution of FISH signals among foci of carcinoma (43,64).

FISH analysis of isolated nuclei reveals a lower frequency of signal loss (mean, 6.9–8.2% in benign tissue and 3–4% in tumors) and reveals a higher frequency of tetrasomy than FISH analysis of tissue sections (66). Differentiation of tetraploid and aneuploid tumors is possible (1,78,80). Because diploid, tetraploid, and aneuploid tumors have different prognoses (52,72), evaluation of isolated nuclei may be the preferred method to define tumor ploidy. FISH analysis of isolated nuclei does not require special training in pathology, and the counting of fluorescence signals is easier than in tissue sections. Thus, large-scale studies can be done by multiple investigators within a reasonable time frame. However, loss of histologic architecture, insufficient hybridization, contamination of benign cells, and the inability to identify intraglandular and intratumoral heterogeneity of chromosomal anomalies of tumors limit the utility of studies of isolated nuclei—especially in the study of carcinogenesis (66).

Table 1 shows that a similar percentage of aneuploid specimens are detected by FISH analysis of isolated nuclei and tissue sections: 44 vs 56%, respectively, with 16 cases of stage $T_3N_0M_0$ prostatic-carcinoma. Other reports using different methods revealed a similar percentage of cases with chromosomal anomalies in prostate cancer *(2,64,66,78,80)*. Takahashi et al. *(78)* observed aneuploidy in 48% of touch preparations from fresh needle biopsies containing prostate cancer. Takahashi et al. *(80)* observed that 56% of paraffin-embedded stage $T_3N_0M_0$ prostate cancer specimens contained chromosomal anomalies in isolated nuclei. Similarly, Qian et al. *(64)* identified chromosomal anomalies in 51% of cancer foci in tissue sections of paraffin-embedded whole-mounted radical prostatectomy specimens. Alers et al. *(2)* reported chromosomal anomalies in 52% of prostate cancer foci with FISH analysis of routine histologic slides. Thus, FISH analysis of isolated nuclei and routine tissue sections from paraffin blocks are reliable methods for the detection of chromosome anomalies in archival tissue of prostate cancer.

A method of FISH analysis of thick sections (20 μm) using confocal microscopy was reported *(81)*. This technique can be used to analyze intact, uncut nuclei while simultaneously maintaining histologic architecture. However, this method is time-consuming and labor-intensive, and is difficult to optimize. New imaging software may facilitate routine application of this novel methodology *(66)*.

3. THE UTILITY OF PCR, CGH, AND MICROARRAYS IN THE DETERMINATION OF GENE AND CHROMOSOME DOSAGE

FISH, PCR, and CGH are commonly used techniques for detecting gene and chromosome dosage in human specimens *(69)*. The recently developed microarray techniques offer the potential to carefully study the complexity of genetic alterations in prostate cancer. Table 2 summarizes the advantages and disadvantages of these techniques.

PCR analysis of microsatellite markers has been very useful for the detection of allelic imbalance in many tumors, especially for the mapping of imbalance of specific chromosomal regions *(23,50,79,88)*. In addition, PCR studies can evaluate a much smaller region of the genome than typical FISH and CGH studies *(20,23,45,47,50,79, 85,88)*. However, PCR analyses are limited by the difficulty of characterizing allelic imbalance as loss or gain, and the analyses are not useful when markers are non-informative *(23,45,50,79,88)*. Fortunately, for the latter problem, closely linked neighboring markers are usually available and informative.

CGH is a relatively new molecular cytogenetic technique used to screen cancer DNA alterations. The significant advantage of CGH is that all chromosome regions can be screened for gains and losses simultaneously *(21,23,45,79)*. However, CGH analyses are limited by the relatively low resolution (the method can only detect deletions greater than 10 Mb in size). In addition, CGH data interpretation requires a trained cytogenetic technologist and requires relatively expensive microscope and computer equipment *(20,21,47,85)*.

Microarrays are newly developed tools to study the genome complexity by providing a systematic survey of DNA or RNA variations *(73)*. Applied to genotyping, microarrays provide the possibility of analyzing alleles at thousands of loci from a hundred DNA samples quickly, allowing the determination of genetic alteration patterns of complex polygenic disorders *(12)*. Applied to mutation screening of disease

Table 1
Distribution of Chromosome Anomalies in Isolated Nuclei vs Tissue Sections of 16 Specimens of Stage T3N0M0 Prostate Cancer

Case	score	% Nuclei with indicated centromere copy number												FISH[a] Ploidy (chromosal anomaly)		Flow cytometric
		Chromosome 7						Chromosome 8								DNA ploidy
		Isolated nuclei			Tissue sections			Isolated nuclei			Tissue sections			Isolated nuclei	Tissue sections	
		0–1	3–8	4	0–1	3–8	4	0–1	3–8	4	0–1	3–8	4			
1	7	4	2	1	31	3	1	3	5	4	22	6	2	Diploid	Diploid	Diploid
2	6	2	3	2	33	2	0	6	3	1	34	3	1	Diploid	Diploid	Diploid
3	5	6	4	3	27	5	0	9	5	1	41	4	0	Diploid	Diploid	Diploid
4	7	3	6	3	22	6	0	7	4	2	35	3	0	Diploid	Diploid	Diploid
5	7	3	23	3	29	14	2	3	26	2	29	19	2	Aneu (+7,+8)	Aneu (+7,+8)	Tetra
6	7	5	47	7	11	32	6	2	4	2	33	3	1	Aneu (+7)	Aneu (+7)	Tetra
7	6	2	24	2	11	30	3	4	42	9	11	38	14	Aneu (+7,+8)	Aneu (+7,+8)b	Tetra
8	9	7	12	1	22	18	2	1	42	12	21	18	4	Aneu (+7,+8)	Aneu (+7,+8)	Tetra
9	8	3	10	4	26	11	1	6	5	1	31	10	2	Aneu (+7)	Aneu (+7,+8)	Tetra
10	9	2	15	5	24	8	2	1	35	15	25	22	7	Aneu (+7,+8)	Aneu (+7,+8)	Tetra
11	6	4	16	4	26	8	0	6	13	6	33	4	0	Aneu (+7,+8)	Aneu (+7)	Tetra
12	8	2	35	22	16	39	16	4	24	19	12	35	11	Tetra (+7,+8)	Tetra?(+7,+8)b	Tetra
13	6	4	8	6	26	17	6	3	15	13	31	10	2	Tetra (+7,+8)	Aneu (+7,+8)	Tetra
14	6	4	13	11	10	40	49	4	17	13	18	35	21	Tetra (+7,+8)	Tetra?(+7,+8)b	Tetra
15	6	2	53	51	12	38	17	2	53	49	14	35	16	Tetra (+7,+8)	Tetra?(+7,+8)b	Aneu
16	6	3	29	22	17	18	6	6	38	22	20	18	12	Tetra (+7,+8)	Aneu (+7,+8)b	Aneu
Mean		3	19	9.3	21	18	5.1	4	21	11.2	26	16	5.4			

Each case contained >70% tumor cells in the region evaluated by FISH.

[a] FISH, fluorescence *in situ* hybridization; Aneu, aneuploid; Tetra, tetraploid; Tetra?, the cases for which FISH analysis of tissue sections cannot distinguish aneuploidy from tetraploidy.

[b] Indicates intratumoral heterogeneity detected by FISH.

Table 2
Summary of Advantages and Disadvantages of FISH, PCR, CGH, and Microarrays[a]

Technique	Advantages	Disadvantages
FISH analysis of interphase cells	1) Can exactly enumerate the copy number of chromosome centromeres and specific chromosomal regions within single cells 2) Easily distinguish chromosomal gain from loss 3) Precisely evaluate tumor cells and assess genetic heterogeneity of cancer foci 4) Study genetic changes within a single lesion or within multiple lesions in a single specimen 5) Compare the alterations between different regions of one chromosome and different chromosomes using FISH with multicolor probes	1) Signal counting is labor-intensive 2) Requires large probes (≥1 kb) that target one locus or at most a few loci at a time 3) Requires compensation for such nuclei truncation when tissue sections are analyzed 4) Loss of morphology and insufficient hybridization in isolated nuclei
PCR-based microsatellite analysis	1) Can detect abnormalities of small region (≤100 bp) 2) Requires small amount of DNA per test and results are usually reproducible 3) Mapping allelic imbalance in one or multiple informative loci of chromosomes 4) Can assess microsatellite instability 5) With microdissection, genetic heterogeneity can be assessed within a single lesion and between different lesions	1) Difficult to distinguish gain from loss 2) Examines small portion of the genome with one probing 3) Is not reliable for detecting homozygous deletion 4) Cannot evaluate noninformative loci
CGH	1) Screen entire genome of cancer DNA at one time 2) Easily distinguish chromosomal gain from loss	1) Only can detect large deletion (≥10 MB) 2) Technique is in early stage of development
Microarrays	1) Provide a systematic survey of DNA or RNA variations 2) Can analyze large number of markers for single or multiple DNA samples quickly 3) Allow the determination of genetic alteration patterns of complex ploygenic disorders 4) Facilitate the measurement of RNA levels for the complete set of transcripts of an organism	1) Technique is still in its infancy 2) The tools remain expensive

[a]FISH, fluorescence *in situ* hybridization; PCR, polymerase chain reaction; CGH, comparative genomic hybridization.

genes, microarrays offer the potential of genetic testing for the disease susceptibility of individuals, or even entire populations *(14)*. Applied to expression analysis, this approach facilitates the measurement of RNA levels for the complete set of transcripts of an organism *(30)*. The new generation of array technologies is still in its infancy. The techniques have become established in only a few areas, and the tools remain expensive.

Importantly, applying different molecular cytogenetics techniques to the same specimens can be extremely useful to clarify the discrepancies observed by a single technique alone *(20,21,23,45,47,50,69,79,85,88)*.

4. THE MOST FREQUENTLY GAINED AND DELETED CHROMOSOMAL REGIONS IN PIN AND CARCINOMA

Prostate carcinogenesis apparently involves multiple genetic changes, such as loss of specific genomic sequences which may be associated with inactivation of tumor suppressor genes and gain of some specific chromosome regions which may be associated with activation of oncogenes *(2,11)*. Tables 3 and 4 summarize results of *in situ* hybridization (ISH) analyses, PCR-based microsatellite analyses, and CGH analyses of paired PIN and carcinoma reported in the English-language literature.

4.1. Gain and Loss of Chromosome 7

Cytogenetic analyses have demonstrated that gain, deletion, and translocation of 7q22-q31 are common in prostate adenocarcinoma *(13,53)*. FISH studies have demonstrated that aneusomy of chromosome 7 is frequent in prostate cancer and is associated with higher tumor grade, advanced pathologic stage, and early patient death from prostate cancer *(1,3,78,80)*. Using PCR analysis of microsatellite markers, we and others have identified frequent imbalance of alleles mapped to 7q31 in prostate and other cancers *(23,50,79,87–89)*. In prostate cancer, allelic imbalance of 7q31 is strongly correlated with tumor aggressiveness, progression, and cancer-specific death *(55,70,78)*. These findings suggest that genetic alterations of the 7 q-arm play an important role in the development of prostate cancer *(23,50,79,87–89)*. However, the allelic imbalance detected by PCR has been assumed to be a result of chromosomal loss or deletion *(50,88)*, while FISH studies have uniformly observed gain of the chromosome 7 centromere *(1,3,64,78,80)*. The resolution of this discrepancy is critically important for the definition of the 7q31 anomalies in prostate cancer.

We undertook a molecular cytogenetic study of 25 prostate specimens with FISH probes for the chromosome 7 centromere and for five loci mapped to 7q31 *(44)*. We found that alterations of chromosome 7, the 7 q-arm, and particularly, 7q31, are common in prostate cancer. Unexpectedly, overrepresentation (gain) of 7q31 was more common than deletion of 7q31 and was strongly correlated with tumor Gleason score *(44)*. We also performed FISH analysis of metaphases from an aphidicolin-induced, chromosome 7 only, somatic-cell hybrid *(44)*. We found that the DNA probe for D7S522 spans the common fragile site FRA7G at 7q31. The coincidence of FRA7G with the region showing the greatest allelic imbalance suggests that the instability in this fragile site may be responsible for both the gains and losses of this region. Our observations have two possible implications. It is possible that overrepresentation of the 7 q-arm, of 7q31, and/or genes in these regions may be important for the development and/or

Table 3
Review of Literature Describing Chromosomal Anomalies in Paired Prostatic Intraepithelial Neoplasia and Carcinoma Specimens Using FISH with Chromosome Centromere-Specific Probes[a]

First Author	Chromosome studied	Tissue material	Number of PIN foci	Number of cancer foci	Chromosome anomalies in PIN		Chromosome anomalies in cancer	
					% foci with any anomaly	The most common anomaly	% foci with any anomaly	The most common anomaly
Macoska (55)	4,7,8,10,Y[b]	5-μm paraffin sections	2	15	50	−10	80	+8,+7
Takahashi (78)	7,8,11,12	Needle biopsy core Touch preparation	3	50	33	+7,+8	48	+7,+8
Alers (2)	1,7,8,10,15,Y	4-μm paraffin sections, with biotin-labeled probes	17	25	12	−Y	52	−Y,+8
Qian (64)	7,8,10,12,Y	5-μm paraffin sections of whole-mount prostates	68	78	50	+8,+10	51	+7,+8
Erbersdobler (35)	7,8,10,17,X	5-μm paraffin sections, with biotin-labeled probes	30	15	57	+8,+X	73	+7,+8
Jenkins (43)	7,8,10,12,Y	5-μm paraffin sections of whole-mount prostates	48	84	62	+8,+10	61	+7,+8

[a]FISH, fluorescence in situ hybridization; PIN, prostatic intraepithelial neoplasia; − or + represent loss or gain of chromosome.
[b]Chromosome Y DNA probe was specific for mid distal Yq (Yq12) region.

Table 4
Review of Literature Describing Genetic Changes in Paired Prostatic Intraepithelial Neoplasia and Carcinoma Specimens Using PCR-Based Microsatellite Analysis, FISH with Region-Specific Probes[a]

First author	Tissue material	Number of PIN foci	Number cancer foci	Genetic changes in informative PIN foci (%)							Genetic changes in informative cancer foci (%)						
				7q	8p	8q	10q	12p	16q	18q	7q	8p	8q	10q	12p	16q	18q
Sakr (70)	PCR, paraffin-embedded tissue	9	29	—	29	—	25	0	20	—	—	29	—	18	0	42	—
Macoska (55)	FISH, PCR, frozen tissue	1	10	—	100	0	—	—	—	—	—	70	43	—	—	—	—
Emmert-Buck (34)	PCR, frozen tissue	54	32	—	63	—	—	—	—	—	—	91	—	—	—	—	—
Jenkins (43)	FISH, paraffin-embedded tissue	48	84	—	—	50	—	—	—	—	—	—	44	—	—	—	—
Bostwick (8)	PCR, paraffin-embedded tissue	84	95	17	41	30	—	—	—	19	30	50	33	—	—	—	52

[a]PCR, polymerase chain reation; FISH, fluorescence *in situ* hybridization; PIN, prostatic intraepithelial neoplasia; —, not studied.

progression of a significant proportion of prostate cancer. Conversely, it is also possible that prostate cancer progression is associated with increased chromosomal fragility, perhaps as a result of other genetic alterations *(44)*. Cui et al. confirmed our results by studying 28 prostate cancer specimens with FISH probes for the chromosome 7 centromere and for five loci mapped to 7q31 *(26)*.

We have previously reported that the frequency of trisomy 7 was much higher in carcinoma than PIN *(64)*. Bostwick et al. observed that allelic imbalance at 7q31 was slightly more frequent in prostate cancer than PIN (30 vs 17%) *(8)*. This indicates that gain of chromosome 7 may play a role in the progression of precursor lesions to carcinoma.

4.2. Loss of 8p and Gain of 8q

The chromosome 8 p-arm is one of the most frequently deleted regions in prostate cancer *(10,34,54,56,57)*. Band 8p22 has been the most intensively studied region *(10,41,54,57)*. The rate of 8p22 loss ranged from 29–50% in PIN, 32–69% in primary tumors, and 65–100% in metastatic cancer *(10,54,57)*. Other frequently deleted 8p regions in prostate cancer include 8p21 and 8p12 *(34,50)*. Emmert-Buck et al. found loss of 8p12-21 in 63% of PIN foci and 91% of cancer foci using microdissected frozen tissue *(34)*. Bostwick et al. detected loss of 8p21-12 in 37% of PIN foci and 46% of cancer foci *(8)*. These findings suggest that more than one tumor suppressor gene may be located on 8p, and inactivation of these tumor suppressor genes may be important for the initiation of prostate cancer. The recently cloned FEZ1 gene, which encodes a leucine zipper protein, may be one candidate tumor suppressor gene at 8p22 *(41)*.

In addition to loss of the 8 p-arm, gain of the 8 q-arm has been reported in prostate cancer *(21,43,54,85)*. Bova et al. found gain of 8q in 11% of primary tumors and 40% of lymph node metastases *(10)*. Van Den Berg et al. found amplification of 8q DNA sequences in 75% of cancers metastatic to lymph nodes *(84)*. Similarly, Visakorpi et al. found gain of 8q far more frequently in locally recurrent cancer than in the primary cancer *(85)*. Cher et al. also detected frequent gain of 8q in metastatic and androgen-independent prostate cancer *(21)*. Using FISH, Qian et al. observed that gain of chromosome 8 was the most frequent chromosomal anomaly in metastatic foci, and the frequency was much higher than in PIN and carcinoma *(64)*. Jenkins et al. identified c-myc gene amplification in 22% of metastatic foci, which was much more frequent than in primary cancer (9%) *(43)*. Bubendorf et al. found c-myc amplification in 11% of hormone-refractory prostate cancers *(15)*. Cribriform PIN and carcinoma also seem to have c-myc amplification *(67)*. Recently, we used dual-probe FISH and DNA probes for 8p22 (the LPL gene), the centromere of 8, and 8q24 (the c-myc gene) to determine the corresponding copy numbers in tumor samples from 144 patients with high-grade pathological stage C prostate carcinoma *(71)*. We found that alterations in c-myc were associated with both systemic progression and patient death. Patients with loss of 8p22 and gain of c-myc had the poorest outcome *(71)*. Together, these data suggest that the 8 q-arm may harbor a gene(s) whose amplification and overexpression may play a key role in the progression and evolution of prostatic carcinoma *(43)*. This gene may be c-myc. Overexpression of the c-myc gene has been found in prostate carcinoma *(16,36)*, and we have previously shown that substantial amplification of the c-myc gene is strongly associated with immunohistochemical evidence of the c-myc protein overexpression

(43). Overexpression of c-myc protein has been hypothesized to cause degradation of p27*kip1*, leading to activation of cyclin E/cyclin-dependent kinase 2 and cell proliferation *(9,75).* It has recently been shown that the level of p27*kip1* is associated with Gleason score, tumor recurrence, and patient survival with prostate carcinoma *(22,24,25,83).* A study using in vivo transduction of prostate cancer cells with antisense c-myc demonstrated that tumor growth was reduced by suppressing c-myc protein *(74).* Thus, these observations suggest that overexpression of c-myc deregulates the control of cell growth, resulting in proliferation of prostate carcinoma cells. This overexpression may be most often mediated through an increased c-myc gene copy number *(43).*

Based on these findings, we hypothesize that the accumulation of chromosome 8 aberrations in prostate carcinoma occurs primarily in three steps (Fig. 1, thick arrows). In the first step, 8p is deleted. Mutation or a small deletion of a gene or genes on 8p that is not detectable by FISH also may take place. Previous studies of 8p loss in PIN and in prostate carcinoma support this hypothesis *(7,45,56,57).* Second, a whole chromosome 8 is gained. Perhaps the chromosome 8 that suffered the first 8p loss is the chromosome that is gained. Third, the 8 q-arm is gained. It is possible that one of the chromosome 8 undergoes isochromosome 8q formation, which will simultaneously delete 8p and gain 8q *(20,61,64,85).*

4.3. Gain and Loss of Other Chromosomal Regions

There is a high frequency of allelic imbalance at 10p and 10q in prostate cancer *(31,38,42).* The most commonly deleted region on the 10 q-arm includes bands 10q23-24, and allelic loss of this region may inactive the MXI-1 gene *(31,38,42).* Recently, another candidate gene in this region has been cloned: PTEN *(51).* All four prostate cancer cell lines have recently been shown to have mutations of this gene *(51).* However, we have observed a low frequency of PTEN deletion by FISH in human prostate cancer specimens (Jenkins, unpublished observations). Trybus et al. mapped the common region of 10p deletion to 10p11.2 *(82).*

Chromosome 16 also has been observed to have frequent allelic imbalance in prostate cancer. Carter et al. observed ~30% allelic imbalance at 16q in clinically localized prostate cancer *(17).* Elo et al. and Latil et al. found a high frequency of allelic imbalance at 16q23-q24 *(33,49).* The most commonly deleted region is located at 16q24.1-q24.2, and this deletion was significantly associated with tumor progression *(33,49).* The frequency of loss of 18q22.1 has been observed to be from 20 to 40% in prostate cancer *(38,61).* Cunningham et al. detected allelic imbalance at 21q22.2-22.3 in 23% of cases of prostate cancer and at 3p25-26 in 20% *(27).* Other regions which demonstrate frequent allelic imbalance include 1q24, 5q12-23, 6q, 13q, 17p31.1, 17q, and the X chromosome *(27).* Loss of 10q, 16q, and 18q has also been reported in PIN *(4,27).* Bostwick et al. found loss of 18q12.2-12.3 was higher in prostate cancer than PIN (52 vs 19%, $p = 0.01$), indicating that this region may harbor a gene whose inactivation may be important for the progression of PIN to carcinoma *(8).*

5. PATHOGENETIC RELATIONSHIP BETWEEN PIN AND CARCINOMA

Since 1992, a small number of molecular biologic studies in PIN has been reported *(2,35,43,64,78).* In earlier studies, only a few PIN foci were analyzed with a limited

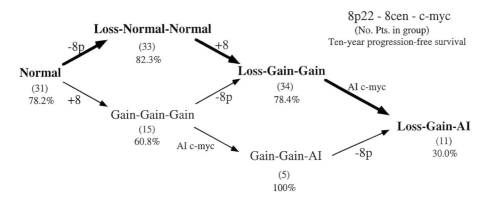

Fig. 1. Possible pathways of chromosome 8 alteration in prostate carcinoma. Thick arrows indicate a potential major pathway and thin arrows indicate a potential minor pathway. –8p, loss of 8p; +8, gain of chromosome 8; additional increase (AI) c-myc, additional increase of the c-myc gene. Loss of 8p and gain of a whole chromosome 8 seem to be the two principal chromosome 8 genetic events in prostate carcinoma. We postulate that the tumors are more prone to have loss of 8p because the frequency of the loss-normal-normal pattern (8p22-8cen-c-myc) (24.3%) (first thick arrow) was higher than that of the gain-gain-gain pattern (10.4%). Next, gain of chromosome 8 (23.6%) is most likely to follow the loss of 8p, resulting in the loss-gain-gain pattern (second thick arrow). Finally, tumors achieve the loss-gain-AI pattern, when they acquire an AI of c-myc (third thick arrow). In the parallel pathway (thin arrows), tumors that initially gain chromosome 8 would also achieve the loss-gain-AI pattern as they lose 8p and acquire an AI of c-myc. Of other combinations with smaller numbers of patients (*see* Table 1), the loss-loss-normal pattern (with two patients) would be included in the major pathway as a variant of loss of 8p, whereas other combinations with an AI of c-myc may not fit these pathways. (Reproduced with permission from ref. *7*).

number of centromere-specific probes *(55,78)*. We previously reported numerical chromosomal anomalies in multiple foci of PIN and carcinoma in 40 whole-mount radical prostatectomy specimens with centromere-specific probes to chromosomes 7, 8, 10, 12, and Y *(64)*. The overall frequency of numeric chromosomal anomalies in PIN and carcinoma foci was remarkably similar *(64)*. To further evaluate the genetic relationship between PIN, primary adenocarcinoma, and lymph node metastases, we studied c-myc gene amplification and numerical chromosomal anomalies in multiple foci of PIN and carcinoma in 25 totally embedded whole-mount radical prostatectomy specimens and 23 matched lymph node metastases *(43)*. Generally, within each prostate, carcinoma foci contained more chromosomal anomalies and extra copies of c-myc than matched PIN foci. The overall frequency of extra c-myc copy-number anomalies and numeric chromosomal anomalies in PIN and carcinoma foci were remarkably similar, suggesting that they share a similar underlying pathogenesis *(43)*. Together with the anatomic association of PIN with cancer that we and others have observed, these findings suggest that PIN is a precursor of carcinoma *(2,43,64)*. However, in some prostates, one or more foci of PIN contained more anomalies than the carcinoma foci *(43,64)*. This indicates that either some PIN foci may have a divergent pathogenesis, that some PIN foci may morphologically progress to cancer more slowly than other PIN foci, or that foci of carcinoma may occasionally be derived from other precursor lesions such as atypical adenomatous hyperplasia *(6)*.

Interestingly, cribriform PIN and cribriform cancer generally exhibited similar anomalies, although the percentage of foci with gain of chromosomes 10 and 12 was higher in cribriform cancer, which support the hypothesis that the cribriform pattern of PIN is closely associated with the cribriform pattern of prostatic carcinoma *(19)*. These findings are important for clarifying the controversy regarding the terminology and grading of the cribriform pattern of prostate cancer.

High-grade PIN and prostatic carcinoma are usually multifocal, indicating a field effect of carcinogenesis *(58,68)*. Our work has demonstrated that extra c-myc copies and chromosomal anomalies can be found in one focus of PIN, while other PIN foci have no apparent FISH anomalies or have other anomalies in whole-mount prostates *(43,64)*. Similar intraglandular genetic heterogeneity was observed in multiple foci of carcinoma *(43,64)*. In general, the dominant focus of carcinoma showed more genetic changes than other smaller foci. However, some small, low-grade tumor foci showed a high level of c-myc amplification and were aneuploid by FISH, while concurrent dominant high-grade tumor foci were normal, indicating that small cancers can have significant alterations. Using PCR, FISH, and DNA ploidy techniques, similar intraglandular heterogeneity has been reported *(39,50,60)*. Thus, the size of a cancer focus and its degree of histologic dedifferentiation does not always reflect the extent of its genetic derangement *(39,43,64)*.

Frequent heterogeneity of genetic change within a single tumor focus (intratumor genetic heterogeneity) of prostate cancer has been reported with molecular genetic techniques *(19,35)*. Using FISH with c-myc regional probes and centromere-specific probes, we observed that 18% of all carcinoma foci and 52% of the dominant (largest) foci showed heterogeneity of c-myc copy number and chromosome number *(43)*. Thus, a subpopulation of cells with additional genetic alterations can develop within an apparently histologically uniform region *(43,64)*. The intraglandular and intratumoral genetic heterogeneity of prostate cancer indicates that, without broad and systematic scrutiny of all preneoplastic and neoplastic foci in a prostate, significant genetic changes will not be detected.

6. THE MOLECULAR BASIS FOR PROSTATE CANCER METASTASIS

The molecular basis for prostate cancer metastasis remains unclear *(21,43,64,70)*. Sakr et al. reported that some lymph node metastases did not share genetic alterations with the primary tumor, but this result may have been caused by incomplete sampling of prostate cancer foci *(70)*. In a previous study, we evaluated c-myc gene dosage and chromosome centromere copy number in a series of carefully mapped multiple primary cancer foci and matched lymph node metastases *(43)*. We found that all 23 metastatic foci showed multiple FISH anomalies. The frequency of c-myc gene amplification and chromosomal aneusomy and the average number of extra c-myc copies and abnormal chromosomes per nucleus were higher than that of the primary tumor, indicating that primary tumor cells with multiple genetic anomalies usually metastasize and/or that metastatic lesions are genetically unstable *(43)*. We also observed that metastases were not necessarily derived from the most abundant clone in the primary tumor *(43,64)*. Indeed, our data indicate that these subpopulations have acquired additional alterations, such as c-myc gene amplification, that are often associated with similar alterations in concomitant metastases *(43)*.

To further investigate the molecular mechanism of metastasis, we carefully evaluated several chromosomal regions by FISH in paired multiple primary carcinomas (119 foci) and corresponding lymph node metastases (114 foci) from 37 patients (Qian et al., submitted for publication). We found that all metastatic foci showed multiple FISH anomalies and usually shared several genetic changes with the paired primary tumors. However, the incidence of +c-myc, simultaneous -8p and +c-myc (possible i(8q) formation), simultaneous +CEP17 and +p53 (possible gain of a whole 17 or a 17 p-arm), and the pattern of -8p, +c-myc, +7q and +p53 were significantly higher in lymph node metastases than in primary tumors (Qian et al., submitted for publication). These findings suggest that additional genetic changes are required for the tumor to metastasize to local lymph nodes, and/or that metastatic lesions are genetically unstable. We also observed that one or more primary tumors usually shared the same FISH alterations as those in corresponding ipsilateral multiple lymph node metastases. This suggests that just a single tumor focus gave rise to the metastatic lesions. Most metastatic lesions had the same alterations as other metastatic lesions within the same patient. However, seven cases had different genetic changes among the multiple metastases. These differences were usually identified in metastases that were located on different sides of the body, indicating that more than one primary tumor focus may give rise to different metastases and/or that metastatic lesions are genetically unstable (Qian et al., submitted for publication). In addition, we found that the metastatic cancer cells within the same lymph node usually have homogeneous histologic characteristics and chromosomal anomalies. This suggests that a single metastasized cancer-cell clone with multiple genetic changes expands quickly within a lymph node.

There may be some other gene (genes) which are involved in triggering the metastases to remote sites *(29,62,86)*. Suzuki et al. found that multiple lymph-node metastases within a patient usually share PTEN gene alterations, although a substantial amount of mutational heterogeneity existed among different remote metastatic sites *(77)*. Further comprehensive study of a large series of patients with multiple remote metastases will be very useful for understanding the molecular basis of prostate cancer metastasis.

7. CONCLUSION

FISH, PCR, and CGH are commonly used techniques for detecting gene and chromosome dosage in human specimens. The recently developed microarray techniques are powerful tools for the study of tumor genome. However, each technique has advantages and disadvantages. Applying different techniques to the same specimens can be extremely useful to clarify discrepancies observed by a single technique, and to further define the role of PIN in prostate carcinogenesis.

The most common genetic alterations in PIN and carcinoma are gain of chromosome 7, particularly 7q31; loss of 8p and gain of 8q; and loss of 10q, 16q, and 18q. Inactivation of tumor suppressor genes and/or overexpression of oncogenes at these regions may be important for the initiation and progression of prostate cancer. These alterations are potential genetic markers for predicting tumor progression and for choosing appropriate therapy.

PIN and prostatic carcinoma foci have a similar proportion of genetic changes, but the foci of carcinoma usually have more alterations. This supports the hypothesis that PIN is the most likely precursor of prostatic carcinoma, and both are influenced by the field change of prostatic carcinogenesis. One or more foci of the primary tumor usually share chromosomal anomalies with associated lymph node metastases, suggesting that often just a single focus of carcinoma gives rise to metastases.

REFERENCES

1. Alcaraz, A., S. Takahashi, J. A. Brown, J. F. Herath, E. Bergstralh, J. Larson-Keller, et al. 1994. Aneuploidy and aneusomy of chromosome 7 detected by fluorescence in situ hybridization are markers of poor prognosis in prostate cancer. *Cancer Res.* **54:** 3998–4002.
2. Alers, C. A., P. J. Krijtenburg, K. J. Vissers, F. T. Bosman, T. H. van der Kwast, and H. Dekken. 1995. Interphase cytogenetics of prostatic adenocarcinoma and precursor lesions: analysis of 25 radical prostatectomies and 17 adjacent prostatic intraepithelial neoplasias. *Genes Chromosomes Cancer* **12:** 241–250.
3. Bandyk, M. G., L. Zhao, and P. Troncoso. 1994. Trisomy 7: a potential cytogenetic markers of human prostate cancer progression. *Genes Chromosomes Cancer* **9:** 19–27.
4. Bergerheim, U. S. R., K. Kunimi, V. P. Collins, and P. Ekman. 1991. Deletion of chromosomes 8, 10, and 16 in human prostatic carcinoma. *Genes Chromosomes Cancer* **3:** 215–220.
5. Blute, M. L., H. Zincke, and G. M. Farrow. 1986. Long-term followup of young patients with stage A adenocarcinoma of the prostate. *J. Urol.* **136:** 840–843.
6. Bostwick, D. G. and J. Qian. 1995. Atypical adenomatous hyperplasia of the prostate: relationship with carcinoma in 217 whole mount radical prostatectomies. *Am. J. Surg. Path.* **19:** 506–518.
7. Bostwick, D. G., A. Pacelli, and A. Lopez-Beltran. 1996. Molecular biology of prostatic intraepithelial neoplasia. *Prostate* **29:** 117–134.
8. Bostwick, D. G., A. Shan, J. Qian, M. Darson, N. J. Maihle, R. B. Jenkins, et al. 1998. Independent origin of multiple foci of prostatic intraepithelial neoplasia. *Cancer* **83:** 1995–2002.
9. Bouchard, C., P. Staller, and M. Eilers. 1998. Control of cell proliferation by Myc. *Trends Cell Biol.* **8:** 202–206.
10. Bova, G. S., B. S. Carter, M. J. G. Bussemakers, M. Emi, Y. Fujiwara, N. Kyprianou, et al. 1993. Homozygous deletion and frequent allelic loss of chromosome 8p22 loci in human prostate cancer. *Cancer Res.* **53:** 3869–3873.
11. Bova, G. S. and W. B. Isaacs. 1996. Review of allelic loss and gain in prostate cancer. *World J. Urol.* **14:** 338–346.
12. Bowtell, D. D. 1999. Options available—from start to finish—for obtaining expression data by microarray. *Nat. Genet.* **21(1 Suppl.):** 25–32.
13. Brothman, A. R., D. M. Peehl, and J. E. McNeal. 1990. Frequency and pattern of karyotypic anomalies in human prostate cancer. *Cancer Res.* **50:** 3795–3803.
14. Brown, P. O. and D. Botstein. 1999. Exploring the new world of the genome with DNA microarrays. *Nat. Genet.* **21(1 Suppl):** 33–37.
15. Bubendorf, L., J. Kononen, P. Koivisto, P. Schraml, H. Moch, T. C. Gasser, et al. 1999. Survey of gene amplifications during prostate cancer progression by high-throughout fluorescence in situ hybridization on tissue microarrays. *Cancer Res.* **59:** 803–806.
16. Buttyan, R., I. S. Sawczuk, M. C. Benson, J. D. Siegal, and C. A. Olsson. 1987. Enhanced expression of the c-myc protooncogene in high-grade human prostate cancers. *Prostate* **11:** 327–337.

17. Carter, B. S., C. M. Ewing, W. S. Ward, B. F. Treiger, T. W. Aalders, J. A. Schalken, et al. 1990. Allelic loss of chromosomes 16q and 10q in human prostate cancer. *Proc. Natl. Acad. Sci. USA* **87:** 8751–8755.

18. Catalona, W. J. 1994. Management of cancer of the prostate. *N. Engl. J. Med.* **331:** 996–1004.

19. Cheng, L., A. Shan, J. C. Cheville, J. Qian, and D. G. Bostwick. 1998. Atypical adenomatous hyperplasia of the prostate: a premalignant lesion? *Cancer Res.* **58:** 389–391.

20. Cher, M. L., D. MacGrogan, R. Bookstein, J. A. Brown, R. B. Jenkins, and R. H. Jensen. 1994. Comparative genomic hybridization, allelic imbalance, and fluorescence in situ hybridization on chromosome 8 in prostate cancer. *Genes Chromosomes Cancer* **11:** 153–162.

21. Cher, M. L., G. S. Bova, D. H. Moore, E. J. Small, P. R. Carroll, S. S. Pin, et al. 1996. Genetic alterations in untreated metastases and androgen-independent prostate cancer detected by comparative genomic hybridization and allelotyping. *Cancer Res.* **56:** 3091–3102.

22. Cheville, J. C., R. V. Lloyd, T. J. Sebo, L. Cheng, L. Erickson, and D. G. Bostwick. 1998. Expression of p27kip1 in prostatic adenocarcinoma. *Mod. Pathol.* **11:** 324–328.

23. Collard, J. G., M. van de Poll, A. Scheffer, E. Roos, A. H. M. Hopman, A. H. M. Geurts van Kessel, et al. 1987. Location of genes involved in invasion and metastasis on human chromosome 7. *Cancer Res.* **47:** 6666–6670.

24. Cordon-Cardo, C., A. Koff, M. Drobnjak, P. Capodieci, I. Osman, and S. S. Millard. 1998. Distinct altered patterns of p27kip1 gene expression in benign prostatic hyperplasia and prostatic carcinoma. *J. Natl. Cancer Inst.* **90:** 1284–1291.

25. Cote, R J., Y. Shi, S. Groshen, A.-C. Feng, C. Cordon-Cardo, and D. Skinner. 1998. Association of p27kip1 levels with recurrence and survival in patients with stage C prostate carcinoma. *J. Natl. Cancer Inst.* **90:** 916–920.

26. Cui, J., D. A. Deubler, L. R. Rohr, X. L. Zhu, T. M. Maxwell, J. E. Changus, et al. 1998. Chromosome 7 abnormalities in prostate cancer detected by dual-color fluorescence in situ hybridization. *Cancer Genet. Cytogenet.* **107:** 51–60.

27. Cunningham, J. M., A. Shan, M. J. Wick, S. K. McDonnell, D. J. Schaid, D. J. Tester, et al. 1996. Allelic imbalance and microsatellite instability in prostatic adenocarcinoma. *Cancer Res.* **56:** 4475–4482.

28. Davidson, D., D. G. Bostwick, J. Qian, P. Wollan, J. E. Osterling, R. Rudders, et al. 1995. Prostatic intraepithelial neoplasia is predictive of adenocarcinoma. *J. Urol.* **154:** 1295–1299.

29. Dong, J. T., P. W. Lamb, C. W. Rinker-Schaeffer, J. Vukanovic, T. Ichikawa, J. T. Isaacs, et al. 1995. KAI1, a metastasis suppressor gene for prostate cancer on human chromosome 11p11.2. *Science* **268:** 884–886.

30. Duggan, D. J., M. Bittner, Y. Chen, P. Meltzer, and J. M. Trent. 1999. Expression profiling using cDNA microarrays. *Nat. Genet.* **21(1 Suppl.):** 10–14.

31. Eagle, L., X. Yin, A. Brothman, B. J. William, N. Atkin, and E. Prochownik. 1995. Mutation of the MXI 1 gene in prostate cancer. *Nat. Genet.* **9:** 249–255.

32. Effert, P. J., A. Neubauer, P. J. Walther, and E. T. Liu. 1992. Alterations of p53 gene are associated with the progression of a human prostate carcinoma. *J. Urol.* **147:** 789–793.

33. Elo, J. P., P. Harkonen, A. P. Kyllonen, O. Lukkarinen, M. Poutanen, R. Vihko, et al. 1997. Loss of heterozygosity at 16q24.1-q24.2 is significantly associated with metastatic and aggressive behavior of prostate cancer. *Cancer Res.* **57:** 3356–3359.

34. Emmert-Buck, M. R., C. D. Vocke, R. O. Pozzatti, P. H. Duray, S. Jennings, C. D. Florence, et al. 1995. Allelic loss on chromosome 8p12-21 in microdissected prostatic intraepithelial neoplasia. *Cancer Res.* **55:** 2959–2962.

35. Erbersdobler, A., N. Gurses, and R. P. Henke. 1996. Numerical chromosomal changes in high-grade prostatic intraepithelial neoplasia (PIN) and concomitant invasive carcinoma. *Pathol. Res. Pract.* **192:** 418–427.

36. Fleming, W. H., A. Hamel, R. MacDonald, E. Ramsey, N. M. Pettigrew, and B. Johnston. 1986. Expression of the c-myc protooncogene in human prostatic carcinoma and benign prostatic hyperplasia. *Cancer Res.* **46:** 1535–1538.

37. Gittes, R. F. 1991. Carcinoma of the prostate. *N. Engl. J. Med.* **324:** 236–245.
38. Gray, I. C., S. M. A. Philips, S. J. Lee, J. P. Neoptolemos, J. Weissenbach, and N. K. Spurr. 1995. Loss of chromosome region 10q23-25 in prostate cancer. *Cancer Res.* **55:** 4800–4803.
39. Greene, D. R., E. Rogers, E. C. Wessels, T. M. Wheeler, S. R. Taylor, R. A. Santucci, et al. 1994. Some small prostate cancers are nondiploid by nuclear image analysis: correlation of deoxyribonucleic acid ploidy status and pathological features. *J. Urol.* **151:** 1301–1307.
40. Isaacs, W. B., G. S. Bova, R. A. Morton, M. J. Bussemaker, J. D. Brooks, and C. M. Ewing. 1995. Molecular genetics and chromosomal alterations in prostate cancer. *Cancer* **75:** 2004–2012.
41. Ishii, H., R. Baffa, S. I. Numata, Y. Murakumo, S. Rattan, H. Inoue, et al. 1999. The FEZ1 gene at chromosome 8p22 encodes a leucine-zipper protein, and its expression is altered in multiple human tumors. *Proc. Natl. Acad. Sci. USA* **96:** 3928–3933.
42. Ittman, M. 1996. Allelic loss on chromosome 10 in prostate adenocarcinoma. *Cancer Res.* **56:** 2143–2147.
43. Jenkins, R. B., J. Qian, M. M. Lieber, and D. G. Bostwick. 1997. Detection of c-myc oncogene amplification and chromosomal anomalies in metastatic prostatic carcinoma by fluorescence *in situ* hybridization (FISH). *Cancer Res.* **57:** 524–531.
44. Jenkins, R. B., J. Qian, H. K. Lee, H. Huang, K. Hirasawa, D. G. Bostwick, et al. 1998. A molecular cytogenetic analysis of 7q31 in prostate cancer. *Cancer Res.* **58:** 759–766.
45. Jenkins, R. B., S. Takahashi, K. A. Delacey, E. Bergstralh, and M. M. Lieber. 1998. Prognostic significance of allelic imbalance of chromosome regions 7q, 8p, 16q, and 18q in stage T3N0M0 prostate cancer. *Genes Chromosomes Cancer* **21:** 131–143.
46. Johansson, J. E., H. O. Adami, S. O. Andersson, R. Bergstrom, L. Holmberg, and U. B. Krusemo. 1992. High 10-year survival rate in patients with early, untreated prostatic cancer. *JAMA* **267:** 2191–2196.
47. Joos, S., U. S. R. Bergerheim, Y. Pan, H. Matsuyama, M. Bentz, S. Dumanir, et al. 1995. Mapping of chromosomal gains and losses in prostate cancer by comparative genomic hybridization. *Genes Chromosomes Cancer* **14:** 267–276.
48. Landis, S. H., T. Murray, S. Bolden, and P. A. Wingo. 1998. Cancer statistics, 1998. *CA Cancer J. Clin.* **48:** 6–29.
49. Latil, A., O. Cussenot, G. Fournier, K. Driouch, L. Lidereau, M. L. Cher, et al. 1994. Comparative genomic hybridization, allelic imbalance, and fluorescence in situ hybridization on chromosome 8 in prostate cancer. *Genes Chromosomes Cancer* **11:** 153–162.
50. Latil, A., O. Cussenot, G. Fournier, J. C. Baron, and R. Lidereau. 1995. Loss of heterozygosity at 7q31 is a frequent and early event in prostate cancer. *Clin. Cancer Res.* **1:** 1385–1389.
51. Li, J., C. Yen, D. Liaw, K. Podsypanina, S. Bose, S. I. Wang, et al. 1997. PTEN, a putative protein tyrosine phosphatase gene mutated in human brain, breast, and prostate cancer. *Science* **275:** 1943–1947.
52. Lieber, M. M., P. A. Murtaugh, G. M. Farrow, R. P. Myers, and H. Zincke. 1995. DNA ploidy and surgically treated prostate cancer: Important independent association with prognosis for patients with prostate carcinoma treated by radical prostatectomy. *Cancer* **75:** 1935–1943.
53. Lundgren, R., N. Mandahl, S. Heim, J. Limon, H. Henrikson, and F. Mitelman. 1992. Cytogenetic analysis of 57 primary prostatic adenocarcinomas. *Genes Chromosomes Cancer* **4:** 16–24.
54. MacGrogan, D. M., A. Levy, D. G. Bostwick, M. Wagner, D. Wells, and R. Bookstein. 1994. Loss of chromosome arm 8p loci in prostate cancer. *Genes Chromosomes Cancer* **10:** 151–159.
55. Macoska, J. A., M. A. Micale, W. A. Sakr, P. D. Benson, and S. R Wolman. 1993. Extensive genetic alterations in prostate cancer revealed by dual PCR and FISH analysis. *Genes Chromosomes Cancer* **8:** 88–97.

56. Macoska, J. A., T. M. Trybus, W. A. Sakr, M. C. Wolf, P. D. Benson, I. J. Powell, et al. 1994. Fluorescence in situ hybridization analysis of 8p allelic loss and chromosome 8 instability in human prostate cancer. *Cancer Res.* **54:** 3824–3830.

57. Macoska, J. A., T. M. Trybus, P. D. Benson, W. A. Sakr, D. J. Grignon, K. D. Wojno, et al. 1995. Evidence for three tumor suppressor gene loci on chromosome 8p in human prostate cancer. *Cancer Res.* **55:** 5390–5395.

58. McNeal, J. E. and D. G. Bostwick. 1986. Intraductal dysplasia: a premalignant lesion of the prostate. *Hum. Pathol.* **17:** 64–71.

59. McNeal, J. E., J. Alroy, I. Leav, E. A. Redwine, F. S. Freiha, and T. A. Stamey. 1988. Immunohistochemical evidence for impaired cell differentiation in the premalignant phase of prostate carcinogenesis. *Am. J. Clin. Path.* **90:** 23–32.

60. Mirchandani, D., J. Zheng, G. J. Miller, A. K. Ghosh, D. K. Shibata, R. J. Cote, et al. 1995. Heterogeneity in intratumor distribution of p53 mutations in human prostate cancer. *Am. J. Pathol.* **147:** 92–101.

61. Nag, A. and R. G. Smith. 1989. Amplification, rearrangement, and elevated expression of c-myc in human prostatic carcinoma cell line LNCaP. *Prostate* **15:** 115–122.

62. Perez-Stable, C., N. H. Altman, P. P. Mehta, L. J. Deftos, and B. A. Roos. 1997. Prostate cancer progression, metastasis, and gene expression in transgenic mice. *Cancer Res.* **57:** 900–906.

63. Pisansky, T. M., S. S. Cha, J. D. Earle, E. D. Durr, T. F. Kozelsky, H. Wieand, et al. 1993. Prostate-specific antigen as a pretherapy prognostic factor in patients treated with radiation therapy for clinically localized prostate cancer. *J. Clin. Oncol.* **11:** 2158–2166.

64. Qian, J., D. G. Bostwick, S. Takahashi, T. J. Borell, J. F. Herath, M. Lieber, et al. 1995. Chromosomal anomalies in prostatic intraepithelial neoplasia and carcinoma detected by fluorescence in situ hybridization. *Cancer Res.* **55:** 5408–5414.

65. Qian, J., R. B. Jenkins, and D. G. Bostwick. 1995. Chromosomal anomalies in atypical adenomatous hyperplasia and carcinoma of the prostate using fluorescence *in situ* hybridization. *Urology* **46:** 837–842.

66. Qian, J., D. G. Bostwick, S. Takahashi, T. J. Borell, J. A. Brown, M. M. Lieber, et al. 1996. Comparison of fluorescence *in situ* hybridization analysis of isolated nuclei and routine histological sections from paraffin-embedded prostatic adenocarcinoma specimens. *Am. J. Pathol.* **149:** 1193–1199.

67. Qian, J., R. B. Jenkins, and D. G. Bostwick. 1997. Detection of chromosomal anomalies and c-myc gene amplification in the cribriform pattern of prostatic intraepithelial neoplasia and carcinoma by fluorescence in situ hybridization. *Mod. Pathol.* **10:** 1113–1119.

68. Qian, J., P. Wollan, and D. G. Bostwick. 1997. The extent and multicentricity of high grade intraepithelial neoplasia in clinically localized prostatic adenocarcinoma. *Hum. Pathol.* **28:** 143–148.

69. Qian, J., R. B. Jenkins, and D. G. Bostwick. 1998. Determination of gene and chromosome dosage in prostatic intraepithelial neoplasia and carcinoma. *Anal. Quant. Cytol. Histol.* **20:** 373–380.

70. Sakr, W. A., J. A. Macoska, P. D. Benson, D. J. Grignon, S. R. Wolman, J. E. Pontes, et al. 1994. Allelic loss in locally metastatic, multisampled prostate cancer. *Cancer Res.* **54:** 3273–3279.

71. Sato, K., J. Qian, J. M. Slezak, M. M. Lieber, D. G. Bostwick, E. Bergstralh, et al. 1999. Clinical significance of alterations of chromosome 8 in high-grade advanced (stage C) prostate carcinoma. *J. Natl. Cancer Inst.* **91:** 1574–1580.

72. Shackney, S. E., C. A. Smith, and B. W. Miller. 1989. Model for the genetic evolution of human solid tumors. *Cancer Res.* **49:** 3344–3354.

73. Southern, E., K. Mir, and M. Shchepinov. 1999. Molecular interactions on microarrays. *Nat. Genet.* **21(1 Suppl.):** 5–9.

74. Steiner, M. S., C. T. Anthony, Y. Lu, and J. T. Holt. 1998. Antisense c-myc retroviral vector suppresses established human prostate cancer. *Hum. Gene Ther.* **9:** 747–755.

75. Steiner, P., A. Philipp, J. Lukas, S. Godden-Kent, M. Pagano, and S. Mittnacht. 1995. Identification of a Myc-dependent step during the formation of active G1 cyclin-cdk 7 complexes. *EMBO J.* **14:** 4814–4826.

76. Stemmermann, G. N., A. M. Nomura, P. H. Chyou, and R. Yatani. 1992. A prospective comparison of prostate cancer at autopsy and as a clinical event: the Hawaii Japanese experience. *Cancer Epidemiol. Biomark. Prev.* **1:** 189–193.

77. Suzuki, H., D. Freije, D. R. Nusskern, K. Okami, P. Cairns, D. Sidransky, et al. 1998. Interfocal heterogeneity of PTEN/MMAC1 gene alterations in multiple metastatic prostate cancer tissue. *Cancer Res.* **58:** 204–209.

78. Takahashi, S., J. Qian, J. A. Brown, A. Alcaraz, D. G. Bostwick, M. M. Lieber, et al. 1994. Potential markers of prostate cancer aggressiveness detected by fluorescence in situ hybridization. *Cancer Res.* **54:** 3574–3579.

79. Takahashi, S., A. Shan, S. R. Ritland, K. Delacey, D. G. Bostwick, M. M. Lieber, et al. 1995. Frequent loss of heterozygosity at 7q31.1 in primary prostate cancer is associated with tumor aggressiveness and progression. *Cancer Res.* **55:** 4114–4119.

80. Takahashi, S., A. Alcaraz, J. A. Brown, T. J. Borell, J. F. Herath, E. J. Bergstralh, et al. 1996. Aneusomies of chromosomes 8 and Y detected by fluorescence in situ hybridization are prognostic markers for pathologic stage C ($pT_3N_0M_0$) prostate carcinoma. *Clin. Cancer Res.* **2:** 137–145.

81. Thompson, C. T., P. E. LeBoit, P. M. Nederlof, and J. W. Gray. 1994. Thick section fluorescence in situ hybridization on formalin-fixed, paraffin-embedded archival tissue provides a histogenetic profile. *Am. J. Pathol.* **144:** 237–243.

82. Trybus, T. M., A. C. Burgess, K. J. Wojno, T. W. Glover, and J. A. Macoska. 1996. Distinct areas of allelic loss on chromosomal regions 10p and 10q in human prostate cancer. *Cancer Res.* **56:** 2263–2267.

83. Tsihlias, T., L. R. Kapusta, G. DeBoer, I. Morava-Protzner, I. Zbieranowski, and N. Bhattacharya. 1998. Loss of cyclin-dependent kinase inhibitor p27kip1 is a novel prognostic factor in localized human prostate adenocarcinoma. *Cancer Res.* **58:** 542–548.

84. Van Den Berg, C., X. Y. Guan, D. Von Hoff, R. B. Jenkins, M. Bitter, C. Griffin, et al. 1995. DNA sequence amplification in human prostate cancer identified by chromosome microdissection: potential prognostic implications. *Clin. Cancer Res.* **1:** 11–18.

85. Visakorpi, T., A. H. Kallioniemi, A. C. Syvanen, E. R. Hyytinen, R. Karhu, T. Tammela, et al. 1995. Genetic changes in primary and recurrent prostate cancer by comparative genomic hybridization. *Cancer Res.* **55:** 342–347.

86. Xu, J., D. Meyers, D. Freije, S. Isaacs, K. Wiley, D. Nusskern, et al. 1998. Evidence for a prostate cancer susceptibility locus on the X chromosome. *Nat. Genet.* **20:** 175–179.

87. Zenklusen, J. C., I. Bieche, R. Lidereau, and C. J. Conti. 1994. $(C-A)_n$ microsatellite repeat D7S522 is the most commonly deleted region in human primary breast cancer. *Proc. Natl. Acad. Sci. USA* **91:** 12,155–12,158.

88. Zenklusen, J. C., J. C. Thompson, P. Troncoso, J. Kagan, and C. J. Conti. 1994. Loss of heterozygosity in human primary prostate carcinoma: a possible tumor suppressor gene at 7q31.1. *Cancer Res.* **54:** 6370–6373.

89. Zenklusen, J. C., J. C. Thompson, A. J. P. Klein-Szanto, and C. J. Conti. 1995. Frequent loss of heterozygosity in human primary squamous cell and colon carcinomas at 7q31.1: evidence for a broad range tumor suppressor gene. *Cancer Res.* **55:** 1347–1350.

9

Genetic Alterations in Prostatic Intraepithelial Neoplasia (PIN)

Paul H. Duray, MD, David K. Ornstein, MD, Cathy D. Vocke, PhD,
Stephen M. Hewitt, MD, PhD, Kristina A. Cole, MD, PhD,
John W. Gillespie, MD, Chad R. Englert, MD,
Emanuel F. Petricoin, PhD, David B. Krizman, PhD,
W. Marston Linehan, MD, and Michael R. Emmert-Buck, MD, PhD

1. INTRODUCTION

Prostatic intraepithelial neoplasia (PIN) is the histologic lesion most strongly associated with prostate cancer, and has been postulated to be a premalignant lesion. However, much of the natural history of PIN remains unknown. A more fundamental understanding of the relationship between PIN and invasive tumors at the molecular level is critically needed, and represents an important future challenge for investigators. This chapter reviews the clinical, pathologic, and genetic studies addressing the relationship between PIN and cancer. The final section presents newly developing techniques and research approaches in molecular pathology and describes how these methods can be used to study PIN.

2. CLINICAL ASPECTS OF PIN

The implementation of widespread PSA-based screening programs has enhanced the ability to diagnose prostate cancer at an early stage, so that in contemporary series more than 60% of prostate cancer patients have organ-confined disease at the time of diagnosis (19,45). The downward-stage migration associated with PSA-based screening programs has resulted in marked improvements in progression-free survival after local therapies (84). Yet prostate cancer results in substantial morbidity, and remains the second leading cause of cancer deaths among American men (55,94,95). Therefore, research efforts aimed at devising effective strategies to prevent prostate cancer are tremendously important. Development of methods to identify men with premalignant lesions and therapies to prevent progression to invasive malignancy should be an effective way to reduce prostate cancer mortality. Currently, alterations in serum total and free PSA levels are the earliest known clinical changes associated with prostate cancer development (37,72,82). However the specificity of early PSA changes is limited, and PSA changes alone are not currently used to direct therapy.

From: *Prostate Cancer: Biology, Genetics, and the New Therapeutics*
Edited by: L. W. K. Chung, W. B. Isaacs, and J. W. Simons © Humana Press Inc., Totowa, NJ

Table 1
Risk of Prostate Cancer on Repeat Biopsy
after Initial Biopsy Demonstrating HGPIN

Series	Year	% Cancer on repeat biopsy
Brawer, et al. *(16)*	1991	57%
Shepherd, et al. *(18)*	1996	47%
Raviv, et al. *(72)*	1996	47.9%
Davidson, et al. *(24)*	1995	35%
Weinstein, et al. *(93)*	1993	75%

There is substantial clinical evidence linking HGPIN to invasive prostate cancer. HGPIN was found in 86% of 195 radical prostatectomy specimens *(67)*. In clinical practice, the finding of HGPIN on needle biopsy of the prostate indicates a significant risk for prostate cancer *(24,49,67,72,78,93)*. Studies shown in Table 1 indicate that cancer will be detected on repeat biopsy in 35–75% of men with isolated HGPIN on initial biopsy. Conversely, isolated LGPIN is not associated with an increased risk of cancer detection on subsequent biopsy. The best predictors of which men with HGPIN will have cancer on subsequent biopsy are the serum PSA level and the digital rectal exam *(99)*; however, HGPIN alone without carcinoma has not been proven to elevate the serum PSA *(2)*. Since the risk of cancer is high regardless of the PSA and rectal exam results, most clinicians recommend rebiopsy of men with isolated HGPIN. Preliminary studies suggest that serum-free/total PSA measurement provides additional predictive information, but it has yet to be determined how the free/total PSA measurement will be used to direct clinical practice in patients with PIN *(50)*. This is an important clinical issue, and improvements in the ability to determine those men with isolated HGPIN and those who also harbor an undiagnosed invasive prostate are needed.

3. HISTOPATHOLOGY OF PIN

PIN is believed to arise in preexisting ducts rather than through formation of new acinar epithelium. This premise is based on histopathologic observation where one consistently observes cell groups exhibiting the cytologic abnormalities that characterize PIN growing adjacent to benign epithelium. In this regard, PIN development appears to follow other models of premalignant epithelial proliferation, such as those seen in colorectal cancer and Barrett's esophagus *(91,98)*. Table 2 summarizes the histopathological criteria that characterize high- and low-grade PIN. Typical benign prostatic glandular epithelial hyperplasia consists of uniform oval nuclei that are small and uniformly chromatic. There should be no conspicuous nucleoli, and the key cytologic element is the small size of the cells. LGPIN shows a background similar to hyperplasia but with scattered larger cells with more prominent nuclei and normal-appearing chromatin. There is some degree of nuclear-size variability, but no striking enlargement of the nucleoli. The key is the presence of larger cells with scattered and isolated nuclear variability. HGPIN is characterized by cell enlargement, cell-shape variability, darkly clumped chromatin with enlarged nucleoli, and one or more nucleoli per nucleus. Most of the cells within the architectural unit (tuft, papilla, cribriform

Table 2
Summary of Diagnostic Features of Prostatic Intraepithelial Neoplasia (PIN)[a]

PIN grade	Nucleoli	Chromatin	Nuclear membrane	Cellularity
1 Low	Absent to rare	No change	Delicate	Mild stratification
2 High	Numerous	Coarse	Thickened	Grouped and crowded
3 High	Approaches 100%	Perinuclear clearing	Thickened, folded	Grouped and overlapped

[a]Modified after Bostwick *(9,10)*.

plate, duct lining) will be similarly abnormal. These populations of PIN cells are readily detectable at low magnification because of the to a discernible dark appearance of the architectural unit in contrast with adjacent normal epithelium or tumor.

The most common architectural form of PIN is the tufted pattern followed closely by the micropapillary unit *(10)*. As the term implies, the abnormal epithelium occupies papillary fronds and is usually depicted as small (micropapillary) papillae (Figs. 1, 2). The tufted architectural pattern shows the PIN cells to be mounded in variable thickness, yielding an undulating epithelial lining (Figs. 3, 4). Alternatively, a ductular structure lined by attenuated one- or two-layered PIN epithelium is called the flat pattern. The last architectural pattern is the cribriform unit, which may be easily confused with the cribriform carcinoma it mimics. Cribriform HGPIN can occur as a standalone unit in prostate needle biopsies, and presents a diagnostic challenge for the pathologist. There are some useful clues to permit separation of cribriform HGPIN from cancer. For example, high molecular-wt keratins are recognized by the antibody 34BE12 and are expressed in basal cells and the basement membrane region of benign prostatic ducts and acini, but are lost in carcinomatous units *(9,16)*. In PIN, the immunostaining for high molecular-wt keratin is retained, but appears as a discontinuous pattern. This may be difficult to discern in some cases, and multiple histologic sections are often required for proper evaluation. The majority of cribriform carcinomas will show more mitoses than cribriform HGPIN, but this quantitation cannot be relied upon in all cases. A practical outcome of future research efforts to delineate the genetic profiles of premalignant lesions and cancer is likely to be the development of additional useful diagnostic markers for problematic cases.

4. ASSOCIATION OF PIN AND PROSTATE CARCINOMA

In 1954 Franks proposed that epithelial hyperplasia was a precursor of prostatic carcinoma *(36)*. A decade later, McNeal described PIN and referred to it as "atypical hyperplasia" *(59)*. Helpap, in a classic description of his experiments with thymidine uptake, suggested that "severe atypical primary hyperplasia is a precancerous lesion" *(44)*. In 1986, McNeal and Bostwick published their landmark paper showing an association between PIN and prostatic adenocarcinoma, followed by a more detailed definition of the term PIN by Bostwick the following year *(9,60)*. Epstein provided further linkage of PIN with organ-confined carcinoma, and multiple studies have now

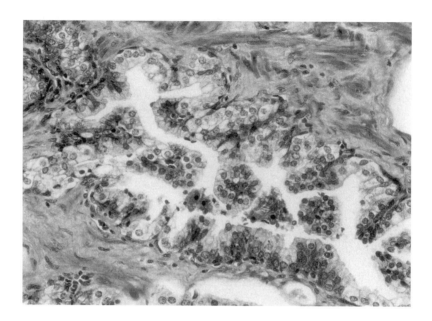

Fig. 1. Photomicrograph of PIN, grade 2–3, showing crowded micropapillae. Magnification is 200×.

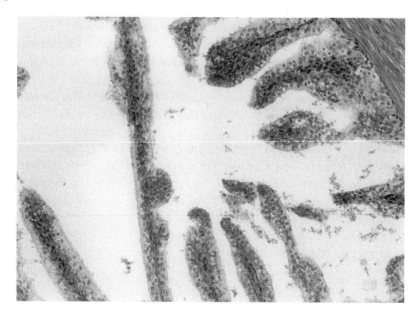

Fig. 2. HGPIN occuring in papillary configuration with elongate, filiform papillae. Magnification is 100×.

described PIN and demonstrated a significant association with adenocarcinoma *(3,11,12,17,24,40,52,67,70,93)*.

The multifocality of PIN within the prostate parallels that of adenocarcinoma and can be traced to the same zones within the gland, thus providing a spatial linkage between the two entities. This relationship has been reported in multiple studies

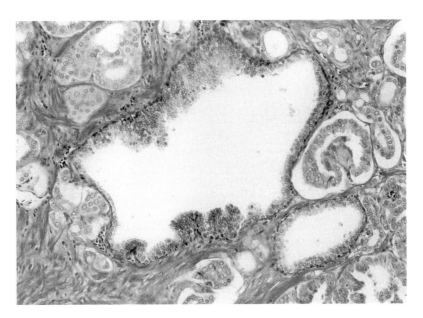

Fig. 3. Tufted form of PIN in a dilated large duct. Note association with surrounding malignant glands. Magnification is 100×.

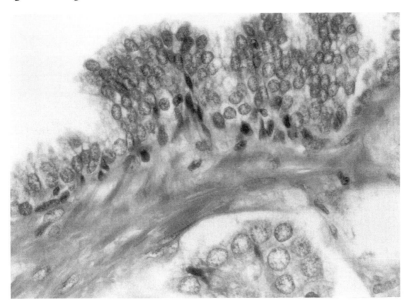

Fig. 4. High-powered view of the LGPIN tufts shown in Fig. 3. Magnification is 400×.

(3,12,66,67). For example, the majority of PIN foci are found in the region of the prostate that is most likely to harbor invasive adenocarcinoma, the peripheral zone *(10,12,52,67)*. Only about one-third of radical prostatectomy specimens have high-grade PIN in both the peripheral and the transition zones, and when carcinoma is found in the transition zone concurrent PIN is usually present. If PIN has developed directly into prostate carcinoma, PIN lesions usually exist in close proximity to malignant glands. In fact, over 80% of carcinoma cases in resected prostates, particularly if

Table 3
**Prevalence (%) of HGPIN and/or Invasive Prostate Cancer
in Autopsy Specimens Based on Age and Race[a]**

	HGPIN		Cancer	
Age	AA	Caucasian	AA	Caucasian
20–29	7	8	8	8
30–39	26	23	31	31
40–49	46	29	43	37
50–59	72	49	46	44
60–69	75	53	70	65
70–79	91	67	81	83

[a]Adapted from Sakr et al., *Eur. Urol*, **30:**138–144, 1996.

prepared by whole mount, harbor high-grade PIN within 2 mm of the carcinomas *(12)*. However, in prostates with a large tumor vol, PIN foci may be overgrown, and thus an association with PIN may not be observed. In the authors' experience, high-grade PIN will parallel carcinoma in whole mounts if the tumor is multifocal and relatively low-volume. This is particularly true for cancers with Gleason scores of 6 and 7, which comprise most of the prostate cases at the NCI. In a significant number of our whole mount prostates (routinely performed at NCI since 1994) sparse, isolated low-volume. infiltrating carcinoma ducts can be found within the fields of grouped PIN units (for additional examples of whole mount studies, *see 12,45,52,66*). When such microscopic tumor foci are found in the anterior prostate, virtually all will be associated with PIN (PH Duray, unpublished observation).

In general, data from autopsy studies supports a precursor-product relationship between PIN and prostate cancer. For example, in a series of 249 autopsy cases, 77% of prostates with HGPIN harbored invasive adenocarcinoma, compared to only 24% without HGPIN *(73)*. Autopsy studies also demonstrate that development of HGPIN predates the development of clinically detectable cancer by 5–10 yr, consistent with the concept that HGPIN is a premalignant lesion *(64)*. Silvestri et al. performed an autopsy study of European men and found an association between HGPIN and carcinoma in the majority of cases *(81)*. However, more recent analyses have revealed that 70% of autopsy cases with histologic evidence of invasive prostate do not have associated HGPIN. In addition, in a series of 62,537 needle biopsies of the prostate, isolated HGPIN was found in only 4.1% of cases, while invasive cancer was found in 38.3% of cases *(64)*. Collectively these findings suggest that a subset of prostate cancers may develop de novo, which does not begin with HGPIN. The discrepancy in the reported prevalence of isolated cancer (without associated HGPIN) among autopsy, surgical, and biopsy series may be partly explained when HGPIN progresses to clinically detectable cancers, and not the latent cancers typically detected in autopsy series. This is further supported by findings in autopsy studies by Sakr et al. (Table 3) that demonstrate a significantly higher prevalence of HGPIN but not latent cancer among African-American men when compared to Caucasian men *(74,75)*.

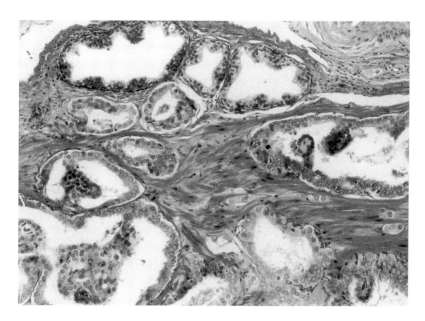

Fig. 5. PIN units showing tufting, papillae, and bridging. Carcinoma is present in apposition to tufted PIN (middle part of the figure). Magnification is 100×.

If HGPIN is a direct precursor of adenocarcinoma, we would expect to find convincing histologic evidence of microinvasive carcinoma emanating from PIN foci and beginning the process of tumor invasion. To examine this question we performed serial sectioning of each of our whole mount radical prostatectomies that show adenocarcinoma within 1–2 mm of HGPIN. Despite extensive study, we have been hard-pressed to document definitive microinvasion from HGPIN lesions (Fig. 5). The overwhelming majority of malignant ducts and acini microscopically close to HGPIN are separate structures in additional sections, or else they are HGPIN "pouches" still attached to the main PIN unit. Ongoing studies have addressed this question, and no firm conclusions can yet be made.

5. GENETIC ALTERATIONS IN PIN

Compared to other common solid tumors, relatively little is known of the molecular events which give rise to prostate cancer development. Even less is known of the molecular alterations that mediate the development of PIN *(15,26,43,46,47,54,56, 61,69)*. Research studies of premalignant lesions are challenging because of the microscopic size of PIN foci and the complex nature of the prostate. Moreover, it is difficult to grow prostate epithelium in culture, thus no well-documented in vitro cell line models of PIN are available for study in the laboratory. However, several areas of current investigation are particularly promising. For example, new rodent models have been created which develop prostate dysplasia and in some instances progress to cancer *(38,39,80)*. These models are likely to be useful tools for basic genetic discoveries as well as important experimental systems for evaluating prostate cancer prevention strategies. A second exciting area of investigation is the search for primary oncogenes and tumor suppressor genes that cause prostate cancer. Several chromosomal arms show frequent alterations in sporadic tumors, and the recent work of Isaacs and Trent has lead to identification of two chromosomal loci that harbor susceptibility genes in a subset of kindreds with familial prostate cancer *(15,83,96)*. Discovery and cloning of the responsible genes at each of these chromosomal regions will permit detailed molecular genetic and biochemical studies of their function during early formation of tumors and premalignant lesions. Another area of active research is based on developing technologies and research methodologies that offer new opportunities to study global mRNA and protein-expression alterations. These approaches can be applied toward identification of the individual genes and collections of genes that mediate the formation of PIN and subsequent transition to cancer (*see* Section 6).

The relationship between PIN and adenocarcinoma at the molecular level has been addressed in several studies using such techiques as microsatellite-based loss of heterozygosity (LOH) analysis, fluorescence in situ hybridization (FISH), comparative genome hybridization (CGH), and DNA methylation studies. In general, these investigations support a link between PIN and carcinoma, as there are a number of abnormalities that are common to both entities. Yet these techniques alone do not provide definitive evidence of such a link; future studies are needed to address this question directly. Moreover, comprehensive molecular and genetic studies of the interrelationship between LGPIN, HGPIN, and cancer have yet to be completed. In an early study, Sakr and Crissman examined LOH on chromosomal arms 8p, 10q, and 16q, and observed significant levels of LOH in PIN and carcinoma in each of these regions *(73)*. The shared allelic loss patterns were the first genetic evidence of a link between PIN and carcinoma. LOH studies in our group revealed a deletion frequency of 63% on chromosome band 8p21 compared with 80% in carcinoma samples from the same group of patients *(29,90)*. Importantly, in 85% of the informative cases containing both PIN and carcinoma, the tumor was associated with at least one potential PIN precursor as determined by loss of the identical alleles (Fig. 6). Shared allelic loss patterns between PIN and adjacent cancer were also reported by Haggman et al. *(41)*. Genome-based studies of tumors utilizing FISH and CGH are consistent with the allelotpying studies *(68,69)*. FISH and CGH detect chromosomal gains more easily than PCR-based analyses, and have revealed that gain of chromosomal arm 8q is the most frequent genetic anomaly in both PIN and carcinoma. This has been postulated to be a result of amplification of the c-myc gene located on chromosome band 8q24. Nelson and colleagues have shown parallel loss of expression of GSTP1 in prostate cancer and PIN caused by hypermethylation of the regulatory region of the gene *(18)*. Thus, similar to clinical and histopathological observations, DNA-based studies support a link between PIN and cancer, but a definitive association between the two has not yet been established.

Studies comparing chromosomal alterations in PIN and cancer suggest that there are differences in allelic deletion profiles between the two, specifically that tumors show additional regions of allelic loss *(29,41,68)*. For example, our work has shown high rates of LOH in PIN and invasive tumors at chromosome band 8p21, but significantly lower rates of LOH in PIN than invasive tumors at band 8p22 and chromosomal arm 16q *(86)*. Similarly, studies by Qian et al. showed lower levels of allelic alterations in PIN than in carcinoma *(68,69)*. In addition to differences between PIN and cancer, genetic heterogeneity among PIN foci based on LOH patterns has been reported *(13)*.

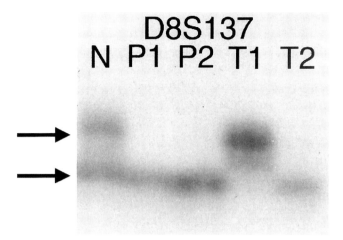

Fig. 6. Denaturing gel showing LOH on chromosome 8p12-21 at marker D8S137 in PIN and prostate carcinoma. Lane N is from normal prostate epithelium and shows the presence of two alleles. Lanes P1 and P2 are from individual PIN foci and show loss of the upper allele. Lane T1 is from cancer region 1 and shows loss of the lower allele. Lane T2 is from cancer region 2 and shows loss of the upper allele.

In our study of chromosome band 8p21 LOH, 11 cases with spatially distinct PIN foci showed distinguishable deletion patterns based on loss of opposite chromosomal arm 8p alleles *(29)*. Sakr et al. also found a high rate of discordance in chromosomal arm 8p loss patterns among PIN lesions within prostatectomy specimens *(73)*.

Thus, based on the clinical, histopathological, and genome-based studies of PIN and prostate cancer, it is possible to construct a simple spatial and temporal model of prostate tumor development and progression. PIN foci develop independently and multifocally within the peripheral zone of the prostate gland approx 5–10 yr before the onset of cancer. This is most commonly associated with inactivation of a gene located at chromosome band 8p21, methylation of the GSTP1 gene promoter and loss of expression, and activation of a gene located on chromosomal arm 8q, possibly c-myc. Subsequent mutations and/or genomic alterations in genes located on chromosomal arms 7q, 13q, and chromosomal band 8p22 result in progression of PIN to invasive tumors. Finally, inactivation of genes located on chromosomal arms 10q (presumably *PTEN*) and 16q allow a metastatic phenotype to emerge and tumor dissemination to occur *(57,86,87)*. In this model, tumor progression proceeds with an orderly accumulation of genomic alterations as has been proposed for other tumor systems *(91)*. Certainly, this is a simplistic view that is far from complete, as only those "genes" altered via chromosomal abnormalities are included. However, this model can serve as a starting point for more detailed studies in the future examining the molecular genetic relationship between PIN and cancer *(see* Section 6.4.).

Gene expression levels of a number of cell-regulatory genes, growth factors, and prostate-specific markers has been examined in PIN and compared with benign prostate epithelium and prostate carcinoma. In many cases, expression of such genes is intermediate in PIN. For instance, levels of prostate specific antigen (PSA) decrease incrementally from benign epithelium to PIN to carcinoma *(14)*. In contrast, prostate specific membrane antigen (PSM) increases incrementally among these tissues *(14)*. Overexpression of p53 is infrequent in organ-confined prostate carcinoma, but is completely absent in high-grade PIN *(48)*. The apoptosis-regulating gene bcl-2 is likewise infrequently expressed in organ-confined carcinoma. However, interestingly, bcl-2 levels are significantly higher in PIN than in either carcinoma or benign prostate tissue. Bax is expressed in all carcinoma and PIN samples. Both the apoptotic and mitotic (Ki-67) indices are intermediate in PIN as compared to benign and malignant tissue *(48)*. Telomerase activity has been detected in a low percentage of PIN foci (16%) compared to carcinomas (69%) *(51)*. c-Met expression is similar in PIN (36%) and latent cancer (33%), but is much more common in clinical disease (81%), and is found in 100% of metastatic lesions *(92)*. In a study examining expression of p27KIP1, the labeling index decreased incrementally from normal tissue (86.4%) through PIN (59.3%) and primary carcinoma (43.5%) to lymph node metastases (7%) *(34)*. There is a trend toward higher expression of membranous EGFR and c-erbB2 and cytoplasmic TGF-alpha, and lower expression of FGF-2 in high-grade PIN and carcinoma than in low-grade PIN or BPH as determined by immunohistochemistry. Staining of cell-proliferation antigen MIB-1 was shown to be increased in HGPIN as compared with LGPIN or BPH *(42)*. Taken together, these gene expression results are consistent with the hypothesis that HGPIN is a premalignant lesion.

Our group has also observed qualitative changes in gene expression in PIN secondary to alterations in transcript splicing. For example, we detected a novel variant of PB39 transcript in a cDNA library derived from PIN cells. PB39 mRNA was previously reported as overexpressed in prostate cancer, but was not known to exist in an alternative splice form *(21)*. Interestingly, based on a search of all cDNA libraries and sequences in dbEST, the novel splice variant is primarily expressed in fetal tissues and tumors, and thus may be associated with the loss of cellular differentiation that occurs during prostate tumor progression *(22)*. PHDhtm and SignalP computer-based analysis of the predicted amino acid sequence of PB39 indicates that the N-terminus contains a srp sequence for a secreted protein. Thus, the protein product of the alternative splice form could potentially serve as a serum marker of early prostate cancer development.

6. FUTURE DIRECTIONS: NEW APPROACHES TO THE STUDY OF PIN

The following section is divided into summaries of some of the new approaches and methodologies being utilized by the Intramural Prostate Cancer Working Group at the NCI to study PIN in the context of prostate tumor progression. Several experimental approaches are briefly described, ranging from tissue-processing methods to high-throughput gene expression platforms to new technology development. The summaries highlight the emphasis placed on the importance of an integrated and cross-disciplinary approach to the study of prostate cancer.

6.1. Tissue Microdissection-Based Analysis of PIN

Molecular analysis studies geared toward an understanding of individual cell types require methods and approaches which permit histopathologically-defined cell types to be selectively studied. This is particularly important for the study of PIN. Therefore, we have found tissue microdissection to be a critical tool in our studies of PIN. The concept of tissue microdissection is quite simple; that is, procuring a specific population of cells from a heterogeneous tissue sample under direct microscopic visualization. However, in practice the approach is technically challenging, and several methods have been developed over the last decade *(6,7,28,35,62,79)*. Our recent approach has been to utilize Laser Capture Microdissection (LCM). LCM is a positive selection method designed to permit simple, fast, and reliable microdissection of tissue sections *(8,30,58)*. The system utilizes an infrared laser integrated into a standard microscope with alignment into the optics subsystem, and relies on the use of a thermoplastic transparent film that lies on the surface of a routinely prepared tissue section on a glass slide. The investigator examines the tissue section microscopically and activates the laser when the desired cells underlie the target. This activates the film with subsequent binding and procurement of the cells of interest. The laser pulse is very short (approx 5 ms); thus, the tissue experiences only a very brief thermal transience, as the heat generated from membrane is rapidly dissipated. LCM allows for visualization and image capturing of each PIN focus as it is microdissected, thus maintaining an accurate record and permitting correlation of histopathology with subsequent molecular results.

6.2. High-Throughput Gene Expression Analysis of PIN

Biomedical research is in the advent of a new era where the integration of high-throughput analysis platforms and information technology are reshaping the way a researcher learns about the nature of biological systems *(1,25,63,71,76,77,89)*. The potential of these platforms for the study of human diseases is exciting, new and technically challenging. Therefore, as a part of the Cancer Genome Anatomy Project (CGAP), we tested the feasibility of performing high-throughput gene expression analysis of prostate tumor progression using expressed tag sequencing (EST) of cDNA libraries as a gene expression platform *(32)* (http://www.ncbi.nlm.nih.gov//ncicgap/). Twelve microdissection-based cDNA libraries were produced from radical prostatectomy specimens from five patients and included normal epithelium, PIN, and cancer (Table 4). A total of 29,183 successful sequences were generated. Unigene clusting algorithms of sequence derived from the microdissected libraries generated 6567 different epithelial genes. By extrapolation, this number represents about 50% of the total number of expected genes, including those expressed at a high level. The majority of genes were observed only once or twice in each library, and the overall diversity (#genes/#sequences) averaged 39.1%—an acceptable value compared to standard methods of library construction from large amounts of RNA. Also, genes known to be highly expressed in prostate epithelium such as PSA were highly represented in the microdissected libraries, suggesting that the libraries are representative of their tissue source of origin.

The sequence information from the prostate libraries has multiple utilities *(85,88)*. For example, we examined the expression levels in normal epithelium, PIN, and cancer using a variety of statistical tests, and found that a subset of ribosomal protein genes were overexpressed in the cancer libraries. This finding is expected in tumor cells, presumably because of the increased requirement for protein synthesis to support cell division *(97)*. Interestingly, these ribosomal protein mRNAs were not increased in libraries from PIN cells. This finding departs from most current theories, which claim that PIN develops because of a marked increase in growth rate. However, based on the present gene expression data set, an alternative hypothesis can be proposed. A decreased

Table 4
Gene Diversity Observed in Twleve Microdissection-Based cDNA Libraries

Library name	Sample type	% Diversity
NCI_CGAP_Pr1	Normal epithelium	35.2
NCI_CGAP_Pr5	Normal epithelium	40
NCI_CGAP_Pr9	Normal epithelium	46.1
NCI_CGAP_Pr11	Normal epithelium	45.2
NCI_CGAP_Pr2	Premalignant lesion	34.9
NCI_CGAP_Pr6	Premalignant lesion	42.6
NCI_CGAP_Pr7	Premalignant lesion	39.1
NCI_CGAP_Pr4	Premalignant lesion	37.8
NCI_CGAP_Pr3	Adenocarcinoma	29.6
NCI_CGAP_Pr8	Adenocarcinoma	42.4
NCI_CGAP_Pr10	Adenocarcinoma	42.6
NCI_CGAP_Pr12	Metastatic adenocarcinoma	33.6
	All microdissected	39.1

rate of cell death as opposed to an increase in cell division mediates the development of PIN. In this scenario, a decreased rate of apoptosis would be an important early event in prostate tumor progression. Certainly, this hypothesis is based on a preliminary data analysis and requires testing in follow-up studies, but it illustrates the potential of global gene expression studies to generate new insights into the fundamental mechanisms underlying the formation of PIN.

6.3. Proteomic Studies of PIN

The phenotype of a given cell type is ultimately determined by the composition and activation status of its proteins. Therefore, quantitative and qualitative proteomic measurement of PIN cells and prostate cancer is an important experimental approach that will complement genomic DNA and gene expression analyses *(4,5,20,26a)*. We have been studying protein profiles of prostate cancer and PIN using LCM and two analysis methods, 2D-PAGE and SELDI *(31)*. Initial 2D-PAGE-based experiments comparing dissected normal epithelial and patient-matched tumors of three cases demonstrated that 98% of the observed proteins were identical between the cell types. However, eight proteins were discovered that showed an identical change (up or downregulation) in each tumor. The identity of these proteins is now being determined. Applying this type of analysis to HGPIN in the future should allow us to identify specific proteins that are over or underexpressed in PIN compared to normal epithelium and cancer. Some limitations of 2D-PAGE analysis of premalignant lesions do exist. For example, at least 40,000 cells are needed in order to analyze the 750 most abundant proteins in the cell. To address this challenge, we are experimenting with methods to efficiently label recovered proteins so that a larger percentage of cellular protein content can be visualized using fewer numbers of cells *(31)*.

Surface Enhanced Laser Desorption Ionization (SELDI) is a new technology that utilizes matrix-assisted laser desorption and time-of-flight analysis to study proteins *(53)*. SELDI is highly sensitive, and is able to analyze a complex milieu of proteins

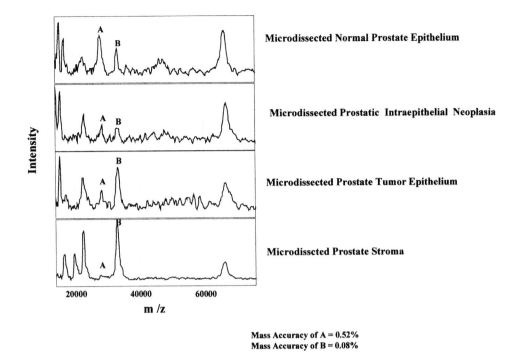

Intensity

20000   40000   60000

m /z

Microdissected Normal Prostate Epithelium

Microdissected Prostatic Intraepithelial Neoplasia

Microdissected Prostate Tumor Epithelium

Microdissected Prostate Stroma

Mass Accuracy of A = 0.52%
Mass Accuracy of B = 0.08%

Fig. 7. Surface enhanced laser desorption ionization (SELDI) analysis of normal prostate epithelium, PIN, cancer and prostate stroma. The relative intensities of the protein peaks labeled **A** and **B** discriminate between each cell type.

either with or without preseparation. Protein profiles can be generated from lysates of 1500 LCM-procured epithelial cells, and proteins as small as 2000 Ka can be reliably detected. Applied to prostate cancer progression, we have found that SELDI protein profiles differ reproducibly among benign and malignant prostate epithelial cells *(65)*. Interestingly, HGPIN cells yield a profile that is intermediate to that of normal and tumor cells (Fig. 7). These initial studies have demonstrated that SELDI will likely be a useful tool in the study of the relationship between PIN and cancer.

6.4. Three-Dimensional Approach to Studying PIN

In order to integrate and synthesize genomic, gene expression, and proteomic data sets in the context of tumor progression, we utilize a whole-mount, three-dimensional approach to the study of prostate cancer *(23)*. This method permits comprehensive analysis of the process of tumor development within individual patients, and allows the physical and molecular relationships between the tumor, premalignant lesions, and normal glands from which they arose to be examined and compared. Studies of prostate tumor progression in three dimensions will allow the relationship between PIN and cancer to be studied in detail at the molecular level. After the primary prostate oncogenes and tumor suppressor genes are identified, it will be possible to analyze the specific mutations that occur in these genes during tumor progression. Thus, investigators will be able to compare and contrast mutations between PIN foci and cancer and "track" mutation patterns in each cell population within individual patients. In comparison with studies such as LOH and CGH that detect gross changes at the genome level, analysis of mutation patterns likely will allow a specific and well-defined relationship between PIN and cancer to be determined.

6.5. 70% Ethanol Fixation and Histopathology of PIN

An important technical issue for molecular studies of clinical prostate samples is the need for improved tissue fixation and embedding strategies that will result in high-quality histologic detail, yet maintain the integrity of macromolecules within the tissue. This is an active area of investigation within the NCI Prostate Group. Diagnostically, it involves maintaining overall orientation of the prostate gland, maximizing evaluable margins for pathological staging, and producing histologic sections of as much of the specimen as practical. From a research perspective, it involves the study the relationship of tumor foci to the surrounding gland, performing serial sections for immunohistochemistry and *in situ* hybridization, and recovery of nucleic acids and proteins from microdissected cell populations.

We have found that fixation of needle biopsies and prostatectomy specimens in 70% aqueous ethanol provides advantages for the study of individual chromatin detail of benign, neoplastic, and PIN cells. There is also excellent concordance between the chromatin and nuclear detail of prostate carcinoma and HGPIN. However, there is a notable difference between Gleason grade 5 nuclei (smaller size and dense chromatin) compared to the expected chromatin of HGPIN. Ethanol-fixed HGPIN nuclei show visibly thicker nuclear membranes (differing from adenosis and hyperplasia), large nucleoli, some with irregular shape, and prominent peri-nucleolar clearing. Cells and nuclei of HGPIN are seen to easily overlap. We have found it comparatively easy to ascertain the frequency of abnormal PIN nuclei and to separate them from antecedent or persistent benign nuclei. Furthermore, ethanol-fixation specimens confirm that LGPIN have scarcely any prominent or abnormally shaped nucleoli. Basal stem cells of PIN units also stand out readily in ethanol fixation. The only pitfall we have encountered thus far is some difficulty with the cytology of posttreatment effects (hormonal or radiation therapy) on prostate carcinoma after ethanol fixation. But in all other situations, ethanol offers an advantage in permitting the study of individual chromatin detail. Ethanol-fixed tissue is suitable for immunohistochemistry as well as *in situ* hybridization, although in some instances it requires modification of the standard protocols designed for formalin-fixed tissue with conditions more closely resembling that of frozen tissue. Additionally, EtOH fixation better preserves the integrity of DNA and mRNA for subsequent microdissection-based studies.

6.6. Developing Technology: Layered Expression Scanning

The molecular study of clinical specimens has evolved substantially over the past decade, resulting mainly from advancements in technology. It is likely that continued improvements in experimental methodologies will be central to future studies of disease processes such as prostate tumor progression. As an example of a technology under development, we have designed a new technique for global expression and proteomic profiling of biological samples called "layered expression scanning." The method combines tissue samples with a high-throughput array approach to provide a simple and rapid method for comprehensive molecular analysis *(33)*. Figure 8 shows

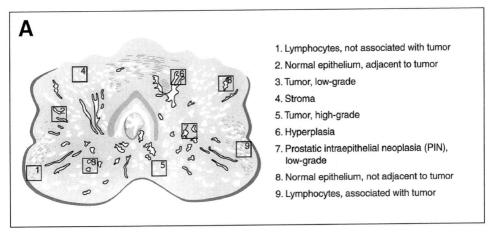

A

1. Lymphocytes, not associated with tumor
2. Normal epithelium, adjacent to tumor
3. Tumor, low-grade
4. Stroma
5. Tumor, high-grade
6. Hyperplasia
7. Prostatic intraepithelial neoplasia (PIN), low-grade
8. Normal epithelium, not adjacent to tumor
9. Lymphocytes, associated with tumor

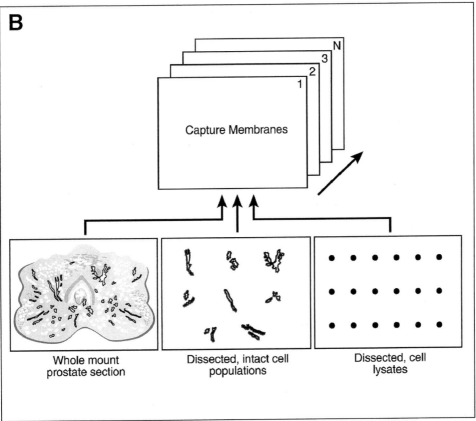

B

Capture Membranes

Whole mount prostate section

Dissected, intact cell populations

Dissected, cell lysates

Fig. 8. Schematic diagram showing the principle of layered expression scanning. (**A**) shows a whole-mount section of prostate from a patient with cancer. Contained within the section are multiple different cell populations and subpopulations, each of biological interest. For example, normal prostate epithelium (2) adjacent to a tumor focus may show a distinct gene expression profile compared to normal epithelium (8) distant from the cancer. Lymphocytes (9) associated with the tumor may show a distinct molecular profile unique to the local environment and/or alter the expression pattern of nearby tumor cells.

the principle of the technique in schematic form. A biological sample (#1-tissue section, #2-dissected cell populations, #3-lysates from cells) is placed adjacent to a set of capture layers, each containing an individual hybridization molecule (antibody or DNA sequence). The specimen(s) is transferred through the membranes and, importantly, the overall two-dimensional architecture and histological relationships within the sample(s) are maintained (Fig. 8B). As the proteins and nucleic acids are transferred, each target molecule specifically hybridizes to the membrane containing its antibody or complementary DNA sequence. After hybridization, each of the membranes are analyzed, providing a measurement of the level of expression of each target molecule in all of the cell types present in the sample.

Figure 8A shows a schematic representation of a whole-mount prostate tissue section from a patient with cancer. Contained within the section are multiple-cell populations of biological interest, including normal epithelium, high and low-grade PIN foci, tumor, stromal components, and important tumor-host interactions such as lymphocytes associated with cancer cells. It is possible to use microdissection to procure any or all of the individual cell populations. However, even with new laser-based methods, this remains a highly labor-intensive task. Investigators are forced to decide which subpopulations of a given cell type to study individually and which ones to pool together for subsequent analysis, as it is not practical to perform many high-throughput molecular studies from every tissue section from each patient in a study. Thus, a critical need in furthering our understanding of the molecular profiles of cells in tissues is an analysis method that permits simultaneous molecular profiling of all cell types present in a histologic section. As layered expression technology progresses, we envision a laboratory method that will meet this need and will have multiple applications for high-throughput molecular profiling of tissue and cell samples.

REFERENCES

1. Abbott, A. 1996. DNA chips intensify the sequence search. *Nature* **379(6564):** 392.
2. Alexander, E. E., J. Qian, P. C. Wollan, R. P. Myers, and D. G. Bostwick. 1996. Prostatic intraepithelial neoplasia does not appear to raise serum PSA concentration. *Urology* **47:** 693–698.
3. Arakawa, A., S. Song, P. T. Scardino, and T. M. Wheeler. 1995. High grade Prostatic Intraepithelial Neoplasia in prostates removed following irradiation failure in the treatment of prostatic carcinoma. *Pathol. Res. Pract.* **191:** 868–872.
4. Anderson, N. and N. G. Anderson. 1998. Proteome and proteomics: new technologies, new concepts, and new words. *Electrophoresis* **19:** 1853–1861.
5. Banks, R., M. J. Dunn, M. A. Forbes, A. Stanley, D. Pappin, T. Naven, et al. 1999. The potential use of laser capture microdissection to selectively obtain distinct populations of cells for proteomic analysis—preliminary findings. *Electrophoresis* **20:** 689–700.
6. Becker, B. K., M. H. Rohrl, and H. Hofler. 1997. Laser-assisted preparation of single cells from stained histological slides for gene analysis. *Histochem. Cell Biol.* **108:** 447–451.
7. Bohm, M. W. I., K. Schutze, and H. Rubben. 1997. Non-contact laser microdissection of membrane-mounted native tissue. *Am. J. Pathol.* **151:** 63–67.
8. Bonner, R., M. R. Emmert-Buck, K. A. Cole, T. Pohida, R. F. Chuaqui, S. R. Goldstein, et al. 1997. Laser capture microdissection: molecular analysis of tissue. *Science* **278:** 1481–1483.
9. Bostwick, D. G. and M. K. Brawer. 1987. Prostatic intraepithelial neoplasia and early invasion in prostate cancer. *Cancer* **59:** 788–794.

10. Bostwick, D. G., M. B. Amin, P. Dundore, W. Marsh, and D. S. Schultz. 1993. Architectural patterns of high grade prostatic intraepithelial neoplasia. *Hum. Pathol.* **24:** 298–310.

11. Bostwick, D. G. 1995. Prostatic intraepithelial neoplasia. The most likely precursor of prostate cancer. *Cancer* **75:** 1823–1836.

12. Bostwick, D. G. and J. Qian. 1995. Atypical adenomatous hyperplasia of the prostate: Relationship with carcinoma in 217 whole mount radical prostatectomies. *Am. J. Surg. Pathol.* **19:** 506–518.

13. Bostwick, D., A. Shan, J. Qian, M. Darson, N. J. Maihle, R. B. Jenkins, et al. 1998. Independent origin of multiple foci of prostatic intraepithelial neoplasia: comparison with matched foci of prostate carcinoma. *Cancer* **83:** 1995–2002.

14. Bostwick, D., A. Pacelli, B. Blute, P. Roche, and G. P. Murphy. 1998. Prostate specific membrane antigen expression in prostatic intraepithelial neoplasia and adenocarcinoma: a study of 184 cases. *Cancer* **82:** 2256–2261.

15. Bova, G. and W. B. Isaacs. 1996. Review of allelic loss and gain in prostate cancer. *World J. Urol.* **14:** 338–346.

16. Brawer, M. K., D. M. Peehl, T. A. Stamey, and D. G. Bostwick. 1985. Keratin immunoreactivity in benign and malignant human prostate. *Cancer Res.* **45:** 3665–3669.

17. Brawer, M. K., S. A. Bigler, O. E. Sohlberg, R. B. Nagle, and P. H. Lange. 1991. Significance of prostatic intraepithelial neoplasia on prostate needle biopsy. *Urology* **38:** 103–107.

18. Brooks, J., M. Weinstein, X. Lin, Y. Sun, S. S. Pin, G. S. Bova, et al. 1998. CG island methylation changes near the GSTP1 gene in prostatic intraepithelial neoplasia. *Cancer Epidemiol. Biomark. Prev.* **7:** 531–536.

19. Catalona, W., D. S. Smith, T. L. Ratliff, and J. W. Basler. 1993. Detection of organ-confined prostate cancer is increased through prostate-specific antigen-based screening. *JAMA* **270:** 948–954.

20. Celis, J., M. Ostergaard, N. A. Jensen, I. Gromova, H. H. Rasmussen, and P. Gromov. 1998. Human and mouse proteomic databases: novel resources in the protein universe. *FEBS Lett.* **430:** 64–72.

21. Chuaqui, R., C. R. Englert, S. Strup, C. D. Vocke, Z. Zhuang, P. H. Duray, et al. 1997. PB39: Identification of a novel gene up-regulated in clinically aggressive human prostate cancer. *Urology* **50:** 302–307.

22. Cole, K., R. F. Chuaqui, K. Katz, S. Pack, Z. Zhuang, C. E. Cole, et al. 1998. cDNA sequencing and analysis of PB39: A novel gene up-regulated in prostate cancer. *Genomics* **51:** 282–287.

23. Cole, K., D. B. Krizman, and M. R. Emmert-Buck. 1999. The genetics of cancer—a 3D model. *Nat. Genet.* **21(1 Suppl.):** 38–41.

24. Davidson, D., D. G. Bostwick, J. Qian, P. C. Wollan, J. E. Oesterling, R. A. Rudders, et al. 1995. Prostatic intraepithelial neoplasia is a risk factor for adenocarcinoma predictive accuracy in needle biopsies. *J. Urol.* **154:** 1295–1299.

25. DeRisi, J., L. Penland, P. O. Brown, M. L. Bittner, P. S. Meltzer, M. Ray, et al. 1996. Use of a cDNA microarray to analyze gene expression patterns in human cancer. *Nat. Genet.* **14:** 457–460.

26. Dong, J., W. B. Isaacs, and J. T. Isaacs. 1997. Molecular advances in prostate cancer. *Curr. Opin. Oncol.* **9:** 101–107.

26a. Dove, A. 1999. Proteomics: translating genomics into products? *Nat. Biotechnol.* **17:** 233–236.

27. Drago, J. R., K. K. Mostofi, and F. Lee. 1989. Introductory remarks and workshop summary. *Urology* **34(Suppl.):** 2,3.

28. Emmert-Buck, M., M. J. Roth, Z. Zhuang, E. Campo, J. Rozhin, B. F. Sloane, et al. 1994. Increased gelatinase A (MMP-2) and cathepsin B activity in invasive tumor regions of human colon cancer samples. *Am. J. Pathol.* **145:** 1285–1290.

29. Emmert-Buck, M., C. D. Vocke, R. O. Pozzatti, P. H. Duray, S. B. Jennings, C. D. Florence, et al. 1995. Allelic loss on chromosome 8p12-21 in microdissected prostatic intraepithelial neoplasia (PIN). *Cancer Res.* **55:** 2959–2962.

30. Emmert-Buck, M., R. F. Bonner, P. D. Smith, R. F. Chuaqui, S. R. Goldstein, Z. Zhuang, et al. 1996. Laser capture microdissection. *Science* **274:** 998–1001.

31. Emmert-Buck, M., J. W. Gillespie, C. P. Paweletz, D. K. Ornstein, V. Basrur, E. Appella, et al. 2000. A strategic approach for proteomic analysis of human tumors. *Mol. Carcin.* **27(3):** 158–165.

32. Emmert-Buck, M. R., R. L. Strausberg, D. B. Krizman, et al. 2000. Molecular profiling of clinical tissue specimens: feasibility and applications. *Am. J. Pathol.* **156(4):** 1109–1115.

33. Englert, C. R., G. Babikova, and M. R. Emmert-Buck. 2000. Layered expression scanning: rapid molecular profiling of tumor samples. *Cancer Res.* **60(6):** 1526–1530.

34. Erdamar, S., G. Yang, J. W. Harper, X. Lu, M. W. Kattan, T. C. Thompson, et al. 1999. Levels of expression of p27KIP1 protein in human prostate and prostate cancer: an immunohistochemical analysis. *Mod. Pathol.* **12:** 751–755.

35. Fearon, E., S. R. Hamilton, and B. Vogelstein. 1987. Clonal analysis of human colorectal tumors. *Science* **238:** 193–197.

36. Franks, L. M. 1954. Atrophy and hyperplasia in the prostate proper. *J. Pathol. Bacteriol.* **98:** 617–621.

37. Gann, P., C. H. Hennekens, and M. J. Stampfer. 1995. A prospective evaluation of plasma prostate-specific antigen for detection of prostatic cancer. *JAMA* **273:** 289–294.

38. Green, J., N. M. Greenberg, J. C. Barrett, C. Boone, R. H. Getzenberg, J. Henkin, et al. 1998. Transgenic and reconstitution models of prostate cancer. *Prostate* **36:** 59–63.

39. Greenberg, N., F. J. DeMayo, M. J. Finegold, D. Medina, W. D. Tilley, J. O. Aspinall, et al. 1995. Prostate cancer in a transgenic mouse. *Proc. Natl. Acad. Sci. USA* **92:** 3439–3443.

40. Haggman, M., J. A. Macoska, K. J. Wojno, and J. E. Oesterling. 1997. The relationship between prostatic intraepithelial neoplasia and prostate cancer: critical issues. *J. Urol.* **158:** 12–22.

41. Haggman, M. J., K. J. Wojno, C. P. Pearsall, and J. A. Macoska. 1997. Allelic loss of 8p sequences in prostatic intraepithelial neoplasia and carcinoma. *Urology* **50:** 643–647.

42. Harper, M., E. Glynne-Jones, L. Goddard, P. Mathews, and R. I. Nicholson. 1998. Expression of androgen receptor and growth factors in premalignant lesions of the prostate. *J. Pathol.* **186:** 169–177.

43. Hayward, S., G. D. Grossfeld, T. D. Tlsty, and G. R. Cunha. 1998. Genetic and epigenetic influences in prostatic carcinogenesis. *Int. J. Oncol.* **13:** 35–47.

44. Helpap, B. 1980. The biologic significance of atypical hyperplasia of the prostate. *Virch. Arch.* **387:** 307–317.

45. Humphrey, P., D. W. Keetch, D. S. Smith, D. L. Shepherd, and W. J. Catalona. 1996. Prospective characterization of pathological features of prostatic carcinomas detected via serum prostate specific antigen based screening. *J. Urol.* **155:** 816–820.

46. Isaacs, W., G. S. Bova, R. A. Morton, M. J. Bussemakers, J. D. Brooks, and C. M. Ewing. 1994. Genetic alterations in prostate cancer. *Cold Spring Harbor Symp. Quant. Biol.* **59:** 653–659.

47. Isaacs, W. 1995. Molecular genetics of prostate cancer. *Cancer Surv.* **25:** 357–379.

48. Johnson, M., M. C. Robinson, C. Marsh, C. N. Robson, D. E. Neal, and F. C. Hamdy. 1998. Expression of Bcl-2, Bax, and p53 in high-grade prostatic intraepithelial neoplasia and localized prostate cancer: relationship with apoptosis and proliferation. *Prostate* **37:** 223–229.

49. Keetch, D., P. Humphrey, D. Stahl, D. S. Smith, and W. J. Catalona. 1995. Morphometric analysis and clinical follow-up of isolated prostatic intraepithelial neoplasia in needle biopsy of the prostate. *J. Urol.* **15:** 347–351.

50. Kilic, S., E. Kukul, A. Danisman, E. Guntekin, and M. Sevuk. 1998. Ratio of free to total prostate-specific antigen in patients with prostatic intraepithelial neoplasia. *Eur. Urol.* **34:** 176–180.

51. Koeneman, K., C. X. Pan, J. K. Jin, J. M. Pyle 3rd, R. C. Flanigan, T. V. Shankey, et al. 1998. Telomerase activity, telomere length, and DNA ploidy in prostatic intraepithelial neoplasia (PIN). *J. Urol.* **160:** 1533–1539.

52. Kovi, J., F. K. Mostovi, M. Y. Heshmat, and J. P. Enterline. 1988. Large acinar atypical hyperplasia and carcinoma of the prostate. *Cancer* **61:** 555–561.

53. Kuwata, H., T. T. Yip, C. L. Yip, M. Tomita, and T. W. Hutchens. 1998. Bactericidal domain of lactoferrin: detection, quantitation, and characterization of lactoferricin in serum by SELDI affinity mass spectrometry. *Biochem. Biophys. Res. Commun.* **245:** 764–773.

54. Lalani, E., A. Stubbs, and G. W. Stamp. 1997. Prostate cancer: the interface between pathology and basic scientific research. *Semin. Cancer Biol.* **8:** 53–59.

55. Landis, S., T. Murray, S. Bolden, and P. A. Wingo. 1999. Cancer statistics, 1999. *Cancer J. Clin.* **49:** 8–31.

56. Latil A. 1998. Genetic aspects of prostate cancer. *Virchows Arch.* **432:** 389–406.

57. Li, J., C. Yen, D. Liaw, K. Podsypanina, S. Bose, S. I. Wang, et al. 1997. PTEN, a putative protein tyrosine phosphatase gene mutated in human brain, breast, and prostate cancer. *Science* **275:** 1943–1947.

58. Luo, L., R. C. Salunga, H. Guo, A. Bittner, K. C. Joy, J. E. Galindo, et al. 1999. Gene expression profiles of laser-captured adjacent neuronal subtypes. *Nat. Med.* **5:** 112–122.

59. McNeal, J. E. 1965. Morphogenesis of prostatic carcinoma. *Cancer* **18:** 1659–1666.

60. McNeal, J. and D. G. Bostwick. 1986. Intraductal dysplasia: a premalignant lesion of the prostate. *Hum. Pathol.* **17:** 64–71.

61. Morton, R. J. and W. B. Isaacs. 1998. Molecular genetics of prostate cancer: clinical applications. *J. Natl. Med Assoc.* **90(11 Suppl.):** S728–731.

62. Moskaluk, C. A. 1997. Microdissection and polymerase chain reaction amplification of genomic DNA from histological tissue sections. *Am. J. Pathol.* **150:** 1547–1552.

63. Nowak, R. 1995. Entering the postgenome era. *Science* **270:** 368–371.

64. Orozco, R., G. O'Dowd, B. Kunnel, M. C. Miller, and R. W. Veltri. 1998. Observations on pathology trends in 62,537 prostate biopsies obtained from urology private practices in the United States. *Urology* **51:** 186–195.

65. Pawletz, C. P., J. W. Gillespie, D. Ornstein, et al. 2000. Rapid protein display profiling of cancer progression directly from human tissue using a protein biochip. *Drug Devel. Res.* **49:** 34–42.

66. Qian, J. and D. G. Bostwick. 1995. The extent and zonal location of prostatic intraepithelial neoplasia and atypical adenomatous hyperplasia: relationship with carcinoma in radical prostatectomy specimens. *Pathol. Res. Pract.* **191:** 860–867.

67. Qian, J., P. Wollan, and D. G. Bostwick. 1997. The extent and multicentricity of high-grade prostatic intraepithelial neoplasia in clinically localized prostatic adenocarcinoma. *Hum. Pathol.* **28:** 143–148.

68. Qian, J., R. B. Jenkins, and D. G. Bostwick. 1998. Determination of gene and chromosome dosage in prostatic intraepithelial neoplasia and carcinoma. *Anal. Quant. Cytol. Histol.* **20:** 373–380.

69. Qian, J., R. B. Jenkins, and D. G. Bostwick. 1999. Genetic and chromosomal alterations in prostatic intraepithelial neoplasia and carcinoma detected by fluorescence in situ hybridization. *Eur. Urol.* **35:** 479–483.

70. Quinn, B. D., K. R. Cho, and J. I. Epstein. 1990. Relationship of severe dysplasia to Stage A (incidental) adenocarcinoma of the prostate. *Cancer* **65:** 2321–2327.

71. Ramsay, G. 1998. DNA chips: state of the art. *Nat. Biotechnol.* **16:** 40–44.

72. Raviv, G., T. Janssen, A. R. Zlotta, F. Descamps, A. Verhest, and C. C. Schulman. 1996. Prostatic intraepithelial neoplasia: influence of clinical and pathological data on the detection of prostate cancer. *J. Urol.* **156:** 1050–1054.

73. Sakr, W., D. J. Grignon, J. D. Crissman, L. K. Heilbrun, B. J. Cassin, J. J. Pontes, et al. 1994. High grade prostatic intraepithelial neoplasia (HGPIN) and prostatic adenocarcinoma between the ages of 20–69: an autopsy study of 249 cases. *In Vivo* **8:** 439–443.

74. Sakr, W., D. J. Grignon, G. P. Haas, L. K. Heilbrun, J. E. Pontes, and J. D. Crissman. 1996. Age and racial distribution of prostatic intraepithelial neoplasia. *Eur. Urol.* **30:** 138–144.

75. Sakr, W. 1999. Prostatic intraepithelial neoplasia: a marker for high-risk groups and a potential target for chemoprevention. *Eur. Urol.* **35:** 474–478.

76. Schena, M., D. Shalon, R. W. Davis, and P. Brown. 1995. Quantitative monitoring of gene expression patterns with a complementary DNA microarray. *Science* **270:** 467–469.

77. Schena, M., R. A. Heller, T. P. Theriault, K. Konrad, E. Lachenmeier, and R. W. Davis. 1998. Microarrays: biotechnology's discovery platform for functional genomics. *Trends Biotechnol.* **16:** 301–306.

78. Shepherd, D., D. W. Keetch, P. A. Humphrey, D. S. Smith, and D. Stahl. 1996. Repeat biopsy strategy in men with isolated prostatic intraepithelial neoplasia on prostate needle biopsy. *J. Urol.* **156:** 460–462.

79. Shibata, D., D. Hawes, Z.-H. Li, A. Hernandez, C. H. Spruck, and P. W. Nichols. 1992. Specific genetic analysis of microscopic tissue after selective ultraviolet radiation fractionation and polymerase chain reaction. *Am. J. Pathol.* **141:** 539–543.

80. Shibata, M.-A., J. M. Ward, D. E. Devor, M. L. Liu, and J. E. Green. 1996. Progression of prostatic intraepithelial neoplasia (PIN) to invasive carcinoma in C3(1)/Tag transgenic mice: histopathologic and molecular alterations. *Cancer Res.* **56:** 4894–4903.

81. Silvestri, F., R. Bussani, N. Pavletic, and F. Bassan. 1995. Neoplastic and borderline lesions of the prostate: autopsy study with epidemiologic data. *Pathol. Res. Pract.* **191:** 908–916.

82. Smith, D., W. J. Catalona, and J. D. Herschman. 1996. Longitudinal screening for prostate cancer with prostate-specific antigen. *JAMA* **276:** 1309–1315.

83. Smith, J., D. Freije, J. D. Carpten, H. Gronberg, J. Xu, S. D. Isaacs, et al. 1996. Major susceptibility locus for prostate cancer on chromosome 1 suggested by a genome-wide search. *Science* **274:** 1371–1374.

84. Stephenson, R. and J. L. Stanford. 1997. Population-based prostate cancer trends in the United States: patterns of change in the era of prostate-specific antigen. *World J. Urol.* **15:** 331–335.

85. Strausberg, R., C. A. Dahl, and R. D. Klausner. 1997. New opportunities for uncovering the molecular basis of cancer. *Nat. Genet.* **15:** 415,416.

86. Strup, S., R. O. Pozzatti, C. D. Florence, M. R. Emmert-Buck, P. H. Duray, L. A. Liotta, et al. 1999. Chromosome 16 allelic loss analysis of a large set of microdissected prostate carcinomas. *J. Urol.* **162:** 590–594.

87. Suzuki, H., D. R. Nusskern, K. Okami, P. Cairns, D. Sidransky, W. B. Isaacs, et al. 1998. Interfocal heterogeneity of PTEN/MMAC1 gene alterations in multiple metastatic prostate cancer tissues. *Cancer Res.* **58:** 204–209.

88. Vasmatzis, G. E. M., U. Brinkmann, B. Lee, and I. Pastan. 1998. Discovery of three genes specifically expressed in human prostate by expressed sequence tag database analysis. *Proc. Natl. Acad. Sci. USA* **95:** 300–304.

89. Velculescu, V., L. Zhang, B. Vogelstein, and K. Kinzler. 1995. Serial analysis of gene expression. *Science* **270:** 484–487.

90. Vocke, C., R. O. Pozzatti, D. G. Bostwick, C. D. Florence, S. B. Jennings, S. E. Strup, et al. 1996. Analysis of 99 microdissected prostate carcinomas reveals high frequency of allelic loss on chromosome 8p12-21. *Cancer Res.* **56:** 2411–2416.

91. Vogelstein, B., E. R. Fearon, and S. R. Hamilton. 1988. Genetic alterations during colorectal-tumor development. *N. Engl. J. Med.* **319:** 525–532.

92. Watanabe, M., K. Fukutome, H. Kato, M. Murata, J. Kawamura, T. Shiraishi, et al. 1999. Progression-linked overexpression of c-Met in prostatic intraepithelial neoplasia and latent as well as clinical prostate cancers. *Cancer Lett.* **141:** 173–178.

93. Weinstein, M. H. and J. I. Epstein. 1993. Significance of high grade prostatic intraepithelial neoplasia on needle biopsy. *Hum. Pathol.* **24:** 624–629.

94. Wingo, P., L. A. Ries, H. M. Rosenberg, D. S. Miller, and B. K. Edwards. 1998. Cancer incidence and mortality, 1973–1995: a report card for the U.S. *Cancer* **82:** 1197–1207.

95. Wingo, P., L. A. Ries, S. L. Parker, and C. W. J. Heath. 1998. Long-term cancer patient survival in the United States. *Cancer Epidemiol. Biomark. Prev.* **7:** 271–282.

96. Xu, J., D. Meyers, D. Freije, S. Isaacs, K. Wiley, D. Nusskern, et al. 1998. Evidence for a prostate cancer susceptibility locus on the X chromosome. *Nat. Genet.* **20:** 175–179.

97. Zhang, L., W. Zhou V. E. Velculescu, S. E. Kern, R. H. Hruban, S. R. Hamilton, et al. 1997. Gene expression profiles in normal and cancer cells. *Science* **276:** 1268–1272.

98. Zhuang, Z., A. O. Vortmeyer, E. J. Mark, R. Odze, M. R. Emmert-Buck, M. J. Merino, et al. 1996. Barrett's esophagus: metaplastic cells with loss of heterozygosity at the APC gene locus are clonal precursors to invasive adenocarcinoma. *Cancer Res.* **56:** 1961–1964.

99. Zlotta, A. and C. C. Schulman. 1999. Clinical evolution of prostatic intraepithelial neoplasia. *Eur. Urol.* **35:** 498–503.

10

Xenograft Models and the Molecular Biology of Human Prostate Cancer

Robert E. Reiter, MD, and Charles L. Sawyers, MD

1. INTRODUCTION

The study of human prostate cancer has historically lagged behind that of other common malignancies such as breast and colon cancer. Although the reasons for this "lag" are multiple, a major obstacle to progress has been the relative lack of human prostate cancer model systems available to study the disease and to test new potential therapeutic strategies. Tissue specimens of primary prostate tumors, although common, are often too small or heterogeneous to be useful for molecular studies. Metastatic specimens are rare. Even when surgical material is available, it has been difficult to establish permanent prostate cancer cell lines. To date, most of the studies in the field of human prostate cancer have focused on just three human prostate cancer cell lines—PC-3, DU-145, and LNCaP. DU-145 and PC-3 do not express prostate specific antigen (PSA) or androgen receptor (AR), raising questions about the relevance of these two cell lines to most cases of clinical prostate cancer. LNCaP is androgen responsive and produces PSA, but it contains a mutation in the androgen receptor which alters ligand specificity and may limit its utility for molecular analysis. More important, it is unlikely that a single PSA-positive cell line can represent the heterogeneous disease we call prostate cancer.

Recently, we and others have addressed the problem of human prostate cancer models by establishing a large number of prostate cancer xenografts. The propagation of prostate cancer tissue samples obtained from patients in immune-deficient mice allows for the expansion of small amounts of starting material and for the enrichment of relatively homogeneous cell populations from heterogeneous tumor cell populations. Xenografts can recapitulate in vivo many of the clinical features of human prostate cancer, such as metastasis and androgen independent progression. These attributes make xenografts excellent models for molecular and genetic analysis, gene discovery, and for testing of new therapeutic strategies based on these molecular discoveries.

2. THE LOS ANGELES PROSTATE CANCER (LAPC) XENOGRAFTS

Over the past 5 years, our group has made a focused effort to develop prostate cancer xenografts by transfer of fresh prostate cancer tissue obtained at surgery directly into immune-deficient SCID mice. To date, we have established more than six independent

From: *Prostate Cancer: Biology, Genetics, and the New Therapeutics*
Edited by: L. W. K. Chung, W. B. Isaacs, and J. W. Simons © Humana Press Inc., Totowa, NJ

prostate cancer xenografts from patients with locally advanced or metastatic prostate cancer. Two of these, LAPC-4 and LAPC-9, have been maintained continuously for more than 2 years by serial passage in SCID mice *(6,17)*. These xenografts can be frozen and reintroduced into SCID mice or dissociated into single-cell suspensions in order to quantify the number of cells being inoculated. One xenograft, LAPC-4, has been successfully established as a cell line in tissue culture *(17)*. The LAPC-4 cell line retains the features of the LAPC-4 xenograft and has been used by a number of investigators in the prostate cancer research community. Explants of LAPC-9 can also be maintained in cell culture for up to 3 mo, but a permanent cell line has not yet been established.

LAPC-4 and LAPC-9 offer several advantages over previous models, which make them suitable for molecular and genetic studies. Like the majority of clinical prostate cancers (and unlike the widely used DU 145 and PC3 cell lines), both xenografts have intact androgen receptor signal transduction pathways. Both express wild-type AR and secrete high levels of the androgen dependent protein PSA. LAPC-4 and LAPC-9 both grow as androgen dependent cancers in male SCID mice, respond to androgen ablation treatment, and eventually progress to a hormone refractory, androgen independent stage. In LAPC-4, androgen ablation results in tumor regression and a decrease in PSA, whereas in LAPC-9 androgen withdrawal reduces PSA without affecting tumor size *(6,17)*.

LAPC-4 and LAPC-9 can be implanted subcutaneously, orthotopically into the mouse prostate, or intratibially. Orthotopic tumors metastasize reproducibly to regional lymph nodes and lung, providing an opportunity to study prostate cancer metastasis. Metastatic deposits can be isolated and propagated to generate sublines with increasing metastatic capabilities. Intratibial injection results in the formation of osteoblastic tumors typical of human prostate cancer. As with metastases, bony tumors can be harvested and reinjected. These bony sublines display an enhanced ability to grow in bone, and are suitable for the study of prostate cancer growth in bone—the major cause of morbidity in men with clinical prostate cancer.

3. CWR22, LUCAP, AND THE NETHERLAND XENOGRAFTS

A number of other groups have also developed prostate cancer xenografts over the past few years (Table 1). Each xenograft has unique properties which provide opportunities to identify the multiple molecular pathways in prostate cancer. In addition, the availability of a diverse group of xenografts provides a more realistic setting in which to test new therapeutic approaches.

3.1. CWR 22

The CWR22 xenograft was established by Pretlow and colleagues by implantation of tissue from a patient with advanced prostate cancer into nude mice *(37)*. Similar to the LAPC xenografts, CWR22 is androgen dependent, regresses after androgen deprivation, and progresses to androgen independence *(21)*. CWR22 expresses both PSA and AR, although CWR22 AR contains a point mutation in codon 874 which renders it sensitive to nonandrogenic ligands, similar to the LNCaP cell line *(32)*. As with LAPC-4, CWR22 has been successfully adapted to growth in tissue culture, although the CWR22 cell line (22Rv1) is androgen independent, whereas LAPC-4 is androgen sensitive *(27)*.

Table 1
Xenograft Models of Prostate Cancer

Name	Derivation	Host system	Androgen sensitivity	Marker	Metastasis	Other
LAPC-3	AI TURP[a]	SCID	AI, low AR	+/–PSA	ND	
LAPC-4	AI LN	SCID	AD, AI subline no AR mutation	PSA, PSCA Her-2/neu	Lung, lymph node (orthotopic)	Cell line, intratibial growth
LAPC-9	AI bone metastasis	SCID	AD, AI subline no AR mutation	PSA, PSCA	Lung, lymph node	Intratibial growth (orthotopic)
LuCAP 23	AI LN	nude	AD, AI sublines	PSA	ND	
CWR22	AD meta-stasis	nude	AD, AI subline AR mutation	PSA, Her-2/neu	ND	
PC-295	AD LN	nude	AD	PSA	ND	Neuroendocrine
PC-310	AD prostate	nude	AD	PSA	ND	
PC-329	AD prostate	nude	AD	PSA	ND	
PC-346	AD TURP	nude	AD	PSA	ND	
PC-324	AI TURP	nude	AI	—	ND	
PC-339	AI TURP	nude	AI	—	ND	
PC-374	AI scrotal metastasis	nude	AI	PSA	ND	

[a]AI, androgen independent; AD, androgen dependent; LN, lymph node; SCID, severe combined immunodeficiency; AR, androgen receptor; PSCA, prostate stem cell antigen; PSA, prostate specific antigen; ND, not done or not reported; TURP, transurethral resection of prostate.

3.2. LuCAP

The LuCAP series of xenografts was recently reported by investigators at the University of Washington. LuCAP 23 was established from independent metastases of a patient who died from prostate cancer (9). Each LuCAP 23 subline exhibits differing degrees of androgen sensitivity, providing a spectrum of biologic behavior to study androgen independent progression (1). As with CWR 22 and LAPC 4 and 9, LuCAP tumors express PSA, again analogous to most cases of human prostate cancer.

3.3. The Netherlands Xenografts

The largest reported series of human prostate cancer xenografts comes from van Weerden et al. at Erasmus Univeristy in the Netherlands. These investigators established seven independent xenografts from primary, locally recurrent, and metastatic tumors (34). All have been passaged more than eight times, indicating that they are genetically stable. Four xenografts (PC-295, PC-310, PC-329 and PC-346) are androgen dependent and regress partially or completely after androgen ablation. Unlike LAPC, CWR22 and LuCAP, these four lines have not been reported to progress to androgen independence, making them somewhat unique reagents to study androgen dependence. PC-295 is also unusual, in that androgen ablation induces neuroendocrine differentiation, a common phenotype associated with androgen independent progression in human prostate cancer (13). The remaining three xenografts (PC-324, PC-339, and PC-374) are androgen independent. PC-324 and PC-339 do not express PSA or

AR, making them possible exemplars of the most advanced forms of hormone refractory human prostate cancer.

4. GENETIC CHARACTERIZATION OF HUMAN PROSTATE CANCER XENOGRAFTS

Carcinogenesis is a complex process characterized by the accumulation of genetic changes. Losses of genetic material are often associated with inactivation of tumor suppressor genes, while regions of chromosomal gain or amplification often signal the presence of oncogenes. Xenografts have been used to identify new regions of chromosomal gain or loss not previously identified, and to pinpoint the minimum regions of change as a means of cloning important prostate cancer genes.

4.1. Chromosome 8p

One of the most frequent genetic abnormalities in prostate cancer is the loss of the short arm of chromosome 8, yet prostate cancer tumor suppressor genes in this region have not yet been clearly identified. One potential clue to the location of a tumor suppressor gene is the finding of a homozygous deletion within this region. Van Alewijk et al. recently identified a small 730-1,320 kb homozygous deletion at 8p12-21 in the PC-133 xenograft, a new xenograft not yet described by the Dutch group *(33)*. Identification of this region may be a first step towards the cloning of a prostate cancer tumor suppressor gene, and is one example of the utility of xenografts.

4.2. Chromosome 12p

The ready supply of large amounts of cancer tissue makes xenografts ideal for cytogenetic studies. We previously reported that LAPC-4 and LAPC-3—two xenografts established from different patients—both contain deletions at chromosome 12p12, a region not previously associated with prostate cancer *(17)*. Kibel and colleagues subsequently identified this same region of loss in a prostate cancer xenograft established from a prostate cancer rib metastasis *(16)*. They also found loss of heterozygosity at 12p12-13 in nine of 19 patients with metastatic prostate cancer, suggesting that this region may harbor an important tumor suppressor gene associated with prostate cancer metastasis. In order to clone this gene, Kibel et al. have mapped the region of homozygous deletion in the prostate xenograft, and demonstrated that this region contains at least two potential candidate genes, CDKN1B and ETV6 *(15)*. These experiments demonstrate the power of xenografts to localize and clone tumor suppressor genes in advanced prostate cancer.

5. XENOGRAFTS FOR THE DEFINITION OF MOLECULAR PATHWAYS IN PROSTATE CARCINOGENESIS

One major focus of current prostate cancer research is to define defects in signal-transduction pathways that lead to prostate cancer. Our strategy has been to use xenografts as reagents to identify and confirm the defective signaling pathways, then move to transgenic and/or knockout mouse models to characterize the functional role of that pathway in a genetically defined system. We also anticipate that the xenografts will become indispensable for testing novel therapies aimed specifically at these signaling defects.

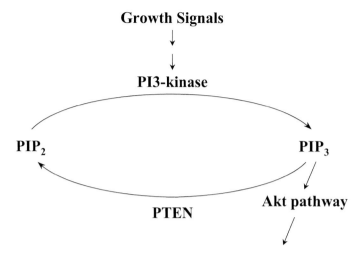

Fig. 1. Regulation of the PI3-kinase/Akt-signaling pathway by PTEN. PI3-kinase is acti-vated by a number of growth-factor receptors that affect proliferation and survival. The pri-mary substrate of PI3-kinase in PIP2, which is converted to PIP3. PIP3 contributes to activation of Akt (also called PKB) by recruiting Akt to the membrane through binding to its pleckstrin homology domain. PTEN is lipid phosphatase that converts PIP3 back to PIP2. Cells that lack PTEN have elevated levels of activated Akt.

5.1. PTEN/Akt

Loss of chromosome 10q is a frequently observed genetic defect in prostate cancer. Recently, the PTEN/MMAC tumor suppressor gene was identified and mapped to chro-mosome 10q23.3 *(18,29)*. PTEN encodes a protein/lipid phosphatase which is mutated or deleted in a range of human cancers. Recent work from our group and others indi-cates that loss of PTEN function occurs in 10–20% of organ-confined and over 50% of advanced prostate cancers, placing it among the most common molecular abnormali-ties reported in human prostate cancer *(5,36,38)*. Fifty percent of LAPC and LuCAP prostate cancer xenografts contain deletions, mutations, or absent expression of PTEN *(38)*. A similar result was recently reported using the Netherlands' xenografts *(36)*. Sixty percent of xenografts either had homozygous deletions or mutations of PTEN. These results confirm the fidelity of xenografts as representations of human prostate cancer, and establish that the signaling pathway regulated by PTEN is critical in prostate cancer. Notably, knockout mice lacking PTEN as a consequence of targeted deletion develop multiple cancers, including prostatic hyperplasia and prostatic intraepithelial neoplasia *(8,22)*.

In our efforts to understand which signaling pathways are regulated by PTEN, we have observed a perfect correlation between the status of PTEN and activation of the serine/threonine kinase Akt *(39)*. This result—together with a series of nearly simulta-neous publications from more than eight groups working on PTEN using different tumor models—has conclusively established that PTEN functions as a negative regula-tor of the PI3-kinase/Akt-signaling pathway *(7,10,12,20,28,30,39)* (Fig. 1). Because PI3-kinase and Akt are known to have oncogenic and/or antiapoptotic functions in various model systems, it is likely that deregulation of this pathway in PTEN-deficient cells is responsible for the cancer phenotype. Future work is focused on defining the role of this signaling pathway using genetically defined mouse models for prostate cancer, and on testing the therapeutic role of drugs that target this pathway.

5.2. Tyrosine Kinase Signaling and Cross-Communication With AR

Prostate epithelial cells utilize androgen as a growth, survival, and differentiation factor. By inference, perturbations in androgen receptor (AR) signaling could play a major role in cancer progression, particularly in patients who relapse after androgen ablation therapy. Strong support for this hypothesis comes from analysis of AR in hormone-refractory cancer, showing AR gene mutation or amplification in 20–40% of cases *(11,31,35)*. Both LNCaP and the CWR22 xenograft bear AR mutations that enable the receptor to be activated by nonandrogenic steroid hormones such as progesterone and estrogen. Another emerging theme is that many hormone-refractory cancers have activated the AR signaling pathway through a ligand-independent mechanism. For example, in cells expressing wild-type AR protein (LAPC-4), we have recently shown that overexpression of the epidermal growth factor receptor (EGFR) family kinase Her-2/neu can activate AR *(6)*.

The concept that nonsteroid receptor signal-transduction pathways can substitute for or synergize with a steroid hormone and activate a nuclear receptor in the setting of hormone deprivation has precedent. The progesterone and estrogen receptors (ER) can be activated independent of hormone by epidermal growth factor (EGF), insulin-like growth factor 1 (IGF-1), and cAMP. The mechanistic details of hormone independent receptor activation are not fully known, but recent findings implicate phosphorylation of the receptor itself, which allows recruitment of accessory proteins into the hormone-receptor transcription complex. The best example is activation of ER by phosphorylation of Ser 118 through the mitogen-activated protein (MAP) kinase pathway *(4,14)*. AR can also become activated in a ligand-independent fashion by IGF-1, EGF, and keratinocyte growth factor. Although compelling, the implication of these observations for human prostate cancer remains unclear.

Her-2/neu, a member of the EGF family of receptor tyrosine kinases which signals through *ras* and MAP kinase pathways, is amplified and overexpressed in 20–30% of human breast and ovarian cancers. Overexpression of Her-2/neu is associated with poor survival in breast cancer patients and has been shown in transgenic models to induce breast cancer. Several recent observations suggest specific interactions between Her-2/neu and ER signaling in breast cancer *(2,19)*. Forced overexpression of Her-2/neu in breast cancer cells activates ER and confers estrogen independent growth, suggesting cross-communication between the Her-2/neu- and ER-signaling pathways.

The LAPC-4 xenograft progresses to androgen independence after androgen ablation and provides a model to study this transition in vivo. Studies of differential gene expression in LAPC-4 revealed a consistent increase in Her-2/neu protein expression in androgen independent tumors, suggesting that overexpression of Her-2/neu may play a role in hormone-refractory progression. Furthermore, forced overexpression of Her-2/neu in androgen dependent prostate cancer cells was sufficient to confer androgen independent growth in vitro and to accelerate androgen independent growth in castrated animals. Her-2/neu overexpression activated the AR signaling pathway in the

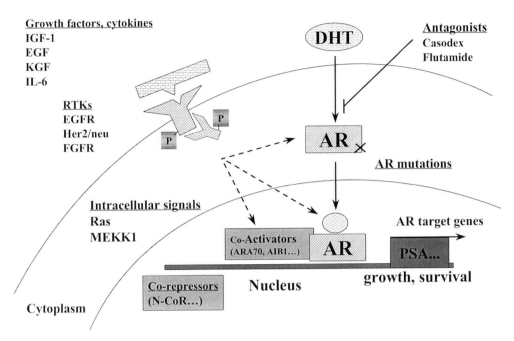

Fig. 2. Mechanisms of ligand-independent androgen receptor activation. Activation of the androgen receptor signaling pathway is a central theme in hormone refractory prostate cancer. This activation can occur through mutations in the androgen receptor which alter specificity for ligands or through upregulation of nonsteroid receptor signaling pathways that activate androgen receptor signaling through unknown mechanisms. Inhibitors of these pathways may have therapeutic utility in hormone refractory prostate cancer. Reprinted with permission from *Cancer and Metastatic Reviews (3)*.

absence of ligand and enhanced the magnitude of AR response in the presence of low levels of androgen. Reconstitution experiments in a heterologous cell type expressing low levels of endogenous AR established that the effects of Her-2/neu on the AR pathway require expression of AR, and are most likely mediated by coactivators or additional transcription factors which function coordinately with AR to activate androgen dependent transcription. These findings demonstrate cross-communication between Her-2/neu and AR-signaling pathways and provide novel mechanistic insight into the clinical problem of androgen independent progression (Fig. 2).

The extent to which Her-2/neu causes androgen independent progression in prostate cancer is unknown. Her-2/neu is expressed in normal prostate basal cells, and has been demonstrated to be expressed or overexpressed in a subset of prostate cancers. Some studies have found an association between Her-2/neu expression and shortened survival, although this finding remains controversial. Most studies, however, have only examined early tumors obtained at the time of radical prostatectomy, rather than the more relevant metastatic or androgen independent tumors. It will be interesting to look at Her-2/neu expression in additional xenografts and advanced prostate cancers. The role of Her-2/neu in androgen independent progression could be tested using Herceptin, a recently developed monoclonal antibody (MAb), which blocks Her-2/neu function and has clinical efficacy in breast cancer. Likewise, it will be important to determine the extent to which the paradigm of Her-2/neu-AR cross-communication can be generalized to other receptor tyrosine kinases, such as IGF-1, KGF and EGF. As stated earlier, previous studies have shown that these tyrosine kinases can activate AR in the absence of ligand. Strategies to inhibit the relevant tyrosine kinases or the point at which they interact with AR may be able to revert androgen independent tumors to androgen dependence.

6. XENOGRAFTS FOR GENE DISCOVERY

One of the advantages of prostate cancer xenografts is that they provide a large and renewable source of tissue for gene discovery. We and others have used xenografts to identify novel genes associated with androgen independent progression, cell surface markers for prostate cancer diagnosis and therapy, and specific gene family members expressed in prostate cancer (i.e., tyrosine kinases, HOX genes, and others).

6.1. Prostate Stem Cell Antigen (PSCA)

The identification of cell surface antigens expressed by prostate cancers is central to the development of new diagnostic and therapeutic strategies. The LAPC-4 xenograft was used to search for novel cell surface proteins upregulated during prostate cancer progression. Prostate stem cell antigen (PSCA) is a glycosylphosphatidylinositol (GPI)-anchored cell surface protein related to the Thy-1/Sca-2 family of hematopoietic stem cell markers *(23)*. In normal male tissues, PSCA mRNA is expressed predominantly by the prostate, although expression has also recently been found in the bladder and stomach. Importantly, PSCA is expressed by more than 80% of prostate cancers and is thus a potential cell surface target in prostate cancer. Our group recently isolated a series of MAbs specific for PSCA. These antibodies recognize PSCA on the cell surface of both normal and malignant prostate cells. Confirming the RNA data, PSCA protein is detected in 84% of primary and 100% of metastatic prostate cancers. When PSCA protein was compared in normal and malignant cells, expression was significantly higher in cancer in 36% of cases. Overexpression correlated with both tumor stage and Gleason score, suggesting that PSCA expression increases with prostate cancer progression. Strikingly, all nine cases of bone metastases examined stained intensely for PSCA, indicating that PSCA may be particularly useful as a target in metastatic prostate cancer.

PSCA maps to chromosome 8q24.2, a region of gene amplification in advanced prostate cancer *(23)*. Recent studies have shown that PSCA is often amplified in cases of locally-advanced prostate cancer, and that this amplification occurs in tandem with c-myc amplification *(25)*. Furthermore, PSCA overexpression correlated with PSCA gene amplification (Fig. 3). Since PSCA and c-myc are coamplified and c-myc is an independent poor prognostic factor in prostate cancer, it is reasonable to infer that PSCA overexpression is a surrogate marker for aggressive disease and a potential target in these tumors.

As noted, xenografts may be useful reagents to test new therapies. LAPC-4 and LAPC-9 both express large amounts of PSCA RNA and protein—particularly LAPC-9, which was established from a bone metastasis. Current efforts are focused upon determining whether MAbs directed against PSCA can prevent or treat LAPC-9 tumor formation or metastasis. Preliminary data have shown that anti-PSCA MAbs can prevent LAPC-9 tumor formation, yet have no effect on non-PSCA-expressing tumors.

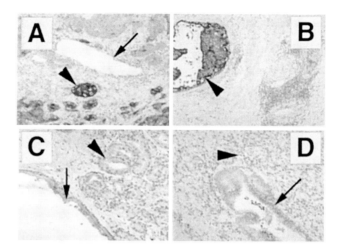

Fig. 3. PSCA protein expression correlates with PSCA copy number in prostate cancer. (**A,B**) tumors (*arrowheads*) from two individuals that were found by FISH analysis to have PCA gene amplification show increased staining relative to adjacent normal tissue (*arrows*); (**C**), tumor without a gain in PSCA copy number (*arrowhead*) expresses equal amounts of PSCA in both normal (*arrow*) and tumor; (**D**), a tumor (*arrowhead*) that has lost one PSCA allele shows decreased PSCA expression compared with adjacent normal tissue (*arrow*).

One of the more intriguing early findings with PSCA was that PSCA mRNA localized in normal prostate to a subset of basal cells *(23)*. Since basal cells are believed to be the progenitors of mature secretory epithelium, it was hypothesized that PSCA may be a marker of prostate stem/progenitor cells. Indeed, PSCA is expressed by a subset of normal prostate epithelial cells in culture *(3)*. These cells coexpress basal and secretory cell cytokeratins, and may represent an intermediate progenitor cell population. Additional work is currently underway to characterize PSCA-positive cells both in humans and in transgenic models using the PSCA promoter as a means of isolating PSCA-positive cells.

6.2. Androgen Independence Genes

Subtractive hybridization of androgen dependent and androgen independent LAPC-4 tumors was performed in order to identify novel genes associated with androgen independent progression *(24)*. A similar strategy achieved success in identifying Her-2/neu as a potential mediator of androgen independent progression. Nine genes were isolated and confirmed to be differentially expressed during the transition of LAPC-4 from androgen dependence to androgen independence. The expression of three of these clones was evaluated in normal and malignant prostate by mRNA *in situ* hybridization. All three genes localized exclusively to basal cells in normal prostate specimens. In addition, strong expression of all three genes could be detected in a majority of androgen independent tumors. These results suggested that androgen independent tumors may be characterized by the expression of genes normally restricted to prostate basal/progenitor cells. Her-2/neu and bcl-2—two other genes upregulated in androgen independent prostate cancer—are also normally expressed by basal cells. We and others have hypothesized that hormone-refractory tumors and normal prostate basal cells, which are androgen independent, may escape androgen withdrawal-induced apoptosis by shared mechanisms *(3)*. Study of genes isolated from androgen independent xenografts may shed new light on the biology of androgen independence.

6.3. Tyrosine Kinases

Tyrosine kinases play central roles in the growth and differentiation of normal cells as well as tumor cells. One example is Her-2/neu, which was fully described earlier. The spectrum of tyrosine kinases expressed and active in prostate carcinogenesis is unknown. The CWR22 xenograft was used to identify these tyrosine kinases using a degenerate reverse-transcriptase PCR approach *(26)*. Eleven tyrosine kinase receptors, 9 nonreceptor kinases, and 7 dual kinases were isolated using this screening technique, including a few previously unidentified genes. One kinase—etk/bmx—has subsequently been studied in more detail, and has been shown to play a potential role in prostate cancer neuroendocrine differentiation. These experiments exemplify the power of xenografts for the identification of potentially important genes in prostate cancer.

7. CONCLUSION

Prostate cancer xenografts are powerful tools for discovery. The recent expansion in the number of xenografts has already led to important new discoveries relevant to the molecular biology of prostate cancer progression. Xenografts provide a renewable, relatively homogeneous population of cancer cells for gene discovery, genetic and molecular analysis, and preclinical trials. Hypotheses generated by experimentation with xenografts can then be correlated with clinical material and tested in transgenic and knockout models. The combination of multiple resources and models should lead to dramatic advances in our ability to prevent and manage prostate cancer in the near future.

REFERENCES

1. Bladou, F., R. Vessella, K. R. Buhler, W. J. Ellis, L. D. True, and P. H. Lange. 1996. Cell proliferation and apoptosis during prostatic tumor xenograft involution and regrowth after castration. *Int. J. Cancer* **67:** 785–790.
2. Bouchard, L., L. Lamarre, P. J. Tremblay, and P. Jolicoeur. 1989. Stochastic appearance of mammary tumors in transgenic mice carrying the MMTV/c-neu oncogene. *Cell* **57:** 931–936.
3. Bui, M. and R. E. Reiter. 1998. Stem cell genes in androgen independent prostate cancer (in process citation). *Cancer Met. Review* **17:** 391–399.
4. Bunone, G., P.-A. Briand, R. J. Miksicek, and D. Picard. 1996. Activation of the unliganded estrogen receptor by EGF involves the MAP kinase pathway and direct phosphorylation. *EMBO J.* **15:** 2174–2183.
5. Cairns, P., K. Okami, S. Halachmi, N. Halachmi, M. Esteller, J. G. Herman, et al. 1997. Frequent inactivation of *PTEN/MMAC1* in primary prostate cancer. *Cancer Res.* **57:** 4997–5000.
6. Craft, N., C. Chhor, C. Tran, A. Belldegrun, J. B. Dekernion, O. N. Witte, et al. 1999. Evidence for clonal outgrowth of androgen independent prostate cancer cells from androgen dependent tumors through a two-step process. *Cancer Res.* **59:** 5030–5036.
7. Davies, M. A., Y. Lu, T. Sano, X. Fang, P. Tang, R. LaPushin, et al. 1998. Adenoviral transgene expression of MMAC/PTEN in human glioma cells inhibits Akt activation and induces anoikis. *Cancer Res.* **58:** 5285–5290.
8. Di Cristofano, A., B. Pesce, C. Cordon-Cardo, and P. P. Pandolfi. 1998. Pten is essential for embryonic development and tumour suppression. *Nat. Genet.* **19:** 348–355.

9. Ellis, W. J., R. L. Vessella, K. R. Buhler, F. Bladou, L. D. True, S. A. Bigler, et al. 1996. Characterization of a novel androgen-sensitive, prostate-specific antigen-producing prostatic carcinoma xenograft: LuCaP 23. *Clin. Cancer Res.* **2:** 1039–1048.

10. Furnari, F. B., H. J. Huang, and W. K. Cavenee. 1998. The phosphoinositol phosphatase activity of PTEN mediates a serum-sensitive G1 growth arrest in glioma cells. *Cancer Res.* **58:** 5002–5008 (Abstract).

11. Gaddipati, J. P., D. G. McLeod, H. B. Heidenberg, L. A. Sesterhenn, M. J. Finger, J. W. Moul, et al. 1994. Frequent detection of codon 877 mutation in the androgen receptor gene in advanced prostate cancers. *Cancer Res.* **54:** 2861–2864.

12. Haas-Kogan, D., N. Shalev, M. Wong, G. Mills, G. Yount, and D. Stokoe. 1998. Protein kinase B (PKB/Akt) activity is elevated in glioblastoma cells due to mutation of the tumor suppressor PTEN/MMAC. *Curr. Biol.* **8:** 1195–1198.

13. Jongsma, J., M. H. Oomen, M. A. Noordzij, et al. 1999. Kinetics of neuroendocrine differentiation in an androgen dependent human prostate xenograft model. *Am. J. Pathol.* **154:** 543–51.

14. Kato, S., H. Endoh, Y. Masuhiro, T. Kitamoto, S. Uchiyama, H. Sasaki, et al. 1995. Activation of the estrogen receptor through phosphorylation by mitogen-activated protein kinase. *Science* **270:** 1491–1494.

15. Kibel, A. S., D. Freije, W. B. Isaacs, et al. 1999. Deletion mapping at 12p12-13 in metastatic prostate cancer. *Genes Chromosomes Cancer* **25:** 270–276.

16. Kibel, A. S., M. Schutte, S. E. Kern, et al. 1998. Identification of 12p as a region of frequent deletion in advanced prostate cancer. *Cancer Res.* **58:** 5652–5655.

17. Klein, K. A., R. E. Reiter, J. Redula, H. Moradi, X. L. Zhu, A. R. Brothman, et al. 1997. Progression of metastatic human prostate cancer to androgen independence in immunodeficient SCID mice. *Nat. Med.* **3:** 402–408.

18. Li, J., C. Yen, D. Liaw, K. Podsypanina, S. Bose, S. I. Wang, et al. 1997. PTEN, a putative protein tyrosine phosphatase gene mutated in human brain, breast, and prostate cancer. *Science* **275:** 1943–1947.

19. Muller, W. J., E. Sinn, P. K. Pattengale, R. Wallace, and P. Leder. 1988. Single-step induction to mammary adenocarcinoma in transgenic mice bearing the activated c-neu oncogene. *Cell* **54:** 105–115.

20. Myers, M. P., I. Pass, I. H. Batty, J. Van der Kaay, J. P. Stolarov, B. A. Hemmings, et al. 1998. The lipid phosphatase activity of PTEN is critical for its tumor suppressor function. *Proc. Natl. Acad. Sci. USA* **95:** 13,513–13,518.

21. Nagabhushan, M., C. M. Miller, T. P. Pretlow, J. M. Giaconia, N. L. Edgehouse, S. Schwartz, et al. 1996. CRW22: the first human prostate cancer xenograft with strongly androgen dependent and relapsed strains both in vivo and in soft agar. *Cancer Res.* **56:** 3042–3046.

22. Podsypanina, K., L. H. Ellenson, A. Nemes, J. Gu, T. Masahito, K. M. Yamada, et al. 1999. Mutation of Pten/Mmac1 in mice causes neoplasia in multiple organ systems. *Proc. Natl. Acad. Sci. USA* **96:** 1563–1568.

23. Reiter, R. E., Z. Gu, T. Watabe, G. Thomas, K. Szigeti, E. Davis, et al. 1998. Prostate stem cell antigen: a cell surface marker overexpressed in prostate cancer. *Proc. Natl. Acad. Sci. USA* **95:** 1735–1740.

24. Reiter, R. E., C. Magi-Galluzzi, H. Hemmati, C. L. Sawyers, M. Loda, and O. N. Witte. 1997. Two genes upregulated in androgen independent prostate cancer are also selectively expressed in the basal cells of normal prostate epithelium. *J. Urol.* **157:** 269A (Abstract).

25. Reiter, R. E., I. Sato, G. Thomas, et al. 2000. Co-amplification of prostate stem cell antigen and myc in locally advanced prostate cancer. *Genes Chrom. Cancer* **27:** 95–103.

26. Robinson, D., F. He, T. Preglow, and H. J. Kung. 1996. A tyrosine kinase profile of prostate carcinoma. *Proc. Natl. Acad. Sci. USA* **93:** 5958–5962.

27. Sramkoski, R. M., T. G. Pretlow, J. M. Giaconia, et al. 1999. A new human prostate carcinoma cell line. *In Vitro Cell Dev. Biol. Anim.* **35:** 403–409.

28. Stambolic, V., A. Suzuki, J. L. de la Pompa, G. M. Brothers, C. Mirtsos, T. Sasaki, et al. 1998. Negative regulation of PKB/Akt-dependent cell survival by the tumor suppressor PTEN. *Cell* **95:** 29–39.

29. Steck, P. A., M. A. Pershouse, S. A. Jasser, W. K. Yung, H. Lin, A. H. Ligon, et al. 1997. Identification of a candidate tumour suppressor gene, MMAC1, at chromosome 10q23.3 that is mutated in multiple advanced cancers. *Nat. Genet.* **15:** 356–362.

30. Sun, H., R. Lesche, D. M. Li, J. Liliental, H. Zhang, J. Gao, et al. 1999. PTEN modulates cell cycle progression and cell survival by regulating phosphatidylinositol 3,4,5,-trisphosphate and Akt/protein kinase B signaling pathway. *Proc. Natl. Acad. Sci. USA* **96:** 6199–6204.

31. Talpin, M. E., G. J. Bubley, T. D. Shuster, M. E. Frantz, A. E. Spooner, G. K. Ogata, et al. 1995. Mutation of the androgen-receptor gene in metastatic androgen independent prostate cancer. *N. Engl. J. Med.* **332:** 1393–1398.

32. Tan, J., Y. Sharief, K. G. Hamil, C. W. Gregory, D. Y. Zang, M. Sar, et al. 1997. Dehydroepiandrosterone activates mutant androgen receptors expressed in the androgen dependent human prostate cancer xenograft CWR22 and LNCaP cells. *Mol. Endocrinol.* **11:** 450–459.

33. van Alewijk, D. C., M. M. van der Weiden, B. J. Eussen, et al. 1999. Identification of a homozygous deletion at 8p12-21 in a human prostate cancer xenograft. *Genes Chromosomes Cancer* **24:** 119–126.

34. van Weerden, W. M., C. M. de Ridder, C. L. Verdaasdonk, J. C. Romijn, T. H. van der Kwast, F. H. Schroder, et al. 1996. Development of seven new human prostate tumor xenograft models and their histopathological characterization. *Am. J. Pathol.* **149:** 1055–1062.

35. Visakorpi, T., E. Hyytinen, P. Koivisto, M. M. Tanner, R. Keinanen, C. Palmberg, et al. 1995. In vivo amplification of the androgen receptor gene and progression of human prostate cancer. *Nat. Genet.* **9:** 401–406.

36. Vlietstra, R. J., D. C. van Alewijk, K. G. Hermans, G. J. van Steenbrugge, and J. Trapman. 1998. Frequent inactivation of PTEN in prostate cancer cell lines and xenografts. *Cancer Res.* **58:** 2720–2723.

37. Wainstein, M. A., F. He, D. Robinson, H. J. Kung, S. Schwartz, J. M. Gianconia, et al. 1994. CWR22: androgen dependent xenograft model derived from a primary human prostatic carcinoma. *Cancer Res.* **54:** 6049–6052.

38. Whang, Y. E., X. Wu, H. Suzuki, R. Reiter, C. Tran, R. L. Vessella, et al. 1998. Inactivation of the tumor suppressor PTEN/MMAC1 in advanced human prostate cancer through loss of expression. *Proc. Natl. Acad. Sci. USA* **95:** 5246–5250.

39. Wu, X., K. Senechal, M. S. Neshat, Y. E. Whang, and C. L. Sawyers. 1998. The PTEN/MMAC1 tumor suppressor phosphatase functions as a negative regulator of the phosphoinositide 3-kinase/Akt pathway. *Proc. Natl. Acad. Sci. USA* **95:** 15,587–15,591.

11

Comprehensive Analyses of Prostate Gene Expression

Peter S. Nelson, MD

1. INTRODUCTION

The development and progression of human prostate cancer is driven by the accumulation of genetic and epigenetic events. A predisposition to certain environmental factors may also contribute to neoplastic growth. To develop rational treatments for this disease, we must identify and understand the specific molecular alterations that influence processes such as proliferation, differentiation, growth-factor response pathways, apoptosis, drug metabolism, DNA replication, DNA repair, adhesion, angiogenesis, and others.

Over the last three decades, the focus of biological investigation has been on the study of individual genes and proteins. This has occurred partly because of the submicroscopic nature and transient existence of relevant molecules and the lack of tools capable of providing a more global, comprehensive view of biological complexity. While great advances have been made in the study of individual molecules and small numbers of molecular interactions, progress has been delayed by the need for a complete inventory of all genes and their cognate proteins relevant for defining normal and disease processes. The completion of the Human Genome Project will provide a foundation for a comprehensive description of this molecular "tool set." More specifically, the tool set required for studies of prostate carcinogenesis is that portion of the human genome used or expressed in the human prostate gland. The subset of genes expressed in a given cell or tissue type such as the prostate may be defined as the *transcriptome*— the dynamic link between the genome, the proteome, and the cellular phenotype of physical characteristics.

Once a transcriptome has been described, the next objective is to understand the relationships of the genes and their protein products in terms of biological pathways, networks, and complex systems in health and disease. With this goal, novel technologies for the comprehensive assessment of genomes and patterns of gene expression have recently been developed. This chapter illustrates the fundamental concepts underlying several of these technologies and describes their application to the study of prostate carcinogenesis.

From: *Prostate Cancer: Biology, Genetics, and the New Therapeutics*
Edited by: L. W. K. Chung, W. B. Isaacs, and J. W. Simons © Humana Press Inc., Totowa, NJ

2. PROSTATE CARCINOMA: THE MOTIVATION FOR COMPREHENSIVE EXPRESSION STUDIES

Carcinoma of the prostate exhibits a wide range of biological variation influenced by genetic, racial, environmental, and other undefined factors. As with many common epithelial cancers, the development of prostate carcinoma is believed to involve an accumulation of genetic damage to critical genes that are important in growth regulation and differentiation. Although genetic alterations in the form of amplifications, deletions, and mutations have frequently been identified in prostate cancers *(21,36)*, the studies of known tumor suppressor genes and oncogenes have yielded inconsistent results *(7,17,26,29,32)*. This implies that:

1. Other as yet unidentified alterations are operative;
2. Significant alterations may be masked by the inherent heterogeneity in normal and neoplastic prostate samples and disease phenotype(s);
3. More sensitive analytical tools and approaches are required; or
4. A more comprehensive approach capable of simultaneous assessment of multiple genetic, epigenetic, and environmental factors is required.

The benefits of identifying molecules with potential roles in mediating critical processes in normal prostatic function and in the development of prostate cancer are relevant for all areas of prostate cancer research. Two genes, prostate specific antigen (PSA) and the androgen receptor (AR), serve to illustrate this point. Both genes play a significant role in the normal physiologic functions of the human prostate. The finding that PSA levels in the serum correlate with the presence of prostate cancer led to the development of PSA assays suitable for screening and monitoring patients with prostate cancer *(8)*. PSA may also be a mediator of prostate cancer growth through interactions with specific endocrine factors *(10,13)*, and may serve as a therapeutic target through vaccine strategies *(23)* and prodrug activation *(15)*. The AR mediates normal essential cellular events involving differentiation, proliferation, and apoptosis. The AR is also an important regulator of prostate cancer growth with the AR pathway currently serving as the major therapeutic target for advanced prostate cancer treatment. Amplifications and mutations of the AR gene have been found in prostate cancers *(14,36)*, and epidemiological studies have shown a correlation between a simple sequence repeat polymorphism in the AR gene and the development of prostate cancer *(31)*.

Despite the considerable biological and clinical importance of these two genes, there remain many unanswered questions and untested hypotheses which have important ramifications for the treatment of prostate cancer. What are the biological activators of PSA? *(33)* What are the other relevant substrates for PSA that could be involved in prostate cancer growth? What are the mediators of the AR pathway? What specific genes are activated or repressed by the androgen receptor? Studies of the rat prostate androgen receptor program indicate that approx 60 genes are upregulated and 10 genes are downregulated by androgens *(37)*. Fewer than one-half of this number of androgen-regulated genes have been identified in the human prostate. A starting point for facilitating studies designed to answer these and other questions is the building of a comprehensive tool set comprised of virtual and physical genetic information derived from the human prostate.

3. THE HUMAN GENOME AND PROSTATE TRANSCRIPTOME

A new five-year plan for the Human Genome Project has emphasized the production of a complete human genome sequence by the end of 2003—two years ahead of previous projections *(11)*. A "working draft" of the human sequence will be produced before the end of 2000 (http://www.ornl.gov/hgmis/project/update.html). In addition to this publicly supported sequencing effort, at least one major private venture will also be submitting large datasets of human genomic sequence into the public domain (http://www.celera.com). The potential applications of these data in biomedical research are tremendous. Possession of the code for every human gene will facilitate the cloning of relevant molecules for individual study. The DNA sequence can often provide information which predicts gene function, structure, regulation, and evolution, and facilitate an understanding of disease states relative to genetic variation.

A more complete understanding of the cellular machinery involved in normal homeostasis and the transformation to malignancy will result from "mining" the human genome for genes and their cognate proteins. Many of these may have direct implications for prostate cancer diagnostic and therapeutic uses. However, much of the genomic data will be in a "raw" sequence format, with little annotation provided. In addition, the tremendous quantities of data—more than 3 billion base pairs of sequence—pose a daunting analysis task. Efficient access to concise and integrated biomedical informatics to support data acquisition, data analysis, and decision making is therefore essential for the timely exploitation of this resource.

One approach to "mining" the human genome is to focus initially on that portion that actually codes for genes: ~3% of the total sequence. The human genome is estimated to comprise approx 100,000 genes *(16)*. To confer developmental and functional specificity, only a fraction of this total is active in a given cell type at a specific point in time. The messenger RNA (mRNA) molecules in a cell or tissue reflect that portion of the genome that is utilized or expressed. Any distinct cell or tissue type is estimated to transcribe between 10,000 and 30,000 different mRNA species *(4)*. A convenient term to describe this repertoire of expressed genes in a cell or tissue is the *transcriptome (35)*. Converting the entire repertoire of cellular mRNAs into a library of cDNAs which are then identified by sequence analysis provides a "snapshot" of transcriptional activity that defines a cellular phenotype or function. For most cDNAs, it is only necessary to sequence <100 nucleotides in order to categorize it as identical or similar to a known gene, or conversely as a novel one (though additional sequence information is often extremely useful for predicting gene function). Thus, the partial sequencing of a cDNA clone generates an identifier, label, or tag that is now commonly referred to as an "Expressed Sequence Tag" or EST.

The systematic categorization of ESTs by clustering and annotation provides a method to define a tissue or cellular transcriptome *(1,24)*. As tumor cells are phenotypically different from their normal counterparts, their set of expressed genes differs in a qualitative (different genes expressed) and quantitative fashion. A thorough understanding of which genes are expressed, to what extent, and under what conditions they are expressed, can provide insights into the processes of homeostasis and carcinogenesis. A database of ESTs (dbEST) *(6)* derived from normal and diseased human tissues has been established at the National Center for Biotechnology Information (NCBI) *(7)*. There are currently more than 2.8 million EST entries in dbEST, including 1.5 million from humans as well as sequences from mouse, nematode, fruit-fly and other species (dbEST release 072399). This database has proven useful for a variety of applications, such as the identification of exons in large tracts of genomic DNA, the identification of human genes homologous to genes in other species ("phylum hopping"), the discovery of new members of gene families involved in human disease, and as a resource for gene-based mapping reagents *(8)*. These ESTs have been assembled into the UniGene collection—a database now comprised of more than 76,000 clusters of sequences, each suggested to represent the transcription products of a distinct human gene (UniGene build 072399). Thus, sequences representing approx 75% of all human genes may be contained in this database.

The National Cancer Institute has initiated an effort termed the Cancer Genome Anatomy Project (CGAP) that aims to use ESTs to establish molecular fingerprints or signatures for common human cancers such as breast, lung, colon, and prostate (http://www.ncbi.nlm.nih.gov/ncicgap/). This project has contributed ESTs to dbEST and the UniGene effort, and also aims to determine the chromosomal locations of many of the novel sequences that are identified. As described here, the further development of this concept with a directed focus on the normal prostate and prostate pathology has established a curated *prostate transcriptome*, in both a virtual and physical (preserved stocks of cDNA clones) format. This project, termed the Prostate Expression Database, is developing a fundamental resource that will facilitate a comprehensive approach for the study of molecular alterations involved in the initiation and progression of prostate cancers.

4. THE PROSTATE EXPRESSION DATABASE: PEDB

The Prostate Expression Database (PEDB) was established as a resource of human prostate gene-expression information to be used by investigators studying normal and neoplastic prostate development *(19)*. PEDB is a curated sequence archive comprising ESTs generated primarily by CGAP and the CaPCURE Genetics Consortium from cDNA libraries representing normal prostate tissues and a wide spectrum of benign and malignant prostate disease states. PEDB currently has >52,000 prostate ESTs that assemble into >17,000 distinct species. The primary PEDB user work sites involve database queries with nucleotide sequence information using the BLAST algorithm *(2)*, and virtual expression analysis using a graphical user interface to perform intra- and interlibrary sequence abundance comparisons. The PEDB also provides links to other relevant WWW resources involving prostate disease, cancer biology, and genomics. The database is available via the World Wide Web (WWW) at http://www.pedb.org.

Further details describing the specific schema, construction, and utilities of PEDB are found at the website and in a recent publication *(19)*. Briefly, software automates an analysis pipeline of sequence submission, masking, clustering, and annotation tasks in conjunction with an Oracle relational database. Public and private ESTs are submitted, quality checked, and masked for vector, *Escherichia coli (E. coli)*, and interspersed repeats. ESTs are clustered with the Contig Assembly Program (CAP2) *(20)*. The consensus sequence from each cluster is used to search three public databases (GenBank, dbEST, and UniGene) using BLAST (http://blast.wustl.edu), and sequence matches are annotated with the appropriate gene identification.

As inventories of ESTs accumulate from a variety of normal and diseased tissues, it becomes possible to compare the expression fingerprints from different tissues using computer algorithms. This Virtual Expression Analysis (VEA), or Digital Differential Display (DDD), has the potential to comprehensively identify genes whose expression differs significantly between multiple tissue types. As described in Section 5, such analyses may identify genes expressed exclusively in specific tissues, or expressed at different stages of neoplastic transformation by comparing, for example, the set of ESTs from normal prostate, prostate intraepithelial neoplasia (PIN), and malignant prostate tissues. Examples of this type of differential expression analysis can be found on the NCI-CGAP (21) and the PEDB *(19)* WWW sites.

5. GENE EXPRESSION STUDIES: BIOINFORMATICS

The application of bioinformatics tools to databases of nucleotide and amino acid sequence information has the potential to rapidly and comprehensively identify specific differences between properly annotated datasets. The essential elements for such analyses include accurate sequence information, the development of software tools for specific database queries, and database elements (sequences) with factual and sufficient annotation. Major advantages of database approaches are that resources can be continually updated with new information, the data is not perishable, and complex comprehensive analyses can be performed with the appropriate software algorithms. The following examples illustrate the practical utility of database resources.

ESTs belong to different cDNA libraries, each of which is prepared from one particular cell type, organ, or tumor. The abundance of specific ESTs, when randomly selected from well-constructed cDNA libraries, provides a rough indication of gene-expression levels. Clustering ESTs into homologous groups, counting the ESTs comprising each group, parsing the EST number into subgroups based on a cell or tissue library source, and then comparing the abundance levels of ESTs in each represented group thus provides a "virtual" method for determining gene expression levels. Several practical demonstrations of this method have been published. A virtual search of 1,137,304 ESTs for genes expressed specifically in human prostate tissue identified four well-described prostate-specific genes and three new uncharacterized prostate-specific genes *(34)*. A less comprehensive method involved the virtual comparison of 6000 ESTs produced from two breast tissue cDNA libraries. This analysis resulted in the identification of a novel breast cancer specific gene, BCSG1, that was confirmed to be upregulated in infiltrating breast cancers using laboratory-based methods *(22)*.

The PEDB website incorporates a Virtual Expression Analysis Tool (VEAT) with a graphical user interface (GUI) developed to view PEDB clusters, annotations, and expression levels. VEAT, written in the Java programming language, provides a virtual inter- and intralibrary analysis of transcript abundance, diversity, and differential expression. Libraries or groups of libraries from normal prostate, primary carcinoma, and metastatic carcinoma or with other specified attributes are selected individually or grouped for comparative analyses. The abundance of each gene or "species" in each

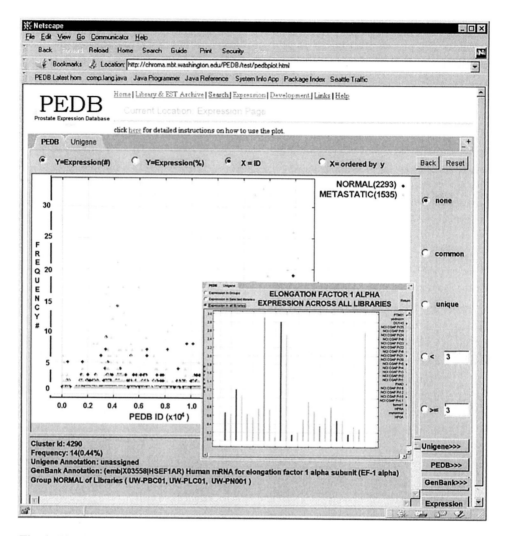

Fig. 1. Viewing gene expression profiles with the Virtual Expression Analysis Tool (VEAT). The abundance profile of ESTs derived from a normal prostate cDNA library (*diamond*) compared with ESTs from a metastatic prostate cDNA library (*triangle*) are compared. The *x*-axis segregates each gene or EST by PEDB identification number. The *y*-axis displays the gene/EST abundance based on the number of times a specific EST appears in the library. Individual datapoints can be selected with the corresponding gene annotation provided in the bottom panel. Gene annotation consists of a cluster or group ID number, the frequency or abundance of the gene in the library, the Unigene Database annotation, and the GenBank Database annotation. Buttons on the bottom right link directly to public database records. Selecting the "expression" button creates a histogram display of the expression level of any gene across all libraries in the PEDB (*inset*).

selected library align to produce a map of gene expression. Genes can also be analyzed for differential expression across all libraries or selected groups of libraries (Fig. 1). The visual output is a dot plot enabling the rapid assessment of differential expression of all represented genes simultaneously with options for user-defined thresholds for expression cut-off *(19)*. The CGAP website has also incorporated a virtual expression tool called Digital Differential Display, designed to determine expression differences between EST datasets. The visual output is similar in format to a "dot-blot" with EST library percentages displayed.

The virtual expression capabilities of PEDB have also been used to develop additional criteria for selecting potential differentially expressed genes identified through laboratory-based investigations. Comprehensive differential screening methods, such as differential display or subtractive hybridization, often produce numerous false-positive clones in addition to bona fide sequences of interest. We employed the virtual expression capabilities of PEDB to evaluate 15 partial cDNAs that exhibited a differential pattern of expression in a model system of increasingly tumorigenic prostate cancer cells. Virtual expression analyses of these sequences determined that one cDNA, subsequently identified as the gene encoding the cell adhesion-related protein Hevin, exhibited a differential EST expression with fewer Hevin ESTs in datasets derived from prostate carcinoma relative to datasets from normal prostate *(25)*. The loss of Hevin expression in metastatic prostate tissues was subsequently confirmed, and recently reported studies of Hevin expression in lung and colon tumors described a downregulation of the Hevin protein in these malignancies *(3)*.

The continued expansion of EST resources derived from additional prostate cDNA libraries representing individual cell types, different metastatic sites, and cancers with different drug resistance profiles will facilitate a complete description of the prostate transcriptome. Additional ESTs will also allow for the application of statistical tools to the data analysis process, thus providing an indication of the significance of virtually-identified differentially expressed sequences.

6. GENE EXPRESSION STUDIES: DNA ARRAYS

Advances in robotics, miniaturization, and informatics have provided new and extremely powerful approaches for DNA analyses. One such approach involves the use of DNA arrays, a method that combines the proven chemistry of nucleic-acid hybridization with advanced automation and image analysis technology to quantitatively monitor changes in the expression of thousands of genes simultaneously. DNA arrays have been described in several configurations, including oligonucleotide arrays *(9)*, microarrays of cDNAs spotted on glass slides *(30)*, and DNAs spotted onto nylon membranes *(27)*. The basic concept is straightforward: DNA representing a particular gene of interest is either spotted (printed) or synthesized onto some type of solid support such as a silicon wafer, glass microscope slide, or nylon membrane. The procedure is repeated in an automated fashion with thousands of genes of interest so that each is deposited in a precise spatial location that allows for the subsequent identification of any particular spot. Annotated nucleotide sequence databases coupled to clone archives are extremely useful resources for designing and constructing array-based experiments. Oligonucleotide arrays are absolutely dependent upon DNA sequence information for oligo design. A limitation on the number of individual elements that can be placed on the area of a given "chip" array places a premium on efficient construction. This is accomplished by eliminating redundancy (maximizing diversity) and incorporating DNA sequences that are relevant for the biological system under study.

We have used the PEDB for the identification and assembly of a nonredundant set of 1500 cDNAs derived from prostate cDNA libraries and constructed microarrays of

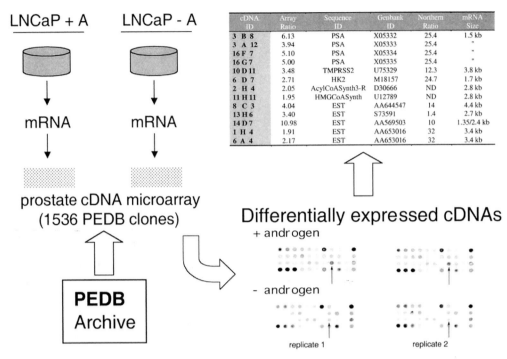

cDNA ID	Array Ratio	Sequence ID	Genbank ID	Northern Ratio	mRNA Size
3 B 8	6.13	PSA	X05332	25.4	1.5 kb
3 A 12	3.94	PSA	X05333	25.4	"
16 F 7	5.10	PSA	X05334	25.4	"
16 G 7	5.00	PSA	X05335	25.4	"
10 D 11	3.48	TMPRSS2	U75329	12.3	3.8 kb
6 D 7	2.71	HK2	M18157	24.7	1.7 kb
2 H 4	2.05	AcylCoASynth3-R	D30666	ND	2.8 kb
11 H 11	1.95	HMGCoASynth	U12789	ND	2.8 kb
8 C 3	4.04	EST	AA644547	14	4.4 kb
13 H 6	3.40	EST	S73591	1.4	2.7 kb
14 D 7	10.98	EST	AA569503	10	1.35/2.4 kb
1 H 4	1.91	EST	AA653016	32	3.4 kb
6 A 4	2.17	EST	AA653016	32	3.4 kb

Fig. 2. Identification of androgen regulated genes in prostate carcinoma using cDNA microarray gene-expression profiling. A cohort of 1536 different cDNAs was selected from the PEDB sequence archive. cDNA inserts were PCR amplified and spotted onto glass microscope slides using a Molecular Dynamics GenII spotting tool. LNCaP prostate cancer cells were either stimulated with androgens V1 (LNCaP + A) or starved of androgens V2 (LNCaP – A) for 72 h. RNA was extracted, converted to cDNA labeled with a fluorescent reporter, and used as probe to simultaneously assess the relative expression levels of the 1536 arrayed genes. The expression of 10 genes increased with androgen stimulation, including the known androgen regulated genes PSA and hK2 as well as two genes involved in lipid metabolism and five uncharacterized cDNAs.

these cDNAs suitable for performing expression studies. These prostate microarrays were used to identify androgen regulated genes in prostate cancer cells (Fig. 2). In addition to the known androgen regulated genes PSA and hK2, we identified 2 genes involved in lipid metabolism, one membrane-bound serine protease, and five uncharacterized genes whose expression was upregulated by androgens in the androgen responsive LNCaP cell line (Fig. 2). A further expansion of this array resource to include the entire prostate transcriptome would allow for the characterization of all genes transcriptionally regulated in the androgen-response program and provide insights into androgen regulated cellular processes.

Technology adapted from the computer industry is driving the evolution of array-based analysis. One process—photolithography—has been used to lay thousands of transistors on a single silicon chip in the construction of microprocessors. Combining photolithography with solid-phase chemical synthesis provides a method for building hundreds of thousands of different short DNA chains (oligonucleotides) on a chip (*21*; Fig. 3). These arrays can also be hybridized with fluorescent probes and analyzed using high-resolution, high-sensitivity detectors. A major advantage with oligonucleotide

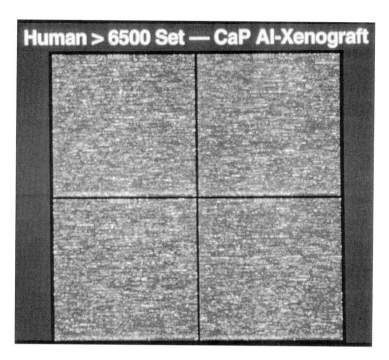

Fig. 3. Affymetrix oligonucleotide array. Oligonucleotides representing >6500 human genes were synthesized on a set of four chips using a photolithographic process. Each gene is represented by 20 oligonucleotide pairs, each with homology to different regions of the targeted gene. More than 65,000 different 25-mer oligonucleotides are present on each chip set. The oligonucleotide array was hybridized with a probe from an androgen independent prostate cancer xenograft and the signal intensities at each oligonucleotide site were quantitated and compared to a second hybridization performed with probe from an androgen dependent prostate cancer xenograft (the second hybridization is not shown). Each bright "dot" is the hybridization signal from a different gene-specific oligonucleotide. Many locations on the array did not hybridize, indicating that these genes are not expressed in the prostate tissue samples. Forty-six genes (2.4% of genes detected) displayed at least a 10-fold difference in expression level between the androgen dependent and the androgen independent tumors.

arrays is the ability to target specific gene sequences and thus avoid regions of repetitive DNA that may lead to spurious cross-hybridization. Gene transcripts with alternatively spliced exons and closely related members of gene families can also be identified. Currently, a limitation of oligo-based methods is the necessity to have knowledge of the DNA sequence of the gene(s) of interest in order to design appropriate oligonucleotides. Genes which have yet to be discovered or sequenced cannot be assessed. However, as the body of genomic information grows through the rapid accumulation of ESTs and the scale-up of the human genome project, this will no longer be an obstacle.

A second process borrowed from the computer industry involves the adaptation of technology currently used in ink-jet printers. Microfabricated ink-jet pumps, such as those found on standard ink-jet printer heads, utilize a piezoelectric element to eject a droplet from an orifice when an electric pulse is applied. Coupling several pumps together, with each pump dispensing different phosphoramidite chemistry reagents (different nucleotide bases) instead of ink, provides a tool to precisely synthesize oligonucleotides directly on a glass slide picoliter drop by picoliter drop. Coupling a moving stage with a computer for precisely firing the pumps to deliver a single drop of reagent to the appropriate location on the slide results in a device capable of synthesizing an array of 100,000 different 25 base oligonucleotides in just over 2 h *(5)*. Ink-jet array devices offer tremendous versatility with the ability to custom-synthesize arrays of different sets of oligos.

7. GENE EXPRESSION STUDIES: PROTEOMICS

While robust comprehensive methods of assessing transcript alterations are now in widespread use, they face a major hurdle because the endpoint for functional genomics analysis and the development of biomedical interventions lies chiefly at the level of the protein rather than the transcript. A major challenge is to establish the relationships between DNA and RNA and their end product, proteins—the actual building blocks and molecular engines of the cell. While nucleic acids are amenable to robust high-throughput analyses, a one-to-one correlation between transcript abundance and protein abundance rarely occurs. In addition, the measurement of a transcript level does not reflect the actual functional status of a given protein that may require for example, a phosphorylation event to be biochemically active.

Large-scale efforts are now underway to analyze the *proteome*, the total protein complement of the genome *(27)*. Analogous to the *transcriptome*, the proteome is a dynamic entity that continually varies to reflect stages of development, differentiation, and response to environmental interactions. Additional levels of proteome complexity are provided by frequent posttranslational modifications that often define functional protein states. A great impediment to proteomics is the lack of an amplifying technology such as the polymerase chain reaction (PCR) that has greatly facilitated the study of DNA and RNA. Thus proteomics research and development has focused on advancing a variety of protein separation, detection, and quantitation methods and techniques for linking proteins to their corresponding gene sequences.

A core technique of proteomics is two-dimensional gel protein electrophoresis (2DE) *(18,28)*. The first dimension separates denatured proteins based upon their isoelectric point charge differences followed by a mass separation through a matrix of polyacrylamide. 2DE is able to determine protein mass and isoelectric point, estimate relative protein abundance, and identify post-translational modifications (isoforms) of intact proteins. This technique remains the highest resolution method for protein separation and is theoretically capable of resolving more than 10,000 proteins and peptides from a complex mixture. However, in current proteomics projects, the total number of proteins identified from 2DE gels is often only a small percentage of the predicted proteome. Figure 4A depicts part of the proteome of the prostate cancer cell line LNCaP. The portion of the proteome displayed includes proteins and peptides with an isoelectric point from pH 3–10. A comparison of the LNCaP proteome under different physiological conditions such as androgen starvation or androgen stimulation can identify molecular alterations at the protein level that correlate with the cellular response to this environmental perturbation. Individual protein spots can be identified either by calculating the theoretical locations of known proteins based upon mass and charge, using specific antibodies for immunodetection, or performing microchemical characterization of spots using microsequencing or mass spectrometry.

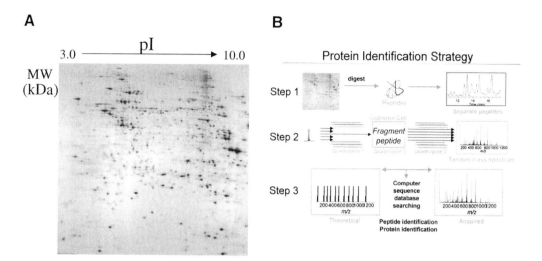

Fig. 4. Gene Expression Studies: Proteomics. (**A**) Two-dimensional gel electrophoresis profile of LNCaP proteins. The first dimension separation resolves the proteins to their isoelectric point between pH 3 and pH 10. The second dimension further separates the proteins based upon their molecular wt and migration rate through a polyacrylamide gel. Protein profiles derived from different cells or tissues are visually compared, and differentially expressed proteins are readily isolated. Individual spots can be identified using mass spectrometry (MS). (**B**) Three-step method for protein identification by MS. Proteins are first resolved by one-dimensional or two-dimensional gel separation methods and digested, and the peptides are separated (*Step 1*). Tandem mass spectra of the peptide mixtures are produced (*Step 2*). Experimental spectra from the protein/peptide of interest are compared against theoretical spectra from protein and nucleic-acid sequence databases to make an identification (*Step 3*).

Mass spectrometry (MS) has evolved to become an indispensable tool for the rapid analysis and identification of proteins and peptides. MS employs an ion source, mass analyzer, and a detector to record a spectra of ion intensity vs the mass to charge ratio of proteins and peptides subjected to analysis (*see* Corthals et al. for an extensive review) *(12)*. Electrospray ionization (ESI) and matrix-assisted laser desorption/ionization (MALDI) have become the preferred methods for the ionization of peptides and proteins because of their effective application on a wide range of proteins. These ionization sources are coupled to mass analyzers such as a time-of-flight (TOF) tube or quadropole analyzer capable of tandem mass spectrometry (MS/MS). Proteins can be digested in a two-dimensional gel using a specific protease, the peptides eluted, and the masses determined through MS. The peptide masses are then used to search protein and nucleic acid databases to determine the identity of the peptide (Fig. 4B).

The identification of proteins is considerably simplified if the protein is already represented in a protein or nucleic acid sequence database. Software algorithms have been devised to automate the correlation of experimental data from MS with theoretical peptide masses and mass spectra for each entry in the database using either enzyme cleavage specificity or the sum of contiguous amino acid residues *(38)*. A major advantage of this MS approach is the ability to assay complex protein mixtures, because each peptide that generates an MS/MS spectrum provides data for an independent database search *(12)*. These methods have been extremely useful for the identification of proteins in organisms where the entire genome is sequenced (e.g., *Saccharomyces cerevisiae, E. coli*). The sequence information provided by ESTs has also greatly facilitated the identification of human proteins by providing partial coding sequence information for tens of thousands of genes far in advance of the completion of the human genome project. The assembly of the complete prostate transcriptome will serve as a valuable resource that will facilitate proteomics research directed toward understanding prostate carcinogenesis.

8. CONCLUSION AND FUTURE DIRECTIONS

The key to understanding human health and disease may be found in the information stored within each cell of the human body as the digital DNA code comprising the genome. Studying the precise regulation of how this information is stored, replicated, and processed has the potential to identify the basic mechanisms underlying the development of cancer. Methods have been developed which permit the examination of genes and their cognate proteins in exquisite detail despite the microscopic nature and often-transient existence of these molecules. Recent technological advances in the biomedical sciences now provide tools for the comprehensive examination of the complex molecular events that occur in normal and cancerous prostate cells.

While great advances have been achieved by investigators studying individual molecules involved in cancer development, the work has been hampered by the lack of a complete "tool set" of all *potential* molecules that are relevant for understanding and defining the cancer process. The completion of the Human Genome Project and the assembly of a virtual and physical prostate transcriptome will provide these resources in a readily accessible format suitable for both small and large-scale experimental applications.

In addition to a myriad of research uses, the potential biomedical applications for array technology and proteomics are numerous. Gene chips are ideal for monitoring the global gene expression fingerprint of a cell, tissue, or organism. Expression profiles change depending upon internal and external perturbations such as aging, infection, or the development of malignancy. Correlating an expression profile with a pathological condition thus may afford a rapid diagnostic test and a means to further classify disease based upon molecular pathology (Fig. 5). Expression profiles may be used to tailor a specific therapy and to monitor the response to treatment. This type of detailed analysis, which deciphers biological networks and pathways of chemical response, can also identify specific molecular derangements that contribute to disease pathogenesis, and thus identify potential targets for therapeutic intervention.

Other probable uses for sequence databases and expression technologies will be the rapid identification of gene mutations in individuals at risk for hereditary diseases, including prostate cancer. Gene chip analysis will be especially useful in cases in which disease-causing mutations can occur at many possible locations within the gene. Oligonucleotide arrays are also likely to be the next genotyping tool. Single nucleotide polymorphisms (SNPs) offer a powerful way to identify genes contributing to polygenic traits, and thousands of these SNPs can be simultaneously detected on genotyping oligo chips. The tremendous amounts of information generated by these "laboratories-

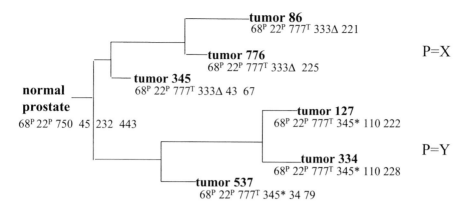

Example: X= progressive phenotype
Y= non-progressive phenotype

Fig. 5. Hypothetical tumor stratification scheme based upon gene expression. Profiles reflecting the expression levels of thousands of genes or proteins from normal prostate and prostate tumors are generated using array-based methods or two-dimensional protein gels. Each gene/protein is given a numerical identifier and clustered or grouped based upon correlations with tumor phenotypic characteristics such as vol, grade, PSA level, ploidy, microvessel density, metastatic site, time to progression, response to therapy, and others. The expression of individual genes or cohorts of genes may then subsequently be used as adjuncts to guide therapeutic interventions. The figure depicts a stratification of 6 prostate tumors that cluster into two distinct groups based upon the expression of a few selected genes. Genes 68 and 22 (P = prostate) define the tissue as prostate (e.g., PSA), and are expressed in all normal and tumor tissues. Gene 777 (T = tumor) is expressed in all prostate tumor tissues, but not in normal prostate. Gene 333 (Δ = progression) is expressed in prostate tumors that progress to metastasize distantly within five yr of diagnosis. Gene 345 (* = nonprogression) is expressed in tumors that do not progress to metastasize within 5 yr of diagnosis.

on-a-chip" will necessitate a continued revolution in the way scientists and physicians view and interpret data. Thus, in addition to the gene chips described here, chips with microcircuits at the heart of every computer will continue to play a vital role in the development and implementation of bioinformatics tools.

ACKNOWLEDGMENT

This work was supported by NIH grant CA75173-01A1 and a gift from the CaPCURE Foundation. The author would like to thank Steven Lasky and Nigel Clegg for critical review of the manuscript, Biaoyang Lin for assistance with cDNA arrays, Yvon Rochon for assistance with 2D gels, and Leroy Hood, David Han and Garry Corthals for helpful discussions.

REFERENCES

1. Adams, M. D., et al. 1995. Initial assessment of human gene diversity and expression patterns based upon 83 million nucleotides of cDNA sequence. *Nature* **377(Suppl. 28):** 3–174.
2. Altschul, S. F., W. Gish, W. Miller, E. W. Myers, and D. J. Lipman. 1990. Basic local alignment search tool. *J. Mol. Biol.* **215:** 403–410.

3. Bendik, I., P. Schraml and C. U. Ludwig. 1998. Characterization of MAST9/Hevin, a SPARC-like protein, that is down-regulated in non-small cell lung cancer. *Cancer Res.* **58:** 626–629.

4. Bishop, J. O., J. G. Morton, M. Rosbash, and M. Richardson. 1974. Three abundance classes in Hela cell messenger RNA. *Nature* **250:** 199–204.

5. Blanchard, A. P., R. J. Kaiser, and L. E. Hood. 1996. High-density oligonucleotide arrays. *Biosensors Bioelectronics* **11:** 687–690.

6. Boguski, M. S., T. M. J. Lowe, and C. M. Tolstoshev. 1993. dbEST-database for "expressed sequence tags." *Nat. Genet.* **4:** 332,333.

7. Brooks, J. D., et al. 1996. An uncertain role for p53 gene alterations in human prostate cancers. *Cancer Res.* **56:** 3814–3822.

8. Catalona, J. J., et al. 1991. Measurement of prostate-specific antigen as a screening test for prostate cancer. *N. Engl. J. Med.* **324:** 1156–1161.

9. Chee, M., et al. 1996. Accessing genetic information with high-density DNA arrays. *Science* **274:** 610–614.

10. Cohen, P., et al. 1992. Prostate-specific antigen (PSA) is an insulin-like growth factor binding protein-3 protease found in seminal plasma. *J. Clin. Endocrinol. Metab.* **75:** 1046–1053.

11. Collins, F. S., et al. 1998. New goals for the U.S. Human Genome Project: 1998-2003. *Science* **282:** 682–689.

12. Corthals, G., S. P. Gygi, R. Aebersold, and S. D. Patterson. 1999. Identification of proteins by mass spectrometry, in *Proteome Research: 2D Gel Electrophoresis and Detection Methods* (T. Rabilloud, ed.) Springer, New York, pp. 197–231.

13. Cramer, S. D., Z. Chen, and D. M. Peehl. 1996. Prostate specific antigen cleaves parathyroid hormone-related protein in the PTH-like domain: inactivation of PTHrP-stimulated cAMP accumulation in mouse osteoblasts. *J. Urol.* **156:** 526–531.

14. Culig, Z., et al. 1997. Androgen receptor gene mutations in prostate cancer. Implications for disease progression and therapy. *Drugs Aging* **10:** 50–58.

15. Denmeade, S. R., et al. 1998. Enzymatic activation of a doxorubicin-peptide prodrug by prostate-specific antigen. *Cancer Res.* **58:** 2537–2540.

16. Fields, C., M. D. Adams, O. White, and J. C. Venter. 1994. How many genes in the human genome? *Nat. Genet.* **7:** 345,346.

17. Gumerlock, P., U. Poonamallee, F. Meyers, and R. W. deVere-White. 1991. Activated ras alleles in human carcinoma of the prostate are rare. *Cancer Res.* **51:** 1632–1637.

18. Hatzimanikatis, V., L. H. Choe, and K. H. Lee. 1999. Proteomics: theoretical and experimental considerations. *Biotechnol. Prog.* **15:** 312–318.

19. Hawkins, V., et al. 1999. PEDB: the Prostate Expression Database. *Nucleic Acids Res.* **27:** 204–208.

20. Huang, X. 1996. An improved sequence assembly program. *Genomics* **33:** 21–31.

21. Isaacs, W. B., et al. 1994. Molecular Biology of Prostate Cancer. *Semin. Oncol.* **21:** 514–521.

22. Ji, H., et al. 1997. Identification of a breast cancer-specific gene, BCSG1, by direct differential cDNA sequencing. *Cancer Res.* **57:** 759–764.

23. Kim, J. J., et al. 1998. Molecular and immunological analysis of genetic prostate specific antigen (PSA) vaccine. *Oncogene* **17:** 3125–3135.

24. Nelson, P. S., et al. 1998. An expressed-sequence-tag database of the human prostate: sequence analysis of 1168 cDNA clones. *Genomics* **47:** 12–25.

25. Nelson, P. S., et al. 1998. Hevin, an antiadhesive extracellular matrix protein, is down-regulated in metastatic prostate adenocarcinoma. *Cancer Res.* **58:** 232–236.

26. Netto, G. J., and P. A. Humphrey. Molecular biologic aspects of human prostatic carcinoma. *Am. J. Clin. Pathol.* **102(Suppl. 1):** S57–S64.

27. Nguyen, C., et al. 1995. Differential gene expresion in the murine thymus assayed by quantitative hybridization of arrayed cDNA clones. *Genomics* **29:** 207–216.

28. O'Farrell, P. H. 1975. High resolution two-dimensional electrophoresis of proteins. *J. Biol. Chem.* **250:** 4007–4021.
29. Peehl, D., N. Wehner, and T. Stamey. 1992. Activated ki-ras oncogene in human prostatic adenocarcinoma. *Prostate* **10:** 281–289.
30. Schena, M., D. Shalon, R. W. Davis, and P. O. Brown. 1995. Quantitative monitoring of gene expression patterns with a complementary DNA microarray. *Science* **270:** 467–470.
31. Stanford, J. L., et al. 1997. Polymorphic repeats in the androgen receptor gene: molecular markers of prostate cancer risk. *Cancer Res.* **57:** 1194–1198.
32. Strohmeyer, T. G. and D. J. Slamon. 1994. Proto-oncogenes and tumor suppressor genes in human urological malignancies. *J. Urol.* **151:** 1479–1497.
33. Takayama, T. K., K. Fujikawa, and E. W. Davie. 1997. Characterization of the precursor of prostate-specific antigen. Activation by trypsin and by human glandular kallikrein. *J. Biol. Chem.* **272:** 21,582–21,588.
34. Vasmatzis, G., M. Essand, U. Brinkmann, B. Lee, and I. Pastan. 1998. Discovery of three genes specifically expressed in human prostate by expressed sequence tag database analysis. *Proc. Natl. Acad. Sci. USA* **95:** 300–304.
35. Velculescu, V. E., et al. 1997. Characterization of the yeast transcriptome. *Cell* **88:** 243–251.
36. Visakorpi, T., et al. 1995. In vivo amplification of the androgen receptor gene and progression of human prostate cancer. *Nat. Genet.* **9:** 401–406.
37. Wang, Z., R. Tufts, R. Haleem, and X. Cai. 1997. Genes regulated by androgen in the rat ventral prostate. *Proc. Natl. Acad. Sci. USA* **94:** 12,999–13,004.
38. Yates, J. R., 3rd. 1998. Database searching using mass spectrometry data. *Electrophoresis* **19:** 893–900.

PART III

CANCER BIOLOGY

12

The Role of the Nuclear Matrix and Cytoskeleton in Cancer

Robert H. Getzenberg, PhD

1. INTRODUCTION

Much of what we know about prostate cancer can be traced back to alterations that occur in the nucleus of the cell. The nucleus is the control center for the cell—it is here that processes such as DNA replication, transcription, and RNA splicing occur. In the prostate, the nucleus is also the site of action of the androgen receptor, which is known to regulate prostatic growth and differentiation. The central question addressed in this chapter is: what is cell structure, and what importance does it have in cancer? This chapter is not meant to provide a comprehensive review of the large and growing body of literature currently available on this topic, but focuses on a number of topics and examples that support the importance of cellular structure in the cancer process.

The central theme of this chapter is the structural components of the nucleus, the nuclear matrix, which was first identified by Berezney and Coffey in 1974 and subsequently has been shown to play a central role in determining nuclear shape, and the structural organization of the nucleus. The nucleus has been linked to a number of phenotypes found in the cancer cell. We currently know a great deal about the nuclear matrix and its role in nuclear organization, as well as tissue and cancer-specific alterations in nuclear matrix proteins that are associated with specific cancer types and have now been applied to the development of novel clinical assays. Finally, we will briefly discuss some of the elements of the cytoskeleton that have been shown to be altered by cancer. As a whole, the studies reviewed in this chapter reveal that cellular and nuclear structure plays an important role in normal cellular processes, and that alterations in these structural components are a fundamental part of cancer pathobiology that can be used to develop novel cancer and tissue-specific markers as well as targets for treatment strategies.

2. NUCLEAR MATRIX

The hallmark of the cancer cell is its abnormal cell and nuclear shape. The term draws its origins from the zodiac symbol of the crab—the cancer cell resembles a crab with rough edges and an uneven profile. A cancerous growth has a tenacious, penetrat-

From: *Prostate Cancer: Biology, Genetics, and the New Therapeutics*
Edited by: L. W. K. Chung, W. B. Isaacs, and J. W. Simons © Humana Press Inc., Totowa, NJ

ing appearance to the naked eye. The abnormal nuclear shape characteristic of cancer cells is determined, at least in part, by the structural framework of the nucleus—the nuclear matrix. The nuclear matrix is the proteinaceous framework of the nucleus that comprises the innermost part of the cell-tissue matrix system extending from the extracellular matrix through the plasma membrane, cytoskeleton, and nuclear envelope. Collectively, these structures form a dynamic continuum of cellular scaffolding that organizes and processes spatial and temporal information for coordination of cell functions *(32)*. Preparations of the nuclear matrix include peripheral lamins, pore constituents, and nucleoprotein complexes, along with a heterogeneous array of other proteins—all resistant to detergents, nucleases, and salt extraction at moderate to high ionic strengths *(7,26)*. The nuclear matrix consists of approx 10% of the nuclear proteins and is virtually devoid of lipids, DNA, and histones *(26)*. As summarized by Getzenberg et al. *(32)*, the nuclear matrix is known to participate in the maintenance of nuclear morphology and DNA organization with recognized specific functions in the synthesis and processing of RNA and in DNA replication. Significantly, specific binding sites for steroid hormone receptors have been localized to the nuclear matrix *(4,5)* strongly suggesting a fundamental role in hormone action. Thus, the nuclear matrix occupies a unique position to determine tissue specificity through regulation of chromatin structure and genomic organization. Evidence to support this hypothesis has been established for male accessory sex tissues *(30)*, and is similarly indicated by matrix-associated gene arrangements in a variety of other organs *(28)*.

The structural components of the nucleus are known to play a central role in the specific topological organization of DNA. DNA in the nucleus is not randomly organized, and although approx 10% of the DNA actually encodes proteins, only specific genes are positioned in a manner that permits the expression of both housekeeping and cell-type-specific genes. The average mammalian somatic cell nucleus contains the linear equivalent of 2 m of DNA packed by a 200,000-fold linear condensation into a 10-μ nucleus. With the use of *in situ* hybridization *(48)*, there is direct evidence for specific three-dimensional organization of the DNA within the nucleus *(14,33)*. Manuelidis and colleagues demonstrated the specific and reproducible compartmentalization of unique chromosomal domains within the nuclei of human central-nervous-system cell lines, and established that functionally distinct cell types have specific patterns of interphase chromosome three-dimensional organization *(46)*. Comparison of the chromosomal topography of human lymphocytes, amniotic fluid cells, fibroblasts, and human cerebral and cerebellar samples have further demonstrated that the topological DNA organization is cell type specific *(3,24)*. The use of confocal microscopy has further enabled the visualization of multiple probes simultaneously, and has confirmed the dynamic and specific cellular localization of specific genes within the nucleus *(43,44)*. The DNA has many forms of higher-order structure, creating a particular pattern of organization that results in the expression of only appropriate tissue-specific genes. In summary, many studies have now demonstrated the specific three-dimensional organization of DNA within the nucleus. Differences in this organization can occur with the same genomic sequence, and are dictated in part by DNA interactions with a tissue-specific nuclear matrix. Nuclear structure is therefore involved in both this topological organization of DNA and the functional aspects which coincide with this organization.

3. NUCLEAR MATRIX AND THE REGULATION OF GENE EXPRESSION

The nuclear matrix is the site of mRNA transcription *(61)*. Active genes have been found to be associated with the nuclear matrix only in cell types in which they are expressed *(28)*. Genes that are not expressed in these cell types are not found to be associated with the nuclear matrix. Recent evidence from our laboratory and others indicates that transcription factors are localized or sequestered on the nuclear matrix, and that this localization may play an important role in the regulation of gene expression *(50,62,66)*. Isomura et al. have identified a 58-kDa protein with putative zinc-finger domains, which they termed RFP. RFP associates with or is a component of the nuclear matrix, binds preferentially to double-stranded and single-stranded DNA, and is involved in the activation of the ret protooncogene *(37)*. Recently, a NMP was identified to be the sequence-specific DNA-binding factor F6 which binds upstream of the cluster region of chicken α-globin genes. This protein belongs to a family of GATA proteins which are the chicken equivalents of the transcription factor NFE-1 *(67)*. Work from the laboratory of Stein and colleagues have examined the regulation of the osteocalcin gene. In the promoter region, they have identified multiple protein-DNA interactions involving two different NMPs. These proteins interact with regions of the gene in proximity to the Vitamin D-responsive sequences. The first nuclear matrix protein that they characterized is termed NMP-1, and is a ubiquitous cell-growth-regulated protein related to the transcription factor ATF. The second protein, termed NMP-2, is a cell type specific protein that recognizes binding sites resembling the consensus site for the CCAAT enhancer binding protein C/EBP, and is localized exclusively on the nuclear matrix *(8)*. Previous work from the Stein laboratory identified two proteins that bound to the nuclear matrix attachment regions upstream of the human H4 histone gene promoter. These proteins were suggested to be from the ATF transcription-factor-binding family *(22)*. As a whole, these results support the concept that transcription factors are localized or sequestered on the nuclear matrix, and that the localization of these factors on the nuclear matrix may play an important role in DNA binding and the specific regulation of gene expression.

Further investigation into the association of active genes with the nuclear matrix has revealed a DNA loop anchorage site in the enhancer regions or intronic sequences of several genes. These sequences have been termed matrix-associated regions (MARs) or scaffold-attached regions (SARs), are usually approx 200 base pairs in length, and are A-T rich, although recent evidence suggests that other sequence types exist *(13)*, and contain topoisomerase cleavage sequences along with other sequences such as polyadenylation signals *(55)*. Although these sequences often have a high degree of homology with topoisomerase II cleavage sequences, only one has been found to actually bind topoisomerase II *(56)*. Recently, MARs have been shown to be A-T rich regions, and to comprise other characteristic regions including T-G-rich motifs and potential Z-DNA as well as polypurine and polypyrimidine blocks *(12)*. MAR sequences have been suggested to play a role in relieving the superhelical strain of the DNA *(11)*.

MARs have also been shown to functionally confer increased transcriptional activity in genes following transfection. These MAR/SAR sequences have been found to be equally distributed between the internal nuclear matrix and the nuclear lamina *(45)*. Classic experiments by Stief and colleagues involved utilizing the matrix-associated DNA sequences of the chicken lysozyme gene and inserting this sequence into a transfectable expression vector. When this reporter system is flanked by the 5′ MAR, its expression is markedly elevated, and is independent of the chromosome position *(63)*. A similar experiment was carried out using the 5′ MAR of the chicken lysozyme gene and a transient transfection system, again demonstrating increased and position-independent transcription of the gene construct *(54)*. To further determine the role of these MARs in gene expression, deletion experiments were carried out to remove the MARs from genes which normally contained these sequences and examining the effect of this deletion on the transcriptional activity of the gene. In the immunoglobulin kappa gene, deletion of the intronic MAR led to a fourfold decrease in expression. When both the intronic MAR and a MAR in the enhancer region were removed from this gene, the expression dropped 11-fold *(10)*. These experiments were then conducted in vivo, and when transgenic animals were produced from these constructs, both of the genes with the intact and deleted MARs were expressed in a tissue specific manner, although those genes with a deleted MAR(s) exhibited only two to threefold less activity *(70)*. These data demonstrate the importance of precise DNA organization, which is necessary for appropriate gene expression. The MARs in the α-globin gene are proposed to be mass binding sites for transcription factors, some of which may be developmental-state-specific, and others which may be ubiquitous *(12)*.

Recently, NMPs which bind to MAR sequences have been identified by a number of laboratories. These nuclear matrix proteins may serve as the attachment points for these matrix-associated DNA sequences, and it is possible that some of these proteins may be responsible for forming DNA loop domains. One of these proteins, termed SATB1, is primarily a tissue-specific MAR-binding protein, found typically in the thymus. In in vitro cotransfection studies, this protein appears to act as a transcription suppressor *(18,20)*. Therefore, these proteins and possibly some of the other MAR-binding proteins identified, may be involved in suppressing the expression of specific genes in a tissue-specific manner. Recent investigations have revealed that calmodulin and other nuclear proteins may participate in the association of MARs with the nuclear matrix *(27)*. Recent evidence from our laboratory has identified the presence of a DNA-binding nuclear matrix protein in the seminal vesicles that may be involved in the tissue specific regulation of genes encoding seminal vesicle secretory proteins *(36)*.

The nuclear matrix plays a central role in RNA processing, and is the site of attachment for products from RNA cleavage and for RNA processing intermediates *(15,69)*. Spliceosome complexes involved in the regulation of RNA splicing are localized to the nuclear matrix. RNA *(35,59)* and ribonucleoprotein particles and fibers *(34,52)* may themselves play an important role in the structure of the nuclear matrix. Newly synthesized heteronuclear RNA and small nuclear RNA are enriched on the nuclear matrix. Additionally, telomeric DNA sequences have been found to be preferentially associated with the nuclear matrix *(19)*, indicating that these attachments may be important in DNA organization.

4. NUCLEAR MATRIX PROTEIN ALTERATIONS AND CANCER

The nuclear matrix plays a central role in determining the shape of the nucleus as well as in nuclear processes. Alterations in nuclear matrix proteins may therefore cause changes in nuclear shape, as well as modifications to the fidelity with which a number of these critical nuclear processes occur. Therefore, changes in the nuclear matrix may result in the phenotypes found in the cancer cell, including altered nuclear shape, genomic instability, and rearrangement and translocation of chromosomes. The nuclear matrix is not a bystander; it appears to play a central role in the cancer process.

While all cell types and physiologic states share the majority of known nuclear matrix proteins (NMPs), some NMPs appear to be unique to certain cell types or states *(51)*. We have previously demonstrated that the protein composition of the nuclear matrix is tissue specific and can serve as a "fingerprint" of each cell and/or tissue type *(28)*. Mitogenic stimulation and the induction of differentiation alter the composition of nuclear matrix proteins and structure *(23,64)*. Differences in NMP composition are also found in a number of human tumors, including prostate *(31,53)*, renal *(41)*, breast *(40)*, colon *(39)*, head and neck *(21,47)*, and bladder *(29)*.

We have studied, and continue to investigate, alterations in nuclear matrix protein composition in prostate cancer. Initially, we examined the NMPs of the normal rat prostate in comparison with rat prostate adenocarcinoma lines from the Dunning model of prostate cancer. We demonstrated that the NMP composition of transformed cell lines differed significantly from their tissue of origin, and while these transformed prostate cell lines were almost entirely composed of a common set of NMPs, there were differences which would distinguish cell lines of different degrees of the transformed phenotype from each another *(31)*. We have been successful in characterizing a number of these nuclear matrix proteins, including the Dunning cancer-associated D-1, -2, and -3. We have isolated sufficient quantities of these proteins to result in their internal peptide sequencing, and will discuss D-2 as an example. We have now identified and sequenced two peptides of D-2, described as D-2-1 and D-2-2. While D-2-1 has no homology with any protein in the databases, D-2-2 has some homology with several proteins, including the human 78 kDa gastrin-binding GBP protein. We have been utilizing purified antipeptide antibodies produced against D-2 to analyze its expression in both prostate cancer cells and tissues. This antibody recognizes the protein in Dunning tumors, but does not find the protein expressed in the normal rat prostate. These studies have demonstrated that the D2-2 antibody only stains microdissected samples of human prostate cancer, but not normal human prostate tissue. To date, although we have increased our sample numbers significantly, staining has been found in adjacent normal prostatic tissue, and we have not identified the expression of D-2 in other tissue or tumor types that we have examined. Therefore, this protein, which has been identified as being associated with prostate cancer in a rat model, detects a protein associated with human prostate cancer.

Currently, a number of reagents have been developed against the two metastatic prostate cancer-specific NMPs, including antibodies and protein sequence data. Our initial antibody to the metastatic prostate cancer-specific NMPs is a polyclonal antibody that was raised against isolated AM-1 gel spots. When the Dunning tumors or cell lines are stained with this antibody, reactivity is found in the metastatic lines, but not in any of the nonmetastatic lines that we have examined. We recently used this antibody to stain human prostatic tissues in order to determine whether the antibody has the potential to separate metastatic and nonmetastatic tumors in humans, as it does in the rat model. Immunoblot and immunohistochemical studies with this antibody raised against the rat AM-1 NMP react with human prostate tumor tissue and provide the evidence that this metastatic disease-specific NMP also exists in human prostate cancer tissues. The anti-AM-1 antibody stains some human prostate cancers, but not normal prostate tissue. We have now screened NMPs from tissues from 13 patients undergoing radical prostatectomy for prostate cancer. Immunoblot analysis reveals that three of the 13 patients (23%) had positive staining only in the tumor, and five (38%) had a significant amount of staining in the tumor with a minimal amount noted in the normal tissues. We are now conducting studies to determine whether positive staining in these patients correlates with disease that has the ability to metastasize. We have been successful in utilizing the previously described anti-AM-1 antibody raised to gel spots in several other experimental approaches. AM-1 expression appears to be prostate specific, and has been detected in cells and tissues by IHC, immunofluorescence, and by immuno-fluorescent confocal microscopy. Immunofluorescence staining was performed to compare this NMP with staining patterns of the other nuclear proteins to formulate an understanding of the function of this protein. The staining of this antibody is nuclear and punctate, and clearly differs from the uniform staining patterns found with an antilamin antibody.

In addition to the antibodies, we recently have been successful in obtaining partial peptide sequences of both the AM-1 and AM-2 proteins. We now have two peptide sequences from AM-1 with no homologies in the database, and we are currently sequencing other peptide peaks from the cleaved AM-1 protein to obtain additional sequences. We also have two peptide sequences to the AM-2 protein. One of the AM-2 peptides has homology with a number of proteins in the NIH nonredundant BLAST protein database, and appears to encode a region similar to that found in the Type II keratin family. The other peptide of AM-2 currently has no homologies in the database. We are now in the process of producing antipeptide antibodies against these peptide sequences as well as developing degenerate oligonucleotides encoding these peptides.

Dr. Alan W. Partin and colleagues completed a study examining the NMP composition in human prostate tissue *(53)*. They compared the NMP patterns for fresh prostate, benign prostatic hyperplasia (BPH), and prostate cancer from 21 men undergoing surgery for clinically localized prostate cancer or BPH. The NMP patterns were compared utilizing the high-resolution gel electrophoresis technique used in the previous studies. In these studies, they identified by mol wt and isoelectric point 14 different proteins that were consistently present or absent among the various tissues. One protein (PC-1)— a M_r 56,000 protein with an isoelectric point of 6.58—appeared in all of 14 nuclear-matrix preparations from different prostate cancer patient specimens and was not detected in normal prostate (0 of 13) or BPH (0 of 14). Studies in other laboratories continue to discern the ability of PC-1 to detect prostate cancer as well as the role of this protein in human disease. A recent analysis of a protein proposed to be PC-1 has shown that it is the nuclear protein B23 or nucleophosmin *(65)*. A recent analysis of nuclear matrix proteins isolated from prostate cancers of varying pathological stages has revealed a 76-kDa protein, YL-1, which appears to be related to aggressive prostate cancer, with significant potential clinical importance *(42)*.

5. NUCLEAR MATRIX: CLINICAL ASSAYS

Matritech Inc., has developed an FDA-approved test that utilizes a nuclear matrix protein (NMP), NMP22, which is identical to the protein NuMA. This NMP is found in the nuclear matrix of all cell types, and is located in the mitotic spindle during mitosis. In a multicenter trial, analysis of the urine of over 1,000 patients previously treated for bladder cancer and being monitored for recurrence of their disease was carried out. The NMP22 test was able to detect all the cases of invasive disease and approx 70% of the cases with localized recurrence *(58)*. Similar results were obtained in a more recent study *(60)*. However, NMP22 is nonspecific for bladder cancer, and can only be utilized to detect recurrence of the disease. This test can also detect other types of cancers, including prostate and renal. Elevated levels of NMP22 are also found in patients with bladder inflammation and other disorders. Matritech has reduced these potential complications by focusing the use of this test on patients who have already been diagnosed with bladder cancer. A recent review of the available data for NMP22, BTA stat, and QUANTICYT computer-assisted dual parameter image analysis reveals that while NMP22 and BTA may be better than cytology alone, these tools are currently inadequate to replace cystoscopy in the determination of recurrent disease *(68)*. The Matritech studies have established a precedent for the presence of NMPs in the urine from even small bladder tumors, and provide support for the concept of utilizing NMPs as diagnostic and/or prognostic markers in cancer.

6. RECENT ADVANCES: EXAMPLE OF CANCER-SPECIFIC NMPS

We now understand a great deal more about cancer-specific NMPs and their use as cancer markers, as well as the functional significance of these proteins. In lieu of presenting a complete analysis of this work, we will focus our discussion on our recent bladder investigations as an example of these studies. Bladder cancer is a significant health problem in the United States and throughout the world. An estimated 53,200 cases will be diagnosed this year in the United States alone *(1)*. When bladder cancer is detected early, the 5-yr survival rate is approx 94%, while patients with metastatic disease, have significantly lower survival rates.

Currently, the only available method for bladder cancer detection is morphological examination of cytology samples or cystoscopic biopsies. This method is accurate for high-grade lesions; however, a significant proportion of bladder tumors (25–45%) are low-grade or well-differentiated, and escape detection upon cytologic examination of exfoliated cells. Cytologic examination cannot detect low numbers of tumor cells, and cannot separate low-grade or well-differentiated cells from their normal counterparts. The diagnostic accuracy of cytology alone for the detection of low-grade transitional carcinoma is between 49 and 64% *(16)*. Repeating the study *(38)* can increase the accuracy of cytology; however, this is a costly and time-consuming practice for both the patient and physician. Development of a sensitive screening assay that could specifically detect bladder carcinoma would significantly facilitate patient management and allow earlier treatment of this disease.

We have recently identified protein components of the nuclear matrix that are able to differentiate human bladder tumors from normal bladder tissue *(29)*. These proteins have not been found in other tumor or tissue types. We sequenced the three most abundant bladder cancer-specific nuclear matrix proteins (BLCA-1, -4 and -6). Here we will focus on one of these nuclear matrix proteins, BLCA-4, that has been sequenced and to which antipeptide antibodies have been generated. Anti-BLCA-4 antibodies can detect BLCA-4 in the bladders of individuals with bladder cancer, but not in those without the disease. In the bladder cancer patient, BLCA-4 is present throughout the bladder (i.e., normal and tumor areas). In age-matched organ donors without bladder cancer, expression of BLCA-4 was not found. Thus, as opposed to the morphologically "normal" areas in the bladders of individuals with bladder cancer, true normal samples from unaffected individuals do not react with the antibody. To date, we have found positive BLCA-4 staining in the 100% of the "normal" tissues from the bladders of patients with bladder cancer. In the corresponding tumor samples, we found expression in 75% of the samples. There were several tumor samples with low levels of expression evident by further exposure of the blots, but these values were not counted as being positive. When the bladders from unaffected individuals were examined, expression was not found in any of the samples examined, even if these blots were overexposed. The association between BLCA-4 and the presence of bladder cancer was highly significant ($p < 2 \times 10^{-4}$, Fisher exact two-sided test).

Our evidence indicates that our anti-BLCA-4 antibody is able to separate individuals with bladder cancer from those without the disease. Further, these data support the presence of a field effect in the bladder, suggesting that even cells that appear to be morphologically normal have undergone alterations. The anti-BLCA-4 antibody is able to identify "normal" tissues in every patient with bladder cancer. It is therefore possible that this antibody may be able to detect very early lesions of bladder cancer, even before morphological alterations occur.

We have developed a urine-based immunoassay to detect BLCA-4 (Fig. 1). In a current study, we have analyzed the BLCA-4 levels in 51 age-matched control individuals without bladder cancer and 54 individuals with bladder cancer. This analysis reveals a specificity of 100% (51/51) (CI = 90.0–100%) and a sensitivity of 96.4% (52/54). All of the control individuals were below our cutoff of 13 established with the first set of three tumor and normal samples. Fifty-two of the 54 urine samples from individuals with bladder cancer were positive. Two were below 13. One had a value of 12.6, which is below our cutoff but above all of the normal samples. The other negative sample was from an individual with CIS who had a value of four. The average value for BLCA-4 in the urine of the 51 normal control individuals was 4.02 ± 4.21 OD U/μg of protein, whereas the average value for individuals with bladder cancer was 43.38 ± 49.07 OD U/μg of protein. The levels are significantly higher in patients with bladder cancer ($p = 2.4 \times 10^{-6}$). Voided urine cytology reports were available in 32 of the patients

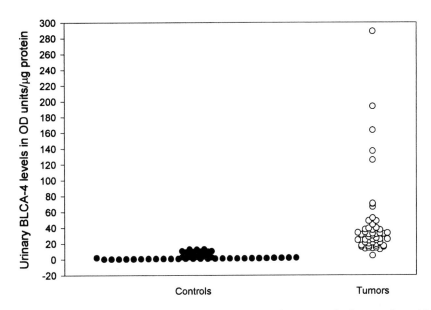

Fig. 1. Distribution of urinary BLCA-4 levels of normal age-matched controls and bladder cancer patients. A cutoff of BLCA-4 levels <13 OD U was established on the first three pairs of normal and tumor samples, and was then utilized prospectively throughout the study. This urine-based immunoassay results in a specificity of 100% (51/51) and a sensitivity of 96.4% (52/54).

with bladder cancer. Of these, 16 patients had positive urine cytology, five were interpreted as suspicious, four we read as atypical and seven were negative. Only two of these 32 patients had a urinary BLCA-4 level below the cutoff of 13 OD U/μg protein. The urine cytology of one of these patients was interpreted as negative, while the other patient was positive. Thus, using urine cytology alone, 16 of 32 patients (50%) would have had an equivocal or negative diagnosis. Of these sixteen patients, BLCA-4 levels were positive in 15 (93.7%). The BLCA-4 levels were also abnormally elevated in 15 of 16 of the individuals with positive urine cytology. BLCA-4 could therefore identify even those individuals in whom bladder cancer is not diagnosed by urine cytology *(41a,41b)*.

7. CYTOSKELETON

The cytoskeletal components of the cell serve an important structural purpose. These consist of the support system and the portion of the tissue matrix system that connects the extracellular matrix with the nuclear matrix. The cytoskeleton is composed of an interacting network of microfilaments (6 nm), microtubules (24 nm), and intermediate filaments (7–11 nm), and interacting proteins that help to modulate their dynamics and function. These filament systems provide the structural conduits from the outside environment to the nucleus. It is now apparent that link many of the connections that the extracellular matrix and the cytoskeleton are known to be altered in cancer. The connections of these filament systems have been associated with alterations in cellular morphology and the tumorigenic phenotype *(57)*.

As described for the nuclear matrix, a few specific examples will be outlined here in order to demonstrate the importance of cytoskeletal structure in the cancer process and to provide a basis for an introduction to these concepts. An example of molecules that help to connect the extraceullular environment to the cytoskeleton is β-catenin. This molecular structure has been shown to interact with cadherins and then with α-catenin, which then directly contacts the microfilaments. Other molecules believed to be important in this process are vinculin and α-actinin *(6)*. In addition to its role in direct interactions between the microfilament and extracellular matrix systems, it has now been shown that β-catenin translocates to the nucleus, where it serves as a transactivator *(6)*. Loss of either of the known catenin family members has been associated with cancer *(25)*. Actin has also been implicated to be involved in the cancer process through its interaction with the Rho GTPase family of signaling molecules. Several members of this family are associated with cell transformation, and also play a role in the reorganization of the actin filaments *(2)*. Actin has also recently been shown to be present in the nuclear matrix, but the functional significance of this remains unclear. *(17)*.

Changes in the protein composition of the intermediate filaments have been associated with transformation. A major intermediate filament family member, the cytokeratins, were shown to give specific patterns in a cell type specific fashion and to exhibit alterations with transformation *(49)*. The intermediate filament family has been shown to interact with the nuclear matrix. Major components of the nuclear matrix, the nuclear lamins, are members of the intermediate filament family. The intermediate filaments located in both the cytoskeleton and nuclear matrix are dynamic and interactive. Lamin B has been shown to associate with cytoskeletal-based intermediate filaments. Therefore, the intermediate filament system may serve as a conduit to transmit information throughout the cell.

8. CONCLUSION

The concept of dynamic reciprocity has been proposed to explain how cell structure is able to serve as a mechanism for a bidirectional flow of information throughout the tissue matrix system *(9)*. The tissue matrix system is indeed a dynamic one, and it is now clear that it serves as a mechanism to transmit signals throughout the cell *(32)*. This chapter briefly describes components of the tissue matrix system that may play a role in the cancer process. We have focused our discussion on the nuclear matrix, the organizing structure of the nucleus that provides a support for its shape as well as nuclear processes including DNA replication, transcription, and RNA splicing. Nuclear matrix proteins have now been identified for a variety of cancer types that are both tissue and tumor type specific. Because of these properties, these NMPs appear to be quite unique, and therefore make ideal candidates as biomarkers as well as targets for treatment strategies. While this concept has existed for several years, it has now become a reality with the recent characterization of several of these NMPs. We now have clinical tests in place which use these changes as their basis. One of these, a bladder cancer-specific NMP, BLCA-4 is described here as an example. We now have the ability to test the functional significance of these proteins to determine their role in the cancer process. In addition to these nuclear matrix proteins, cytoskeletal alterations are clearly found in cancer cells, which reflect more than just changes in the shape of the cell. Shape is function, and data is now available to show that alterations in these cytoskeletal components may be active participants in transformation. Structural alterations are clearly a central component of the cancer process. Although we have had this knowledge for many years, we now understand more about how structure is involved in cellular regulation, and how alterations in these processes may lead to cancer.

REFERENCES

1. Greenlee, R. T., T. Murray, S. Bolden, and P. A. Wingo. 2000. Cancer Statistics 2000. *Cancer J. Clin.* **50:** 7–33.
2. Apenström, P. Effectors for the Rho GTPases. 1999. *Cell Biology.* **11:** 95–102.
3. Arnoldus, E. P. J., A. C. B. Peters, G. T. A. M. Bots, A. K. Raap, and M. van der Ploeg. 1989. Somatic pairing of chromosome 1 centromeres in interphase nuclei of human cerebellum. *Hum. Genet.* **83:** 231–234.
4. Barrack, E. R. 1987. Steroid hormone receptor localization in the nuclear matrix: interaction with acceptor sites. *J. Steroid Biochem.* **27:** 115–121.
5. Barrack, E. R. and D. S. Coffey. 1980. The specific binding of estrogens and androgens to the nuclear matrix of sex hormone responsive tissues. *J. Biol. Chem.* **255:** 7265–7275.
6. Ben-Ze'ev, A. and B. Geiger. 1998. Differential molecular interactions of β-catenin and plakoglobin in adhesion, signaling and cancer. *Cell Biol.* **10:** 629–639.
7. Berezney, R. and D. S. Coffey. 1974. Identification of a nuclear protein matrix. *Biochem. Biophys. Res. Commun.* **60:** 1410–1417.
8. Bidwell, J. P., A. J. van Wijnen., E. G. Fey, S. Dworetzky, S. Penman, J. L. Stein, et al. 1993. Osteocalcin gene promoter-binding factors are tissue-specific nuclear matrix components. *Proc. Natl. Acad. Sci. USA* **90:** 3162–3166.
9. Bissell, M. J., V. M. Weaver, S. A. Lelièvre, F. Wang, O. W. Petersen, and K. L. Schmeichel. 1999. Tissue structure, nuclear organization, and gene expression in normal and malignant breast. *Cancer Res.* **59:** 1757s–1764s.
10. Blasquez, V. C., M. Xu, S. C. Moses, and W. T. J. Garrard. 1989. Immunoglobulin kappa gene expression after stable integration. I. Role of the intronic MAR and enhancer in plasmacytoma cells. *Biol. Chem.* **264:** 21,183–21,189.
11. Bode, J., Y. Kohwi, L. Dickinson, T. Joh, D. Klehr, C. Mielke, et al. 1992. Biological significance of unwinding capability of nuclear matrix-associating DNAs. *Science* **255:** 195–197.
12. Boulikas, T. 1993. Homeodomain protein binding sites, inverted repeats, and nuclear matrix attachment regions along the human-globin gene complex. *J. Cell. Biochem.* **52:** 23–26.
13. Boulikas, T. and C. F. Kong. 1993. A novel class of matrix attached regions (MARs) identified by random cloning and their implications in differentiation and carcinogenesis. *Int. J. Oncol.* **2:** 325–330.
14. Carter, K. C. and J. B. Lawrence. 1991. DNA and RNA within the nucleus: how much sequence-specific spatial organization? *J. Cell. Biochem.* **47:** 124–129.
15. Carter, K. C., D. Bowman, W. Carrington, K. Fogarty, J. A. McNeill, F. S. Fey, et al. 1993. A three-dimensional view of precursor messenger RNA metabolism within the mammalian nucleus. *Science* **259:** 1330–1335.
16. Case, R. A. M., M. E. Hosker, D. B. McDonald, and J. T. Pearson. 1954. Tumors of the urinary bladder in workmen engaged in the British chemical industry. Role of aniline, benzidine, alpha-naphtylamine and beta-naphtylamine. *Br. J. Ind. Med.* **11:** 75–104.
17. Club, B. H. and M. Locke. 1998. Peripheral nuclear matrix actin forms perinuclear shells. *J. Cell Biochem.* **70:** 240–251.
18. De Belle, I., S. Cai, and T. Kohwi-Shigematsu. 1998. The genomic sequences bound to Special AT-rich sequence binding protein 1 (SATB1) in vivo in Jurkat T cells are tightly

associated with the nuclear matrix at the bases of the chromatin loops. *J. Cell Biology* **141:** 335–348.

19. de Lange, T. 1992. Human telomeres are attached to the nuclear matrix. *EMBO J.* **11:** 717–724.

20. Dickinson, L. A., T. Joh, Y. Kohwi, and T. Kohwi-Shigematsu. 1992. A tissue-specific MAR/SAR DNA-binding protein with unusual binding site recognition. *Cell* **70:** 631–645.

21. Donat, T. L., W. Sakr, J. E. Lehr, and K. J. Pienta. 1996. Nuclear matrix protein alteration in intermediate biomarkers in squamous cell carcinoma of the head and neck. *Otolaryngol.— Head Neck Surg.* **127:** 609–622.

22. Dworetkzky, S. I., K. L. Wright, E. G. Fey, S. Penman, J. B. Lian, J. L. Stein, et al. 1993. Sequence-specific DNA-binding proteins are components of a nuclear matrix-attachment site. *Proc. Natl. Acad. Sci. USA* **89:** 4178–4182.

23. Dworetzky, S. I., E. G. Fey, S. Penman, J. B. Lian, J. L. Stein, and G. S. Stein. 1990. Progressive changes in the protein composition of the nuclear matrix during rat osteoblast differentiation. *Proc. Natl. Acad. Sci. USA* **87:** 4605–4609.

24. Emmerich, P., P. Look, A. Jauch, A. H. N. Hopman, J. Wiegant, M. J. Higgins, et al. 1989. Double *in situ* hybridization in combination with digital image analysis: a new approach to study interphase chromosome topography. *Exp. Cell Res.* **181:** 126–140.

25. Ewing, C. M., N. Ru, R. A. Morton, J. C. Robinson, M. Wheelock, K. R. Johnson, et al. 1995. Chromosome 5 suppresses tumorigenicity of PC3 prostate cancer cells: correlation with re-expression of alpha catenin and restoration of E-cadherin function. *Cancer Res.* **55:** 4813–4817.

26. Fey, E. G., P. Bangs, C. Sparks, and P. Odgren. 1991. The nuclear matrix: defining structural and functional roles. *Crit. Rev. Eukaryot. Gene Exp.* **1:** 127–144.

27. Fishel, B. R., A. O. Sperry, and W. T. Garrard. 1993. Yeast calmodulin and a conserved nuclear protein participate in the in vivo binding of a matrix association region. *Proc. Natl. Acad. Sci. USA* **90:** 5623–5627.

28. Getzenberg, R. H. 1994. The nuclear matrix and the regulation of gene expression: tissue specificity. *J. Cell. Biochem.* **55:** 22–31.

29. Getzenberg, R. H., B. R. Konety, T. A. Oeler, M. M. Quigley, A. Hakam, M. Becich, et al. 1996. Bladder cancer associated nuclear matrix proteins. *Cancer Res.* **56:** 1690–1694.

30. Getzenberg, R. H., K. J. Pienta, E. Y. W. Huang, and D. S. Coffey. 1991. Identification of nuclear proteins in the cancer and normal rat prostate. *Cancer Res.* **51:** 6514–6520.

31. Getzenberg, R. H., K. J. Pienta, E. Y. W. Huang, and D. S. Coffey. 1991. Identification of nuclear proteins in the cancer and normal rat prostate. *Cancer Res.* **51:** 6514–6520.

32. Getzenberg, R. H., K. J. Pienta, and D. S. Coffey. 1990. The tissue matrix: cell dynamics and hormone action. *Endocr. Rev.* **11:** 399–417.

33. Haaf, T. and M. Schmid. 1991. Chromosome topology in mammalian interphase nuclei. *Exp. Cell Res.* **192:** 325–332.

34. Harris, S. G. and M. C. Smith. 1988. SnRNP coreprotein enrichment in the nuclear matrix. *Biochem. Biophys. Res. Commun.* **152:** 1383–1387.

35. He, D., J. A. Nickerson, and S. Penman. 1990. Core filaments of the nuclear matrix. *J. Cell Biol.* **110:** 569–580.

36. Horton, M. J. and R. H. Getzenberg. 1999. Rat seminal vesicle secretory protein SVS-II binds DNA with a preference for 5′ regulatory regions of secretory protein genes: presence among components of the nuclear matrix. *J. Androl.* **20:** 267–279.

37. Isomura, T., K. Tamiya-Koizumi, M. Suzuki, S. Yoshida, M. Taniguchi, M. Matsuyama, et al. 1992. RFP is a DNA binding protein associated with the nuclear matrix. *Nucleic Acids Res.* **20:** 5305–5310.

38. Kantor, A. F., P. Hartge, R. N. Hoover, A. Narayana, J. W. Sullivan, and J. F. Fraumeni Jr. 1984. Urinary tract infections and the risk of bladder cancer. *Am. J. Epidemiol.* **119:** 510–515.

39. Keesee, S. K., M. D. Meneghini, R. P. Szaro, and Y. J. Wu. 1994. Nuclear matrix proteins in human colon cancer. *Proc. Natl. Acad. Sci. USA* **91**: 1913–1916.

40. Khanuja, P. S., J. E. Lehr, H. D. Soule, S. K. Gehani, A. C. Noto, S. Choudhury, et al. 1993. Nuclear matrix proteins in normal and breast cancer cells. *Cancer Res.* **53**: 3394–3398.

41. Konety, B. R., A. K. Nangia, T. S. T. Nguyen, B. N. Veitmeier, R. Dhir, J. Acierno, et al. 1998. Identification of nuclear matrix protein alterations associated with renal cell carcinoma. *J. Urol.* **159**: 1359–1363.

41a. Konety, B. R., T-S. T. Nguyen, R. Dhir, R. S. Day et al. 2000. Detection of bladder cancer using a novel nuclear matrix protein, BLCA-4. *Clin. Cancer Res.* **6**: 2618–2625.

41b. Konety, B. R., T-S. T. Nguyen, G. Brehes, A. Sholder et al. 2000. Clinical usefulness of the novel marker BLC-4 for the detection of bladder cancer. *J. Urol.* **164**: 634–639.

42. Lakshmanan, Y., E. N. P. Subong, and A. W. Partin. 1998. Differential nuclear matrix protein expression in prostate cancers: correlation with pathological stage. *J. Urol.* **159**: 1354–1358.

43. Lichter, P. and D. C. Ward. 1990. Is non-isotopic *in situ* hybridization finally coming of age? *Nature (London)* **345**: 93–94.

44. Lichter, P., C.-J. C. Tang, K. Call, G. Hermanson, G. A. Evans, D. Housman, et al. 1990. High-resolution mapping of human chromosome 11 by *in situ* hybridization with cosmid clones. *Science* **247**: 64–69.

45. Luderus, M. E. E., A. de Graaf, E. Mattia, J. L. den Blaauwen, M. A. Grande, L. de Jong, et al. 1992. Binding of matrix attachment regions to Lamin B_1. *Cell* **70**: 949–959.

46. Manuelidis, L. and J. J. Borden. 1988. Reproducible compartmentalization of individual chromosome domains in human CNS cells revealed by *in situ* hybridization and three-dimensional reconstruction. *Chromosoma* **96**: 397–410.

47. McCaffrey, J. D., M. Gapany, R. A. Faust, A. T. Davis, G. L. Adams, and K. L. Ahmed. 1997. Nuclear matrix proteins as malignant markers in squamous cell carcinoma of the head and neck. *Arch. Otolaryngol. Head Neck Surg.* **123**: 283–288.

48. McNeil, J. A., C. V. Johnson, K. C. Carter, R. H. Singer, and J. B. Lawrence. 1991. Localizing DNA and RNA within nuclei and chromosomes by fluorescence *in situ* hybridization. *Genet. Anal. Tech. Appl.* **8**: 41–58.

49. Moll, R., W. W. Franks, D. L. Schiller, B. Geiger, and R. Krepler. 1982. The catalog of human cytokeratins: patterns of expression in normal epithelia, tumors and cultured cells. *Cell* **31**: 11–24.

50. Nardozza, T. A., M. M. Quigley, and R. H. Getzenberg. 1996. Association of transcription factors with the nuclear matrix. *J. Cell. Biochem.* **61**: 467–477.

51. Nickerson, J. A. 1998. Nuclear dreams: the malignant alteration of nuclear architecture. *J. Cell. Biochem.* **70**: 172–180.

52. Nickerson, J. A., G. Krochmalnic, K. M. Wan, and S. Penman. 1989. Chromatin architecture and nuclear RNA. *Proc. Natl. Acad. Sci. USA* **86**: 177–181.

53. Partin, A. W., R. H. Getzenberg, M. J. Carmichael, D. Vindivich, J. Yoo, J. Epstein, and D. S. Coffey. 1993. Nuclear matrix protein patterns in human benign prostatic hyperplasia and prostate cancer. *Cancer Res.* **53**: 744–746.

54. Phi-Van, L., J. P. von Kries, W. Ostertag, and W. H. Stratling. 1990. The chicken lysozyme 5′ matrix attachment region increases transcription from a heterologous promoter in heterologous cells and dampens position effects on the expression of transfected genes. *Mol. Cell. Biol.* **10**: 2302–2307.

55. Roberge, M. and S. M. Gasser. 1992. DNA loops: structural and functional properties of scaffold-attached regions. *Mol. Microbiol.* **6**: 419–423.

56. Sander, M., T. S. Hsieh, A. Udvardy, and P. Schedl. 1987. Sequence dependence of *Drosophila topoisomerase II* in plasmid relaxation and BND binding. *J. Mol. Biol.* **194**: 219–229.

57. Schwab, E. D. and K. J. Pienta. 1997. Explaining aberrations of cell structure and cell signaling in cancer using complex adaptive systems, in *Advances in Molecular and Cell Biology* (Bittar, E. E. and R. H. Getzenberg, eds.), Jai Press Inc., Greenwich, CT, pp. 207–247.

58. Soloway, M. S., J. V. Briggman, G. A. Carpinito, G. W. Chodak, P. A. Church, D. L. Lamm, et al. 1996. Use of a new tumor marker, urinary NMP22, in the detection of occult or rapidly recurring transitional cell carcinoma of the urinary tract following surgical treatment. *J. Urol.* **156:** 363–367.

59. Spector, D. L. 1990. Higher order nuclear organization: three-dimensional distribution of small nuclear ribonucleoprotein particles. *Proc. Natl. Acad. Sci. USA* **87:** 147–151.

60. Stampfer, D. S., G. A. Carpinito, J. Rodriguez-Villanueva, L. W. Willsey, C. P. Dinney, H. B. Grossman, et al. 1998. Evaluation of NMP22 in the detection of transitional cell carcinoma of the bladder. *J. Urol.* **159:** 394–398.

61. Stein, G. S., A. J. van Wijnen, J. L. Stein, J. B. Lian, S. Pockwinse, and S. McNeil. 1998. Interrelationships of nuclear structure and transcriptional control: functional consequences of being in the right place at the right time. *J. Cell. Biochem.* **70:** 200–212.

62. Stenoien, D., Z. D. Sharp, C. L. Smith, and M. A. Mancini. 1998. Functional subnuclear partitioning of transcription factors. *J. Cell. Biochem.* **70:** 213–221.

63. Stief, A., D. M. Winter, W. H. Stratling, and A. E. Sippel. 1989. A nuclear DNA attachment element mediates elevated and position-independent gene activity. *Nature (London)* **341:** 343–345.

64. Stuurman, N., R. van Driel, L. de Jong, A. M. L. Meijne, and J. van Renswoude. 1989. The protein composition of the nuclear matrix of murine P19 embryonal carcinoma cells is differentiation-state dependent. *Exp. Cell Res.* **180:** 460–466.

65. Subong, E. N., M. J. Shue, J. I. Epstein, J. V. Briggman, P. K. Chan, and A. W. Partin. 1999. Monoclonal antibody to prostate cancer nuclear matrix protein (PRO:4-216) recognizes nucleophosmin/B23. *Prostate* **39:** 98–304.

66. van Wijnen, A. J., J. P. Bidwell, E. G. Fey, S. Penman, J. B. Lian, J. L. Stein, et al. 1993. Nuclear matrix association of multiple sequence-specific DNA binding activities related to SP-1, ATF, CCAAT, C/EBP, OCT-1, and AP-1. *Biochemistry* **32:** 8397–8402.

67. Vassetzky, Y. S., C. V. De Moura Gallo, A. N. Bogdanova, S. V. Razin, and K. Scherrer. 1993. The sequence-specific nuclear matrix binding factor F6 is a chicken GATA-like protein. *Mol. Gen. Genet.* **238:** 309–314.

68. Wiener, H. G., C. H. Mian, A. Haitel, A. Pycha, G. Schatzl, and M. Marberger. 1998. Can urine bound diagnostic tests replace cystoscopy in the management of bladder cancer? *J. Urol.* **159:** 1876–1880.

69. Xing, Y., C. V. Johnson, P. R. Dobner, and J. B. Lawrence. 1993. Higher level organization of individual gene transcription and RNA splicing. *Science* **259:** 1326–1330.

70. Xu, M., R. E. Hammer, V. C. Blasquez, S. L. Jones, and W. T. Garrard. 1989. Immunoglobulin kappa gene expression after stable integration. II. role of the intronic *mar* and enhancer in transgenic mice. *J. Biol. Chem.* **264:** 21,190–21,195.

13

The Role of Cell Adhesion Molecules in Prostate Development and Carcinogenesis

Jer-Tsong Hsieh, PhD

1. INTRODUCTION

In the multicellular organism, the formation and maintenance of the structure and function of tissues require specific communication and regulated three-dimensional organization between each cell type and extracellular signals. Cell adhesion molecules (CAMs) have been shown to be one of the key components controlling embryonic development and organization of multicellular organisms. In contrast, aberrant expression of CAMs is often associated with tumorigenesis in many neoplasms. For example, decreased expression of E-cadherin, which is predominantly expressed in epithelial cells, is associated with the progression of several types of neoplasm *(6,15,19,44)*. Giancotti and Ruoslahti *(21)* have demonstrated that increasing expression of $\alpha_5\beta_1$ integrin by gene transfection can reduce tumorigenicity of Chinese hamster ovary cells in vivo.

Cell adhesion was recognized during embryonic cell reorganization about 40 yr ago *(24)*. However, 20 yr later, the first characterization of a CAM molecule was undertaken by Beug et al. *(3)* by raising a specific antibody. Currently, at least 50 different CAMs have been identified, and can be divided into four major families based on their protein structure (Fig. 1). The immunoglobulin (Ig) superfamily, a calcium independent CAM, is composed of variable numbers of Ig-like repeats (ranging from 4–6 U) on the ligand-binding domain and fibronectin-like repeats (up to 5 U) on the extracellular domain, transmembrane domain, and intracellular domain (except N-CAM). The cadherin family, a calcium dependent CAM, contains 3–5 internal repeats on the extracellular domain, transmembrane domain, and intracellular domain. All integrins consist of two noncovalently associated subunits—α and β, that are typical transmembrane proteins. Integrins are the major receptor for many extracellular matrices. For selectins, the extracellular domain contains three different domains: a calcium dependent lectin domain, an epidermal growth factor-like domain, and a variable number of repeats homologous to complement regulatory protein. This chapter summarizes recent progress regarding the role of CAMs in prostate biology, and discusses the potential application of CAMs in prostate cancer management.

From: *Prostate Cancer: Biology, Genetics, and the New Therapeutics*
Edited by: L. W. K. Chung, W. B. Isaacs, and J. W. Simons © Humana Press Inc., Totowa, NJ

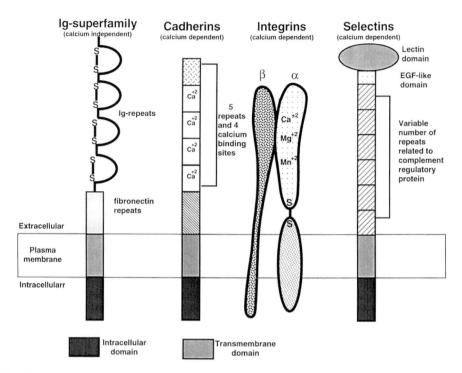

Fig. 1. Major class of cell-adhesion molecules (CAMs). Structurally, CAMs can subdivided into four major types: Ig-superfamily, cadherin, integrins, and selectins. Homophilic interactions are often associated with either Ig-superfamily or cadherins. The ligands for integrins are extracellular matrix. Selectins can bring to carbohydrate moieties of membrane protein.

2. IG SUPERFAMILY

2.1. C-CAM1

The CAMs containing four Ig-like loops in the extracellular domain are the largest members of the CAMs. These molecules have a homophilic interaction. Recently, we studied C-CAM1, an epithelial CAM with a molecular wt of 105,000. C-CAM1 is highly homologous to BGP1, a biliary glycoprotein that crossreacts with antibodies against carcinoembryonic antigen (CEA) *(50)*. C-CAM1 was originally identified by Ocklind and Obrink *(38)* by monitoring the ability of papain-solubilized plasma membrane components to neutralize the inhibition of cell aggregation by antibodies generated against cell surface proteins. In our recent study, we demonstrated that the expression of C-CAM1 in rat ventral prostatic epithelium was repressed by androgen *(25)*. A similar regulatory pattern was also observed in the seminal vesicle (SV), but not in other organs (the liver and kidney), suggesting that regulation of C-CAM1 expression by androgen is tissue specific.

During human prostate development, the spatial-tempo expression of C-CAM1 correlates with basal cell differentiation. It is known that the human prostate arises from the urogenital sinus and the vesicourethral components of the cloaca as solid buds. The bud stage (20–30 wk gestation) is characterized by the appearance of solid cellular buds at the ends of ducts without a recognizable lumen. C-CAM1 can be detected in the multiple cell layers of the acinar bud of a 30-wk fetal prostate, but not the surrounding stromal component *(34)*. By 36 wk, when tubular morphogenesis of the epithelial bud has occurred, the staining of C-CAM1 is localized predominantly in the basal cell layer of these tubular structures. In a 13-yr-old juvenile prostate, C-CAM1 can be clearly found in the basal cell layer of all glands examined *(34)*. The basal cell in the prostate has been suggested to represent a stem cell population from different studies *(4,11,30,68)*. Therefore, we believe that C-CAM1 may play an important role in controlling prostate development. On the other hand, we have studied a series of benign and malignant human prostate tissues, including prostatic intraepithelial neoplasia (PIN). In both benign prostatic hyperplasia (BPH) and PIN, an overall decrease in C-CAM1 staining was detected. Also, C-CAM1 was not detected in well, moderately, and poorly-differentiated carcinoma *(34)*. These results indicate that there is an inverse correlation between C-CAM1 expression and clinical grades of prostate cancer, suggesting that loss of C-CAM1 expression is an early event in the development of prostate cancer. Similarly, several investigators *(23,49,53)* showed that decreased C-CAM1 expression is found in several other tumor types.

To examine the functional role of C-CAM1 in the prostate tumor, we transfected the C-CAM1 expression vector into the human metastatic prostate cancer cell line PC-3. The C-CAM1-expressing clones had a significantly reduced in vitro growth compared to that of the control cells. These clones formed significantly fewer colonies in soft agar in three independent experiments. Furthermore, an in vivo tumorigenic assay was carried out using these transfected cells. The outcome clearly demonstrated that expression of C-CAM1 could markedly suppress the tumorigenicity of PC-3 cells *(26)*. Alternatively, another approach to our study of the tumor suppressive role of C-CAM1 in prostate carcinogenesis was to reduce its expression in a nontumorigenic prostatic epithelial cell line (i.e., NbE) using an antisense expression vector. In vivo tumorigenic data indicated that antisense clones could induce tumors in nude mice while the parental cells remained nontumorigenic *(26)*. Western blot indicated that the levels of C-CAM1 were significantly (10- to 100-fold) lower in all six sublines than in the parental cells *(26)*. These results are consistent with the reduced expression of C-CAM1 in malignant cells seen in human prostate specimens, indicating that C-CAM1 is a potent tumor suppressor occuring in early events of prostate carcinognesis.

Little is known about the functional domain(s) of C-CAM1 in modulating its tumor suppression activity in prostate cancer. As shown in Fig. 2, our data *(27)* indicated that both the first Ig domain and the tyrosine phosphorylation site (i.e., amino acid 488) did not play any significant role in modulating the suppression function of C-CAM1 in vivo. Interestingly, H458 lost half the strength of tumor suppression function, suggesting that the C-terminal sequences (i.e., the 61 amino acids adjacent to amino acid 458), including the ARH domain, may be needed to retain the tumor suppression function of C-CAM1. Nevertheless, this study indicated that these four amino acids containing a potential Ser/The phosphorylation site are crucial for maintaining the tumor suppression function of C-CAM1 (Fig. 2). Similar results were observed in breast cancer cells *(40)*. Based on these results, we hypothesized that C-CAM1 protein phosphorylation modulated by protein kinase A may be important in suppressing prostate cancer growth. The intracellular domain of C-CAM1 may also interact with other soluble factors to

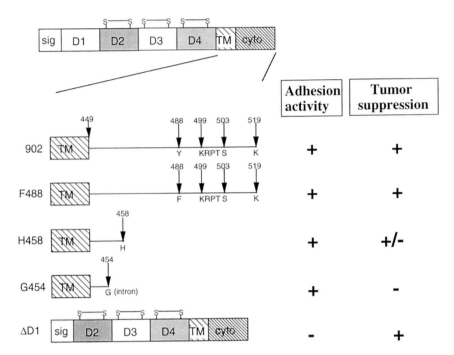

Fig. 2. The summary of structural functional relationship of C-CAM1 molecule. We generated recombinant adenovirus carrying either a full-length cDNA (i.e., 902) or a series of C-CAM1 mutants as follows: F488 (Tyr-488 of C-CAM1 was changed to phenylalanine); H458 (deletion of intracellular domain to the His-458 position); Gly 454 (deletion of intracellular domain to the Gly-454 position); ΔD1 (the first Ig domain deletion); sig, signal peptide; D1, first Ig domain; D2, second Ig domain; D3, third Ig domain; TM, transmembrane domain, cyto: cytoplasmic domain.

transduce its negative signal. An 80-kDa protein was recently identified as a potential interactive protein correlated with growth inhibitory activity *(41)*. The potential interactive proteins associated with C-CAM1 warrant further investigation.

We further explored the possibility of applying C-CAM1 as a potential therapeutic agent for developing prostate cancer gene therapy using an adenoviral delivery system. We found that the delivery of a single dose of C-CAM adenovirus was able to repress the growth of PC-3-induced tumors in nude mice for at least 3 wk. Therefore, we believe that C-CAM1 is a potential candidate for human prostate cancer therapy.

2.2. DCC

Deletion in colon carcinoma (DCC) *(18)* shares a similar Ig-like structure with C-CAM1 and was first cloned from colon carcinoma cells as a potential tumor suppressor gene. Recent studies demonstrated that DCC is a receptor for netrin, a critical factor involved in central nervous system development *(7,35)*. Interestingly, data from a knockout mouse model indicates that the loss of DCC is lethal during fetal development because the littermate has an impairment in the axonal formation of the spinal cord *(17)*. In addition to its physiological role, DCC is often found to be missing in various cancers, including prostate, bladder and colon *(22,10)*. Recently, we established a recombinant adenoviral expression system with a high efficiency of gene delivery into target cells. With this technique, we have demonstrated that the expression of DCC can induce apoptosis in a variety of cancer cell lines *(8)*. The timing of the appearance of the apoptotic phenotype coincided with the cleavage of poly(ADP-ribose) polymerase (PARP), which is the substrate of caspases and is a hallmark of the biochemical pathway of apoptosis *(8)*. DCC-induced apoptosis can not be abrogated by the antagonistic effect of Bcl-2 , suggesting that a different apoptotic signal induced by DCC is operated via a Bcl-2 independent pathway *(8)*.

2.3. CD44

CD44 (85 kDa) also belongs to the Ig-superfamily of CAMs and participates in specific cell-cell and cell-extracellular matrix interactions such as hyaluronic acid and osteopontin *(69,70)*. The expression of CD44 is considered to be a unique maker for the basal-cell population in the human prostate gland *(39)*. Furthermore, down-regulation of the CD44 mRNA, as well as protein levels, correlates with acquisition of metastatic ability of the Dunning tumor system *(20)*. It appears that CD44 can function as a metastatic suppressor *(20)*. Recent study indicates that hypermethylation of the CD44 gene is often detected in metastatic human prostate cancer specimens compared to their normal counterparts *(42)*.

3. CADHERIN

The cadherin family is subdivided into at least three types, including E-, P-, and N-cadherin, and each cadherin has a unique tissue distribution. E-cadherin (or L-CAM) is present in virtually all types of epithelial cells, although E-cadherin expression is also found in glia and some types of neurons. P-cadherin is expressed in both the basal and lower layers of stratified epithelia and in the mesothelium. N-cadherin is predominantly associated with neuronal tissue and cells of mesodermal origin.

In a normal prostate gland, E-cadherin is localized in the lateral side of luminal epithelia. However, in a Dunning prostate tumor, Bussemaker et al. *(3)* demonstrated that there is an inverse correlation of E-cadherin mRNA and metastatic ability of tumor cells, suggesting that E-cadherin may be involved in tumor progression by disrupting cell-cell communication. A possible cause of altered E-cadherin expression may be the loss of heterozygosity at the 16.1q chromosome band, which is often detected in human prostate cancer *(62,66)*. Clinically, decreased or absent E-cadherin expression in prostate cancer is associated with tumor grade, advanced clinical stage, and poor survival *(9,51,54,66,67)*. The regulation of E-cadherin gene expression in prostate cancer is still not fully understood; however, some evidence indicates that hyper-methylation of the E-cadherin promoter region in cancer cells may reduce its gene expression.

In some cases, not every patient with normal E-cadherin expression had a better survival, suggesting that the downstream effector of E-cadherin may be impaired in these cancer cells. It is known that E-cadherin can form a complex with catenin proteins that serve as an anchor point to the microfilament cytoskeleton *(42,52,65)*. There are three major catenins based on their SDS-PAGE: α (102 kDa), β (88 kDa) and γ (82 kDa). The α-catenin serves as a bridge between E-cadherin and β-catenin which will connect with the microfilament cytoskeleton. Morton et al. *(48)* demonstrated that loss of α-catenin expression in E-cadherin-positive human prostate cancer cells (i.e.,

PC-3 cell) is caused by homozygous deletion. Clinically, about 25% of prostate cancer specimens analyzed have loss of heterozygosity in the α-catenin gene (5q21–22) *(46)*. To evaluate the role of α-catenin in prostate cancer progression, increased expression of α-catenin in PC-3 cells results in the suppression of tumorigenicity in a thymic mouse by microcell-mediated transfer of the entire chromosome 5 *(16)*.

On the other hand, altered β-catenin expression can disassemble the adherent junction that can make the cell become more invasive *(60)*. Recent data *(55,61)* indicate that a potential tumor suppressor APC can stabilize β-catenin through a specific interaction. Furthermore, β-catenin can form a complex with a specific transcription factor of TCF/LEF-1 (T cell factor/lymphoid enhancer factor-1) family *(12,28)*. This complex can associate with the 5′ end of the E-cadherin gene and also can activate several genes involved in cell proliferation *(2,14)*, further suggesting that β-catenin may be involved in cancer progression. In the case of γ-catenin, levels of protein have been found to correlate with the tumorigenicity of several tumor types. Transfection of γ-catenin into tumor cells significantly decreases their tumorigenicity in vivo. A recent immunostaining study *(47)*, using 45 prostate cancer specimens obtained from radical prostatectomy, indicates that aberrant expression of three types of catenin are associated with capsular invasion, although the significant relationship is retained only for β-and γ-catenin when restricted to moderately differentiated (Gleason score 5–7) tumors. Therefore, the functional role of both β- and γ-catenin in prostate cancer progression warrants further investigation.

P-cadherin is present in the cell-cell boundary of the basal epithelia of the normal prostate gland *(63)*, suggesting that P-cadherin can be a potential basal cell marker. The expression of P-cadherin is downregulated in PIN tissue and is absent in cancer lesions ranging from well to poorly-differentiated tumors *(31)*. Soler et al. *(59)* further observed that all P-cadherin-positive cells are negative for prostate-specific antigen (PSA). In addition to the loss of P-cadherin expression in the majority of prostate cancer cells, some tumors that are P-cadherin positive are frequently located close to ejaculatory ducts and are negative for PSA, suggesting that P-cadherin may be a useful diagnostic marker for patients with low levels of PSA.

4. INTEGRIN

Integrins were initially defined based on the structural homology between leukocyte adhesion receptors and cell-surface glycoproteins involved in extracellular matrix recognition *(29)*. Structurally, integrins are heterodimers composed of two transmembrane glycoproteins, termed α and β, which remain noncovalently associated. A single β subunit that could associate with a specific group of subunits led to the initial classification of integrin into at least three subfamilies: β1 or Very Late Activation antigens (VLA) (β1: α1–α8); β2 or leukocyte-specific integrins (β2: αL, αM, αX); β3 or cytoadhesins (β3: αV, gpIIb) *(56)*.

Current understanding of integrin-mediated signal transduction is focused on the characterization of focal adhesion kinase (FAK) *(32)*, a novel cytoplasmic tyrosine kinase. FAK has a central tyrosine kinase domain, a cytoplasmic domain that can interact with paxillin, and an amino acid terminal that may interact with integrin. FAK-mediated tyrosine phosphorylation of paxillin leads to a change in cytoskeleton organization. FAK or other effector proteins are also involved in the signaling pathway leading to cell proliferation *(32)*.

The normal prostate basal cells express several integrins (extracellular matrix receptors, including α 2, 3, 4, 5, 6, v, β1, and β4 that are adjacent to the basal lamina *(13,58)*. The integrin α6β4 is associated with hemidesmosomal-like structures. Although hemidesmosomal proteins and the α3β1 and α6β1 integrins (laminin receptors) are still detectable in the early PIN lesions, the expression of the integrins α2, α4, α5, αv, and β4 is lost in carcinoma *(1,13,64)*. The α3β1 and α6β1 integrins remain associated with invasive carcinoma, where integrin expression is diffuse in the plasma membrane and not restricted to the basal aspects of the cell *(13)*. Also, the α6β1 integrin became a potential candidate for conferring the invasive phenotype of prostatic carcinoma when it was tested in a SCID mouse model system *(13)*. It is likely that blockage of the expression or function of α6β1 or laminin and/or preventing the loss of β4 would be essential steps in confining the carcinoma to the prostate gland.

Prostatic carcinoma cells have a propensity to metastasize to bone, and it is believed that this phenomenon may be promoted by the adhesion of metastatic cells to bone matrix made by osteoblasts. Kostenuik et al. *(37)* developed an in vitro model of bone matrix by isolating the substratum deposited by human osteoblast-like U2OS cells. They were able to demonstrate that this adhesion appears to be mediated by the interaction of α2β1 integrin on PC-3 cells with matrix-derived collagen. The stimulation of this adhesion by TGF-β suggests that the coexpression of TGF-β and type I collagen in bone may synergistically facilitate the adhesion of metastatic cells to bone matrix proteins and thereby increase their localization in the skeleton.

5. SELECTIN

The selectins are the recently merging members of CAM family. The three known members of this family (L-, E-, and P-selectin) mediate the binding of leukocytes to endothelial cells, and are involved in the homing of lymphocyte to lymph node, as well as the extravasation of neutrophilic granulocytes into inflamed tissue. Unlike other normally expressed CAMs such as E-cadherin, which are lost, E-selectin is altered and overexpressed in metastatic melanoma tumors *(43)*. Also, it has been reported that there is upregulation of oligosaccharide sialyl Le(x), a selectin isoform, in hormone-resistant prostate cancer *(57)*. However, several groups of investigators *(5,43)* have studied the potential role of selectins in prostate cancer progression from either prostate cancer cell lines or cancer specimens. Their data have concluded that selectins are not detected in human prostate cancer cell lines, including metastatic PC-3 and DU145. Also, the serum levels of selectin from prostate cancer patients do not show any significant difference from that of normal individuals.

6. CONCLUSION

Morphologically, prostatic epithelia can be divided into subtypes: columnar glandular epithelia and cuboid basal epithelia. Androgen deprivation induces apoptosis of the luminal prostatic epithelium, leading to degeneration of the prostate gland. In contrast, the basal epithelial cells are more resistant to the apoptotic effects of androgen deprivation. Animal studies demonstrate that following castration-induced degeneration, the prostate regrows to its preprogrammed size in response to exogenous androgen regardless of the dosage and schedule of androgen administration, suggesting that the basal cells may represent the stem cell population *(11,30,68)*. Apparently, CAMs play an important role in prostate development and glandular morphorgenesis. For example, C-CAM1 can be detected in the basal cell population from as early as the acini bud stage of gestation, suggesting that C-CAM1 may be one of the key CAMs for controlling the recognition between basal cells during prostate development *(34)*. This is further evidenced by the consistent expression of C-CAM1 in normal basal cells throughout adulthood *(34)*. In addition to C-CAM1, P-cadherin *(63)* and E-cadherin *(66)* are detected in different cell types, suggesting that there may be a unique cell–cell contact within the same cell compartment. Also, the basal epithelia contact with the extracellular matrix through the integrins (such as $\alpha6\beta1$) on the their basal membrane *(13)*. The coordination between each type of CAM constitutes the architectural integrity and physiologic activity of normal prostate gland.

In contrast to normal cells, malignant cells often lose contact inhibition and anchorage-dependent growth, and become mobile and invasive. These changes are caused by alteration of CAMs. Ig-superfamily and cadherins generally participate in cell–cell communication, leading to contact inhibition. Loss of integrin will render cancer cells anchorage-independent, and they may acquire invasiveness. However, expression of certain integrin molecules (such as $\alpha3\beta1$ and $\alpha6\beta1$) on the surface of cancer cells may facilitate their metastatic potential to distant sites. Therefore, the impact of CAMs on the cancer phenotype during prostate cancer progression may be very dynamic. More detailed studies are essential to evaluate the role of CAM during the natural history of prostate cancer progression.

7. PERSPECTIVE

Receptors that mediate adhesion interactions—including the Ig-superfamily, cadherins, integrins and selectins—have long been recognized for their important role in cell structure and architecture. However, it becomes quite clear that adhesion receptors also participate in key signal transduction processes that regulate cell growth and cell differentiation. For example, integrin can interact with FAK and other effectors to elicit a signaling pathway leading to cell growth. Interaction between E-cadherin and catenin proteins plays an important role in supporting cell architecture. Although the pathways mediated by the Ig-superfamily are still unclear, the intracellular domain of C-CAM1, containing both Ser/Thr and tyrosine phosphorylation sites, was found to be able to interact with a cytosolic protein (80 kDa) that may be involved in the cascade of tumor inhibition. Therefore, further investigation into the underlying mechanisms of CAMs can help us understand the potential interaction between different CAMs, and also the possible relationship with growth factor receptor.

Prostate cancer is a multifocal disease, and each focus may have a distinct phenotype and genetic profile that often impacts invasiveness and metastatic potential. It is conceivable that changing every CAM expression in each focus will affect the natural history of each tumor. To analyze each focus for any given CAM expression, tissue-chip technology can offer a rapid screening for more than 1000 tissue sections in a single slide *(36)*. Also, it is crucial to analyze the profile of the entire CAM expression during prostate cancer progression. Currently, DNA microarry technology can rapidly achieve this goal *(33)*. The outcome of these studies should help us to refine the tools of diagnosis and select a better therapeutic target.

REFERENCES

1. Allen, M. V., G. J. Smith, R. Juliano, S. J. Maygarden, and J. L. Mohler. 1998. Downregulation of the beta4 integrin subunit in prostatic carcinoma and prostatic intraepithelial neoplasia. *Hum. Pathol.* **29:** 311–318.
2. Behrens, J., J. P. von Kries, M. Kuhl, L. Bruhn, D. Wedlich, R. Grosschyedl, et al. 1996. Functional interaction with transcription factor LEF-1. *Nature* **382:** 638–642.
3. Beug, H., F. E. Katz, and G. Gerisch. 1973. Dynamics of antigenic membrane sites relating to cell aggregation in *Dictyostelium discoideum. J. Cell. Biol.* **56:** 647–658.
4. Bonkohoff, H. and K. Remberger. 1996. Differentiation pathways and histogenetic aspects of normal and abnormal prostatic growth: a stem cell model. *Prostate* **28:** 98–106.
5. Brayton, J., Z. Qing, M. N. Hart, J. C. VanGilder, and Z. Fabry. 1998. Influence of adhesion molecule expression by human brain microvessel endothelium on cancer cell adhesion. *J. Neuroimmunol.* **89:** 104–112.
6. Bussemakers, M. J., R. J. van Moorselaar, L. A. Giroldi, T. Ichikawa, J. T. Isaacs, M. Takeichi, et al. 1992. Decreased expression of E-cadherin in the progression of rat prostate cancer. *Cancer Res.* **52:** 2916–2922.
7. Chan, S. S-Y., H. Zheng, M. W. Su, R. Wilk, M. T. Killeen, E. M. Hedgecock, et al. 1996. UNC-40, a *C. elegans* homolog of DCC (Deleted in Colorectal Cancer), is required in motile cells responding to UNC-6 netrin cues. *Cell* **87:** 187–195.
8. Chen, Y. Q., J. T. Hsieh, R. C. Pong, B. Fang, and F. Yao. 1999. Induction of apoptosis and G2/M cell cycle arrest by DCC. *Oncogene* **18:** 2747–2757.
9. Cheng, L., M. Nagabbushan, T. P. Prelow, S. B. Amini, and T. G. Prelow. 1996. Expression of E-cadherin in primary and metastatic prostate cancer. *Am. J. Pathol.* **148:** 1375–1380.
10. Cho, K. R. and E. R. Fearon. 1995. DCC: linking tumor suppressor genes and altered cell surface interactions in cancer? *Eur. J. Cancer* **31A:** 1055–1060.
11. Coffey, D. S. and P. C. Walsh. 1990. Clinical and experimental studies of benign prostatic hyperplasia. *Urol. Clin. N. Am.* **17:** 461–475.
12. Cox, R. T. and M. Peifer. 1998. Wingless signaling: the inconvenient complexities of life. *Curr. Biol.* **8:** R140–144.
13. Cress, A. E., I. Rabinovitz, W. Zhu, and R. B. Nagle. 1995. The alpha 6 beta 1 and alpha 6 beta 4 integrins in human prostate cancer progression. *Cancer Metastasis Rev.* **14:** 219–228.
14. Daniel, J. M. and A. B. Reynolds. 1997. Tyrosine phosphorylation and cadherin/catenin function. *BioEssays* **19:** 883–891.
15. Edelman, G. M. and K. L. Crossin. 1991. Cell adhesion molecules: Implication for a molecular histology. *Annu. Rev. Biochem.* **60:** 155–190.
16. Ewing, C. M., K. Ru, R. A. Morton, J. C. Robinson, M. J. Wheelock, K. R. Johnson, et al. 1995. Chromosome 5 suppresses tumorigenicity of PC-3 prostate cancer cells: correlation with re-expression of α-catenin and restoration of E-cadherin function. *Cancer Res.* **55:** 4813–4817.
17. Fazeli, A., S. L. Dickinson, M. L. Hermiston, R. V. Tighe, R. G. Steen, C. G. Small, et al. 1997. Phenotype of mice lacking functional deleted in colorectal cancer (DCC) gene. *Nature* **386:** 796–804.
18. Fearon, E. R., K. R. Cho, J. M. Nigro, S. E. Kern, J. W. Simons, J. M. Ruppert, et al. 1990. Identification of a chromosome 18q gene that is altered in colorectal cancers. *Science* **247:** 49–56.
19. Frixen, U. H., J. Behrens, M. Sachs, G. Eberle, B. Voss, A. Warda, et al. 1991. E-cadherin-mediated cell-cell adhesion prevents invasiveness of human carcinoma cells. *J. Cell Biol.* **113:** 173–185.

20. Gao, A., W. Lou, J. T. Doong, and J. T. Isaacs. 1997. CD44 is a metastasis suppressor gene for prostatic cancer located on human chromosome 11p13. *Cancer Res.* **57:** 846–849.

21. Giancotti, F. G. and E. Ruoslahti. 1990. Elevated levels of the $\alpha_5\beta_1$ fibronectin receptor suppress the transformed phenotype of Chinese hamster ovary cells. *Cell* **60:** 849–859.

22. Hedrick, L., K. R. Cho, E. R. Fearon, T. C. Wu, K. W. Kinzler, and B. Vogelstein. 1994. DCC gene product in cellular differentiation and colorectal tumorigenesis. *Genes Dev.* 1174–1183.

23. Hixson, D., K. D. McEntire, and B. Obrink. 1985. Alterations in the expression of a hepatocyte cell adhesion molecule by transplantable rat hepatocellular carcinomas. *Cancer Res.* **45:** 3742–3749.

24. Holtfreter, J. 1948. Significant of the cell membrane in embryonic process. *Ann. NY Acad. Sci.* **49:** 709–760.

25. Hsieh, J. T. and S-H. Lin. 1994. Androgen regulation of cell adhesion molecule (CAM) gene expression in rat prostate during organ degeneration: C-CAM belongs to a new class of androgen-repressed genes associated with enriched stem/amplifying cell population after prolonged castration. *J. Biol. Chem.* **269:** 3711–3716.

26. Hsieh, J. T., W. Luo, W. Song, Y. Wang, D. Kleinerman, N. T. Van, et al. 1995. Tumor suppressive role of an androgen-regulated epithelial cell adhesion molecule (C-CAM) in prostate carcinoma cell revealed by sense and antisense approaches. *Cancer Res.* **55:** 190–197.

27. Hsieh, J. T., K. Early, R. C. Pong, Y. Wang, N. T. Van, and S-H. Lin. 1999. Structural analysis of C-CAM1 molecule for its tumor suppression function in prostate cancer cells. *Prostate* **41:** 31–38.

28. Huber, O., R. Korn, J. McLaughlin, M. Oshugi, B. G. Hermann, and R. Kemler. 1996. Localization of β-catenin by interaction with transcription factor LEF-1. *Mech. Dev.* **59:** 3–11.

29. Hynes, R. O. 1987. Integrins: family of cell surface receptors. *Cell* **48:** 549–554.

30. Issacs, J. T. and D. S. Coffey. 1989. Etiology and disease process of benign prostatic hyperplasia. *Prostate* **(Suppl.)2:** 33–50.

31. Jarrard, D. F., R. Paul, A. von Bokhoven, S. H. Nguyen, G. S. Bova, M. J. Wheelock, et al. 1997. *Clin. Cancer. Res.* **3:** 2121–2128.

32. Juliano, R. 1996. Cooperation between soluble factors and integrin-mediated cell anchorage in the control of cell growth and differentiation. *BioEssays* **18:** 911–917.

33. Khan, J., M. L. Bittner, Y. Chen, P. S. Meltzer, and J. M. Trent. 1999. DNA microarray technology: the anticipated impact on the study of human disease. *Biochim. Biophys. Acta* **1423:** M17–M28.

34. Kleinerman, D., P. Troncoso, S-H. Lin L. L. Pisters, E. R. Sherwood, T. Brooks, et al. 1995. Consistent expression of an epithelial cell adhesion molecule (C-CAM) in human prostate development and in prostate carcinoma: implication as a tumor suppressor. *Cancer Res.* **55:** 1215–1220.

35. Kolodziej, P. A., L. C. Timpe, K. J. Mitchell, S. R. Fried, C. S. Goodman, L. Y. Jan, et al. 1996. Frazzled encodes a Drosophila member of the DCC immunoglobulin subfamily and is required for CNS and motor axon guidance. *Cell* **87:** 197–204.

36. Kononen, J., L. Bubendorf, A. Kallioniemi, M. Barlund, P. Schraml, S. Leighton, et al. 1998. Tissue microarrays for high-throughput molecular profiling of tumor specimens. *Nat. Med.* **4:** 844–847.

37. Kostenuik, P. J., O. Sanchez-Sweatman, F. W. Orr, and G. Singh. 1996. Bone cell matrix promotes the adhesion of human prostatic carcinoma cells via the alpha 2 beta 1 integrin. *Clin. Exp. Metastasis* **14:** 19–26.

38. Lin, S-H. and G. Guidotti. 1989. Cloning and expression of a cDNA coding for a rat liver plasma membrane ecto-ATPase. *J. Biol. Chem.* **264:** 14,408–14,414.

39. Liu, A. Y., L. D. True, L. LaTray, P. S. Nelson, W. J. Ellis, R. L. Vessella, et al. 1997. Cell-cell interaction in prostate gene regulation and cytodifferentiation. *Proc. Natl. Acad. Sci. USA* **94:** 10,705–10,710.

40. Luo, W., C. G. Wood, K. Early, M. Hung, and S-H. Lin. 1997. Suppression of tumorigenicity of breast cancer cells by an epithelial cell adhesion molecule (C-CAM1): the adhesion and growth suppression are mediated by different domain. *Oncogene* **14:** 1697–1704.

41. Luo, W., K. Early, V. Tantingco, D. C. Hixson, T. C. Liang, and S-H. Lin. 1998. Association of an 80 kDa protein with C-CAM1 cytoplasmic domain correlates with C-CAM1-mediated growth inhibition. *Oncogene* **16:** 1141–1147.

42. Lou, W., D. Krill, R. Dhir, M. J. Becich, J-T. Dong, H. F. Frierson, et al. 1999. Methylation of the CD44 metastasis suppressor gene in human prostate cancer. *Cancer Res.* **59:** 2329–2331.

43. Lynch, D. F., W. Hassen, M. A. Clements, P. F. Schellhammer, and G. Wright. 1997. Serum levels of endothelial and neural cell adhesion molecules in prostate cancer. *Prostate* **32:** 214–220.

44. Matsuura, K., J. Kawanishi, S. Fuji, M. Imamura, S. Hirano, M., Takeichi. et al. 1992. Altered expression of E-cadherin in gastric cancer tissues and carcinomatous fluid. *Br. J. Cancer* **66:** 1122–1130.

45. McCrea, P. D. and B. Gumbiner. 1991. Purification of a 92KDa cytoplasmic protein tightly associated with the cell-cell adhesion molecule E-cadherin (uvomorulin) characterization and extractability of the protein complex from the cell cytostructure. *J. Biol. Chem.* **266:** 4514–4520.

46. McPherson, J. D., R. A. Morton, C. M. Ewing, J. J. Wasmuth, J. Overhauser, A. Nagafuchi, et al. 1994. Assignment of the human α-catenin gene to chromosome 5q21–q22. *Genomics* **19:** 188–190.

47. Morita, N., H. Uemura, K. Tsumatani, M. Cho, Y. Hirao, E. Okajima, et al. 1999. E-cadherin and α-, β-, and γ-catenin expression in prostate cancers: correlation with tumor invasion. *Br. J. Cancer* **79:** 1879–1883.

48. Morton, R. A., C. M. Ewing, A. Nagafuchi, S. Tsukita, and W. B. Isaacs. 1993. Reduction of E-cadherin levels and deletion of the α-catenin gene in human prostate cancer cells. *Cancer Res.* **53:** 3585–3590.

49. Neumaier, M., S. Paululat, A. Chan, and P. Matthaes. 1993. Biliary glycoprotein, a potential human cell adhesion molecule, is down-regulated in colorectal carcinomas. *Proc. Natl. Acad. Sci. USA* **90:** 10,744–10,748.

50. Ocklind, C. and B. Obrink. 1982. Intercellular adhesion of rat hepatocytes: identification of a cell surface glycoprotein involved in the initial adhesion process. *J. Biol. Chem.* **257:** 6788–6795.

51. Otto, T., K. Rembrink, M. Goepel, M. Meyer-Schwickerath, and H. Rubben. 1993. E-cadherin: a marker for differentiation and invasiveness in prostatic carcinoma. *Urol. Res.* **21:** 359–362.

52. Ozawa, M., H. Baribault, and R. Kemler. 1990. The cytoplasmic domain of the cell adhesion molecule uvomorulin associates with three independent proteins structurally related in different species. *EMBO J.* **8:** 1711–1717.

53. Rosenberg, M., P. Nédellec, S. S. Jothy, D. Fleiszer, C. Turbide, and N. Beauchemin. 1993. The expression of mouse biliary glycoprotein, a carcinoembryonic antigen-related gene, is down-regulated in malignant mouse tissues. *Cancer Res.* **53:** 4938–4945.

54. Ross, J. S., H. L. Figge, H. X. Bui, A. D. del Rosario, H. A. G. Fisher, T. Nazeer, et al. 1994. E-cadherin expression in prostatic carcinoma biopsies: correlation with tumor grade, DNA content, pathologic stage and clinical outcome. *Mod. Pathol.* **7:** 833–841.

55. Rubinfeld, B., B. Souza, I. Albert, O. Muller, S. H. Chamberlain, F. R. Masiarz, et al. 1993. Association of APC gene product with beta-catenin. *Science* **262:** 1731–1734.

56. Sanchez-Madrid, F. and A. L. Corbi. 1992. Lekocyte integrins: structure, function and regulation of their activity. *Semin. Cell Biol.* **3:** 199–210.
57. Satoh, M., K. Numahata, S. Kawamura, S. Saito, and S. Orikasa. 1998. Lack of selectin-dependent adhesion in prostate cancer cells expressing sialyl Le(x). *Int. J. Urol.* **5:** 86–91.
58. Schwartz, M. A. 1993. Signaling by integrins: implications for tumorigenesis. *Cancer Res.* **53:** 1503–1506.
59. Soler, A. P., G. D. Harner, K. A. Knudson, F. X. McBreatry, E. Grujic, H. Salazar, et al. 1997. Expression of P-cadherin identifies prostate-specific-antigen-negative cells in epithelial tissues of male sexual accessory organs and in prostatic carcinomas. *Am. J. Pathol.* **151:** 471–478.
60. Sommers, C. L., E. P. Gelmann, R. Kemler, P. Cowin, and S. W. Byers. 1994. Alterations in beta-catenin phosphorylation and plakoglobin expression in human breast cancer cells. *Cancer Res.* **54:** 3544–3552.
61. Su, L. K., B. Vogelstein, and K. W. Kinzler. 1993. Association of the APC tumor suppressor protein with catenins. *Science* **262:** 1734–1737.
62. Suzuki, H., A. Komiya, M. Emi, H. Kuramochi, T. Shiraishi, R. Yatani, et al. 1996. Three distinct commonly deleted regions of chromosome arm 16q in human primary and metastatic prostate cancers. *Genes Chromosomes Cancer* **17:** 225–233.
63. Takeichi, M. 1991. Cadherin cell adhesion receptor as a morphogenetic regulator. *Science* **251:** 1451–1455.
64. Trikha, M., E. Raso, Y. Cai, Z. Fazakas, S. Paku, A. T. Porter, et al. 1998. Role of alphaII(b)beta3 integrin in prostate cancer metastasis. *Prostate* **35:** 185–192.
65. Tsukita, S., S. A. Tsukita, A. Nagafuchi, and S. Yonemura. 1992. Molecular linkage between cadherins and actin filaments in cell-cell adherens junction. *Curr. Opin. Cell Biol.* **4:** 834–839.
66. Umbas, R., J. A. Schalken, T. W. Aalders, B. S. Carter, H. F. Karthaus, H. E. Schaafsma, et al. 1992. Expression of the cellular adhesion molecule E-cadherin is reduced or absent in high-grade prostate cancer. *Cancer Res.* **52:** 5104–5109.
67. Umbas, R., W. B. Isaacs, D. P. Bringuier, H. E. Schaafsma, H. F. Karthaus, G. O. Oosterhof, et al. 1994. Decreased E-cadherin expression is associated with poor prognosis in patients with prostate cancer. *Cancer Res.* **54:** 3929–3933.
68. Verhagen, A. P. M., T. W. Aalders, F. C. S. Ramaekers, F. M. J. Debruyne, and J. A. Schalken. 1988. Differential expression of keratins in the basal and luminal compartments of rat prostatic epithelium during degeneration and regeneration. *Prostate* **13:** 25–38.
69. Weber, G. F., S. Ashkar, M. Glimcher, and H. Cantor. 1996. Receptor-ligand interaction between CD44 and osteopontin (Eta-1). *Science* **271:** 509–512.
70. Welsh, C. F., D. Zhu, and L. Y. Bourguignon. 1995. Interaction of CD44 variant isoforms with hyaluronic acid and the cytoskeleton in human prostate cancer cells. *J. Cell Physiol.* **164:** 605–612.

14

Ligand Dependent and Independent Activation of the Androgen Receptor

Gloria R. Mora, PhD, and Donald J. Tindall, PhD

1. INTRODUCTION

Androgens play a pivotal role in the embryonic development, growth, and function of many tissues within male species. The cells of these tissues are influenced by androgens through the binding and resultant conformational changes in the androgen receptor (AR). The importance of the role played by ARs in the life of androgen dependent tissues is evidenced in the genetic diseases that produce alterations in the AR, resulting in alterations in the male phenotype. Most of the available knowledge regarding the function of androgens and the role of AR has been obtained from studies of the prostate gland. These studies have elucidated the importance of androgens in the maintenance of homeostasis. The prostate provides a physiologic tissue model of AR action. The study of prostate cancer also provides a pathophysiologic model for the investigation of androgens and AR. Androgen ablation therapies in prostate cancer take advantage of the continued requirement of the androgen–AR relationship in the immortalized tumor cells. Unfortunately, these therapies often fail with time, and the disease progresses to an androgen refractory and/or androgen independent stage. Recent studies have begun to pull back the veil regarding the pathophysiology of these refractory cells and the role of AR in their growth.

Because of the frequent use in the scientific community of terms to define androgenic responses in prostate cells, we must begin by establishing our definitions. Normal prostate cells contain ARs and require androgens to survive. Therefore, these cells are defined as *androgen dependent*. Cancer cells, at least initially, also require androgens to survive. These cancer cells contain functional ARs, and therefore respond to hormonal ablation therapies. These cells are defined as *androgen sensitive*. The three terms *androgen refractory*, *androgen insensitive*, and *androgen independent* have been used to describe prostate cancer cells that no longer require androgens for their growth and/or survival. We define *androgen independent* cells as those cells that lack a functional AR because of genetic alterations, and no longer require androgens to survive. Consequently, these cells do not respond to hormonal ablation therapies. *Androgen refractory* cells are defined as those cells that contain functional AR, but do not require the presence of androgens for their proliferation. The role of AR in these androgen

From: *Prostate Cancer: Biology, Genetics, and the New Therapeutics*
Edited by: L. W. K. Chung, W. B. Isaacs, and J. W. Simons © Humana Press Inc., Totowa, NJ

refractory cells remains an open question, and the evidence for an active role by AR is only suggestive. Thus, while the classical function of the AR in androgen action has been very well explored and described by many investigators in the last 30 yr, an alternative role for AR in mediating nonandrogenic responses has only recently been recognized.

The literature addressing the theme of this chapter is extensive. An exhaustive review of the topic is unnecessary in this context, and interested readers should refer to the more extensive reviews available from this laboratory *(78,89)* and others *(7,21,69,121)*. The goal of this chapter is to provide a highlighted review of the current knowledge regarding the function of AR in the presence and absence of ligand. This chapter also addresses some of the unanswered questions regarding the role for AR in prostate cancer beyond its classical ligand dependent action.

2. LIGAND DEPENDENT ACTIVATION OF THE ANDROGEN RECEPTOR

2.1. Androgens and the Prostate

Testosterone and the adrenal androgens (which constitute only 5–10% of the circulating androgens) are shepherded through the systemic circulation by plasma-binding proteins *(118)*. The most important of these is sex hormone binding globulin (SHBG), which binds androgens with high affinity *(47)*. After release from the binding proteins, androgens diffuse freely across the plasma membranes of prostate cells *(84)*. Through enzymatic action, androgens are rapidly converted into the most potent metabolite 5α-DHT, which is the major androgen in the prostate of men *(127)*, dogs *(42)*, and rodents *(9)*. Two 5α-reductase isoenzymes, type 1 and type 2, have been characterized according to their tissue-specific expression and biochemical parameters *(122)*. The two 5α-reductase isoenzymes have a differential localization in prostate cells: Type 1 isoenzyme is expressed in the luminal secretory epithelial cells, while the Type 2 isoenzyme is expressed in the basal epithelial and stromal cells *(2)*. 5α-DHT is responsible for prostate-gland development, growth, and secretory activity *(85,140)*. A balance is reached between 5α-reductase and the androgen-inactivating enzymes (dehydrogenases and sulfotransferases), which convert testosterone and 5α-DHT into metabolites with low physiological activity *(45,131)*.

2.2. Androgen Receptor Structure

The steroid receptor superfamily of nuclear proteins includes, among others, receptors for steroids, thyroid hormones, vitamin D$_3$, *cis*- and *trans*-retinoic acid, ecdisone, and orphan receptors, whose physiological ligands are not yet known *(135)*. These proteins share a cognate structure, well characterized domains, and mode of action— i.e., binding to specific DNA sequences as ligand-receptor complexes to regulate the transcription of target genes. The A/B amino terminal domain, variable in length and sequence, contains specific transactivation regulatory amino acid sequences. This domain of approx 500 amino acids arises from exon 1 in the human AR gene *(77)* and is polymorphic in healthy individuals because of homopolymeric stretches of glutamine (12–31 residues, starting at amino acid -58) and glycine (approx 24 residues starting at amino acid -448). The biological function of these motifs is unclear; however, a longer stretch of glutamines results in lower AR transactivation *(13)*. Interestingly, data from the epidemiological Massachusetts Male Aging Study involving 882 men found that individuals with shorter CAG repeats have lower serum testosterone levels *(72)*. The authors found that testosterone levels decreased by 0.74% ± 0.36% for each CAG repeat decrement. Shorter CAG repeats have also been associated with an increased risk of developing prostate cancer *(41)*. Moreover, race may be a determinant of CAG length and prostate cancer risk, since there is an inverse relationship between the incidence of prostate cancer and CAG repeats in African-American, non-Latino whites, and Asians *(123)*. Deletion and mutational analyses of the amino terminal domain have demonstrated that this domain, by itself, has no transcriptional activity *(147)*. However, based on transient transfection assays, the amino terminal domain does contain specific sequences required for modulation of transcriptional activity. This is denoted as an activation function (AF) for the nuclear receptors. For AR, these sequences have been grouped into two separate units—AF1 and AF5. Whereas AF1 (amino acids 100–370) is active in the full-length, ligand-activated AR, AF5 (amino acids 360–385) has been shown to be constitutively active in deletion mutants that lack the ligand-binding domain *(58)*. The studies of Gordon et al. *(43)*, based on chimeric proteins of AR and glucocorticoid receptor (GR), have demonstrated a steroid specificity function for the amino terminal domain. Thus, this domain provides the selective responsiveness and recognition between these two steroids in cells which coexpress AR and GR.

The DNA binding, or C domain, is highly conserved in length and sequence (≈70 amino acids). It is located in the center of the molecule and contains nine conserved cysteines. Based on crystallographic and NMR data of GR *(48,49,93)* and estrogen receptors (ER) *(124)*, eight of the cysteine residues are coordinated tetrahedrically with zinc to form DNA binding structures that direct the interaction with the major groove at the hormone response elements (HREs). The AR, GR, mineralocorticoid receptor (MR), and progesterone receptor (PR) can be grouped together based on their sequence homology at the DNA binding domain, and the same imperfect palindrome acts as a DNA acceptor site *(46)*. The absence of a unique DNA sequence and the well conserved binding domain indicate that DNA binding specificity and defined steroid responsiveness is a complex mechanism involving additional steroid-specific factors. In this regard, the receptor accessory factor (RAF) has been identified as a ≈130 kDa protein that interacts directly with receptor-DNA binding complexes and enhances the binding to AREs of receptor fragments containing an intact DNA binding domain *(80)*. The interaction of RAF is specific with a GR fragment and a truncated rat and human AR (containing approx 100 amino acids from the amino terminal domain, the entire DNA binding domain and hinge region, and approx 50 amino acids from the carboxy terminal domain). This interaction does not occur with a PR fragment. In addition, a specific ARE sequence is required, since enhancement of binding has not been observed using an estrogen response element. It should be noted that RAF has been purified to near homogeneity and corresponds to insulin degrading enzyme (IDE) *(79)*. Insulin effectively competes with AR or GR for interaction with IDE, suggesting a potential interaction between the insulin and steroid signaling pathways.

The carboxy terminal domain is also conserved between members of the nuclear receptors. In addition to creating a hydrophobic pocket for ligand binding, the carboxy terminal domain contains sequences for binding heat-shock proteins (HSP), coregulatory proteins (denoted as AF-2), and also sequences involved in receptor dimerization *(57,94,147)*. While androgens bind to this region with high affinity, other ligands bind with a relatively lower affinity. The physiological implications are discussed in specific situations in the following sections. Ligand binding regulates the distribution of AR between cytoplasm and nucleus. Prior to cloning of the AR *(17,92)*, biochemical studies showed that unbound AR was mainly a cytoplasmic protein (probably because of the lower affinity of AR with the "nuclear acceptor" sites), and that the ligand induced a nuclear translocation. When antibodies became available, immunohistochemistry demonstrated that the AR remains in the nucleus regardless of the absence of ligand *(55,125)*. However, in the studies of Jenster et al. *(59)*, transient transfection of a full-length AR expression vector in the absence of androgen resulted in a cell line-specific distribution of the AR, and the ligand induced a nuclear localization regardless of the cell type. Thus, the in vivo intracellular localization in cells continuously exposed to androgens is more likely to be cytoplasmic only transiently after neosynthesis, and it might well be a cell-specific event dependent on more than just the presence of the ligand. The region required for nuclear import has been identified by deletion mutagenesis in two reports *(59,128)*. The sequences overlap and are localized in the hinge region between the DNA and hormone-binding domains.

A hormone-dependent molecular interaction between the domains at each end of the AR molecule has been described *(35,81,82)*. These findings, based on protein-protein interaction assays, have suggested an antiparallel orientation of AR-ligated dimers, since no interaction was observed between two steroid-binding domains at physiological concentration of androgens *(82)*. Two regions in the amino terminal domain responsible for this interaction have been identified, one near to the amino terminus and the other immediately adjacent to the DNA binding domain *(82)*. Val-889 and Arg-752 in the ligand-binding domain are also important *(81)*.

The AR, one of the largest proteins in the nuclear receptor superfamily, is encoded by a single gene located on a highly conserved region of the mammalian X chromosome at Xq11-12 *(8,129)*. The gene spans over 90 kb, and lacks TATA and CAAT sequences (134). Instead, it contains pur/pyr and GC box SP1-binding sites *(18)*, has eight exons to generate a mRNA of ≈10 kb, and has a protein of ≈917–919 amino acids with a predicted molecular wt of ≈99 kDa *(91)*. AR usually appears as a 110–112 doublet in denaturing gel electrophoresis. Interestingly, 2 yr before the cloning of the AR gene, chromatography assays had predicted an identical molecular wt for the monomeric subunit *(60)*. The expression of the AR mRNA is regulated by a number of factors, including hypermethylation of the AR gene promoter *(56)*, growth factor dependent pathways *(52)* and ligand concentration, a phenomenon known as autoregulation *(132)*. Autoregulation of the AR mRNA has been shown in several rat tissues *(11,100,132)*, LNCaP prostate cancer cells *(73)* and in T47D breast cancer cells *(73)*. This effect requires a functional AR *(114)*, and in LNCaP cells this downregulation is mediated through a decrease in transcription initiation *(141)*. Our unpublished data using a 6-kb fragment of the AR gene promoter has suggested that androgens do not downregulate the AR promotor activity through specific *cis*-acting element(s). Moreover, we have found that this effect is not active in androgen independent cells. These observations suggest that downregulation is cell-specific and is consistent with the upregulation of the AR mRNA in PC3 cells (prostate cancer cells that do not contain AR) transiently transfected with a recombinant AR *(27)*. The data also suggest that downregulation requires additional proteins (through a protein–protein dependent mechanism), which are present only in AR-positive cells, and agrees with a previous report *(71)*. In addition to androgens altering the AR mRNA levels, in most cases androgens increase or maintain the AR protein levels. Earlier data from castrated animals demonstrated the importance of the ligand in stabilizing the AR protein *(117)*. This concept has been extended to a ligand-induced decrease in the rate of receptor degradation *(67)* and a ligand dependent increase in translation *(99)*.

2.3. Androgens, Antiandrogens, and Alternative Ligands for the Androgen Receptor

Testosterone and 5α-DHT are the best known ligands for the AR. However, a number of related molecules can bind to the AR with various levels of affinity. When the binding affinity of a number of steroid molecules relative to 5α-DHT was measured in purified AR from rat prostate *(15)*, testosterone had a relative affinity of 84%, progesterone: 24%, 5α-androstane-3α, 17β-diol (or 3α-androstanediol, a 5α-DHT metabolite): 17%, 17β -estradiol: 7% and cortisol: 1%. Studies by Zhou et al. *(148)* have suggested that the lower relative binding affinity (or higher dissociation) of testosterone compared to 5α-DHT relates directly with AR protein stability. Their findings, using a transfected recombinant AR in monkey kidney COS-1 cells, showed that testosterone at physiological concentrations, within 0.1 and 5 nM, dissociates from AR three times faster than 5α-DHT, and that AR degradation was twice as fast when testosterone was the ligand. Therefore the prostate, in which the predominant androgen is 5α-DHT, has a stable AR protein and is more likely in a protected conformational structure. This is particularly true in the nucleus where the concentration of 5α-DHT can be as high as 250 nM *(10)*.

The development of synthetic ligands with either agonistic or antagonistic properties has further emphasized the importance of the ligand in the structure and activity of the AR. The synthetic androgen R1881 (methyltrienolone, 17β-hydroxy-17α-methylestra-4,9,11-trien-3-one) binds with high affinity to the AR (Kd: 1.5 nM) *(103)*. Mibolerone (7α,17α-dimethyl-17β-hydroxy-4-estren-3-one) also binds with high affinity (Kd: 2.3 nM); however, it is more chemically stable and circumvents the problem of R1881 binding to PR *(103)*. Of clinical interest has been the development of drugs that antagonize the action of androgens directly by competitively inhibiting their binding to the AR or indirectly by altering androgen synthesis, uptake, and metabolism. Two types of antiandrogens are currently used: steroidal and nonsteroidal. The steroidal cyproterone acetate (CPA) was the first antiandrogen used clinically. However, because of a variety of side effects related to its steroidal nature, such as progestational properties and the suppression of the gonadotrophin-releasing hormone, it has had limited use *(40)*. The nonsteroidal drugs flutamide, hydroxyflutamide (OHFLU), and nilutamide (anandron, RU 23908) act directly on androgen target tissues by inhibiting binding of androgens to AR. However, they also inhibit the negative feedback of androgens in the central nervous system, leading to an increase in LHRH secretion and ultimately a greater stimulus for further androgen secretion by the testis *(40)*. Thus, these agents usually require combined use with medical or surgical castration. Casodex (bicalutamide, ICI 176,334), a nonsteroidal antiandrogen, has no reported activity at the hypothalamic-pituitary-gonadal axis, and is currently in clinical trials in patients with both early and advanced prostate cancer *(70)*. All these compounds bind to the AR, although with a much lower affinity than that of natural or synthetic androgens (i.e, 0.1–0.4%, compared to 100% for R1881), and all, with the exception of casodex, have shown agonistic properties at high concentrations both in vitro *(144)* and in vivo *(130)*. Three new nonsteroidal antiandrogens (RU 56187, RU 57073, and RU 59063) that have high affinity for the AR have been described *(133)*. Their affinities are approximately three times that of testosterone, and effectively block the growth of androgen dependent tissues in rats. To date, there is no information regarding the clinical use of these new compounds.

Although synthetic or natural androgens and antiandrogens bind to the AR, the induced-conformational changes appear to be distinct *(62,74)*. This conclusion was drawn from limited proteolytic studies of AR complexed with different ligands in which a differential pattern of AR-digested fragments was observed. Complementing this conclusion of an alternative structure, Kemppainen et al. *(66)* have shown that although high-affinity androgens promote an interaction between the amino and carboxyl terminal domains at nanomolar concentrations, the antiandrogens CPA or OHFLU at concentrations up to 1 μM do not promote an interaction between these two domains. Likewise, in the same report, medroxy-progesterone, a weak androgen that binds the AR and promotes low androgenic effects in vivo does not promote an interaction between domains as do the high-affinity ligands.

The potential binding of other molecules to the AR, particularly C19 steroids from adrenal origin becomes important during the progression of prostate cancer, in which hormonal ablation therapies preserve the pituitary-adrenal axis *(116)*. In addition, mutations of the AR gene—as described in advanced prostate cancer—can give rise to AR proteins with altered structure and increase binding affinity to adrenal androgens and related molecules. An example of this possibility was shown by Culig et al. *(25)* in their identification of a mutant AR (Val 715→Met) from an androgen independent prostate tumor, which in cotransfection and transactivation experiments is activated by adrenal androgens and progesterone. Moreover, the AR Val 715 and the AR Met 730 (Val 730→Met) can both be activated by high concentrations of OHFLU *(109)* and can transactivate the PSA promoter in the presence of androgen metabolites *(26)*. Perhaps the most well-characterized mutant AR is the one present in LNCaP androgen sensitive prostate cancer cells. A single point mutation results in the substitution of threonine 868 by alanine and a promiscuous binding of progesterone, estradiol, and OHFLU *(136,137)*. Moreover, the increased binding affinity for OHFLU correlates with an increase in stability of the mutant AR *(65)*.

2.4. Androgen Receptor Activation

The theory that the AR needs to be activated in a ligand dependent manner before it can bind DNA and activate transcription of target genes has been extensively studied. From earlier work in AR purification and studies of the physicochemical properties of the receptor, it was obvious that the process of activation required additional factors.

The activation process was represented by the "transformation" of AR in two physically different forms—the 8-9S and the 4-5S. The 8-9S form binds androgen with high-affinity and DNA with low affinity. The 4-5S form represents the converse: a high DNA-binding-affinity form *(16,30)*. In the absence of ligand, AR remains in a functionally inactive state bound to chaperone HSP and other less well-characterized proteins *(38,94)*. Using antibodies against HSP90, it was shown that under nonactivating conditions HSP90 interacted with the 8-9S AR complex, while in a high salt buffer the AR in a 5S form was not bound to HSP90 *(94)*. Indeed, Fang et al. *(37)* using a yeast model that expressed the HSP90 protein because of the mutant temperature-sensitive gene *hsp82*, showed that HSP90 binds to AR and actively participates in maintaining the AR in a high-affinity binding state for the ligand, and loss of HSP90 function resulted in a lower ligand dependent transactivation. In contrast, other studies have shown no changes in hormone binding affinity regardless of the presence or the absence of HSP90 *(105)*.

Thus, upon ligand binding, the transformation process involves changes in the conformation of the receptor and the chaperone proteins, receptor dimerization, and binding of AR complexes to ARE to regulate the rate of transcription of androgen target genes. The administration of androgens to castrated rats, or to prostate cells grown in the absence of androgens, has revealed a number of androgen-regulated genes in the prostate gland. Among others, androgens upregulate the expression of the rat probasin *(64)*, the rat androgen-binding protein *(28)*, the prostate specific antigen (PSA) *(146)*, the human glandular kallikrein-1 (hKLL2) *(146)*, the cell cycle genes CDK2, CDK4, and CKIp16 *(90)*, and the homeobox gene NKX3.1 *(112)*. Androgens downregulate the expression of the early growth-response gene α *(4)*, the prostatic acid phosphatase *(51)* and the AR mRNA *(114)*. In CV1 cells (cotransfected with the rAR) androgens induce a negative regulation of a CAT reporter containing the promotor of the rat low-affinity neurotrophin receptor (p75) *(61)*. Interestingly, the downregulatory effect does not involve direct binding of the AR to *cis* elements in the p75 promoter, suggesting that negative regulation of transcription by androgens may not require direct interaction with DNA sequences, which is consistent with our unpublished observations of androgens downregulating the AR mRNA.

The AR is a phosphoprotein, as are all steroid receptors. With regard to the activation process, although ligand dependent phosphorylation might be involved, the AR has been shown to be both phosphorylated in an androgen dependent *(76)* and in an androgen independent manner *(75)*. Kuiper et al. *(75)* showed that in denaturing gels of total lysates of LNCaP cells prepared in the absence of androgens, the neosynthesized 110 kDa AR is rapidly converted into a phosphorylated 112 kDa protein. In isolated fractions, this phosphorylated receptor is found predominantly in the cytosol *(76)*. When these cells were exposed to R1881, the phosphorylated form in cytosol increased 1.8-fold, and a phosphorylated form in the nucleus could be detected *(76)*, even though no changes were observed in total AR protein. Moreover, the ratio of phosphate to AR was identical in the cytoplasmic and nuclear fractions, indicating that no net changes in receptor phosphorylation takes place during transformation. Recently, Wang et al. *(138)* found that 5α-DHT treatment of LNCaP cells results in an increase in the ratio of phosphorylated/dephosphorylated AR with only a moderate increase in total AR protein content (1.5-fold). This effect was mimicked (to a lesser extent) by other receptor agonists such as 17β estradiol and OHFLU, but not by antagonists such as casodex. The latter data suggest that changes in the phosphorylation ratio could be an index of agonistic vs antagonistic activity. Kempainnen et al. *(67)*, using a recombinant AR in COS cells, have also shown a phosphorylated form of AR in the absence of androgens. However, in contrast to the previous observations, R1881 induced a net increase in AR protein by three to fivefold (caused by enhanced AR half-life) and increased AR phosphorylation by two to fourfold. Thus, no net changes in the phosphorylation state of AR were observed when related to protein content. From these studies, the conclusion could be drawn that in the absence of ligand the receptor is phosphorylated, and—while dependent on the system (the mutant receptor in LNCaP cells vs the recombinant receptor in COS cells)—androgens alter AR protein stability and increase AR phosphorylation. However, androgens do not appear to cause a change in the phosphorylation state of the active nuclear AR protein. Nevertheless, the role of phosphorylation in relation to receptor activation is yet to be precisely determined, and it cannot be ruled out that androgens could cause a redistribution of the phosphorylation sites in the AR molecule during activation. Even so, phosphorylation appears to play an active role in AR transactivation, and may distinguish agonists from antagonists. From the potential phosphorylation sites, phosphorylation at serines at 650 *(147)*, 641 *(5)*, and 653 *(5)*, located in the hinge region, have been shown to be required for transcriptional activity of the human AR.

Research suggests that phosphorylation indirectly mediates AR transactivation. Cotreatment of androgens with activators of protein kinase A *(115)* and protein kinase C *(31)* synergize with the AR transcriptional activity. However, our laboratory has shown that forskolin (activator of protein kinase A) had no effect on the mibolerone-dependent AR transactivation of the PSA gene in LNCaP cells, whereas the 12-O-tetradecanoyl-phorbol-13-acetate phorbol ester (a PKC activator) repressed the transcription of PSA *(1)*. However, Block et al. *(5)* demonstrated that forskolin treatment of LNCaP cells results in a decrease in R1881-induced phosphorylation of AR at residues 641 and 653, and a less transcriptionally active AR. One of the possible explanations for the discrepancy on the forskolin effect is the different interval of time treatment (9 h vs 24 h) and the ligand employed in these experiments.

The androgen dependent transactivation (dependent or independent of phosphorylation) involves the regulation of and interaction with accessory proteins. Coregulatory proteins, by definition, do not bind to specific DNA sequences. They bind nuclear receptors, and are believed to act as adapters between the AF domains and the basal transcription machinery *(36)*. Although a number of coregulatory proteins have been identified, the AR appears to be unique because it seems to require AR-specific coactivators. Herein, we will emphasize the coregulatory molecules involved in modulation of AR transactivation (for information on coregulatory molecules involved in modulating other receptors, *see* refs. *36* and *126*). When Yeh and Chang *(142)* used a GAL4-AR fusion protein containing the AR carboxy terminal domain as a bait in a yeast-two hybrid screening system, the associated protein 70 (ARA$_{70}$), was identified and shown to interact with AR in a ligand dependent manner. This interaction resulted in an enhanced AR transactivation by 10-fold in the presence of 5α-DHT. This response was receptor specific, since ARA_{70} increased only by twofold the transcriptional activity of GR, PR and ER. ARA_{70} is ubiquitously expressed with the exception of the DU145 prostate cancer cell line, which does not express AR. In more recent studies, AR_{70} has been shown to interact in a ligand independent manner with the peroxisome proliferator-activated receptor γ (PPARγ), a member of the nuclear receptor family *(50)*. This receptor regulates the transcription of genes involved in lipid metabolism, and AR_{70} potentiates the transcriptional activity of PPARγ, which is enhanced by the ligand. Interestingly, when AR, PPARγ and AR_{70} are coexpressed in DU145 cells, AR significantly reduces the transcriptional activity of PPARγ, suggesting a potential interaction and competition between AR and PPARγ transcriptional signaling pathways. In addition, antiandrogens promote the interaction of AR_{70} to AR in a dose-dependent manner *(95)*, and the activation of AR target genes by OHFLU requires AR_{70} *(144)*, suggesting that the agonistic activity of antiandrogens may require the presence of AR_{70}. In subsequent studies, two other AR specific coactivators have been identified: ARA54 *(63)* and ARA55 *(39)*. ARA54 enhances the transcriptional activity of wild-type AR transfected in DU-145 cells as well as mutant ARs. In particular, ARA54 enhances the transactivation activity of the LNCaP mutant AR in the presence of estradiol or OHFLU, suggesting that coregulatory proteins such as ARA54 can mediate the promiscuous activation of mutant ARs. The retinoblastoma (Rb) tumor suppressor protein has been shown to interact with and increase the transcriptional activity of AR *(145)*. The physical interaction of AR and Rb is not androgen dependent, although androgens are required for the AR transactivation and the coactivation properties of Rb. AR_{70} can further enhance the effect of Rb and—while the interacting region for AR_{70} is located at the ligand-binding domain—Rb does not interact with this domain. The precise site of interaction of Rb within the amino terminal or DNA binding domain has not been described. A nuclear protein kinase termed ANPK (AR-interacting nuclear protein kinase) has been shown to interact with the zinc-finger region of the AR in an androgen dependent manner, and to increase AR transcriptional activity *(97)*. Interestingly, a testis-specific coregulatory protein for AR termed ARIP3 (AR interacting protein 3) also associates with the zinc-finger region of the AR and modulates its transcriptional activity *(98)*. ARIP3 has also been shown to facilitate the androgen dependent interaction between the two ends of the AR molecule *(98)*.

In searching for coregulatory proteins that interact with the AF1 domain at the amino terminal domain of steroid receptors (SR), Lanz et al. *(83)* have identified the SR RNA activator (SRA). This novel coactivator acts as an RNA transcript to enhance the ligand dependent transcriptional activity of AR, PR, ER, PPARγ, thyroid receptor, and retinoic acid receptor. Further characterization, based on gel-filtration chromatography and immunoprecipitation, have defined SRA as a ribonucleoprotein complex with SR coactivator 1 (SRC-1), an extensively characterized general coactivator for SR that binds poorly to AR *(34)*. Interestingly, with the advent and application of sophisticated molecular biology techniques, the original hypothesis suggesting that SR associate with RNA or ribonucleoproteins proposed by several laboratories *(53,107,120)* in the 1980s has developed into a theory with supportive data. Another recently described AR coactivator is Ubc9, an enzyme shown to covalently link the ubiquitin-like protein SUMO-1 (small ubiquitin-related modifier) to target proteins *(32)*. SUMO-1 conjugation is involved in targeting of proteins to or within the nucleus. In COS cells transiently transfected with a recombinant AR, Ubc9 increases its transcriptional activity in an androgen dependent manner *(111)*. Participating amino acid residues lie within the nuclear localization signal (residues: 629–633). Mutations that abrogate the ability of Ubc9 to transfer SUMO-1 do not affect its AR coactivating ability, suggesting that androgen dependent coactivation of AR by Ubc9 does not involve a SUMO-1-AR interaction. In addition, AR has been shown to increase its transcriptional activity through a ligand dependent interaction with the transcription intermediary factor 2 (TIF-2) *(3)*, the small nuclear RING finger protein (SNURF) *(96)*, and the Tat interacting protein 60 (Tip60) *(6)*.

The second group of coregulatory molecules for SR involves the corepressors. These proteins, although less studied than those participating in transcriptional activation, are critical to SR action and regulation of transcription. Cyclin D1, a regulatory molecule of cyclin dependent kinase 4 and 6, is a ligand dependent activator of the ER *(106)*, and has been shown to interact directly with the AR in a ligand dependent manner to decrease its transcriptional activity *(68)*. This physical interaction is specific for cyclin D1, since cyclin E or A are ineffective, and cyclin D3 is less able to repress AR transactivation. The effect of cyclin D1 is independent of its cell-cycle regulatory function *(68)*.

3. LIGAND INDEPENDENT ACTIVATION OF THE ANDROGEN RECEPTOR

A subject of current interest, particularly in the development of androgen refractory prostate cancer, is the androgen independent activation of AR. For example, the recurrent refractory CWR22 prostatic-tumor xenograft expresses a number of well-known AR target genes, such as PSA, hK2, and Nkx3.1 *(44)*. Studies suggest that ligand independent pathways in refractory cells maintain the AR transcriptional activity, and/ or AR target genes are activated in an AR independent manner. The discussion in Section 3. indicates that AR may be active in regulating the transcription of these genes in refractory cells. This related work is reviewed according to the molecule and/or pathway involved.

3.1. The IL-6 and Her-2/Neu Tyrosine Kinase Pathways

HER-2/neu (*erb*B2) is a member of the epidermal growth factor (EGF) tyrosine kinase receptor family *(12)*. HER-2/neu levels are higher in androgen independent sublines derived from the LAPC-4 xenograft than to the androgen dependent lines *(20)*. Craft et al. *(20)* showed that stable transfection of HER-2/neu in LNCaP cells produces an androgen refractory phenotype and an increase in the tumor formation rate when inoculated in a castrated host. HER-2/neu also caused an increase in PSA synthesis and secretion, and acted synergistically with androgens to increase AR activity. Furthermore, Yeh et al. *(143)* have revealed that HER-2/neu can enhance by threefold the androgen independent AR transactivation of a PSA-CAT reporter when cotransfected with AR and AR_{70} in DU-145 cells. This effect was synergized by very low levels of androgens (10^{-10}-10^{-11} 5α-DHT), and was not abolished by OHFLU. The specific

MAPKK inhibitor PD98059 inhibited the Her-2/neu-induced AR transactivation, suggesting that the MAP signaling transduction pathway may also be involved. Notably, most hormonal ablation therapies do not diminish serum androgen levels to zero. In the report by Qiu et al. *(113)* IL-6 has been identified as an upstream activator of Her-2/neu. In the latter report, IL-6 treatments on the androgen sensitive LNCaP cells, the androgen independent DU-145 cells, and the androgen refractory CWR22 cells, cultured in serum-free medium, causes the activation of HER-2/neu by inducing the formation of a complex between HER-2/neu and the tyrosine phosphorylated IL-6 receptor subunit gp130. This association induces the intrinsic Her-2/neu tyrosine activity and subsequent MAPK activation, an effect associated with cell proliferation.

LNCaP and the androgen independent DU-145 and PC3 cells have been shown to express IL-6 receptor, while only the androgen independent cells secrete IL-6 *(108)*. In addition, Il-6 decreases the growth of LNCaP cells, an effect associated with a G1 arrest *(102)*. IL-6 has no effect on growth of androgen independent cells. However, when cells were incubated with an IL-6 neutralizing antibody, only the growth of androgen independent cells was affected *(19,108)*. These data indicate that growth of androgen sensitive cells is regulated by exogenous IL-6, perhaps from stromal cells, while the growth of independent cells correlates directly to their own synthesis and secretion of IL-6. Therefore, as suggested previously *(108)*, IL-6 acts as a paracrine growth factor in sensitive cells and as an autocrine growth factor in independent cells.

Hobisch et al. *(54)* have shown that IL-6 increases, in a ligand independent manner, the AR transactivation in DU-145 cells cotransfected with AR and an ARE_2CAT reporter. A synergistic effect was observed in cotreatments of IL-6 with low concentration of androgen (10 pM)—an effect that is AR-mediated, as casodex inhibited the response. The inhibitors of PK-A, PK-C and MAPKK also eliminated the effect of IL-6, suggesting that these three pathways are involved in the IL-6-induced AR transactivation. When LNCaP cells (cultured with 10 p*M* R1881 or without androgens) were treated with IL-6, the synthesis and secretion of PSA increased *(54)*, with a concomitant increase in AR protein levels *(88)*. Likewise, stably transfection of Her-2/neu in LNCaP cells increased their proliferation rate, as well as the synthesis and secretion of PSA without an increase in AR protein levels *(143)*. The AR mediates the response of IL-6, as casodex was inhibitory in combination with 10 p*M* R1881 *(143)*.

From the data presented here, it appears that IL-6 and Her-2/neu may be involved in activating AR in a ligand independent manner. A simplistic cascade of events would include activation of IL-6 receptor (this effect could be autocrine and/or paracrine), which in turn activates Her-2/neu tyrosine phosphorylation and precipitates a cascade of events involving PKA, PKC, and MAPK pathways that eventually cause phosphorylation of AR and/or coregulatory proteins—or formation of AR coactivator complexes, involved in ligand independent transactivation of AR target genes such as PSA.

3.2. Luteinizing Hormone Releasing Hormone

Luteinizing Hormone Releasing Hormone (LHRH) is a hypothalamic decapeptide essential for the synthesis and release of pituitary gonadotropins. LHRH agonists have been used primarily in hormonal ablation therapies to induce chemical castration by downregulation of the pituitary-testicular axis. Evidence of a local synthesis of LHRH-like peptides and the expression of LHRH binding sites in peripheral tissues suggest paracrine and autocrine effects. LNCaP cells synthesize LHRH and express LHRH receptors, and LHRH agonists have been shown to inhibit their proliferation *(86)*. Androgen sensitive LNCaP cells are characterized by a slower growth rate when cultured in a steroid-free medium. Under these conditions, LHRH antagonists increase cell proliferation, suggesting that LHRH plays an inhibitory role *(87)*. The inhibitory growth effect has also been observed in DU145 cells, where LHRH agonists reduce the effect of EGF-dependent phosphorylation of the EGF receptor *(101)*.

The role of LHRH in modulating AR activity has been suggested by experiments where LHRH increased the AR transactivation in DU-145 cells transiently transfected with AR, in a ligand independent manner *(22)*. In this study, LHRH together with a low concentration of androgens synergizes the AR transcriptional activity. The signal transduction events of LHRH involve the generation of the second messenger cAMP. When db cAMP was used in these experiments, it mimicked the LHRH response. Interestingly, in LNCaP cells, db cAMP—but not LHRH analogs—synergize with low concentration of androgens to increase PSA secretion *(22)*, suggesting that direct receptor activation in these cells is not required.

3.3. Sex Hormone Binding Globulin

As described previously, SHBG is the carrier of sex steroid hormones. However, additional evidence suggests that SHBG is more than just a passive carrier *(110)*. SHBG receptors (SHBGR) have been identified in androgen target cells. In LNCaP cells, SHBG binds to SHBGR and subsequently induces cAMP synthesis *(118)*. The concept of certain steroids binding SHBG and altering intracellular pathways without entering the cells has been well-documented and presented in the review by Rosner et al. *(119)*.

While there is no direct evidence of SHBG effecting androgen refractory cells, the findings of Ding et al. *(33)* are quite provocative. Using the prostate of dogs castrated for 7 d, it was demonstrated that estradiol and 3-α diol (the 5α-DHT metabolite) required the formation of the SHBG ligand receptor complex to increase the synthesis of cAMP and of prostate arginine esterase (AE), the canine equivalent of PSA *(33)*. This effect was blocked by OHFLU, suggesting that unligated AR is involved in activating AE synthesis.

3.4. Growth Factors

The importance of growth factors in prostate cancer became evident with the study of Chan et al. *(14)*, in which serum levels of the insulin growth factor 1 (IGF-1) directly correlated with the risk of prostate cancer. Most growth factors and their receptors are found in the prostate *(23,139)*. Moreover, IGF-1 has been shown to be a strong activator of AR transcriptional activity in DU-145 cells *(24)*. In addition, IGF-1 stimulates the secretion of PSA in LNCaP cells cultured in serum-free medium *(24)*. Casodex eliminates the effects of IGF-1 on AR transactivation and PSA secretion, thus demonstrating that these responses are AR-mediated.

3.5. PKA and PKC Pathways

The data presented here indicate that the involvement of the PKA signaling pathway in ligand independent activation of AR is incontrovertible. Moreover, forskolin increases the AR transactivation in CV-1 cells transiently transfected with a recombinant AR in a ligand independent manner *(104)*. This ligand independent effect was 73% of that caused by the synthetic androgen R1881, and was blocked both by a specific PKA inhibitor and antiandrogens. The total AR levels were not altered by forskolin treatment, and only a small increase was evident in the nuclear levels.

The human breast cancer T47D cell line does contain AR, although to a lesser extent than in prostate cells. Phorbol ester (a PKC activator) in the absence of androgens is capable of increasing the transcriptional activity of a recombinant AR in T47D cells *(29)*. However, db cAMP does not activate unbound AR, indicating that PKA is not involved in the ligand independent activation of AR in T47D cells. These studies indicate that the host cell may direct the preferential pathway of ligand independent activation of AR, and more likely, in prostate cells both PKA and PKC pathways are involved.

4. CONCLUSION

Progression from hormone sensitive to hormone refractory tumors often occurs following hormonal ablation therapy. Within these defiant tumors, a clone of cells develops that propagates in the absence of testicular androgens, although they contain AR and express AR dependent genes, such as PSA. The hypothesis that the AR itself mediates the progression to a refractory state raises several pertinent questions. What is the stimulus (or the stimuli) inducing this change? Do genetic alterations take place in AR? More evidence suggests that AR remains as the wild-type receptor, since AR mutations represent the minority of tumors and the frequency of mutations in prostate cancer is low. Therefore, if this is a wild-type receptor, how is it able to resist the absence of androgens, considering that the stability of this protein has been widely demonstrated to be dependent on the ligand? What type of AR is present in refractory cells? Is there a more resistant receptor that can be promiscuously activated by other molecules beyond its natural ligand, and does this promiscuous resistant AR define resistant disease?

To answer these questions, additional research is needed and crucial experiments are required. Such experiments must include the inactivation of AR in refractory cells. Would these cells maintain their hardy refractory phenotype, or would they progressively die? If the latter were the case, we would surmise that AR is crucial to maintain the refractory phenotype. The biochemical characteristics of AR in refractory cells also need to be described. Is this receptor a more resilient version with a longer half-life and a different conformational structure? Many questions remain unanswered.

The clinical relevance of ligand independent activation of the AR is just beginning to be acknowledged. Clinicians were initially cautious when the agonistic properties of antiandrogens were discovered, prompting the development of more potent antiandrogens. The discovery that adrenal androgens activate AR has motivated the pursuit of alternative hormonal manipulations to block this source of androgens to prostate cancer cells. Perhaps blocking AR in refractory cells will be the gene therapy strategy for refractory prostate cancer for the 21st century and beyond.

REFERENCES

1. Andrews, P. E., C. Y. Young, B. T. Montgomery, and D. J. Tindall. 1992. Tumor-promoting phorbol ester down-regulates the androgen induction of prostate-specific antigen in a human prostatic adenocarcinoma cell line. *Cancer Res.* **52:** 1525–1529.
2. Berman, D. M. and D. W. Russell. 1993. Cell-type-specific expression of rat steroid 5 alpha-reductase isozymes. *Proc. Natl. Acad. Sci. USA* **90:** 9359–9363.
3. Berrevoets, C. A., P. Doesburg, K. Steketee, J. Trapman, and A. O. Brinkmann. 1998. Functional interactions of the AF-2 activation domain core region of the human androgen receptor with the amino-terminal domain and with the transcriptional coactivator TIF2 (transcriptional intermediary factor2). *Mol. Endocrinol.* **12:** 1172–1183.
4. Blok, L. J., M. E. Grossmann, J. E. Perry, and D. J. Tindall. 1995. Characterization of an early growth response gene, which encodes a zinc finger transcription factor, potentially involved in cell cycle regulation. *Mol. Endocrinol.* **9:** 1610–1620.
5. Blok, L. J., P. E. de Ruiter, and A. O. Brinkmann. 1998. Forskolin-induced dephosphorylation of the androgen receptor impairs ligand binding. *Biochemistry* **37:** 3850–3857.
6. Brady, M. E., D. M. Ozanne, L. Gaughan, I. Waite, S. Cook, D. E. Neal, et al. 1999. Tip60 is a nuclear hormone receptor coactivator. *J. Biol. Chem.* **274:** 17,599–17,604.
7. Brinkmann, A. O., L. J. Blok, P. E. de Ruiter, P. Doesburg, K. Steketee, C. A. Berrevoets, et al. 1999. Mechanisms of androgen receptor activation and function. *J. Steroid Biochem. Mol. Biol.* **69:** 307–313.
8. Brown, C. J., S. J. Goss, D. B. Lubahn, D. R. Joseph, E. M. Wilson, F. S. French, et al. 1989. Androgen receptor locus on the human X chromosome: regional localization to Xq11–12 and description of a DNA polymorphism. *Am. J. Hum. Genet.* **44:** 264–269.
9. Bruchovsky, N. and J. D. Wilson 1968. The conversion of testosterone to 5-alpha-androstan-17-beta-ol-3-one by rat prostate in vivo and in vitro. *J. Biol. Chem.* **243:** 2012–2021.
10. Bruchovsky, N., P. S. Rennie, and A. Vanson. 1975. Studies on the regulation of the concentration of androgens and androgen receptors in nuclei of prostatic cells. *Biochim. Biophys. Acta* **394:** 248–266.
11. Burgess, L. H. and R. J. Handa. 1993. Hormonal regulation of androgen receptor mRNA in the brain and anterior pituitary gland of the male rat. *Mol. Brain Res.* **19:** 31–38.
12. Carraway, K. L. 3rd and S. J. Burden. 1995. Neuregulins and their receptors. *Curr. Opinion Neurobiol.* **5:** 606–612.
13. Chamberlain, N. L., E. D. Driver, and R. L. Miesfeld. 1994. The length and location of CAG trinucleotide repeats in the androgen receptor N-terminal domain affect transactivation function. *Nucleic Acids Res.* **22:** 3181–3186.
14. Chan, J. M., M. J. Stampfer, E. Giovannucci, P. H. Gann, J. Ma, P. Wilkinson, et al. 1998. Plasma insulin-like growth factor-I and prostate cancer risk: a prospective study. *Science* **279:** 563–566.
15. Chang, C. H., D. R. Rowley, and D. J. Tindall. 1983. Purification and characterization of the androgen receptor from rat ventral prostate. *Biochemistry* **22:** 6170–6175.
16. Chang, C. H., D. R. Rowley, T. J. Lobl, and D. J. Tindall. 1982. Purification and characterization of androgen receptor from steer seminal vesicle. *Biochemistry* **21:** 4102–4109.
17. Chang, C. S., J. Kokontis, and S. T. Liao. 1988. Molecular cloning of human and rat complementary DNA encoding androgen receptors. *Science* **240:** 324–326.
18. Chen, S., P. C. Supakar, R. L. Vellanoweth, C. S. Song, B. Chatterjee, and A. K. Roy. 1997. Functional role of a conformationally flexible homopurine/homopyrimidine domain

of the androgen receptor gene promoter interacting with Sp1 and a pyrimidine single strand DNA-binding protein. *Mol. Endocrinol.* **11:** 3–15.

19. Chung, T. D., J. J. Yu, M. T. Spiotto, M. Bartkowski, and J. W. Simons. 1999. Characterization of the role of IL-6 in the progression of prostate cancer. *Prostate* **38:** 199–207.

20. Craft, N., Y. Shostak, M. Carey, and C. L. Sawyers. 1999. A mechanism for hormone-independent prostate cancer through modulation of androgen receptor signaling by the HER-2/neu tyrosine kinase. *Nat. Med.* **5:** 280–285.

21. Cude, K. J., S. C. Dixon, Y. Guo, J. Lisella, and W. D. Figg. 1999. The androgen receptor: genetic considerations in the development and treatment of prostate cancer. *J. Mol. Med.* **77:** 419–426.

22. Culig, Z., A. Hobisch, A. Hittmair, M. V. Cronauer, C. Radmayr, J. Zhang, et al. 1997. Synergistic activation of androgen receptor by androgen and luteinizing hormone-releasing hormone in prostatic carcinoma cells. *Prostate* **32:** 106–114.

23. Culig, Z., A. Hobisch, M. V. Cronauer, C. Radmayr, A. Hittmair, J. Zhang, et al. 1996. Regulation of prostatic growth and function by peptide growth factors. *Prostate* **28:** 392–405.

24. Culig, Z., A. Hobisch, M. V. Cronauer, C. Radmayr, J. Trapman, A. Hittmair, et al. 1994. Androgen receptor activation in prostatic tumor cell lines by insulin-like growth factor-I, keratinocyte growth factor, and epidermal growth factor. *Cancer Res.* **54:** 5474–5478.

25. Culig, Z., A. Hobisch, M. V. Cronauer, A. C. Cato, A. Hittmair, C. Radmayr, et al. 1993. Mutant androgen receptor detected in an advanced-stage prostatic carcinoma is activated by adrenal androgens and progesterone. *Mol. Endocrinol.* **7:** 1541–1550.

26. Culig, Z., J. Stober, A. Gast, H. Peterziel, A. Hobisch, C. Radmayr, et al. 1996. Activation of two mutant androgen receptors from human prostatic carcinoma by adrenal androgens and metabolic derivatives of testosterone. *Cancer Detect. Prev.* **20:** 68–75.

27. Dai, J. L. and K. L. Burnstein. 1996. Two androgen response elements in the androgen receptor coding region are required for cell-specific up-regulation of receptor messenger RNA. *Mol. Endocrinol.* **10:** 1582–1594.

28. Danzo, B. J., S. N. Pavlou, and H. L. Anthony. 1990. Hormonal regulation of androgen-binding protein in the rat. *Endocrinology* **127:** 2829–2838.

29. Darne, C., G. Veyssiere, and C. Jean. 1998. Phorbol ester causes ligand independent activation of the androgen receptor. *Eur. J. Biochem.* **256:** 541–549.

30. de Boer, W., M. Lindh, J. Bolt, A. Brinkmann, and E. Mulder. 1986. Characterization of the calf uterine androgen receptor and its activation to the deoxyribonucleic acid-binding state. *Endocrinology* **118:** 851–861.

31. de Ruiter, P. E., R. Teuwen, J. Trapman, R. Dijkema, and A. O. Brinkmann. 1995. Synergism between androgens and protein kinase-C on androgen-regulated gene expression. *Mol. Cell. Endocrinol.* **110:** R1–6.

32. Desterro, J. M., J. Thomson, and R. T. Hay. 1997. Ubch9 conjugates SUMO but not ubiquitin. *FEBS Lett.* **417:** 297–300.

33. Ding, V. D., D. E. Moller, W. P. Feeney, V. Didolkar, A. M. Nakhla, L. Rhodes, et al. 1998. Sex hormone-binding globulin mediates prostate androgen receptor action via a novel signaling pathway. *Endocrinology* **139:** 213–218.

34. Ding, X. F., C. M. Anderson, H. Ma, H. Hong, R. M. Uht, P. J. Kushner, et al. 1998. Nuclear receptor-binding sites of coactivators glucocorticoid receptor interacting protein 1 (GRIP1) and steroid receptor coactivator 1 (SRC-1): multiple motifs with different binding specificities. *Mol. Endocrinol.* **12:** 302–313.

35. Doesburg, P., C. W. Kuil, C. A. Berrevoets, K. Steketee, P. W. Faber, E. Mulder, et al. 1997. Functional in vivo interaction between the amino-terminal, transactivation domain and the ligand binding domain of the androgen receptor. *Biochemistry* **36:** 1052–1064.

36. Edwards, D. P. 1999. Coregulatory proteins in nuclear hormone receptor action. *Vitam. Horm.* **55:** 165–218.

37. Fang, Y., A. E. Fliss, D. M. Robins, and A. J. Caplan. 1996. Hsp90 regulates androgen receptor hormone binding affinity in vivo. *J. Biol. Chem.* **271:** 28,697–28,702.
38. Froesch, B. A., S. Takayama, and J. C. Reed. 1998. BAG-1L protein enhances androgen receptor function. *J. Biol. Chem.* **273:** 11,660–11,666.
39. Fujimoto, N., S. Yeh, H. Y. Kang, S. Inui, H. C. Chang, A. Mizokami, et al. 1999. Cloning and characterization of androgen receptor coactivator, ARA55, in human prostate. *J. Biol. Chem.* **274:** 8316–8321.
40. Furr, B. J. 1995. Casodex: preclinical studies and controversies. *Ann. NY Acad. Sci.* **761:** 79–96.
41. Giovannucci, E., M. J. Stampfer, K. Krithivas, M. Brown, D. Dahl, A. Brufsky, et al. 1997. The CAG repeat within the androgen receptor gene and its relationship to prostate cancer. *Proc. Natl. Acad. Sci. USA* **94:** 3320–3323 (published erratum appears in *Proc. Natl. Acad. Sci. USA* **94:** 8272, 1997).
42. Gloyna, R. E., P. K. Siiteri, and J. D. Wilson. 1970. Dihydrotestosterone in prostatic hypertrophy. II. The formation and content of dihydrotestosterone in the hypertrophic canine prostate and the effect of dihydrotestosterone on prostate growth in the dog. *J. Clin. Investig.* **49:** 1746–1753.
43. Gordon, D. A., N. L. Chamberlain, F. A. Flomerfelt, and R. L. Miesfeld. 1995. A cell-specific and selective effect on transactivation by the androgen receptor. *Exp. Cell Res.* **217:** 368–377.
44. Gregory, C. W., K. G. Hamil, D. Kim, S. H. Hall, T. G. Pretlow, J. L. Mohler, et al. 1998. Androgen receptor expression in androgen independent prostate cancer is associated with increased expression of androgen-regulated genes. *Cancer Res.* **58:** 5718–5724.
45. Gurpide, E. 1978. Enzymatic modulation of hormonal action at the target tissue. *J. Toxicol. Envir. Health* **4:** 249–268.
46. Ham, J., A. Thomson, M. Needham, P. Webb, and M. Parker. 1988. Characterization of response elements for androgens, glucocorticoids and progestins in mouse mammary tumour virus. *Nucleic Acids Res.* **16:** 5263–5276.
47. Hammond, G. L. 1990. Molecular properties of corticosteroid binding globulin and the sex-steroid binding proteins. *Endocr. Rev.* **11:** 65–79.
48. Hard, T., E. Kellenbach, R. Boelens, B. A. Maler, K. Dahlman, L. P. Freedman, et al. 1990. Solution structure of the glucocorticoid receptor DNA-binding domain. *Science* **249:** 157–160.
49. Hard, T., E. Kellenbach, R. Boelens, R. Kaptein, K. Dahlman, J. Carlstedt-Duke, et al. 1990. 1H NMR studies of the glucocorticoid receptor DNA-binding domain: sequential assignments and identification of secondary structure elements. *Biochemistry* **29:** 9015–9023.
50. Heinlein, C. A., H. Ting, S. Yeh, and C. Chang. 1999. Identification of ARA70 as a ligand-enhanced coactivator for the peroxisome proliferator-activated receptor. *J. Biol. Chem.* **274:** 16,147–16,152.
51. Henttu, P. and P. Vihko. 1992. Steroids inversely affect the biosynthesis and secretion of human prostatic acid phosphatase and prostate-specific antigen in the LNCaP cell line. *J. Steroid Biochem. Mol. Biol.* **41:** 349–360.
52. Henttu, P. and P. Vihko. 1993. Growth factor regulation of gene expression in the human prostatic carcinoma cell line LNCaP. *Cancer Res.* **53:** 1051–1058.
53. Hiipakka, R. A. and S. Liao. 1988. Steroid receptor recycling and interaction of receptor with RNA. *Am. J. Clin. Oncol.* **11(Suppl. 2):** S18–22.
54. Hobisch, A., I. E. Eder, T. Putz, W. Horninger, G. Bartsch, H. Klocker, et al. 1998. Interleukin-6 regulates prostate-specific protein expression in prostate carcinoma cells by activation of the androgen receptor. *Cancer Res.* **58:** 4640–4645.
55. Husmann, D. A., C. M. Wilson, M. J. McPhaul, W. D. Tilley, and J. D. Wilson. 1990. Antipeptide antibodies to two distinct regions of the androgen receptor localize the recep-

tor protein to the nuclei of target cells in the rat and human prostate. *Endocrinology* **126:** 2359–2368.

56. Izbicka, E., J. R. Macdonald, K. Davidson, R. A. Lawrence, L. Gomez, and D. D. Hoff. 1999. 5,6 Dihydro-5′-azacytidine (DHAC) restores androgen responsiveness in androgen-insensitive prostate cancer cells. *Anticancer Res.* **19:** 1285–1292.

57. Jenster, G., H. A. van der Korput, C. van Vroonhoven, T. H. van der Kwast, J. Trapman, and A. O. Brinkmann. 1991. Domains of the human androgen receptor involved in steroid binding, transcriptional activation, and subcellular localization. *Mol. Endocrinol.* **5:** 1396–1404.

58. Jenster, G., H. A. van der Korput, J. Trapman, and A. O. Brinkmann. 1995. Identification of two transcriptional activation units in the N-terminal domain of the human androgen receptor. *J. Biol. Chem.* **270:** 7341–7346.

59. Jenster, G., J. Trapman, and A. O. Brinkmann. 1993. Nuclear import of the human androgen receptor. *Biochem. J.* **293:** 761–768.

60. Johnson, M. P., C. Y. Young, D. R. Rowley, and D. J. Tindall. 1987. A common molecular weight of the androgen receptor monomer in different target tissues. *Biochemistry* **26:** 3174–3182.

61. Kallio, P. J., H. Poukka, A. Moilanen, O. A. Janne, and J. J. Palvimo. 1995. Androgen receptor-mediated transcriptional regulation in the absence of direct interaction with a specific DNA element. *Mol. Endocrinol.* **9:** 1017–1028.

62. Kallio, P. J., O. A. Janne, and J. J. Palvimo. 1994. Agonists, but not antagonists, alter the conformation of the hormone-binding domain of androgen receptor. *Endocrinology* **134:** 998–1001.

63. Kang, H. Y., S. Yeh, N. Fujimoto, and C. Chang. 1999. Cloning and characterization of human prostate coactivator ARA54, a novel protein that associates with the androgen receptor. *J. Biol. Chem.* **274:** 8570–8576.

64. Kasper, S., P. S. Rennie, N. Bruchovsky, P. C. Sheppard, H. Cheng, L. Lin, et al. 1994. Cooperative binding of androgen receptors to two DNA sequences is required for androgen induction of the probasin gene. *J. Biol. Chem.* **269:** 31,763–31,769.

65. Kemppainen, J. A. and E. M. Wilson. 1996. Agonist and antagonist activities of hydroxyflutamide and Casodex relate to androgen receptor stabilization. *Urology* **48:** 157–163.

66. Kemppainen, J. A., E. Langley, C. I. Wong, K. Bobseine, W. R. Kelce, and E. M. Wilson. 1999. Distinguishing androgen receptor agonists and antagonists: distinct mechanisms of activation by medroxyprogesterone acetate and dihydrotestosterone. *Mol. Endocrinol.* **13:** 440–454.

67. Kemppainen, J. A., M. V. Lane, M. Sar, and E. M. Wilson. 1992. Androgen receptor phosphorylation, turnover, nuclear transport, and transcriptional activation. Specificity for steroids and antihormones. *J. Biol. Chem.* **267:** 968–974.

68. Knudsen, K. E., W. K. Cavenee, and K. C. Arden. 1999. D-Type cyclins complex with the androgen receptor and inhibit its transcriptional transactivation ability. *Cancer Res.* **59:** 2297–2301.

69. Kokontis, J. M. and S. Liao. 1999. Molecular action of androgen in the normal and neoplastic prostate. *Vitam. Horm.* **55:** 219–307.

70. Kolvenbag, G. J., G. R. Blackledge, and K. Gotting-Smith. 1998. Bicalutamide (Casodex) in the treatment of prostate cancer: history of clinical development. *Prostate* **34:** 61–72.

71. Kopp, H., J. R. W. Masters, W. Wieland, F. Hofstaedter, and R. Buettner. 1993. Differentielle Regulation des Androgenrezeptor-Promoters in hormonsensitiven und-resistenten Prostatakarzinomzellen. [Differential regulation of androgen receptor promoter in hormone-sensitive and -insensitive prostate carcinoma cells]. [German] *Verhandlungen der Deutschen Gesellschaft fur Pathologie* **77:** 129–132.

72. Krithivas, K., S. M. Yurgalevitch, B. A. Mohr, C. J. Wilcox, S. J. Batter, M. Brown, et al. 1999. Evidence that the CAG repeat in the androgen receptor gene is associated with the age-related decline in serum androgen levels in men. *J. Endocrinol.* **162:** 137–142.

73. Krongrad, A.., C. M. Wilson, J. D. Wilson, D. R. Allman, and M. J. McPhaul. 1991. Androgen increases androgen receptor protein while decreasing receptor mRNA in LNCaP cells. *Mol. Cellular Endocrinol.* **76:** 79–88.

74. Kuil, C. W. and E. Mulder. 1994. Mechanism of antiandrogen action: conformational changes of the receptor. *Mol. Cell. Endocrinol.* **102:** R1–5.

75. Kuiper, G. G., P. E. de Ruiter, and A. O. Brinkmann. 1992. Androgen receptor heterogeneity in LNCaP cells is caused by a hormone independent phosphorylation step. *J. Steroid Biochem. Mol. Biol.* **41:** 697–700.

76. Kuiper, G. G., P. E. de Ruiter, J. Trapman, W. J. Boersma, J. A. Grootegoed, and A. O. Brinkmann. 1993. Localization and hormonal stimulation of phosphorylation sites in the LNCaP-cell androgen receptor. *Biochem. J.* **291:** 95–101.

77. Kuiper, G. G., P. W. Faber, H. C. van Rooij, J. A. van der Korput, C. Ris-Stalpers, P. Klaassen, et al. 1989. Structural organization of the human androgen receptor gene. *J. Mol. Endocrinol.* **2:** R1–4.

78. Kumar, M. V. and D. J. Tindall. 1998. Transcriptional regulation of the steroid receptor genes. *Prog. Nucleic Acid Res. Mol. Biol.* **59:** 289–306.

79. Kupfer, S. R., E. M. Wilson, and F. S. French. 1994. Androgen and glucocorticoid receptors interact with insulin degrading enzyme. *J. Biol. Chem.* **269:** 20,622–20,628.

80. Kupfer, S. R., K. B. Marschke, E. M. Wilson, and F. S. French. 1993. Receptor accessory factor enhances specific DNA binding of androgen and glucocorticoid receptors. *J. Biol. Chem.* **268:** 17,519–17,527.

81. Langley, E., J. A. Kemppainen, and E. M. Wilson. 1998. Intermolecular NH2-/carboxyl-terminal interactions in androgen receptor dimerization revealed by mutations that cause androgen insensitivity. *J. Biol. Chem.* **273:** 92–101.

82. Langley, E., Z. X. Zhou, and E. M. Wilson. 1995. Evidence for an anti-parallel orientation of the ligand-activated human androgen receptor dimer. *J. Biol. Chem.* **270:** 29,983–29,990.

83. Lanz, R. B., N. J. McKenna, S. A. Onate, U. Albrecht, J. Wong, S. Y. Tsai, et al. 1999. A steroid receptor coactivator, SRA, functions as an RNA and is present in an SRC-1 complex. *Cell* **97:** 17–27.

84. Lasnitzki, I., H. R. Franklin, and J. D. Wilson. 1974. The mechanism of androgen uptake and concentration by rat ventral prostate in organ culture. *J. Endocrinol.* **60:** 81–90.

85. Lesser, B. and N. Bruchovsky. 1973. The effects of testosterone, 5 dihydrotestosterone and adenosine 3′, 5′ monophosphate on cell proliferation and differentiation on rat prostate. *Biochim. Biophys. Acta* **308:** 426–437.

86. Limonta, P., D. Dondi, R. M. Moretti, R. Maggi, and M. Motta. 1992. Antiproliferative effects of luteinizing hormone-releasing hormone agonists on the human prostatic cancer cell line LNCaP. *J. Clin. Endocrinol. Metabol.* **75:** 207–212.

87. Limonta, P., R. M. Moretti, D. Dondi, M. M. Marelli, and M. Motta. 1994. Androgen dependent prostatic tumors: biosynthesis and possible actions of LHRH. *J. Steroid Biochem. Mol. Biol.* **49:** 347–350.

88. Lin, D. L. and E. T. Keller. 1999. Mechanism of interleukin-6 promotion of androgen receptor function in prostate cancer cells. Proceedings of the International Prostate Cancer Meeting, Iowa City, IA.

89. Lindzey, J., M. V. Kumar, M. Grossman, C. Young, and D. J. Tindall. 1994. Molecular mechanisms of androgen action. *Vitam. Horm.* **49:** 383–432.

90. Lu, S., S. Y. Tsai, and M. J. Tsai. 1997. Regulation of androgen dependent prostatic cancer cell growth: androgen regulation of CDK2, CDK4, and CKI p16 genes. *Cancer Res.* **57:** 4511–4516.

91. Lubahn, D. B., D. R. Joseph, M. Sar, J. Tan, H. N. Higgs, R. E. Larson, et al. 1988. The human androgen receptor: complementary deoxyribonucleic acid cloning, sequence analysis and gene expression in prostate. *Mol. Endocrinol.* **2:** 1265–1275.

92. Lubahn, D. B., D. R. Joseph, P. M. Sullivan, H. F. Willard, F. S. French, and E. M. Wilson. 1988. Cloning of human androgen receptor complementary DNA and localization to the X chromosome. *Science* **240:** 327–330.

93. Luisi, B. F., W. X. Xu, Z. Otwinowski, L. P. Freedman, K. R. Yamamoto, and P. B. Sigler. 1991. Crystallographic analysis of the interaction of the glucocorticoid receptor with DNA. *Science* **352:** 497–505.

94. Marivoet, S., P. Van Dijck, G. Verhoeven, and W. Heyns. 1992. Interaction of the 90-kDa heat shock protein with native and in vitro translated androgen receptor and receptor fragments. *Mol. Cell. Endocrinol.* **88:** 165–174.

95. Miyamoto, H., S. Yeh, G. Wilding, and C. Chang. 1998. Promotion of agonist activity of antiandrogens by the androgen receptor coactivator, ARA70, in human prostate cancer DU145 cells. *Proc. Natl. Acad. Sci. USA* **95:** 7379–7384.

96. Moilanen, A. M., H. Poukka, U. Karvone, M. Hakli, O. A. Janne, and J. J. Palvimo. 1998. Identification of a novel RING finger protein as a coregulator in steroid receptor-mediated gene transcription. *Mol. Cell. Biol.* **18:** 5128–5139.

97. Moilanen, A. M., U. Karvonen, H. Poukka, O. A. Janne, et al. 1998. Activation of androgen receptor function by a novel nuclear protein kinase. *Mol. Biol. Cell* **9:** 2527–2543.

98. Moilanen, A. M., U. Karvonen, H. Poukka, W. Yan, J. Toppari, O. A. Janne, and J. J. Palvimo. 1999. A testis-specific androgen receptor coregulator that belongs to a novel family of nuclear proteins. *J. Biol. Chem.* **274:** 3700–3704.

99. Mora, G. R. and V. B. Mahesh. 1999. Autoregulation of the androgen receptor at the translational level: testosterone induced accumulation of the ARmRNA in the rat ventral prostate polyribosomes. *Steroids* **64:** 587–591.

100. Mora, G. R., G. S. Prins, and V. B. Mahesh. 1996. Autoregulation of androgen receptor protein and messenger RNA in rat ventral prostate is protein synthesis dependent. *J. Steroid Biochem. Mol. Biol.* **58:** 539–549.

101. Moretti, R. M., M. M. Marelli, D. Dondi, A. Poletti, L. Martini, M. Motta, et al. 1996. Luteinizing hormone-releasing hormone agonists interfere with the stimulatory actions of epidermal growth factor in human prostatic cancer cell lines, LNCaP and DU 145. *J. Clin. Endocrinol. Metabol.* **81:** 3930–3937.

102. Mori, S., K. Murakami-Mori, and B. Bonavida. 1999. Interleukin-6 induces G1 arrest through induction of p27(Kip1), a cyclin-dependent kinase inhibitor, and neuron-like morphology in LNCaP prostate tumor cells. *Biochem. Biophys. Res. Commun.* **257:** 609–614.

103. Murthy, L. R., M. P. Johnson, D. R. Rowley, C. Y. Young, P. T. Scardino, and D. J. Tindall. 1986. Characterization of steroid receptors in human prostate using mibolerone. *Prostate* **8:** 241–253.

104. Nazareth, L. V. and N. L. Weigel. 1996. Activation of the human androgen receptor through a protein kinase A signaling pathway. *J. Biol. Chem.* **271:** 19,900–19,907.

105. Nemoto, T., Y. Ohara-Nemoto, and M. Ota. 1992. Association of the 90-kDa heat shock protein does not affect the ligand-binding ability of androgen receptor. *J. Steroid Biochem. Mol. Biol.* **42:** 803–812.

106. Neuman, E., M. H. Ladha, N. Lin, T. M. Upton, S. J. Miller, J. DiRenzo, et al. 1997. Cyclin D1 stimulation of estrogen receptor transcriptional activity independent of cdk4. *Mol. Cell. Biol.* **17:** 5338–5347.

107. Ohara-Nemoto, Y., T. Nemoto, and M. Ota. 1988. Ribonucleic acid association with androgen receptor from rat submandibular gland. *J. Steroid Biochem.* **29:** 27–31.

108. Okamoto, M., C. Lee, and R. Oyasu. 1997. Interleukin-6 as a paracrine and autocrine growth factor in human prostatic carcinoma cells in vitro. *Cancer Res.* **57:** 141–146.

109. Peterziel, H., Z. Culig, J. Stober, A. Hobisch, C. Radmayr, G. Bartsch, et al. 1995. Mutant androgen receptors in prostatic tumors distinguish between amino acid-sequence requirements for transactivation and ligand binding. *Int. J. Cancer* **63:** 544–550.

110. Porto, C. S., M. F. Lazari, L. C. Abreu, C. W. Bardin, and G. L. Gunsalus. 1995. Receptors for androgen-binding proteins: internalization and intracellular signalling. *J. Steroid Biochem. Mol. Biol.* **53:** 561–565.

111. Poukka, H., P. Aarnisalo, U. Karvonen, J. J. Palvimo, and O. A. Janne. 1999. Ubc9 interacts with the androgen receptor and activates receptor-dependent transcription. *J. Biol. Chem.* **274:** 19,441–19,446.

112. Prescott, J. L., L. Blok, and D. J. Tindall. 1998. Isolation and androgen regulation of the human homeobox cDNA, NKX3.1. *Prostate* **35:** 71–80.

113. Qiu, Y., L. Ravi, and H. J. Kung. 1998. Requirement of ErbB2 for signalling by interleukin-6 in prostate carcinoma cells. *Nature* **393:** 83–85.

114. Quarmby, V. E., W. G. Yarbrough, D. B. Lubahn, F. S. French, and E. M. Wilson. 1990. Autologous down-regulation of androgen receptor messenger ribonucleic acid. *Mol. Endocrinol.* **4:** 22–28.

115. Rana, S., D. Bisht, and P. K. Chakraborti. 1999. Synergistic activation of yeast-expressed rat androgen receptor by modulators of protein kinase-A. *J. Mol. Biol.* **286:** 669–681.

116. Reese, D. M. and E. J. Small. 1999. Secondary hormonal manipulations in hormone refractory prostate cancer. *Urol. Clin. N. Am.* **26:** 311–321.

117. Robel, P., B. Eychenne, J. P. Blondeau, I. Jung-Testas, M. T. Groyer, C. Mercier-Bodard, et al. 1983. Androgen receptors in rat and human prostate. *Horm. Res.* **18:** 28–36.

118. Rosner, W. 1990. The functions of corticosteroid-binding globulin and sex hormone-binding globulin: recent advances. *Endocrine Rev.* **11:** 80–91.

119. Rosner, W., D. J. Hryb, M. S. Khan, A. M. Nakhla, and N. A. Romas. 1998. Sex hormone-binding globulin mediates steroid hormone signal transduction at the plasma membrane. *J. Steroid Biochem. Mol. Biol.* **69:** 481–485.

120. Rowley, D. R., R. T. Premont, M. P. Johnson, C. Y. Young, and D. J. Tindall. 1986. Properties of an intermediate-sized androgen receptor: association with RNA. *Biochemistry* **25:** 6988–6995.

121. Roy, A. K., Y. Lavrovsky, C. S. Song, S. Chen, M. H. Jung, N. K. Velu, et al. 1999. Regulation of androgen action. *Vitam. Horm.* **55:** 309–352.

122. Russell, D. W., D. M. Berman, J. T. Bryant, K. M. Cala, D. L. Davis, C. P. Landrum, et al. 1994. The molecular genetics of steroid 5 alpha-reductases. *Recent Prog. Horm. Res.* **49:** 275–284.

123. Sartor, O., Q. Zheng, and J. A. Eastham. 1999. Androgen receptor gene CAG repeat length varies in a race-specific fashion in men without prostate cancer. *Urology* **53:** 378–380.

124. Schwabe, J. W., D. Neuhaus, and D. Rhodes. 1990. Solution structure of the DNA-binding domain of the oestrogen receptor. *Nature* **348:** 458–461.

125. Shan, L. X., M. C. Rodriguez, and O. A. Janne. 1990. Regulation of androgen receptor protein and mRNA concentrations by androgens in rat ventral prostate and seminal vesicles and in human hepatoma cells. *Mol. Endocrinol.* **4:** 1636–1646.

126. Shibata, H., T. E. Spencer, S. A. Onate, G. Jenster, S. Y. Tsai, M. J. Tsai, et al. 1997. Role of co-activators and co-repressors in the mechanism of steroid/thyroid receptor action. *Recent Prog. Horm. Res.* **52:** 141–164 (discussion 164,165).

127. Siiteri, P. K. and J. D. Wilson. 1970. Dihydrotestosterone in prostatic hypertrophy. I. The formation and content of dihydrotestosterone in the hypertrophic prostate of man. *J. Clin. Investig.* **49:** 1737–1745.

128. Simental, J. A., M. Sar, M. V. Lane, F. S. French, and E. M. Wilson. 1991. Transcriptional activation and nuclear targeting signals of the human androgen receptor. *J. Biol. Chem.* **266:** 510–518.

129. Spencer, J. A., J. M. Watson, D. B. Lubahn, D. R. Joseph, F. S. French, E. M. Wilson, et al. 1991. The androgen receptor gene is located on a highly conserved region of the X chromosomes of marsupial and monotreme as well as eutherian mammals. *J. Hered.* **82:** 134–139.

130. Steinsapir, J., G. Mora, and T. G. Muldoon. 1991. Effects of steroidal and non-steroidal antiandrogens on the androgen binding properties of the rat ventral prostate androgen receptor. *Biochim. Biophys. Acta* **1094:** 103–112.
131. Strott, C. A. 1996. Steroid sulfotransferases. *Endocrine Rev.* **17:** 670–697.
132. Tan, J. A., D. R. Joseph, V. E. Quarmby, D. B. Lubahn, M. Sar, F. S. French, et al. 1988. The rat androgen receptor: primary structure, autoregulation of its messenger ribonucleic acid, and immunocytochemical localization of the receptor protein. *Mol. Endocrinol.* **2:** 1276–1285.
133. Teutsch, G., F. Goubet, T. Battmann, A. Bonfils, F. Bouchoux, E. Cerede, et al. 1994. Non-steroidal antiandrogens: synthesis and biological profile of high-affinity ligands for the androgen receptor. *J. Steroid Biochem. Mol. Biol.* **48:** 111–119.
134. Tilley, W. D., M. Marcelli, and M. J. McPhaul. 1990. Expression of the human androgen receptor gene utilizes a common promoter in diverse human tissues and cell lines. *J. Biol. Chem.* **265:** 13,776–13,781.
135. Tsai, M. J. and B. W. O'Malley. 1994. Molecular mechanisms of action of steroid/thyroid receptor superfamily members. *Annu. Rev. Biochem.* **63:** 451–486.
136. Veldscholte, J., C. A. Berrevoets, C. Ris-Stalpers, G. G. Kuiper, G. Jenster, J. Trapman, et al. 1992. The androgen receptor in LNCaP cells contains a mutation in the ligand binding domain which affects steroid binding characteristics and response to anti-androgens. *J. Steroid Biochem. Mol. Biol.* **41:** 665–669.
137. Veldscholte, J., C. Ris-Stalpers, G. G. Kuiper, G. Jenster, C. Berrevoets, E. Claassen, et al. 1990. A mutation in the ligand binding domain of the androgen receptor of human LNCaP cells affects steroid binding characteristics and response to anti-androgens. *Biochem. Biophys. Res. Commun.* **173:** 534–540.
138. Wang, L. G., X. M. Liu, W. Kreis, and D. R. Budman. 1999. Phosphorylation/dephosphorylation of androgen receptor as a determinant of androgen agonistic or antagonistic activity. *Biochem. Biophys. Res. Commun.* **259:** 21–28.
139. Ware, J. L. 1993. Growth factors and their receptors as determinants in the proliferation and metastasis of human prostate cancer. *Cancer Metastasis Rev.* **12:** 287–301.
140. Wilson, J. D. 1978. Sexual differentiation. *Annu. Rev. Physiol.* **40:** 279–306.
141. Wolf, D. A., T. Herzinger, H. Hermeking, D. Blaschke, and W. Horz. 1993. Transcriptional and posttranscriptional regulation of human androgen receptor expression by androgen. *Mol. Endocrinol.* **7:** 924–936.
142. Yeh, S. and C. Chang. 1996. Cloning and characterization of a specific coactivator, ARA70, for the androgen receptor in human prostate cells. *Proc. Natl. Acad. Sci. USA* **93:** 5517–5521.
143. Yeh, S., H. K. Lin, H. Y. Kang, T. H. Thin, M. F. Lin, and C. Chang. 1999. From HER2/Neu signal cascade to androgen receptor and its coactivators: a novel pathway by induction of androgen target genes through MAP kinase in prostate cancer cells. *Proc. Natl. Acad. Sci. USA* **96:** 5458–5463.
144. Yeh, S., H. Miyamoto, and C. Chang. 1997. Hydroxyflutamide may not always be a pure antiandrogen (letter). *Lancet* **349:** 852,853.
145. Yeh, S., H. Miyamoto, K. Nishimura, H. Kang, J. Ludlow, P. Hsiao, et al. 1998. Retinoblastoma, a tumor suppressor, is a coactivator for the androgen receptor in human prostate cancer DU145 cells. *Biochem. Biophys. Res. Commun.* **248:** 361–367.
146. Young, C. Y., P. E. Andrews, and D. J. Tindall. 1995. Expression and androgenic regulation of human prostate-specific kallikreins. *J. Androl.* **16:** 97–99.
147. Zhou, Z. X., C. I. Wong, M. Sar, and E. M. Wilson. 1994. The androgen receptor: an overview. *Recent Prog. Horm. Res.* **49:** 249–274.
148. Zhou, Z. X., M. V. Lane, J. A. Kemppainen, F. S. French, and E. M. Wilson. 1995. Specificity of ligand dependent androgen receptor stabilization: receptor domain interactions influence ligand dissociation and receptor stability. *Mol. Endocrinol.* **9:** 208–218.

15

Tyrosine Kinases and Cellular Signaling in Prostate Cancer

Hsing-Jien Kung, PhD, Clifford G. Tepper, PhD, and Ralph W. deVere White, MD

1. INTRODUCTION

There is very strong evidence that tyrosine kinases are involved in the growth and metastasis of prostate cancer *(65,152,165)*. Tyrosine kinases also play key roles in modulating tumor sensitivity to radiation- and chemical-induced apoptosis. Thus, there is hope that they may play an important role in the response of metastatic prostate cancer to hormonal intervention as well as to other chemotherapeutic approaches *(78)*. Their potential importance as targets for intervention is indicated by the FDA approval of the HER2/Neu-directed therapy, Herceptin, for breast cancer therapy and current clinical trials investigating its effectiveness for prostate cancer *(140)*. Presently, because of screening, 80% of prostate cancers are found while still localized to the gland. If we had the ability to determine which cancers would not metastasize, treatment could be given on an individual basis. Presently, prostate specific antigen (PSA) and tumor grade are the best markers we have. While being generally good clinical indicators, they lack specificity for the individual patient. There are a number of indications that tyrosine kinases may be valuable as prognostic markers in these situations *(65,152,165)*.

It has been estimated that there are about 1000–2000 protein kinases in the human genome; of these, 100 to 200 (i.e., 10%) are tyrosine kinases *(59)*. At present, there are 85 human tyrosine kinases identified in the GenBank database, and based on the relatively slow rate of discovery in the past few years, 100 is a better approximation to the total number of tyrosine kinases encoded by the human genome. In a given cell at a given stage, it is reasonable to assume that there are 30–50 tyrosine kinases expressed—a number large enough to provide characteristic tissue-specific patterns, but small enough to be identified in a simple screening. The hope for tyrosine kinases as prognostic markers rests with the fact that the identification of a stage-specific expression pattern will be identified in prostate cancer cells while they remain localized to the gland.

From: *Prostate Cancer: Biology, Genetics, and the New Therapeutics*
Edited by: L. W. K. Chung, W. B. Isaacs, and J. W. Simons © Humana Press Inc., Totowa, NJ

2. A TYROSINE KINASE PROFILE OF PROSTATE CANCER

In an effort to identify one or more novel biomarkers, an effective tyrosine kinase display approach was developed to identify all or nearly all tyrosine kinases expressed in prostate cancer using a single RT-PCR reaction and visualized in a single polyacrylamide gel. The approach takes advantage of common invariable motifs present in the catalytic domain of the great majority of tyrosine kinases (for example, DFG and DVW motifs in subdomains VII and IX, respectively). Degenerate primers based on reverse translation of these highly conserved sequence motifs are used to generate RT-PCR products of tyrosine kinases, and the resulting amplicons can be sequenced by traditional means—or better yet, subjected to restriction enzyme digestions so that the resulting fragments of different sizes reflect individual kinases. In the latter approach, the identities of the tyrosine kinases can be "read" directly from the gel, saving the time-consuming steps of cloning and sequencing. The band intensity corresponds well to the level of expression of a given kinase. When samples from normal and tumor tissues are compared, overexpressed tyrosine kinases can be readily identified. The first comprehensive tyrosine kinase profile was constructed from an androgen-sensitive, prostate specific antigen (PSA)-releasing prostate cancer xenograft CWR22. Table 1 summarizes the data derived from the display approach, as well as direct sequencing of the amplicons *(118)*. There are 20 receptor-tyrosine kinases and 12 nonreceptor tyrosine kinases. Among the receptor kinases, three (ErbB1, 2, and 3) come from the epidermal growth factor receptor (EGFR) family, and four (EphA1, A2, A4 and B4) from the Eph family. In addition to the Eph family of kinases, there are several cell adhesion molecule-related receptor kinases expressed in this CaP xenograft: Sky and Nyk, which carry neural cell adhesion molecule (NCAM)-like domains; the discoidin domain receptor tyrosine kinases Ddr1 and 2; and RET, which contains a cadherin domain. The presence of EGFR (ErbB1) nerve growth factor receptor (NGFR, trkA) *(39,49)*, fibroblast growth factor (FGFR) *(33,51,125,127)*, and insulin-like growth factor I receptor (IGFR) *(85,112)* are consistent with literature reports describing the responses of prostate cancer cells to these ligands. Among the nonreceptor tyrosine kinases represented, the src family contains three members (src, yes, and lck), and the related src-B family member Frk. The initial profile data also revealed several novel kinases, unknown at the time of discovery, but subsequently cloned: Nyk/Mer, an NCAM-related receptor tyrosine kinase *(53,80)*, and Etk/Bmx, a pleckstrin homology (PH) domain-containing tyrosine kinase *(114,144)*. The former has an elevated expression in CaP, compared to normal prostate epithelial cells, and the latter is expressed at a higher level in LNCaP than in other cell lines, and is implicated in IL-6 induced neuroendocrine differentiation. It is also noteworthy that trkA, trkC, and RET receptor kinases are expressed in CWR22 and LNCaP. This finding was initially surprising, as these kinases are known to be associated primarily with neuronal tissues, but is consistent with the idea that some of the prostate epithelial cells, especially when devoid of hormonal control, have neuroendocrine properties and can be trans-differentiated into such a lineage. RET has recently been shown to be overexpressed in high-grade CaP and high-grade PIN, but not in low-grade samples *(34)*. This finding suggests that RET may play a significant role in CaP progression, and raises the interesting possibility that high-grade CaPs are derived directly from high-grade PIN. Over-

Table 1
Tyrosine Kinase Profile in CWR22 CaP Xenograft

Receptor TK		Nonreceptor TK	
Family	Members	Family	Members
EGFR	ErbB1	*Src*	src
	ErbB2		yes
	ErbB3		lck
Eph	EphA1	*CSK*	Csk
	EphA2		
	EphA4	*Src-B*	Frk
	EphB4		
		JAK	JAK1
UFO/Axl	Sky/Tyro3		tyk2
	Nyk/mer		
		Abl	abl
Ddr	Ddr1		arg
	Ddr2		
		Btk	Etk/Bmx
PDGFR	PDGFR		
		FAK	FAK
FGFR	FGFR2		
	FGFR4	*ZAP70*	Syk
InR	IGFR		
MET	MET		
	Ron		
RET	RET		
NGFR	trkA		
	trkC		

all, the CWR22 tyrosine kinase profile described here is typical for all CaPs studied, although there is a greater similarity of the tyrosine kinase profiles between the two androgen sensitive models—CWR22 and LNCaP—than those of the androgen insensitive lines.

A number of ligands that transmit signals through receptor tyrosine kinases have been implicated in prostate cancer transformation and progression. This chapter focuses on the EGF receptor family of kinases and the signals transmitted by these receptors. The involvement of FGFR and NGFR families is briefly discussed to serve as a reference for further discussion. The literature citations are representative, and are not meant to be inclusive.

3. THE FIBROBLAST GROWTH FACTOR (FGF) RECEPTOR FAMILY OF TYROSINE KINASES

FGF-2 or basic FGF (bFGF), FGF-7 or keratinocyte growth factor (KGF), FGF-8, and FGF-9 are strong mitogens for prostate cells, and their production is associated with benign prostatic hyperplasia and CaP development *(35,52,71,103,121,146)*. Both FGF-2 *(142)* and FGF-7 *(160)* are provided by the stromal cells under normal conditions, but

FGF-2 expression in prostate epithelial cells is downregulated by androgen *(131)*. However, during the development of prostate cancer, alternative splicing of the FGFR2 locus leads to a switch in the expression of FGF receptor 2 isoforms from FGFR2(IIIb) to FGFR2(IIIc), with a concomitant shift in affinity from FGF-7 to FGF-2. An important event following this is the upregulation of FGF2 expression resulting in the establishment of an autocrine loop *(160)*, rendering the cells stromal-independent and androgen-independent *(17)*. In general, the FGF family of growth factors is viewed as progression factors for CaP. The observation that FGF-2 expression is regulated by androgen in prostate epithelial cells suggests that the molecular events leading to hormonal independence may occur at a much earlier stage than presently thought, and further implicates it as a critical factor to consider in relation to androgen ablative therapy *(131)*.

4. THE NERVE GROWTH FACTOR (NGF) RECEPTOR FAMILY OF TYROSINE KINASES

NGF has two receptors: the high-affinity receptor, trkA, and the low-affinity gp75NGFR. TrkA is a tyrosine kinase that serves to transduce NGF-induced differentiation and survival signals, whereas gp75NGFR tends to induce apoptosis. In the normal prostate, gp75NGFR is expressed in the epithelial cells, whereas the ligand NGF is expressed in the stroma *(109)*. The expression of gp75NGFR is reduced in prostate carcinomas and is completely absent in malignant CaP cell lines, Tsu-pr1, DU145, PC3, and LNCaP. Thus, there is an inverse correlation of expression of the gp75NGFR and CaP development. Consistent with its negative role in CaP progression is the finding that artificial expression of gp75NGFR in the Tsu-pr1 cell line results in NGF-induced apoptosis *(108)*. In contrast to the low-affinity receptor, trkA seems to be expressed in the majority of CaPs and all four CaP cell lines, and is a positive growth modulator for CaPs. NGF treatment of these cells stimulates their growth *(6)* and inhibitors of the NGF/trkA pathway inhibit CaP growth *(38,50)*. It is interesting that while NGF/trkA-induced signaling in neuronal cells results in neuronal differentiation, neuroendocrine differentiation in CaP is induced by agents such as interleukin-6 (IL-6) and forskolin, but not by NGF *(6,102)*. NGF also fails to induce the growth of normal prostate cells, and a recent finding suggests that the difference in the biological behaviors between tumor and normal cells cannot be attributed to mutations of trkA *(50)*, but more likely to the presence or absence of gp75NGFR. In two other studies, it was shown that NGF induces the invasiveness of DU145 *(49)* and hormone independence of Tsu-pr1 *(39)*. Thus, NGF plays a dual role in prostate cancer, depending on the repertoire of the receptors present in the cells: trkA behaves as a positive regulator for growth and tumor progression, whereas p75NGFR acts as an apoptosis inducer.

5. THE ErbB/EGF-RECEPTOR FAMILY OF TYROSINE KINASES

Among receptor kinases, the ErbB/EGF-receptor family is most frequently implicated in human malignancies. There are four members in this family—ErbB1, ErbB2, ErbB3, and ErbB4 *(25,73,110)*. The majority of prostate carcinomas express ErbB1, ErbB2, and ErbB3, but little or no ErbB4 *(118)*. ErbB1 is the EGF receptor, and frequently has been found overexpressed in tumors of epithelial origin. Amplification of ErbB1/EGFR has not been detected in CaP, but overexpression of this receptor is common. In nearly all CaP cell lines or tissues surveyed, an autocrine loop of TGF-α/EGF and ErbB1/EGFR exists, thus replacing the requirement for the normal stromal-derived ligand *(23,84,94,132,147)*. Inhibition of ErbB1/EGFR autocrine loop or the kinase activity of the receptor prevents the growth of CaP cells, indicating an essential role of ErbB1/EGFR in their growth *(12,118)*. Interestingly, such an inhibition also affects the actions of IGF-I and protein kinase A (PKA), indicating a general role for ErbB1/EGFR signaling in CaP growth *(112)*.

ErbB2, also called Neu (for the rat homolog) or HER2 (Human EGF Receptor 2), is the second member of this family, and figures prominently in human malignancies. The ErbB2 gene is amplified and overexpressed in 20–30% of primary breast cancers, and correlates with a poor prognosis. However, a humanized mouse monoclonal antibody (MAb) against ErbB2/HER2—Herceptin—exploits this feature as a novel molecular target, and has shown promise in clinical trials as an anti-breast cancer therapeutic agent, alone or in combination with standard chemotherapeutics *(104)*. Unlike breast carcinoma, genomic amplification of ErbB2 is rarely observed in prostate cancer *(13,45,74,88,153)*, but there are noteworthy exceptions *(122–124,134)*. The expression of both ErbB2 and 3 is either low or undetectable on normal prostate luminal epithelial cells, but is prevalent in prostate adenocarcinoma *(82)*. Accordingly, the expression of ErbB2 is considered to be an early event of CaP transformation *(96)*. The level of ErbB2 expression does not seem to vary significantly among CaPs of different histological grade *(57,76)*, although overexpression of ErbB2 in primary prostatic tissue predicts poor survival *(46,93)*. In addition, elevated serum levels of ErbB2 seem to correlate with progression of the disease status *(5a,93a)* and association of ErbB2 overexpression with the occurrence of metastatic disease has also been reported *(122)*. Further strong evidence for ErbB2 as an important factor in CaP metastasis was provided experimentally by the demonstration that in vitro transfection of rat prostatic epithelial cells with an oncogenic ErbB2 mutant (i.e. *Neu* mutation) resulted in metastatic tumors after orthotopic injection into nude mice *(87,166)*.

ErbB3, the third family member, is a kinase-impaired receptor, and requires dimerization with other family members to become an active signal transducer *(58)*. ErbB3 is expressed in the majority of primary and metastatic CaPs *(55,77,96,111,118)*. The ligand for ErbB3—heregulin (HRG) or neuregulin (NRG)—is reported to be expressed in 36% of CaPs analyzed by Leung et al. *(77)*, and the autocrine loop of HRG/ErbB3 appears to be associated with less favorable prognosis in advanced CaPs. By contrast, Lyne et al. *(82)* and Grasso et al. *(55)* found that HRG expression was absent in CaP specimens, three established CaP cell lines (LNCaP, DU145, PC3), and one xenograft (CWR22). However, HRG is expressed in an immortalized, nontumorigenic prostate epithelial cell line *(55)*, and is expressed in 100% of stroma, 100% of basal epithelial cells, and 58% of luminal cells in normal and benign hyperplastic prostatic tissue *(82)*. The latter studies suggest a downregulation of HRG and a concomitant loss of this autocrine loop during tumor progression, consistent with its growth arrest and differentiation effect on CaP cell lines.

In the next section we discuss the signaling events elicited by growth factors such as TGF-α/EGF and HRG, and by cytokines such as IL-6, as they pertain to CaP biology. Depending on the partners, and the individual receptors they associate with, they channel very different signals, with profoundly different biological outcomes.

6. TYROSINE KINASE SIGNALS
THROUGH GROWTH FACTOR RECEPTORS

6.1. EGF/TGF-α Signals: Growth, Androgen Independence, Survival, and Invasion

Among the peptide growth factors, the action of EGF and TGF-α on prostate growth have been most extensively analyzed. There is a preponderance of evidence suggesting the involvement of EGF/TGF-α in the growth of prostate epithelial cells, and the autocrine loop of TGF-α/EGFR found in virtually all prostate cancer cells plays a significant part in their uncontrolled growth. Addition of EGFR-blocking antibody or specific inhibitors of the EGFR kinase *(12,167)* diminishes the growth of CaP. Inclusion of exogenous EGF and TGF-α in growth media further increases the growth rate of the prostate cancer cells, and this effect is synergistic with androgen. In the CWR22 xenograft model, the conversion from androgen-sensitive to the relapsed form (CWR22R) correlates with increased expression of TGF-α, indicating that the TGF-α/EGFR autocrine loop may override the requirement for androgen *(95)*. EGF/TGF-α stimulation of LNCaP induces tyrosine phosphorylation of EGFR/ErbB1, ErbB2, and ErbB3, with ErbB1 being the strongest. Homo and heterodimer formation of ErbB1/ErbB1, ErbB1/ErbB2, and ErbB1/ErbB3 dimers are all detected. Functionally, however, it appears that the ErbB1/ErbB1 homodimer is the most important. Using a LNCaP cell line where ErbB2 is functionally knocked out by the transfection of a single-chain antibody gene directed against ErbB2, it was shown that ErbB2 is dispensable for most of the EGF/TGF-α induced growth phenotypes *(54)*. Under these conditions, phosphorylation of ErbB3 is significantly reduced, indicating that ErbB2 mediates ErbB3 phosphorylation. Since only the growth properties of the ErbB2 "knockout" cells were studied, the role of ErbB2 and ErbB3 in other EGF-induced functions such as migration or survival have yet to be defined.

Intracellular signals are transmitted from membrane-associated tyrosine kinases to serine kinases or lipid kinases, and eventually to transcriptional factors through phosphorylation cascades. ErbB1/EGFR signals through several pathways in prostate cancer cells: Shc/mitogen-activated protein kinase (MAPK) *(18,56,112)*, phosphatidylinositol 3-kinase (PI3K)/Akt, phospholipase C-γ (PLC-γ)/protein kinase C (PKC), p21-activated kinase (PAK)/Jun N-terminal kinase (JNK), and the signal transducers and activators of transcription (STATs) *(55)*. The prevailing model is that upon ligand binding, homo- or heterodimers of the cognate receptors are formed, leading to transphosphorylation and activation of the intrinsic kinase activity. The active kinase is phosphorylated at the tyrosine residues which serve as anchor sites for a number of substrates with *src* homology 2 (SH2) and phosphotyrosine binding (PTB) domains, resulting in the phosphorylation of these substrates. Different substrates define the engagement of different pathways, although there is strong evidence that these pathways are interconnected and tend to modulate one another. A combination of the signal outputs from individual pathways defines the eventual phenotypes of the receptor activation. In subsequent sections, we review what is known about the signals involved in the growth, hormone-independent growth, survival, and motility induced by EGF/TGF-α. Except in cases of motility and invasion, where DU145 is a better model, the experi-

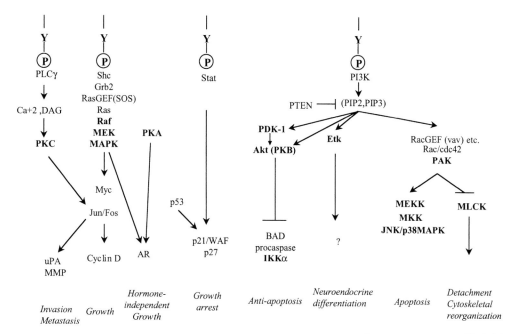

Fig. 1. Summary of the putative signal transduction pathways of prostate cancer cells initiated by tyrosine phosphorylations. Arrows indicate activation of downstream substrates. T-shaped bars indicate inactivations. The highlighted molecules are tyrosine or seirine kinases. The nomenclatures are described in the text. The data is based primarily on the studies of the erbB family of kinases.

mental data were principally derived from LNCaP studies. A summary diagram of the various signal transduction pathways is shown in Fig. 1.

6.2. The Growth Signals

Among the various pathways listed above, MAPK seems to be the most important in channeling the growth signals and the initial transformation of the cells. An early clue that attests to the importance of this pathway for growth and transformation comes from the fact that both *ras* and *raf*, which lie upstream in the pathway, are potent oncogenes and growth stimulators in a variety of cell types. In prostate cancer cells, mutations of *ras* or *raf* are rarely found, yet heightened activation of MAPK is detected in high-grade and hormone-independent CaP *(18)*. The TGF-α/ErbB autocrine loop found in most of the advanced CaP almost certainly contributes to the persistent activation of MAPK. Other overexpressed tyrosine kinases, such as RET and NYK, may also play a significant role. These receptors presumably activate MAPK through the well-defined Shc/Grb2/SOS/*ras*/*raf*/MEK pathway (Fig. 1) *(32,42,75,81,106,151)*. Although there are several upstream activators of MAPK, how MAPK drives the growth pathway is still not entirely clear. It has been reported that MAPK is able to phosphorylate c-Myc and Elk. Elk—an Ets-like transcriptional factor—is known to augment the expression of the AP-1 complex components fos, jun, and jun B. Both the AP-1 complex and c-Myc are known to activate cyclin D, thus propelling cells toward *S* phase.

Furthermore, Chen et al. recently showed that ectopic overexpression of cyclin D stimulates constitutive growth and tumorigenicity of LNCaP *(20)*. Perry et al. demonstrated that EGF activates cyclin D1 in LNCaP *(107)*, lending support to the above model. The same group further demonstrated that EGF-induced activation of cyclin D1 expression was dependent upon PKC. This finding seems reasonable, since EGF is known to activate PLC-γ, which in turn induces intracellular calcium elevations and produces diacylglycerol (DAG), two agonists for PKC, which is an activator of AP-1 complex. Activation of the AP-1 complex by the MAPK and PKC pathways follows two different phosphorylation cascades which are expected to be synergistic. It seems reasonable to propose that the elevated expression of cyclin D1—because of the combined action of MAPK and PKC pathways—plays an important role in EGF/TGF-α induced growth of LNCaP. It is noteworthy that LNCaP has wild-type p53 and Rb genes, making the overexpression of cyclin D1 necessary to overcome the actions of these cell-cycle gatekeepers. However, LNCaP carries a mutant PTEN which encodes a phosphatase specific for the product of PI3K, phosphatidylinositol 3,4,5-trisphosphate *(150)*. Deficiency of PTEN is believed to augment PI3K activity, which confers survival through Akt activation. However, at least one recent report implicates PTEN in G1 growth arrest and points to an unrecognized function of Akt in cell cycle progression *(117)*. This indicates that PTEN mutation may also contribute to the aggressive growth properties of LNCaP, although the mechanism is less clear.

6.3. The Survival Signals

The phosphatidylinositol 3-kinase pathway has recently attracted a great deal of attention because of its diverse effects. PI3K is a lipid kinase which catalyzes reactions to engender 3′-phosphoinositides (Fig. 1). These lipid moieties bind a class of molecules bearing PH domains, which translocate them to the cytoplasmic membrane and often alter their conformation. Akt/protein kinase B (PKB), a serine/threonine kinase involved in antiapoptosis, is one such substrate whose translocation to the membrane allows it to be phosphorylated and activated by 3-phosphoinositide-dependent protein kinase-1 (PDK1), another PH domain containing serine/threonine kinase activated by PI3K. A direct inhibitory effect on the cell death machinery has been demonstrated by phosphorylation of Bad *(31,37)* and procaspase-9 by active Akt *(15)*, inactivating their proapoptotic functions. Recruitment of the PI3K/Akt pathway can also have a cytoprotective effect via activation of nuclear factor-kappa B (NF-κB) and subsequent upregulation of an antiapoptotic transcriptional program *(101,120)*. Akt can mediate degradation of the NF-κB inhibitor IκB by interacting with, phosphorylating, and activating IκB kinase (IKK). IKK, in turn, phosphorylates IκB and targets it for degradation. NF-κB is then liberated and permitted to be translocated to the nucleus. This scheme is postulated to be the molecular basis of PI3K's ability to function as a survival factor. Recent studies by Lin et al. *(79)* and Carson and Weber *(16)* provide direct evidence that PI3K plays a significant role in sustaining survival of LNCaP, based on the observation that the PI3K inhibitors, wortmannin and LY294002, induce a high level of LNCaP cell death. These apoptotic effects can be partially rescued by treatment with EGF, which is known to activate PI3K—presumably via the activation of the ErbB1/ErbB3 heterodimer *(79)*. Interestingly, the Akt activity is not restored (since the

PI3K inhibitor is still present), and the authors postulate the existence of Akt-independent survival signals channeled by PI3K. ErbB3 carries multiple PI3K binding sites, and is particularly effective in forming a multimolecular complex with PI3K involving at least five additional tyrosine phosphorylated species *(54)*. It is conceivable that PI3K, with its multiple protein-protein interaction domains, may impart signal transduction by serving as an adaptor molecule without invoking lipid kinase activity.

Counteracting PI3K is the lipid phosphatase PTEN/MMAC1, originally discovered as a tumor suppressor gene for a number of cancers, including prostate cancers—up to 60% of which are defective in structure or expression of this gene *(150)*. This phosphatase removes a phosphate from the 3′ site of phosphatidyl polyphosphates, particularly phosphatidylinositol 3,4,5-trisphosphate, thereby diminishing the activating signal for Akt. Indeed, prostate cancers such as LNCaP lacking PTEN/MMAC1 have a constitutively high level of activated Akt *(155)*, which may account for the unusual durability of this cell line in harsh conditions. LNCaP, while growth-arrested, can survive long-term in serum-free and androgen-free conditions.

A new PI3K effector, Etk/Bmx, has recently been identified in prostate cancer cells *(114,118)*. Etk/Bmx is a tyrosine kinase that carries a PH domain at the N-terminus and belongs to the Btk family. Etk is the only member of the Btk family that is expressed in prostate cells such as LNCaP. In a manner similar to Akt, it was shown that Etk is able to protect CaP from thapsigargin or radiation-induced apoptosis *(159)*. While the molecular nature of this protective effect remains unclear, this finding demonstrates that there are other potential effectors of PI3K in antiapoptosis. STAT1,3, and 5 have also been shown to be phosphorylated and activated by Etk/Bmx *(128)*, and their connections to the protective effect of Etk are being examined.

6.4. The Hormone Independence Signals

LNCaP requires androgen for growth. The autocrine loop of TGF-α/EGFR existing in this cell line is apparently insufficient to override the hormone dependence. However, the addition of exogenous EGF or IGF-1 can induce LNCaP growth in the absence of synthetic androgen *(28)*. This suggests that either the EGF signal can activate the androgen receptor (AR) pathway in the absence of androgen (i.e., EGF and androgen in the same pathway), or EGF induces an independent growth pathway, obviating the need for androgen (i.e., EGF and androgen are in parallel pathways) or both. At least one report has indicated that the androgenic growth signal requires the interaction between amphiregulin and EGFR *(135)*, suggesting that the EGFR pathway lies downstream of the androgen pathway. Recent demonstrations that the MAPK pathway is able to activate androgen receptor transcriptional activity in the absence of its ligand *(1,27,162)* support this theory. While in the latter studies, the authors utilized overexpressed ErbB2 as a source for MAPK activation, ErbB2 is activated by EGF through heterodimerization with ErbB1, and as described here, EGF is a potent activator of MAPK. Thus, it is likely that EGF or TGF-α induced androgen-independent growth of LNCaP also follow the same pathways. In support of a role for ErbB2 in the conversion of prostate cancer cells into a hormone-independent state is the finding that prostatic acid phosphatase which diminishes ErbB2 activity restores hormone-sensitivity of a variant LNCaP line refractory to hormone induction *(90)*. If MAPK is the key factor involved in activating AR in the absence of androgen, one would predict that MAPK agonists other than ErbB family members should also be able to convert hormone sensitive cells to refractory status—a theory which has not yet been tested. On the other hand, it is equally likely that MAPK is only one of the several pathways activated by ErbB1 or ErbB2 which contribute to AR activation. In the latter case, not all agonists that activate MAPK would induce AR independence. How does MAPK activate the transcriptional activity of AR? Chen et al. found that the target for the phosphorylation cascade is AR itself at a site where phosphorylation would strengthen the interaction with cofactors such as ARA50 or ARA70. These factors presumably enhance the DNA binding or transactivation function of the unliganded AR in a manner similar to the liganded AR. There is also evidence that PKA or elevated cAMP level activates AR in the absence of ligand *(126)*. While this is probably the result of direct phosphorylation of AR by PKA *(126)*, there are at least two reports indicating a synergy between PKA and ErbB1 in the activation of MAPK in LNCaP *(18,112)* which may contribute to the androgen independent activation of AR.

6.5. The Motility and Invasion Signals

EGF is known to induce cell motility, detachment, and invasion of cancer cells. As these processes are dependent upon the cell type and the extracellular matrix used, it is therefore difficult to generalize. For instance, EGF or TGF-α seems to have little effect on the cytoskeletal structure, motility, or invasiveness of LNCaP cells, although it promotes chemomigration of Tsu-pr1 cells *(116)* and motility of DU145 cells *(148)*. In the case of DU145, the activation of PLC-γ seems to be crucial in the migratory properties of the cell, presumably through the activation of PKC and the mobilization of calcium *(149)*. The same authors also showed that disassembly of focal adhesions—a step linked to migration—involves the MAPK pathway *(158)*. In other cell types, growth-factor-induced cell migration often involves the PI3K pathway and small GTPases such as rac1/rhoA/cdc42.

In addition to cell motility, invasion requires the release of proteinases to digest the extracellular matrix. In prostate cancer, EGF induces the release of matrilysin and urokinase (uPA), two molecules strongly implicated in the invasion process *(43,44,67, 115,143)*. The pathway leading to uPA activation involves AP-1, and thus probably includes MAPK and JNK as its effectors *(154)*.

7. HEREGULIN (HRG) SIGNALS: GROWTH ARREST, CYTOSKELETAL REORGANIZATION, AND APOPTOSIS

EGF and TGF-α are involved in many aspects of prostate cancer progression by engaging with ErbB family receptors, primarily ErbB1 and ErbB2. However, ErbB3 and ErbB4 are the high-affinity receptors for heregulin, a polypeptide ligand that has varying effects on different prostate cancer cell lines *(14)*. HRG was also identified as neuregulin (NRG) and Neu differentiation factor (NDF), among other names, but will be referred to as HRG in this chapter *(64,86,105)*. Since ErbB4 is not usually expressed in CaP, HRG functions in this cell type primarily through activation of ErbB3/ErbB2, and to a lesser extent, through ErbB3/ErbB1 heterodimers. Under these conditions, an ErbB3/ErbB3 homodimer may also form, but would be unproductive, as ErbB3 is

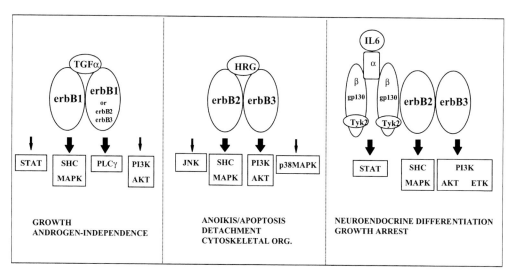

Fig. 2. Schematic representation of key ErbB-mediated signal transduction pathways induced by TGF-α, HRG, and IL-6 in LNCaP prostate cancer cells. Signaling is initiated by ErbB receptor heterodimerization induced by direct ligand binding (i.e., TGF-α, HRG) or indirectly via association with the activated IL-6 receptor. Activation of the intrinsic ErbB tyrosine kinase activity leads to tyrosine phosphorylation of intracytoplasmic domains, recruitment of proteins containing SH2 or PTB domains, and propagation of the signal. Well-characterized signaling pathways in this system are annotated in boxes and the relative strengths of each pathway are indicated by the thickness of the arrows.

kinase-impaired and requires other kinase-active receptors to transphosphorylate it. Indeed, using a LNCaP cell line that has ErbB2 knocked out by the ErbB2 antibody gene-trapping technique, the signaling ability of HRG is completely eliminated *(54)*. Thus, in prostate cancer cells, ErbB2 is a vital component of the HRG signal machinery, and the ErbB2/ErbB3 heterodimer is the principal component activated by HRG. Expression analysis of HRG provides an interesting contrast to that of EGF/TGF-α: HRG is highly expressed in normal prostate epithelial cells—especially basal cells and stromal cells—but at low or undetectable levels in prostate cancer cells *(55,82)*. None of the commonly used CaP cell lines express HRG, whereas an immortalized, normal prostate-epithelial cell line does (MLC-SV40). This suggests that NDF may serve a differentiation or antiproliferative role in prostate cancer cells, as it does in some of the breast cancer cell lines *(29,145)*.

Some of the intracellular signals such as MAPK—which are induced by HRG and by EGF/TGF-α—are similar, but others are different, and have distinct biological consequences. Some of the notable differences are summarized here (Fig. 2). For instance, after HRG treatment, PI3K is assembled into an "activation complex," which can be differentiated from that induced by EGF/TGF-α based upon the tyrosine-phosphorylated band patterns present in the complexes. In addition, HRG treatment activates p38MAPK and JNK, but not PLC-γ and STATs *(55)*. Akt is activated only moderately over the already high background of constitutive activity in LNCaP.

7.1. The Growth Arrest Signals

LNCaP grows well in media containing androgen and serum. In the presence of HRG, the growth rate declines, indicating that HRG transmits a dominant growth-arrest signal *(55,82)*. Addition of the MEK inhibitor PD98059 does not restore growth of LNCaP treated with HRG, nor does the addition of a PI3K inhibitor (LY294002). These results are somewhat difficult to interpret, because LY294002 induces apoptosis even in the absence of HRG. How does HRG induce growth arrest? Bacus et al. *(7)* demonstrated that HRG induces the expression of p53 and p21WAF1, a CyclinD/CDK2 inhibitor, in LNCaP. Yu et al. *(163)* also showed that ErbB2 overexpression upregulates the transcription of p21WAF1. The accumulation of p21 may be one reason that cells go into quiescence. Consistent with this concept is the finding that PDGF treatment of prostate cancer cells results in the induction of p21WAF1 expression, G1 arrest, and the sensitization toward radiation-induced apoptosis *(70)*. Additionally, tamoxifen-induced apoptosis of PC3 and DU145 apparently involves the upregulation of p21WAF1 expression *(119)*, as does cell-cycle inhibition of DU145 induced by type-I interferon alpha *(62)*. Thus, p21WAF1 may be a common mediator of growth arrest in prostate cancer cells.

7.2. The Cytoskeletal Reorganizaton and Detachment Signals

In addition to growth arrest, treatment of LNCaP with HRG induces immediate, cytoskeletal rearrangements characterized by the formation of filopodia, lamellopodia, and stress fibers. A distinct morphological change accompanies this by an alteration in cell shape to a more rounded appearance from the slender shape assumed by typical epithelial cells *(54)*. This is followed by detachment of cells from the plate. Specific inhibitor experiments have indicated that this process depends on PI3K rather than MAPK. The involvement of PI3K in shaping the cytoskeletal structure has been well-documented in other systems, and is thought to engage rac/rho/Cdc42 *(133)*. Rac and Cdc42 are small *ras*-like, RhoA family GTPases with an approximate molecular mass of 21 kDa, and are often referred to as p21 small G proteins. This family of GTPases is known to induce filopodia, lamellipodia, and the disassembly of stress fibers, counteracting the action of RhoA, which contributes to stress fiber assembly. Rac and Cdc42 are activated by guanine exchanger factors (GEF) such as vav, which contain PH domains and thus are effectors for PI3K *(2,83)*. This may explain why PI3K inhibition prevents cell-shape changes and detachment. Rac and Cdc42 activate several kinases, including p21-activated kinases (PAKs) *(137)*, which comprise a family of kinases that share homology in their kinase domains to yeast Ste-20-like kinases. At least three members have been cloned from mammalian cells. Interestingly, a dual role for PAK exists—it is involved in cytoskeletal reorganization and cell movement by phosphory-lating myosin light-chain kinase *(30,130,136)*, and it is able to mediate apoptosis through the activation of JNK and p38 MAP kinases *(24,91)* (Fig. 1).

7.3. The Anoikis/Apoptosis Signals

The detached cells soon undergo apoptosis through a process referred to as anoikis *(47)*. It has been postulated that anoikis involves MEKK and either one of the stress-activated kinases, JNK or p38MAPK *(48)*, although an alternative mechanism may be responsible *(69)*. The activation of JNK and p38MAPK in LNCaP by HRG, but not by EGF is consistent with this hypothesis. Apoptosis induced this way must be able to offset the antiapoptotic effect of Akt activity, which is constitutively present in this cell type. p38MAPK activation is known to induce differentiation and apoptosis in several cell types, thereby providing additional support for this as a mechanism of cell death in this system *(97,157,164)*. Perhaps most germane to the present discussion is the report that in the breast cancer cell line SKBR3, HRG induces apoptosis through p38 activation and subsequent apoptosis *(29)*.

8. TYROSINE KINASE SIGNALS THROUGH A CYTOKINE RECEPTOR

8.1. IL-6 Signals: Hormone Independence, Growth Arrest, and Neuroendocrine Differentiation

Few interleukins are implicated in CaP progression; one that has drawn considerable attention is IL-6. Originally identified as a regulator of immune and inflammatory responses, IL-6 has now been recognized as a key factor involved in the growth and metastasis of several types of neoplasms *(61)*. IL-6 has a two-component receptor—the p80 α-subunit which binds IL-6 and the gp130 β-subunit which is the actual signal transducer and is shared with other cytokine receptors such as oncostatin M (OM), leukemia inhibitory factor (LIF), and interleukin-11 (IL-11) *(60)*. Both components of the IL-6 receptor are expressed in all prostate cancer specimens and cell lines surveyed, indicating a role for IL-6 in CaP biology *(139)*. However, this role is complex. In androgen-dependent cells such as LNCaP, dihydrotestosterone (DHT) suppresses IL-6 expression through a mechanism of androgen receptor-mediated repression of NF-κB activity *(68)*. Addition of exogenous IL-6 to this cell line inhibits growth and induces neuroendocrine differentiation *(36,114)*. By contrast, IL-6 functions as a growth factor for androgen independent CaP cell lines, DU145 and PC3, increasing their growth rate *(100)* and colony-formation potential, and conferring resistance to certain chemotherapeutic agents and tumor necrosis factor (TNF)-mediated cell death *(9,21,98)*. The IL-6 autocrine loop is present in all androgen independent CaP cells, but not in dependent lines *(21)*, suggesting that the IL-6 autocrine loop may be functionally linked to the androgen independent phenotype. These observations, coupled with the finding that the level of circulating IL-6 is elevated in metastatic prostatic carcinoma *(3,4)* implicate IL-6 in CaP progression. While this view seems to be at odds with the antiproliferative effect of IL-6 in androgen dependent cells such as LNCaP, it should be noted that neuroendocrine differentition results in the release of neurotrophins which facilitate the survival and chemomigration of the surrounding CaP cells.

8.2. Hormone Independent Growth and Antiapoptosis Signals

IL-6 is a strong inducer of growth and survival of androgen-independent DU145 and PC3 *(10,11)*. Among the signals triggered by IL-6, MAPK is likely to be responsible for the growth response and PI3K for drug and apoptosis resistance, by analogy to the action of EGF. Since PC3 and DU145 do not express androgen receptors, the IL-6-induced growth and survival signals must pass through an androgen receptor independent pathway. Interestingly, if the androgen receptor status is artificially restored by transfection into DU145, IL-6 is able to stimulate androgen receptor dependent gene transcripton (e.g., a reporter gene driven by the androgen-response element (ARE)) in the absence of androgen *(63)*. This could be inhibited by the nonsteroidal androgen-receptor antagonist bicalutamide (Casodex), indicating that IL-6 indeed mediates its activation through the androgen receptor. The authors have further demonstrated that this activation requires the activities of PKC, PKA, and MAPK. In the AR-positive cell line LNCaP, IL-6 is able to induce transcription from the PSA promoter in the absence of androgen (Dr. Li-Fen Lee, personal communication). Since PSA promoter activation is critically dependent upon AR activity, the experiment described serves as confirmation of the ability of IL-6 to activate the androgen receptor. This is an intriguing finding which suggests that IL-6 may facilitate the initial transition of a prostate cancer cell from hormone dependence to independence by acting as a pseudo-activator. Eventually, in the case of DU145 and PC3, androgen receptor expression is lost and the androgen receptor independent IL-6 pathway takes over. Since AR is known to suppress the transcription of the IL-6 gene *(68)*, the loss of AR further increases the expression of IL-6, setting up a permanent autocrine loop. Oncostatin M, which, like IL-6, activates gp130, is also capable of stimulating the growth of DU145 *(11)*. In this case, STAT3 activation is required. This suggests that although diverse ligands interacting with similar receptors leads to an identical phenotype, diversification of signal transduction pathways contributes to CaP tumor progression and increases the likelihood for selection of aggressive phenotypes.

8.3. The Growth Arrest and Neuroendocrine Differentiation Signals

In contrast to the strong growth stimulation of DU145 and PC3, IL-6 inhibits the growth of LNCaP and induces neuroendocrine (NE) differentiation *(114)*. The acquisition of cells with NE characteristics has been reported to be an early marker for development of androgen independence of prostate cancers, and tumor cell populations have been reported to become enriched for NE cells following long-term antiandrogen therapy *(22,40,99)*. It has been suggested that these NE cells function as a paracrine source of factors to support androgen independent growth of the surrounding cancer cells. NE cells are identified by neurite outgrowth, the presence of neurosecretory granules, and their ability to express a wide variety of neuronal-specific markers such as chromogranin A, neurospecific enolase, and a number of potentially mitogenic neuropeptide hormones, including parathyroid hormone-related peptide, bombesin, serotonin, calcitonin, and others *(26)*. Increased serum levels of chromograinin A are found to correlate well with the acquisition of androgen independence and CaP progression. Although NE cells are nonmitotic, proliferating carcinoma cells have been found in close proximity to them. These observations suggest that NE differentiation of prostate cells is associated with progression of CaP towards an androgen independent state. The origin of NE cells in CaP is not entirely clear, although it has been suggested that they are derived from either prostate stem cells or prostate epithelial cells through transdifferentiation. The fact that some prostate cancer cell lines, such as LNCaP, can undergo NE differentiation suggests that at least a subset of NE cells is derived from prostate epithelial cells. In addition to IL-6 *(114)*, a number of diverse stimuli have been described to induce NE phenotypes of prostate cancer cells. These include the cytokines IL-1 and IL-2 *(41)*, long-term serum/androgen starvation *(138)*, and elevation of intracellular cyclic AMP (cAMP) levels *(26)*. A variety of physiological and pharmacological agents can increase cAMP levels, such as epinephrine, forskolin (adenylate cyclase activator), and the cAMP analog dibutyryl cAMP *(8,26)*. Interestingly, withdrawal of forskolin and epinephrine from LNCaP cells induces the loss of neuritic processes and the reacquisition of a morphology typical of untreated cells, indicating that NE differentiation is reversible and that the affected cells were arrested in growth, but not terminally differentiated and senescent. In the IL-6-induced differentiation model system, treated LNCaP cells were shown to be growth arrested at the G1/S boundary *(92,114)*. This growth arrest apparently involves the activation of p27 at the transcriptional level, but is independent of SHP2 association with IL-6R *(72,92)*. Since it has been demonstrated that elevated cAMP levels can potentiate IL-6 signal transduction, cross-communication between the cAMP and IL-6 pathways may further augment NE differentiation *(19)*. An even more dynamic and aggressive environment can conceivably be established after malignant prostatic neuroendocrine begins secreting mitogenic neuropeptides, which can also contribute to cAMP elevation.

What are the signal pathways which lead to neuroendocrine differentiation of LNCaP cells? The studies of IL-6 *(114)* and cAMP agonists *(26)* have provided insight into this process. In the case of cAMP elevation, it is expected that PKA is involved, and indeed forced expression of a dominant-negative mutant of PKA blocks the differentiation process (M. Cox and S. Parsons, personal communication). PKA activates CREB and ATF, and these transcriptional factors are likely to be responsible for activating the genes involved in neuroendocrine differentiation. Yet, in LNCaP, PKA also activates the MAPK pathway via Rap1, which leads to jun/fos activation *(18)*. Thus, a combination of these bZIP proteins may be involved in this phenotype. The mechanism whereby IL-6 induces NE was more obscure. Early studies in PC12—a rat pheochromocytoma cell line which can be induced by IL-6 to undergo neuronal differentiation—revealed the role of the PI3K pathway in this process *(89,141,156,161)*. When LNCaP was treated with IL-6, the MAPK, JAK/STAT3 and PI3K pathways were all strongly activated *(114)* (Fig. 2). In addition, a PH-domain containing tyrosine kinase, Etk/Bmx, was also activated, and serves as an effector molecule for PI3K. This is understandable, since the PH domain interacts with 3′-phosphoinositides, metabolic products of PI3K *(129)*. By analogy to Btk and Itk, close cousins of Etk, 3′-phosphoinositide binding unfolds this family of proteins, exposing their kinase domains and translocating them to the cytoplasmic membrane where they can be activated by *src*-like kinases *(5)*. That Etk/Bmx is crucial for IL-6-induced neuroendocrine differentiation was demonstrated by the differentiation-resistant phenotype acquired by LNCaP cells stably transfected with a dominant-negative Etk expression construct *(114)*. A key question raised by this study was: What transmits the high level of tyrosine phosphorylation signal, considering that IL-6 receptor itself is not a tyrosine kinase? Jak family kinases known to be activated by cytokine are possible candidates. Tyk2 is indeed activated in IL-6 treated LNCaP cells, but more intriguingly, ErbB2 and ErbB3 are also activated *(113)* (Fig. 2). ErbB1—the only other receptor tyrosine kinase in this family expressed in LNCaP cells—is not activated, indicating the specificity of this cross-communication. Furthermore, ErbB2 forms a stable complex with the gp130 subunit of the IL-6 receptor in an IL-6 dependent manner. This suggests that IL-6 activation of ErbB kinases occurs through direct engagement, and that ErbB2 and Tyk2 both contribute to the elevation of tyrosine phosphorylation induced by IL-6 in LNCaP. Using the ErB2-trapping approach described here (i.e., single-chain antibody expression construct) to functionally knock out ErbB2, it was shown that both ErbB3 and MAPK activation require ErbB2 engagement. This example illustrates how a cytokine receptor can diversify its signal through engagement with receptor tyrosine kinases, which may help explain the complex and pleiotropic phenotypes induced by IL-6. Consistent with a role for ErbB2 in neuroendocrine differentiation is the demonstration that prostatic neuroendocine cells with dendritic appearance and chromogranin A expression express ErbB2 *(66)*. These findings indicate that at least the PKA and PI3K/Etk pathways are involved in the neuroendocrine differentiation of LNCaP. Most likely, other pathways such as MAPK or STAT3 also contribute to this phenotype.

9. CONCLUSION

Tyrosine kinases play significant roles in cellular signaling in prostate cancer. They respond to growth factors as well as to cytokines. The widely recognized pathways such as MAPK, PI3K, PLC-γ, and STATs are activated by multiple inducers, and clearly participate in the signaling (Fig. 1). Yet these pathways do not tell the whole story, and the final outcome depends not only on the combination of multiple pathways, but on their relative intensities. By design, our studies have focused on signals mediated by ErbB kinases. Fig. 2 provides a summary of the various signal pathways outlined in this chapter. Whereas TGF-α/EGF is a strong growth stimulator for all CaP cells thus far studied, HRG induces anoikis and apoptosis. These two diametrically opposite phenotypes nevertheless share overlapping signals. For instance, both TGF-α and HRG activate SHC/MAPK (thick arrows) strongly and PI3K to varying degrees. By contrast, PLC-γ is solely induced by TGF-α, and p38MAPK by HRG. The latter signals thus may be responsible for the particular phenotypes induced by individual growth factors. A comparison of HRG and IL-6 signal pathways offers another intriguing scenario. Here, both involve an ErbB2/ErbB3 complex—one activated by HRG from outside and the other activated by complex formation with IL-6 receptor from within. Again, common signals associated with ErbB2 and ErbB3, such as MAPK and PI3K, are induced. Yet the biological consequences are profoundly different. The likelihood that the Tyk2/STAT pathway contributes to the unique neuroendocrine phenotype needs further examination. How and whether it is related to the cAMP agonist-induced neuroendocrine phenotype are also worth exploring. Prostate cancer offers a complex, yet fascinating biological system to dissect key signal molecules involved in cell fate determination. A full understanding of these pathways is important for scientific study, and may benefit strategies to modify the tumor behavior (e.g., to make tumors more prone to apoptosis and enhance sensitivity to therapy). The success of Herceptin may herald the use of antityrosine kinase antibodies or inhibitors as general anticancer agents. Future intervention strategies may also include potentiating the toxicity of Herceptin through a combination with heregulin, as well as disruption of autocrine growth factor/receptor loops. In light of recent findings, it will also be critical to consider the interplay of androgen receptor signaling with the pathways discussed in the design of tyrosine kinase-based therapies. For all these reasons, and to explore the possibility of uncovering potential tumor markers, the study of tyrosine kinases and cellular signaling in prostate cancer promises to be a flourishing area of research in the new millennium.

REFERENCES

1. Abreu-Martin, M. T., A. Chari, A. A. Palladino, N. A. Craft, and C. L. Sawyers. 1999. Mitogen-activated protein kinase 1 activates androgen receptor-dependent transcription and apoptosis in prostate cancer. *Mol. Cell Biol.* **19:** 5143–5154.
2. Adam, L., R. Vadlamudi, S. B. Kondapaka, J. Chernoff, J. Mendelsohn, and R. Kumar. 1998. Heregulin regulates cytoskeletal reorganization and cell migration through the p21-activated kinase-1 via phosphatidylinositol-3 kinase. *J. Biol. Chem.* **273:** 28,238–28,246.
3. Adler, H. L., M. A. McCurdy, M. W. Kattan, T. L. Timme, P. T. Scardino, and T. C. Thompson. 1999. Elevated levels of circulating interleukin-6 and transforming growth factor-beta1 in patients with metastatic prostatic carcinoma. *J. Urol.* **161:** 182–187.
4. Akimoto, S., A. Okumura, and H. Fuse. 1998. Relationship between serum levels of interleukin-6, tumor necrosis factor-alpha and bone turnover markers in prostate cancer patients. *Endocr. J.* **45:** 183–189.
5. Andreotti, A. H., S. C. Bunnell, S. Feng, L. J. Berg, and S. L. Schreiber. 1997. Regulatory intramolecular association in a tyrosine kinase of the Tec family. *Nature* **385:** 93–97.
5a. Arai, Y., T. Yoshiki, and O. Yoshida. 1997. c-erbβ-2 oncoprotein: a potential biomarker of advanced prostate cancer. *Prostate* **30:** 195–201.
6. Angelsen, A., A. K. Sandvik, U. Syversen, M. Stridsberg, and H. L. Waldum. 1998. NGF-beta, NE-cells and prostatic cancer cell lines. A study of neuroendocrine expression in the human prostatic cancer cell lines DU-145, PC-3, LNCaP, and TSU-pr1 following stimulation of the nerve growth factor-beta. *Scand. J. Urol. Nephrol.* **32:** 7–13.
7. Bacus, S. S., Y. Yarden, M. Oren, D. M. Chin, L. Lyass, C. R. Zelnick, et al. 1996. Neu differentiation factor (Heregulin) activates a p53-dependent pathway in cancer cells. *Oncogene* **12:** 2535–2547.
8. Bang, Y. J., F. Pirnia, W. G. Fang, W. K. Kang, O. Sartor, L. Whitesell, et al. 1994. Terminal neuroendocrine differentiation of human prostate carcinoma cells in response to increased intracellular cyclic AMP. *Proc. Natl. Acad. Sci. USA* **91:** 5330–5334.
9. Borsellino, N., A. Belldegrun, and B. Bonavida. 1995. Endogenous interleukin 6 is a resistance factor for *cis*-diamminedichloroplatinum and etoposide-mediated cytotoxicity of human prostate carcinoma cell lines. *Cancer Res.* **55:** 4633–4639.
10. Borsellino, N., A. Belldegrun, and B. Bonavida. 1995. Endogenous interleukin 6 is a resistance factor for *cis*-diamminedichloroplatinum and etoposide-mediated cytotoxicity of human prostate carcinoma cell lines. *Cancer Res.* **55:** 4633–4639.
11. Borsellino, N., B. Bonavida, G. Ciliberto, C. Toniatti, S. Travali, and N. D'Alessandro. 1999. Blocking signaling through the Gp130 receptor chain by interleukin-6 and oncostatin M inhibits PC-3 cell growth and sensitizes the tumor cells to etoposide and cisplatin-mediated cytotoxicity. *Cancer* **85:** 134–144.
12. Bos, M., J. Mendelsohn, Y. M. Kim, J. Albanell, D. W. Fry, and J. Baselga. 1997. PD153035, a tyrosine kinase inhibitor, prevents epidermal growth factor receptor activation and inhibits growth of cancer cells in a receptor number-dependent manner. *Clin. Cancer Res.* **3:** 2099–2106.
13. Bubendorf, L., J. Kononen, P. Koivisto, P. Schraml, H. Moch, T. C. Gasser, et al. 1999. Survey of gene amplifications during prostate cancer progression by high-throughput fluorescence *in situ* hybridization on tissue microarrays (published erratum appears in *Cancer Res.* 1999 Mar. 15;59(6):1388). *Cancer Res.* **59:** 803–806.

14. Burden, S. and Y. Yarden. 1997. Neuregulins and their receptors: a versatile signaling module in organogenesis and oncogenesis. *Neuron* **18**: 847–855.

15. Cardone, M. H., N. Roy, H. R. Stennicke, G. S. Salvesen, T. F. Franke, E. Stanbridge, et al. 1998. Regulation of cell death protease caspase-9 by phosphorylation. *Science* **282**: 1318–1321.

16. Carson, J. P., G. Kulik, and M. J. Weber. 1999. Antiapoptotic signaling in LNCaP prostate cancer cells: a survival signaling pathway independent of phosphatidylinositol 3′-kinase and Akt/protein kinase B. *Cancer Res.* **59**: 1449–1453.

17. Carstens, R. P., J. V. Eaton, H. R. Krigman, P. J. Walther, and M. A. Garcia-Blanco. 1997. Alternative splicing of fibroblast growth factor receptor 2 (FGF-R2) in human prostate cancer. *Oncogene* **15**: 3059–3065.

18. Chen, T., R. W. Cho, P. J. Stork, and M. J. Weber. 1999a. Elevation of cyclic adenosine 3′,5′-monophosphate potentiates activation of mitogen-activated protein kinase by growth factors in LNCaP prostate cancer cells. *Cancer Res.* **59**: 213–218.

19. Chen, T., R. W. Cho, P. J. Stork, and M. J. Weber. 1999b. Elevation of cyclic adenosine 3′,5′-monophosphate potentiates activation of mitogen-activated protein kinase by growth factors in LNCaP prostate cancer cells. *Cancer Res.* **59**: 213–218.

20. Chen, Y., L. A. Martinez, M. LaCava, L. Coghlan, and C. J. Conti. 1998. Increased cell growth and tumorigenicity in human prostate LNCaP cells by overexpression to cyclin D1. *Oncogene* **16**: 1913–1920.

21. Chung, T. D., J. J. Yu, M. T. Spiotto, M. Bartkowski, and J. W. Simons. 1999. Characterization of the role of IL-6 in the progression of prostate cancer. *Prostate* **38**: 199–207.

22. Cohen, R. J., G. Glezerson, and Z. Haffejee. 1991. Neuro-endocrine cells-a new prognostic parameter in prostate cancer. *Br. J. Urol.* **68**: 258–262.

23. Connolly, J. M. and D. P. Rose. 1990. Production of epidermal growth factor and transforming growth factor-alpha by the androgen-responsive LNCaP human prostate cancer cell line. *Prostate* **16**: 209–218.

24. Coso, O. A., M. Chiariello, J. C. Yu, H. Teramoto, P. Crespo, N. Xu, et al. 1995. The small GTP-binding proteins Rac1 and Cdc42 regulate the activity of the JNK/SAPK signaling pathway. *Cell* **81**: 1137–1146.

25. Coussens, L., T. L. Yang-Feng, Y. C. Liao, E. Chen, A. Gray, J. McGrath, et al. 1985. Tyrosine kinase receptor with extensive homology to EGF receptor shares chromosomal location with neu oncogene. *Science* **230**: 1132–1139.

26. Cox, M. E., P. D. Deeble, S. Lakhani, and S. J. Parsons. 1999. Acquisition of neuroendocrine characteristics by prostate tumor cells is reversible: implications for prostate cancer progression. *Cancer Res.* **59**: 3821–3830.

27. Craft, N., Y. Shostak, M. Carey, and C. L. Sawyers. 1999. A mechanism for hormone-independent prostate cancer through modulation of androgen receptor signaling by the HER-2/neu tyrosine kinase (see comments). *Nat. Med.* **5**: 280–285.

28. Culig, Z., A. Hobisch, M. V. Cronauer, C. Radmayr, J. Trapman, A. Hittmair, et al. 1994. Androgen receptor activation in prostatic tumor cell lines by insulin-like growth factor-I, keratinocyte growth factor, and epidermal growth factor. *Cancer Res.* **54**: 5474–5478.

29. Daly, J. M., M. A. Olayioye, A. M. Wong, R. Neve, H. A. Lane, F. G. Maurer, et al. 1999. NDF/heregulin-induced cell cycle changes and apoptosis in breast tumour cells: role of PI3 kinase and p38 MAP kinase pathways. *Oncogene* **18**: 3440–3451.

30. Daniels, R. H., P. S. Hall, and G. M. Bokoch. 1998. Membrane targeting of p21-activated kinase 1 (PAK1) induces neurite outgrowth from PC12 cells. *EMBO J.* **17**: 754–764.

31. Datta, S. R., H. Dudek, X. Tao, S. Masters, H. Fu, Y. Gotoh, et al. 1997. Akt phosphorylation of BAD couples survival signals to the cell-intrinsic death machinery. *Cell* **91**: 231–241.

32. Davis, R. J. 1995. Transcriptional regulation by MAP kinases. *Mol. Reprod. Dev.* **42:** 459–467.
33. Davol, P. A. and A. R. J. Frackelton. 1999. Targeting human prostatic carcinoma through basic fibroblast growth factor receptors in an animal model: characterizing and circumventing mechanisms of tumor resistance. *Prostate* **40:** 178–191.
34. Dawson, D. M., E. G. Lawrence, G. T. MacLennan, S. B. Amini, H. J. Kung, D. Robinson, et al. 1998. Altered expression of RET proto-oncogene product in prostatic intraepithelial neoplasia and prostate cancer (see comments). *J. Natl. Cancer Inst.* **90:** 519–523.
35. De Bellis, A., C. Crescioli, C. Grappone, S. Milani, P. Ghiandi, G. Forti, et al. 1998. Expression and cellular localization of keratinocyte growth factor and its receptor in human hyperplastic prostate tissue. *J. Clin. Endocrinol. Metab.* **83:** 2186–2191.
36. Degeorges, A., R. Tatoud, F. Fauvel-Lafeve, M. P. Podgorniak, G. Millot, P. de Cremoux, et al. 1996. Stromal cells from human benign prostate hyperplasia produce a growth-inhibitory factor for LNCaP prostate cancer cells, identified as interleukin-6. *Int. J. Cancer* **68:** 207–214.
37. del Peso, L., M. Gonzalez-Garcia, C. Page, R. Herrera, and G. Nunez. 1997. Interleukin-3-induced phosphorylation of BAD through the protein kinase Akt. *Science* **278:** 687–689.
38. Delsite, R. and D. Djakiew. 1996. Anti-proliferative effect of the kinase inhibitor K252a on human prostatic carcinoma cell lines. *J. Androl.* **17:** 481–490.
39. Delsite, R. and D. Djakiew. 1999. Characterization of nerve growth factor precursor protein expression by human prostate stromal cells: a role in selective neurotrophin stimulation of prostate epithelial cell growth. *Prostate* **41:** 39–48.
40. di Sant'Agnese, P. A. and A. T. Cockett. 1996. Neuroendocrine differentiation in prostatic malignancy. *Cancer* **78:** 357–361.
41. Diaz, M., M. Abdul, and N. Hoosein. 1998. Modulation of neuroendocrine differentiation in prostate cancer by interleukin-1 and -2. *Prostate Suppl.* **8:** 32–36.
42. Downward, J., R. Riehl, L. Wu, and R. A. Weinberg. 1990. Identification of a nucleotide exchange-promoting activity for p21ras. *Proc. Natl. Acad. Sci. USA* **87:** 5998–6002.
43. Evans, C. P., F. Elfman, S. Parangi, M. Conn, G. Cunha, and M. A. Shuman. 1997. Inhibition of prostate cancer neovascularization and growth by urokinase-plasminogen activator receptor blockade. *Cancer Res.* **57:** 3594–3599.
44. Festuccia, C., F. Guerra, S. D'Ascenzo, D. Giunciuglio, A. Albini, and M. Bologna. 1998. In vitro regulation of pericellular proteolysis in prostatic tumor cells treated with bombesin. *Int. J. Cancer* **75:** 418–431.
45. Fournier, G., A. Latil, Y. Amet, J. H. Abalain, A. Volant, P. Mangin, et al. 1995. Gene amplifications in advanced-stage human prostate cancer. *Urol. Res.* **22:** 343–347.
46. Fox, S. B., R. A. Persad, N. Coleman, C. A. Day, P. B. Silcocks, and C. C. Collins. 1994. Prognostic value of c-erbB-2 and epidermal growth factor receptor in stage A1 (T1a) prostatic adenocarcinoma. *Br. J. Urol.* **74:** 214–220.
47. Frisch, S. M. and H. Francis. 1994. Disruption of epithelial cell-matrix interactions induces apoptosis. *J. Cell Biol.* **124:** 619–626.
48. Frisch, S. M., K. Vuori, D. Kelaita, and S. Sicks. 1996. A role for Jun-N-terminal kinase in anoikis; suppression by bcl-2 and crmA. *J. Cell Biol.* **135:** 1377–1382.
49. Geldof, A. A., M. A. De Kleijn, B. R. Rao, and D. W. Newling. 1997. Nerve growth factor stimulates in vitro invasive capacity of DU145 human prostatic cancer cells. *J. Cancer Res. Clin. Oncol.* **123:** 107–112.
50. George, D. J., H. Suzuki, G. S. Bova, and J. T. Isaacs. 1998. Mutational analysis of the TrkA gene in prostate cancer. *Prostate* **36:** 172–180.
51. Giri, D., F. Ropiquet, and M. Ittmann. 1999. Alterations in expression of basic fibroblast growth factor (FGF) 2 and its receptor FGFR-1 in human prostate cancer. *Clin. Cancer Res.* **5:** 1063–1071.

52. Gleave, M., J. T. Hsieh, C. A. Gao, A. C. von Eschenbach, and L. W. Chung. 1991. Acceleration of human prostate cancer growth in vivo by factors produced by prostate and bone fibroblasts. *Cancer Res.* **51:** 3753–3761.

53. Graham, D. K., T. L. Dawson, D. L. Mullaney, H. R. Snodgrass, and H. S. Earp. 1994. Cloning and mRNA expression analysis of a novel human protooncogene, c-mer (published erratum appears in Cell Growth Differ 1994 Sep;5(9):1022). *Cell Growth Differ.* **5:** 647–657.

54. Grasso, A. W. 1999. Neuregulin-induced signaling and cell biology in the LNCaP human prostate carcinoma cell line. Ph.D. Thesis

55. Grasso, A. W., D. Wen, C. M. Miller, J. S. Rhim, T. G. Pretlow, and H. J. Kung. 1997. ErbB kinases and NDF signaling in human prostate cancer cells. *Oncogene* **15:** 2705–2716.

56. Gresham, J., P. Margiotta, A. J. Palad, K. D. Somers, P. F. Blackmore, G. L. J. Wright, et al. 1998. Involvement of Shc in the signaling response of human prostate tumor cell lines to epidermal growth factor. *Int. J. Cancer* **77:** 923–927.

57. Gu, K., A. M. Mes-Masson, J. Gauthier, and F. Saad. 1996. Overexpression of her-2/neu in human prostate cancer and benign hyperplasia. *Cancer Lett.* **99:** 185–189.

58. Guy, P. M., J. V. Platko, L. C. Cantley, R. A. Cerione, and K. L. Carraway. 1994. Insect cell-expressed p180erbB3 possesses an impaired tyrosine kinase activity. *Proc. Natl. Acad. Sci. USA* **91:** 8132–8136.

59. Hanks, S. K. and T. Hunter. 1995. Protein kinases 6. The eukaryotic protein kinase superfamily: kinase (catalytic) domain structure and classification. *FASEB J.* **9:** 576–596.

60. Heinrich, P. C., I. Behrmann, G. Muller-Newen, F. Schaper, and L. Graeve. 1998. Interleukin-6-type cytokine signalling through the gp130/Jak/STAT pathway. *Biochem. J.* **334 (Pt 2):** 297–314.

61. Hirano, T., K. Nakajima, and M. Hibi. 1997. Signaling mechanisms through gp130: a model of the cytokine system. *Cytokine Growth Factor Rev.* **8:** 241–252.

62. Hobeika, A. C., W. Etienne, P. E. Cruz, P. S. Subramaniam, and H. M. Johnson. 1998. IFNgamma induction of p21WAF1 in prostate cancer cells: role in cell cycle, alteration of phenotype and invasive potential. *Int. J. Cancer* **77:** 138–145.

63. Hobisch, A., I. E. Eder, T. Putz, W. Horninger, G. Bartsch, H. Klocker, et al. 1998. Interleukin-6 regulates prostate-specific protein expression in prostate carcinoma cells by activation of the androgen receptor. *Cancer Res.* **58:** 4640–4645.

64. Holmes, W. E., M. X. Sliwkowski, R. W. Akita, W. J. Henzel, J. Lee, J. W. Park, et al. 1992. Identification of heregulin, a specific activator of p185erbB2. *Science* **256:** 1205–1210.

65. Humphrey, P. A., X. Zhu, R. Zarnegar, P. E. Swanson, T. L. Ratliff, R. T. Vollmer, et al. 1995. Hepatocyte growth factor and its receptor (c-MET) in prostatic carcinoma. *Am. J. Pathol.* **147:** 386–396.

66. Iwamura, M., K. Koshiba, and A. T. Cockett. 1998. Receptors for BPH growth factors are located in some neuroendocrine cells. *Prostate Suppl.* **8:** 14–17.

67. Jarrard, D. F., B. F. Blitz, R. C. Smith, B. L. Patai, and D. B. Rukstalis. 1994. Effect of epidermal growth factor on prostate cancer cell line PC3 growth and invasion. *Prostate* **24:** 46–53.

68. Keller, E. T., C. Chang, and W. B. Ershler. 1996. Inhibition of NF-κβ activity through maintenance of IκBα levels contributes to dihydrotestosterone-mediated repression of the interleukin-6 promoter. *J. Biol. Chem.* **271:** 26,267–26,275.

69. Khwaja, A. and J. Downward. 1997. Lack of correlation between activation of Jun-NH2-terminal kinase and induction of apoptosis after detachment of epithelial cells. *J. Cell Biol.* **139:** 1017–1023.

70. Kim, H. E., S. J. Han, T. Kasza, R. Han, H. S. Choi, K. C. Palmer, et al. 1997. Platelet-derived growth factor (PDGF)-signaling mediates radiation-induced apoptosis in human prostate cancer cells with loss of p53 function. *Int. J. Radiat. Oncol. Biol. Phys.* **39:** 731–736.

71. Kitsberg, D. I. and P. Leder. 1996. Keratinocyte growth factor induces mammary and prostatic hyperplasia and mammary adenocarcinoma in transgenic mice. *Oncogene* **13:** 2507–2515.

72. Kortylewski, M., P. C. Heinrich, A. Mackiewicz, U. Schniertshauer, U. Klingmuller, K. Nakajima, et al. 1999. Interleukin-6 and oncostatin M-induced growth inhibition of human A375 melanoma cells is STAT-dependent and involves upregulation of the cyclin-dependent kinase inhibitor p27/Kip1. *Oncogene* **18:** 3742–3753.

73. Kraus, M. H., P. Fedi, V. Starks, R. Muraro, and S. A. Aaronson. 1993. Demonstration of ligand-dependent signaling by the erbB-3 tyrosine kinase and its constitutive activation in human breast tumor cells. *Proc. Natl. Acad. Sci. USA* **90:** 2900–2904.

74. Kuhn, E. J., R. A. Kurnot, I. A. Sesterhenn, E. H. Chang, and J. W. Moul. 1993. Expression of the c-erbB-2 (HER-2/neu) oncoprotein in human prostatic carcinoma. *J. Urol.* **150:** 1427–1433.

75. Kyriakis, J. M., H. App, X. F. Zhang, P. Banerjee, D. L. Brautigan, U. R. Rapp, et al. 1992. Raf-1 activates MAP kinase-kinase. *Nature* **358:** 417–421.

76. Latil, A., J. C. Baron, O. Cussenot, G. Fournier, L. Boccon-Gibod, A. Le Duc, et al. 1994. Oncogene amplifications in early-stage human prostate carcinomas. *Int. J. Cancer* **59:** 637,638.

77. Leung, H. Y., J. Weston, W. J. Gullick, and G. Williams. 1997. A potential autocrine loop between heregulin-alpha and erbB-3 receptor in human prostatic adenocarcinoma. *Br. J. Urol.* **79:** 212–216.

78. Levitzki, A. and A. Gazit. 1995. Tyrosine kinase inhibition: an approach to drug development. *Science* **267:** 1782–1788.

79. Lin, J., R. M. Adam, E. Santiestevan, and M. R. Freeman. 1999. The phosphatidylinositol 3′-kinase pathway is a dominant growth factor-activated cell survival pathway in LNCaP human prostate carcinoma cells. *Cancer Res.* **59:** 2891–2897.

80. Ling, L. and H. J. Kung. 1995. Mitogenic signals and transforming potential of Nyk, a newly identified neural cell adhesion molecule-related receptor tyrosine kinase. *Mol. Cell. Biol.* **15:** 6582–6592.

81. Lowenstein, E. J., R. J. Daly, A. G. Batzer, W. Li, B. Margolis, R. Lammers, et al. 1992. The SH2 and SH3 domain-containing protein GRB2 links receptor tyrosine kinases to ras signaling. *Cell* **70:** 431–442.

82. Lyne, J. C., M. F. Melhem, G. G. Finley, D. Wen, N. Liu, D. H. Deng, et al. 1997. Tissue expression of neu differentiation factor/heregulin and its receptor complex in prostate cancer and its biologic effects on prostate cancer cells in vitro. *Cancer J. Sci. Am.* **3:** 21–30.

83. Ma, A. D., A. Metjian, S. Bagrodia, S. Taylor, and C. S. Abrams. 1998. Cytoskeletal reorganization by G protein-coupled receptors is dependent on phosphoinositide 3-kinase gamma, a Rac guanosine exchange factor, and Rac. *Mol. Cell. Biol.* **18:** 4744–4751.

84. MacDonald, A. and F. K. Habib. 1992. Divergent responses to epidermal growth factor in hormone sensitive and insensitive human prostate cancer cell lines. *Br. J. Cancer* **65:** 177–182.

85. Manes, S., M. Llorente, R. A. Lacalle, C. Gomez-Mouton, L. Kremer, E. Mira, et al. 1999. The matrix metalloproteinase-9 regulates the insulin-like growth factor-triggered autocrine response in DU-145 carcinoma cells. *J. Biol. Chem.* **274:** 6935–6945.

86. Marchionni, M. A., A. D. Goodearl, M. S. Chen, O. Bermingham-McDonogh, C. Kirk, M. Hendricks, et al. 1993. Glial growth factors are alternatively spliced erbB2 ligands expressed in the nervous system (see comments). *Nature* **362:** 312–318.

87. Marengo, S. R., R. A. Sikes, P. Anezinis, S. M. Chang, and L. W. Chung. 1997. Metastasis induced by overexpression of p185neu-T after orthotopic injection into a prostatic epithelial cell line (NbE). *Mol. Carcinog.* **19:** 165–175.

88. Mark, H. F., D. Feldman, S. Das, H. Kye, S. Mark, C. L. Sun, et al. 1999. Fluorescence in situ hybridization study of HER-2/neu oncogene amplification in prostate cancer. *Exp. Mol. Pathol.* **66:** 170–178.

89. Marz, P., T. Herget, E. Lang, U. Otten, and S. Rose-John. 1997. Activation of gp130 by IL-6/soluble IL-6 receptor induces neuronal differentiation. *Eur. J. Neurosci.* **9:** 2765–2773 (published erratum appears in *Eur. J. Neurosci.* 1998 May;10(5):1936).

90. Meng, T. C. and M. F. Lin. 1998. Tyrosine phosphorylation of c-ErbB-2 is regulated by the cellular form of prostatic acid phosphatase in human prostate cancer cells. *J. Biol. Chem.* **273:** 22,096–22,104.

91. Minden, A., A. Lin, F. X. Claret, A. Abo, and M. Karin. 1995. Selective activation of the JNK signaling cascade and c-Jun transcriptional activity by the small GTPases Rac and Cdc42Hs. *Cell* **81:** 1147–1157.

92. Mori, S., K. Murakami-Mori, and B. Bonavida. 1999. Interleukin-6 induces G1 arrest through induction of p27(Kip1), a cyclin-dependent kinase inhibitor, and neuron-like morphology in LNCaP prostate tumor cells. *Biochem. Biophys. Res. Commun.* **257:** 609–614.

93. Morote, J., I. De Torres, C. Caceres, C. Vallejo, S. J. Schwartz, and J. Reventos. 1999. Prognostic value of immunohistochemical expression of the c-erbB-2 oncoprotein in metastasic prostate cancer. *Int. J. Cancer* **84:** 421–425.

93a. Myers, R. B., D. Brown, D. K. Oelschlager, J. W. Waterbor, M. E. Marshall, S. Srivastava, C. R. Stockard, D. A. Urban, and W. E. Grizzle. 1996. Elevated serum levels of p105(erbB-2) in patients with advanced-stage prostate adenocarcinoma. *Int. J. Cancer* **69:** 398–402.

94. Myers, R. B., J. E. Kudlow, and W. E. Grizzle. 1993. Expression of transforming growth factor-alpha, epidermal growth factor and the epidermal growth factor receptor in adenocarcinoma of the prostate and benign prostatic hyperplasia. *Mod. Pathol.* **6:** 733–737.

95. Myers, R. B., D. Oelschlager, U. Manne, P. N. Coan, H. Weiss, and W. E. Grizzle. 1999. Androgenic regulation of growth factor and growth factor receptor expression in the CWR22 model of prostatic adenocarcinoma. *Int. J. Cancer* **82:** 424–429.

96. Myers, R. B., S. Srivastava, D. K. Oelschlager, and W. E. Grizzle. 1994. Expression of p160erbB-3 and p185erbB-2 in prostatic intraepithelial neoplasia and prostatic adenocarcinoma (see comments). *J. Natl. Cancer Inst.* **86:** 1140–1145.

97. Nagata, Y. and K. Todokoro. 1999. Requirement of activation of JNK and p38 for environmental stress-induced erythroid differentiation and apoptosis and of inhibition of ERK for apoptosis. *Blood* **94:** 853–863.

98. Nakajima, Y., A. M. DelliPizzi, C. Mallouh, and N. R. Ferreri. 1996. TNF-mediated cytotoxicity and resistance in human prostate cancer cell lines. *Prostate* **29:** 296–302.

99. Noordzij, M. A., W. M. van Weerden, C. M. A. de Ridder, T. H. van der Kwast, F. H. Schroder, and G. J. van Steenbrugge. 1996. Neuroendocrine differentiation in human prostatic tumor models. *Am. J. Pathol.* **149:** 859–871.

100. Okamoto, M., C. Lee, and R. Oyasu. 1997. Interleukin-6 as a paracrine and autocrine growth factor in human prostatic carcinoma cells in vitro. *Cancer Res.* **57:** 141–146.

101. Ozes, O. N., L. D. Mayo, J. A. Gustin, S. R. Pfeffer, L. M. Pfeffer, and D. B. Donner. 1999. NF-kappaB activation by tumour necrosis factor requires the Akt serine-threonine kinase (see comments). *Nature* **401:** 82–85.

102. Paul, A. B., E. S. Grant, and F. K. Habib. 1996. The expression and localisation of beta-nerve growth factor (beta-NGF) in benign and malignant human prostate tissue: relationship to neuroendocrine differentiation. *Br. J. Cancer* **74:** 1990–1996.

103. Peehl, D. M. and J. S. Rubin. 1995. Keratinocyte growth factor: an androgen-regulated mediator of stromal-epithelial interactions in the prostate. *World J. Urol.* **13:** 312–317.

104. Pegram, M., S. Hsu, G. Lewis, R. Pietras, M. Beryt, M. Sliwkowski, et al. 1999. Inhibitory effects of combinations of HER-2/neu antibody and chemotherapeutic agents used for treatment of human breast cancers. *Oncogene* **18:** 2241–2251.

105. Peles, E., S. S. Bacus, R. A. Koski, H. S. Lu, D. Wen, S. G. Ogden, et al. 1992. Isolation of the neu/HER-2 stimulatory ligand: a 44 kd glycoprotein that induces differentiation of mammary tumor cells. *Cell* **69:** 205–216.

106. Pelicci, G., L. Lanfrancone, F. Grignani, J. McGlade, F. Cavallo, G. Forni, et al. 1992. A novel transforming protein (SHC) with an SH2 domain is implicated in mitogenic signal transduction. *Cell* **70:** 93–104.

107. Perry, J. E., M. E. Grossmann, and D. J. Tindall. 1998. Epidermal growth factor induces cyclin D1 in a human prostate cancer cell line. *Prostate* **35:** 117–124.

108. Pflug, B. and D. Djakiew. 1998. Expression of p75NTR in a human prostate epithelial tumor cell line reduces nerve growth factor-induced cell growth by activation of programmed cell death. *Mol. Carcinog.* **23:** 106–114.

109. Pflug, B. R., M. Onoda, J. H. Lynch, and D. Djakiew. 1992. Reduced expression of the low affinity nerve growth factor receptor in benign and malignant human prostate tissue and loss of expression in four human metastatic prostate tumor cell lines. *Cancer Res.* **52:** 5403–5406.

110. Plowman, G. D., J. M. Culouscou, G. S. Whitney, J. M. Green, G. W. Carlton, L. Foy, et al. 1993. Ligand-specific activation of HER4/p180erbB4, a fourth member of the epidermal growth factor receptor family. *Proc. Natl. Acad. Sci. USA* **90:** 1746–1750.

111. Poller, D. N., I. Spendlove, C. Baker, R. Church, I. O. Ellis, G. D. Plowman, et al. 1992. Production and characterization of a polyclonal antibody to the c-erbB-3 protein: examination of c-erbB-3 protein expression in adenocarcinomas. *J. Pathol.* **168:** 275–280.

112. Putz, T., Z. Culig, I. E. Eder, C. Nessler-Menardi, G. Bartsch, H. Grunicke, et al. 1999. Epidermal growth factor (EGF) receptor blockade inhibits the action of EGF, insulin-like growth factor I, and a protein kinase A activator on the mitogen-activated protein kinase pathway in prostate cancer cell lines. *Cancer Res.* **59:** 227–233.

113. Qiu, Y., L. Ravi, and H.-J. Kung. 1998. Requirement of ErbB2 for signaling by interleukin-6 in prostate carcinoma cells. *Nature* **393:** 83–85.

114. Qiu, Y., D. Robinson, T. G. Pretlow, and H. J. Kung. 1998. Etk/Bmx, a tyrosine kinase with a pleckstrin-homology domain, is an effector of phosphatidylinositol 3′-kinase and is involved in interleukin 6-induced neuroendocrine differentiation of prostate cancer cells. *Proc. Natl. Acad. Sci. USA* **95:** 3644–3649.

115. Quax, P. H., A. C. de Bart, J. A. Schalken, and J. H. Verheijen. 1997. Plasminogen activator and matrix metalloproteinase production and extracellular matrix degradation by rat prostate cancer cells in vitro: correlation with metastatic behavior in vivo. *Prostate* **32:** 196–204.

116. Rajan, R., R. Vanderslice, S. Kapur, J. Lynch, R. Thompson, and D. Djakiew. 1996. Epidermal growth factor (EGF) promotes chemomigration of a human prostate tumor cell line, and EGF immunoreactive proteins are present at sites of metastasis in the stroma of lymph nodes and medullary bone. *Prostate* **28:** 1–9.

117. Ramaswamy, S., N. Nakamura, F. Vazquez, D. B. Batt, S. Perera, T. M. Roberts, et al. 1999. Regulation of G1 progression by the PTEN tumor suppressor protein is linked to inhibition of the phosphatidylinositol 3-kinase/Akt pathway. *Proc. Natl. Acad. Sci. USA* **96:** 2110–2115.

118. Robinson, D., F. He, T. Pretlow, and H. J. Kung. 1996. A tyrosine kinase profile of prostate carcinoma. *Proc. Natl. Acad. Sci. USA* **93:** 5958–5962.

119. Rohlff, C., M. V. Blagosklonny, E. Kyle, A. Kesari, I. Y. Kim, D. J. Zelner, et al. 1998. Prostate cancer cell growth inhibition by tamoxifen is associated with inhibition of protein kinase C and induction of p21(waf1/cip1). *Prostate* **37:** 51–59.

120. Romashkova, J. A. and S. S. Makarov. 1999. NF-kappaB is a target of AKT in anti-apoptotic PDGF signalling (see comments). *Nature* **401:** 86–90.

121. Ropiquet, F., P. Berthon, J. M. Villette, G. Le Brun, N. J. Maitland, O. Cussenot, et al. 1997. Constitutive expression of FGF2/bFGF in non-tumorigenic human prostatic epithelial cells results in the acquisition of a partial neoplastic phenotype. *Int. J. Cancer* **72:** 543–547.

122. Ross, J. S., T. Nazeer, K. Church, C. Amato, H. Figge, M. D. Rifkin, et al. 1993. Contribution of HER-2/neu oncogene expression to tumor grade and DNA content analysis in the prediction of prostatic carcinoma metastasis. *Cancer* **72:** 3020–3028.

123. Ross, J. S., C. Sheehan, A. M. Hayner-Buchan, R. A. Ambros, B. V. Kallakury, R. Kaufman, et al. 1997. HER-2/neu gene amplification status in prostate cancer by fluorescence *in situ* hybridization. *Hum. Pathol.* **28:** 827–833.

124. Ross, J. S., C. E. Sheehan, A. M. Hayner-Buchan, R. A. Ambros, B. V. Kallakury, R. P. J. Kaufman, et al. 1997. Prognostic significance of HER-2/neu gene amplification status by fluorescence *in situ* hybridization of prostate carcinoma. *Cancer* **79:** 2162–2170.

125. Russell, P. J., S. Bennett, A. Joshua, Y. Yu, S. R. Downing, M. A. Hill, et al. 1999. Elevated expression of FGF-2 does not cause prostate cancer progression in LNCaP cells. *Prostate* **40:** 1–13.

126. Sadar, M. D. 1999. Androgen-independent induction of prostate-specific antigen gene expression via cross-talk between the androgen receptor and protein kinase A signal transduction pathways. *J. Biol. Chem.* **274:** 7777–7783.

127. Saez, C., A. C. Gonzalez-Baena, M. A. Japon, J. Giraldez, D. I. Segura, J. M. Rodriguez-Vallejo, et al. 1999. Expression of basic fibroblast growth factor and its receptors FGFR1 and FGFR2 in human benign prostatic hyperplasia treated with finasteride. *Prostate* **40:** 83–88.

128. Saharinen, P., N. Ekman, K. Sarvas, P. Parker, K. Alitalo, and O. Silvennoinen. 1997. The Bmx tyrosine kinase induces activation of the Stat signaling pathway, which is specifically inhibited by protein kinase Cdelta. *Blood* **90:** 4341–4353.

129. Salim, K., M. J. Bottomley, E. Querfurth, M. J. Zvelebil, I. Gout, R. Scaife, et al. 1996. Distinct specificity in the recognition of phosphoinositides by the pleckstrin homology domains of dynamin and Bruton's tyrosine kinase. *EMBO J.* **15:** 6241–6250.

130. Sanders, L. C., F. Matsumura, G. M. Bokoch, and P. de Lanerolle. 1999. Inhibition of myosin light chain kinase by p21-activated kinase (see comments). *Science* **283:** 2083–2085.

131. Saric, T. and S. A. Shain. 1998. Androgen regulation of prostate cancer cell FGF-1, FGF-2, and FGF-8: preferential down-regulation of FGF-2 transcripts. *Growth Factors* **16:** 69–87.

132. Scher, H. I., A. Sarkis, V. Reuter, D. Cohen, G. Netto, D. Petrylak, et al. 1995. Changing pattern of expression of the epidermal growth factor receptor and transforming growth factor alpha in the progression of prostatic neoplasms. *Clin. Cancer Res.* **1:** 545–550.

133. Schoenwaelder, S. M. and K. Burridge. 1999. Bidirectional signaling between the cytoskeleton and integrins. *Curr. Opin. Cell Biol.* **11:** 274–286.

134. Schwartz, S. J., C. Caceres, J. Morote, I. De Torres, J. M. Rodriguez-Vallejo, J. Gonzalez, et al. 1999. Gains of the relative genomic content of erbB-1 and erbB-2 in prostate carcinoma and their association with metastasis. *Int. J. Oncol.* **14:** 367–371.

135. Sehgal, I., J. Bailey, K. Hitzemann, M. R. Pittelkow, and N. J. Maihle. 1994. Epidermal growth factor receptor-dependent stimulation of amphiregulin expression in androgen-stimulated human prostate cancer cells. *Mol. Biol. Cell* **5:** 339–347.

136. Sells, M. A., J. T. Boyd, and J. Chernoff. 1999. p21-activated kinase 1 (Pak1) regulates cell motility in mammalian fibroblasts. *J. Cell Biol.* **145:** 837–849.

137. Sells, M. A., U. G. Knaus, S. Bagrodia, D. M. Ambrose, G. M. Bokoch, and J. Chernoff. 1997. Human p21-activated kinase (Pak1) regulates actin organization in mammalian cells. *Curr. Biol.* **7:** 202–210.

138. Shen, R., T. Dorai, M. Szaboles, A. E. Katz, C. A. Olsson, and R. Buttyan. 1997. Transdifferentiation of cultured human prostate cells to a neuroendocrine cell phenotype in a hormone-depleted medium. *Urol. Res.* **3:** 67–75.

139. Siegsmund, M. J., H. Yamazaki, and I. Pastan. 1994. Interleukin 6 receptor mRNA in prostate carcinomas and benign prostate hyperplasia. *J. Urol.* **151:** 1396–1399.

140. Slamon, D. J. 1998. Addition of Herceptin (humanized anti-HER2 antibody) to first line chemotherapy for HER 2 overexpressiong matastatic breast cancer (HER2+/MBC) mark-

edly increases anticancer activity: a randomized, multinational controlled phrase III trial. *Progr. Proc. Am. Soc. Clin. Oncol.* **17.**

141. Sterneck, E., D. R. Kaplan, and P. F. Johnson. 1996. Interleukin-6 induces expression of peripherin and cooperates with Trk receptor signaling to promote neuronal differentiation in PC12 cells. *J. Neurochem.* **67:** 1365–1374.

142. Story, M. T., B. Livingston, L. Baeten, S. J. Swartz, S. C. Jacobs, F. P. Begun, et al. 1989. Cultured human prostate-derived fibroblasts produce a factor that stimulates their growth with properties indistinguishable from basic fibroblast growth factor. *Prostate* **15:** 355–365.

143. Sundareshan, P., R. B. Nagle, and G. T. Bowden. 1999. EGF induces the expression of matrilysin in the human prostate adenocarcinoma cell line, LNCaP (in process citation). *Prostate* **40:** 159–166.

144. Tamagnone, L., I. Lahtinen, T. Mustonen, K. Virtaneva, F. Francis, F. Muscatelli, et al. 1994. BMX, a novel nonreceptor tyrosine kinase gene of the BTK/ITK/TEC/TXK family located in chromosome Xp22.2. *Oncogene* **9:** 3683–3688.

145. Tan, M., R. Grijalva, and D. Yu. 1999. Heregulin beta1-activated phosphatidylinositol 3-kinase enhances aggregation of MCF-7 breast cancer cells independent of extracellular signal-regulated kinase. *Cancer Res.* **59:** 1620–1625.

146. Tanaka, A., A. Furuya, M. Yamasaki, N. Hanai, K. Kuriki, T. Kamiakito, et al. 1998. High frequency of fibroblast growth factor (FGF) 8 expression in clinical prostate cancers and breast tissues, immunohistochemically demonstrated by a newly established neutralizing monoclonal antibody against FGF 8. *Cancer Res.* **58:** 2053–2056.

147. Tillotson, J. K. and D. P. Rose. 1991. Density-dependent regulation of epidermal growth factor receptor expression in DU 145 human prostate cancer cells. *Prostate* **19:** 53–61.

148. Turner, T., P. Chen, L. J. Goodly, and A. Wells. 1996. EGF receptor signaling enhances in vivo invasiveness of DU-145 human prostate carcinoma cells. *Clin. Exp. Metastasis* **14:** 409–418.

149. Turner, T., M. V. Epps-Fung, J. Kassis, and A. Wells. 1997. Molecular inhibition of phospholipase cgamma signaling abrogates DU-145 prostate tumor cell invasion. *Clin. Cancer Res.* **3:** 2275–2282.

150. Vlietstra, R. J., D. C. van Alewijk, K. G. Hermans, G. J. van Steenbrugge, and J. Trapman. 1998. Frequent inactivation of PTEN in prostate cancer cell lines and xenografts. *Cancer Res.* **58:** 2720–2723.

151. Vojtek, A. B., S. M. Hollenberg, and J. A. Cooper. 1993. Mammalian *ras* interacts directly with the serine/threonine kinase Raf. *Cell* **74:** 205–214.

152. Ware, J. L. 1993. Growth factors and their receptors as determinants in the proliferation and metastasis of human prostate cancer. *Cancer Metastasis Rev.* **12:** 287–301.

153. Watanabe, M., T. Nakada, and H. Yuta. 1999. Analysis of protooncogene c-erbB-2 in benign and malignant human prostate. *Int. Urol. Nephrol.* **31:** 61–73.

154. Wilson, C. L. and L. M. Matrisian. 1996. Matrilysin: an epithelial matrix metalloproteinase with potentially novel functions. *Int. J. Biochem. Cell Biol.* **28:** 123–136.

155. Wu, X., K. Senechal, M. S. Neshat, Y. E. Whang, and C. L. Sawyers. 1998. The PTEN/MMAC1 tumor suppressor phosphatase functions as a negative regulator of the phosphoinositide 3-kinase/Akt pathway. *Proc. Natl. Acad. Sci. USA* **95:** 15,587–15,591.

156. Wu, Y. Y. and R. A. Bradshaw. 1996. Induction of neurite outgrowth by interleukin-6 is accompanied by activation of Stat3 signaling pathway in a variant PC12 cell (E2) line. *J. Biol. Chem.* **271:** 13,023–13,032.

157. Xia, Z., M. Dickens, J. Raingeaud, R. J. Davis, and M. E. Greenberg. 1995. Opposing effects of ERK and JNK-p38 MAP kinases on apoptosis. *Science* **270:** 1326–1331.

158. Xie, H., M. A. Pallero, K. Gupta, P. Chang, M. F. Ware, W. Witke, et al. 1998. EGF receptor regulation of cell motility: EGF induces disassembly of focal adhesions inde-

pendently of the motility-associated PLCgamma signaling pathway. *J. Cell Sci.* **111 (Pt 5):** 615–624.

159. Xue, L. Y., Y. Qiu, J. He, H. J. Kung, and N. L. Oleinick. 1999. Etk/Bmx, a PH-domain containing tyrosine kinase, protects prostate cancer cells from apoptosis induced by photodynamic therapy or thapsigargin. *Oncogene* **18:** 3391–3398.

160. Yan, G., Y. Fukabori, G. McBride, S. Nikolaropolous, and W. L. McKeehan. 1993. Exon switching and activation of stromal and embryonic fibroblast growth factor (FGF)-FGF receptor genes in prostate epithelial cells accompany stromal independence and malignancy. *Mol. Cell Biol.* **13:** 4513–4522.

161. Yao, R. and G. M. Cooper. 1995. Requirement for phosphatidylinositol-3 kinase in the prevention of apoptosis by nerve growth factor. *Science* **267:** 2003–2006.

162. Yeh, S., H. K. Lin, H. Y. Kang, T. H. Thin, M. F. Lin, and C. Chang. 1999. From HER2/Neu signal cascade to androgen receptor and its coactivators: a novel pathway by induction of androgen target genes through MAP kinase in prostate cancer cells. *Proc. Natl. Acad. Sci. USA* **96:** 5458–5463.

163. Yu, D., T. Jing, B. Liu, J. Yao, M. Tan, T. J. McDonnell, et al. 1998. Overexpression of ErbB2 blocks Taxol-induced apoptosis by upregulation of p21Cip1, which inhibits p34Cdc2 kinase. *Mol. Cell* **2:** 581–591.

164. Zetser, A., E. Gredinger, and E. Bengal. 1999. p38 mitogen-activated protein kinase pathway promotes skeletal muscle differentiation. Participation of the Mef2c transcription factor. *J. Biol. Chem.* **274:** 5193–5200.

165. Zhau, H. E., L. L. Pisters, M. C. Hall, L. S. Zhao, P. Troncoso, A. Pollack, et al. 1994. Biomarkers associated with prostate cancer progression. *J. Cell Biochem. Suppl.* **19:** 208–216.

166. Zhau, H. Y., J. Zhou, W. F. Symmans, B. Q. Chen, S. M. Chang, R. A. Sikes, et al. 1996. Transfected neu oncogene induces human prostate cancer metastasis. *Prostate* **28:** 73–83.

167. Zi, X., A. W. Grasso, H. J. Kung, and R. Agarwal. 1998. A flavonoid antioxidant, silymarin, inhibits activation of erbB1 signaling and induces cyclin-dependent kinase inhibitors, G1 arrest, and anticarcinogenic effects in human prostate carcinoma DU145 cells. *Cancer Res.* **58:** 1920–1929.

16

Molecular Pathways Underlying Prostate Cancer Progression

The Role of Caveolin-1

Timothy C. Thompson, PhD, Terry L. Timme, PhD, Likun Li, PhD, Chengzen Ren, MS, Alexei Goltsov, PhD, Salahaldin Tahir, PhD, and Guang Yang, MD, PhD

1. INTRODUCTION

In recent years, efforts to detect and treat prostate cancer have increased dramatically throughout the United States, resulting in approximately a threefold increase in the reported incidence of the disease and a dramatic rise in the number of radical prostatectomies and irradiation therapy treatments *(20,24)*. The incidence of prostate cancer has begun to decline (a probable result of saturation by prostate cancer screening), and age-adjusted mortality from prostate cancer (as well as other malignancies) has also declined by approx 5% from 1990 to 1995 *(20,39)*. Unfortunately, the mortality rate remains exceedingly high—a somewhat surprising condition in light of the increased utilization of potentially curative treatment modalities over the last decade. One possible explanation for the low impact of prostate cancer therapy thus far is that occult metastases were present at the time of treatment. The treatments currently used for presumably localized disease are indeed exclusively local treatments that are designed to ablate the primary tumor either surgically or through radiation. Metastatic disease at the time of treatment would therefore continue to progress. The reported failure rate, within 5 yr as indicated by rising prostate specific antigen levels for patients undergoing radical prostatectomy, ranges from 20% *(30)* to 57% *(55)*, indicating the presence of either local tumor recurrence and/or occult metastasis at the time of treatment. The assessment of prostate cancer in regard to stage of disease is complicated by the lack of reliable, specific tests that differentiate localized disease from early metastatic disease, and the highly complex presentation of the local tumor. Localized prostate cancer is exceedingly slow-growing, and exhibits a remarkable degree of morphologic complexity and histologic heterogeneity. Although a prominent index of cancer is typically present, it has long been recognized that prostate cancer is multifocal, usually contains more than one histological grade, and is often juxtaposed and admixed with other benign pathology such as benign prostatic hyperplasia (BPH). The

From: *Prostate Cancer: Biology, Genetics, and the New Therapeutics*
Edited by: L. W. K. Chung, W. B. Isaacs, and J. W. Simons © Humana Press Inc., Totowa, NJ

malignant potential is currently most often assessed by the grading system proposed by Gleason *(11)*. Yet examination of radical prostatectomy specimens of nonpalpable cancers has revealed that up to 45% of high-grade tumors (Gleason grade 4 or 5) were less than 1 cm^3 in vol *(7)*. These clinical data highlight the possibility that highly aggressive disease may present early as small tumors, and does not necessarily develop in a predictable fashion from low-grade tumors *(52)*. The results of other studies also indicate that although there is a general relationship of tumor volume with metastatic progression, relatively small tumors confined to the prostate may also seed metastases *(32,34)*. These clinical observations have been supported by the results of in vivo experiments indicating that metastases do not necessarily originate from the most abundant clone of the malignant cells at the primary site *(47)*. Overall, the complex morphologic patterns, histologic heterogeneity, and early manifestations of high malignant potential preclude a straightforward assessment of the metastatic potential of localized prostate cancer.

Interestingly, available data thus far suggests that the genetic alterations that occur in prostate cancer do not give rise to extensive clonal expansion at the primary tumor site. Therefore, genetic alterations that predispose to metastasis may also be low-frequency occurrences in primary prostate cancer. Yet one would expect that genetic alterations relevant to the metastatic process would be represented at a higher frequency in metastatic lesions. This pattern has been demonstrated for p53 alterations in primary vs metastatic prostate cancer. Mutations in metastatic prostate cancer have been shown to be significantly higher in metastatic lesions when compared to primary tumors from the same patient, supporting a specific role for p53 in the development of metastatic prostate cancer (reviewed in ref. *49*). Because p53 is a transcription factor, alterations in function for the p53 gene product could lead to multiple changes in gene expression that affect potential metastatic activities such as growth arrest, apoptosis, and angiogenesis *(46,49)*. Another example of this type of pattern is the observation that complete inactivation of the tumor suppressor gene PTEN/MMAC1 *(23,40)* is more common in prostate cancer metastases relative to primary tumors *(41)*. PTEN/MMAC1 has been identified as a phosphatidylinositol 3, 4, 5-triphosphatase *(25)*, and through this activity PTEN appears to negatively regulate protein kinase B/AKT and possibly other signaling pathways *(38)*. PTEN can also regulate cellular motility and matrix interactions through focal adhesion kinases *(43)*. An additional specific genetic alteration that has been identified as being specifically associated with metastatic prostate cancer is amplification and overexpression of c-*myc*. Early studies reported overexpression of c-*myc* in prostate cancer at the mRNA level *(2,9)* and more recent analysis of human tissues using *in situ* molecular biology techniques have demonstrated that the c-*myc* gene is amplified at higher frequencies in metastatic tissues relative to their primary tumor counterparts *(1,17)*. It is remarkable that two of these metastasis-related genetic alterations, i.e., p53 mutation and PTEN/MMAC1 inactivation, impart antiapoptotic activities. This suggests that inactivation of apoptotic pathways and/or activation of survival pathways may be critical determinants of the metastatic phenotype.

Although DNA sequence alterations are of primary consideration in understanding the molecular mechanisms underlying cell transformation and malignant progression, recent technical advances in the analysis of large pools of mRNA have dramatically expanded the conceptual framework regarding the molecular profiling of cancer *(33)*. Indeed, recent efforts in gene expression profiling using differential display, SAGE, and microarray analysis have provided indications that alterations in gene expression patterns are highly common in malignant tissues (reviewed in ref. *42*). Efforts are underway in many laboratories to elucidate gene expression patterns in primary tumor vs metastatic human prostate cancer specimens, yet these studies face considerable technical challenges because of the complex pathology and heterogeneity of prostate cancer. Indeed, the molecular changes leading to metastasis in one clone of cells may be obscured by various molecular events occurring simultaneously in cells that are in the same tumor, but not in the metastatic pathway.

2. A MODEL SYSTEM FOR STUDYING PROSTATE CANCER PROGRESSION

The development of a model system that would allow for direct comparisons between "metastatic progenitor cells" and their fully competent metastatic derivatives would maximize the identification of metastasis-related genes by differential screening methods. To implement such a system, we derivatized and extended the in vivo metastatic mouse prostate reconstitution (MPR) mouse model system to an in vitro set of primary tumor and metastasis-derived cell lines used in combination with molecular methods such as differential display-PCR (DD-PCR). Early passage clonal cell lines were generated from primary and metastatic tumors initiated in p53 mutant fetal prostate tissues with Zipras/myc-9, a recombinant retroviral vector encoding the *ras* and *myc* oncogenes *(47,48)*. The clonal relationship of the metastatic progenitor cell with the metastatic derivative cell was confirmed by Southern blotting techniques that identify unique Zipras/myc-9 cDNA junction fragments *(47)*. These clonally matched pairs of cells originated in identical genetic backgrounds, and were used at low passage to collect RNA for use in DD-PCR. Clonally related cell lines derived from primary tumors and their metastases were subsequently tested for metastatic activities in vivo using an orthotopic model *(12)*. Interestingly, in initial studies using these cell lines, we found that sc and orthotopic tumors produced by cell lines derived from metastatic lesions usually grew less rapidly, but demonstrated greater spontaneous metastatic potential than their matched counterpart cell lines derived from the parental primary tumor *(12)*. Overall, this comparison-based model system effectively controls for genetic alterations that are unrelated to the metastatic process, and can be used to identify metastasis-related genes for further validation in human prostate cancer tissue and by functional analysis.

3. IDENTIFICATION OF CAVEOLIN-1 AS A METASTASIS-RELATED GENE IN PROSTATE CANCER

The derivitized MPR model system described here has led to the identification of numerous candidate metastasis-related genes for prostate cancer. One of the sequences identified as being upregulated in metastatic mouse prostate cancer using this system encoded mouse caveolin-1 *(54)*. Caveolins are major structural proteins of caveolae—specialized plasma membrane invaginations that are abundant in smooth muscle cells, adipocytes, and endothelium, and mediate signal transduction activities and molecular transport *(13)*. Initial studies based on our detection of caveolin-1 overexpression using DD-PCR investigated caveolin-1 expression in a large number of primary and metastatic pairs of cell lines derived from the MPR model system. The results indicated that caveolin-1 protein was elevated in metastasis-derived cells relative to their matched primary tumor counterparts *(54)*. We further analyzed human prostate cancer cell lines for caveolin-1 expression, and determined that caveolin-1 was highly expressed in three of four prostate cancer cell lines analyzed. Interestingly, caveolin-1 was not readily detected in the androgen-responsive LNCaP cell line. To further determine the extent of caveolin-1 expression in human metastatic prostate cancer, a series of prostate cancer tissues obtained from primary and metastatic tumors were stained for caveolin-1 using immunohistochemistry. The results indicated that overexpression of caveolin-1 was associated with metastatic progression as primary tumors from prostate cancer patients with lymph node metastases, as well as metastatic lesions *per se*, were positive for caveolin-1 at high frequencies relative to localized tumors and normal glandular epithelium, which demonstrated very low to nondetectable levels of caveolin-1 protein *(54)*.

The functional significance of caveolin-1 overexpression in metastatic prostate cancer was initially explored using metastatic androgen insensitive mouse prostate cancer cell lines. A series of stably transfected antisense caveolin-1 cell lines were generated that showed reduced levels of caveolin-1 protein relative to vector controls in parental cells. Surprisingly, these cell lines were sensitive to castration therapy in vivo, and orthotopic prostate cancer tumors with these cells regressed following castration, whereas vector control clones and parental cells did not *(28)*. Interestingly, when a representative antisense caveolin-1 clone was grown orthotopically in castrated males in vivo, cells isolated from the resulting tumors were androgen insensitive and demonstrated high caveolin-1 and androgen receptor expression. A novel in vitro model system was also used to investigate the response of antisense caveolin-1 clones to hormone withdrawal. The antisense caveolin-1 clones underwent significant apoptosis in the absence of testosterone, whereas vector control clones and parental cell lines did not. Re-expression of relatively high levels of caveolin-1 with a recombinant adenoviral vector in a representative antisense cell line converted these androgen sensitive cells to the androgen insensitive phenotype in vitro, confirming the association of caveolin-1 protein with androgen insensitivity *(28)*.

4. SIGNIFICANCE OF CAVEOLIN-1 OVEREXPRESSION IN PROSTATE CANCER

Caveolin-1 is a protein constituent of caveolae, which play a highly specialized role in the differentiated phenotype of smooth muscle, endothelial cells and adipocytes (reviewed in ref. *13*). In addition to structural functions, caveolae have been shown to mediate signal transduction activities and molecular transport in a cell type specific fashion. Thus far, our laboratory has demonstrated that caveolin-1 is associated with the metastatic phenotype, and is a candidate gene for the androgen-resistant phenotype in prostate cancer. The development of these complex prostate cancer phenotypes is often discussed and studied independently, and no definitive link has yet been established between them. However, our data raises the question of whether some degree of androgen resistance is an inherent characteristic of the metastatic phenotype in prostate cancer and contributes in some way to its development. Interestingly, two papers published after our reports provided correlative evidence that caveolin-1 is also associated with the drug-resistant phenotype. A multiple drug-resistant human colon-carcinoma cell line and a adriamycin-resistant human breast cancer cell line demonstrated significant caveolin-1 upregulation independent of P-glycoprotein expression *(21)*. Independently, significant caveolin-1 upregulation was also reported in taxol and epithilone B-resistant lung carcinoma cell lines and a vinblastine-resistant ovarian cancer cell line *(53)*. These data linking caveolin-1 overexpression with drug resistance are congruent with our data associating caveolin-1 upregulation with androgen resistance. Indeed, as we have proposed *(45)*, these observations suggest a possible overlapping common protective/survival function for caveolin-1 in regard to androgen and drug resistance.

Remarkably, caveolin-1 can also induce growth suppression of some transformed cells *(5,22)* and in general, metastasis-derived mouse prostate cancer cells that overexpress caveolin-1 have a slower growth rate in vitro and in vivo than primary tumor-derived mouse prostate cancer cells that have lower levels of caveolin-1 *(12)*. However, arguments for an explicit tumor suppressor role for caveolin-1 appear tenuous at this time. The caveolin-1 gene has been mapped to human chromosome 7q31.1 which has been reported as a frequent site of loss of heterozygosity in multiple tumor types such as prostate cancer *(6,16)*. However, in prostate cancer, this chromosomal region often has amplification or gain of genetic material when evaluated by either comparative genomic hybridization or fluorescent *in situ* hybridization *(29)*. Furthermore, mutation analysis of the caveolin-1 gene in a large set of mouse and human prostate cancer cell lines *(16)* (and Ren et al., unpublished observations) failed to identify mutations consistent with tumor suppressor activity.

Specific information is only beginning to emerge regarding caveolin-1 overexpression in the natural history of prostate cancer, and possibly other malignancies *(54)*—yet certain concepts and themes can be considered. Because increased frequencies of caveolin-1-positive prostate cancer cells were found within the lymph nodes of patients who had not been treated with anti-androgen therapy, it can be inferred that these cells were not selected by conditions generated by extrinsic hormone manipulation, but by "normal" conditions in the metastatic pathway. Our experimental results also indicate that mouse prostate cancer cells with high caveolin-1 levels are more resistant to androgen ablation-induced apoptosis *(28)*. As a whole, the results of these studies suggest that coselection for the metastatic and androgen resistant phenotypes based on common properties in the metastatic and castration-induced environment can occur *(45)*. Following castration, levels of testosterone are abruptly and dramatically reduced within the prostate to exceedingly low levels *(19)*. Reduced testosterone can lead to protease-mediated loss of normal cell–cell and cell–matrix interactions *(44)* and alterations in the patterns of expression for multiple-growth factors *(4)*, including EGF *(14)* in prostate tissues. Reduced intraprostatic blood flow also occurs upon castration *(35)*. Metastatic cells seeded into either the lymphatics or general vasculature from the prostatic environment may encounter similar environmental stresses that exist within the prostate gland following castration. In the vascular compartment various plasma proteins bind steroids *(3)* so that when metastatic cells enter, they may be exposed to an abrupt reduction in free testosterone as well as significant alterations in polypeptide growth-factor levels. The loss of appropriate cell–cell and cell–matrix interactions also occurs during metastatic seeding of cells into the vasculature. Hypoxic conditions may also be encountered at various points in the metastatic pathway. It is conceivable, therefore, that cells that escape the prostate during metastatic progression are selected for survival based on properties that overlap with those necessary for survival in the castrated environment.

As discussed here, our recent data indicate that caveolin-1 expression suppresses apoptotic cell death in the absence of testosterone in androgen sensitive mouse prostate cancer cells in vitro and that androgen ablation can lead to selection for the outgrowth of caveolin-1 positive, androgen insensitive mouse prostate cancer cells in vivo *(28)*. These results raise the question of whether testosterone levels can regulate the expression of caveolin-1. Since normal luminal prostate epithelial cells (generally believed to be the direct precursors of malignant cells) have very low caveolin-1 levels *(54)*, and a significant fraction of both human and mouse prostate cancer lymph node metastases that occurred in intact males were shown to express caveolin-1 *(54)*, it seems likely that prostate cancer cells acquire the capacity to upregulate caveolin-1 at some point during the process of transformation/metastatic progression in the presence of physiologically normal testosterone levels. However, surgical castration leads to the outgrowth of caveolin-1 positive, androgen-insensitive mouse prostate cancer cells, suggesting complex regulation of caveolin-1 by testosterone in vivo. Although direct stimulatory effects of testosterone on caveolin-1 gene expression may occur, it seems likely that additonal regulatory pathways for caveolin-1 gene expression are involved in prostate cancer. Although recent studies have failed to demonstrate that gene methylation is involved in caveolin-1 expression in prostate cancer *(16)*, this possibility needs further study. It is also conceivable that polypeptide growth factors regulate caveolin-1 expression in prostate cancer cells. Previous studies have documented that specific growth factors can modulate caveolin-1 protein levels in NIH3T3 cells *(10)*, yet additional studies are required to determine the effects of growth factors on caveolin-1 expression in prostate cancer. Interestingly, one of the candidate growth factors for regulation of caveolin-1 expression basic fibroblast growth factor (FGF-2), is under androgenic control in prostate cancer cells *(56)*, and is expressed in prostatic stromal cells *(27)*. A better understanding of the molecular mechanisms underlying caveolin-1 expression in prostate cancer cells is needed. Fuller investigations of the downstream effects of caveolin-1 in cancer cells are also of critical importance.

5. CAVEOLIN-1 AS A SURVIVAL FACTOR IN PROSTATE CANCER

Specific molecular activities associated with caveolin-1/caveolae may provide a mechanistic link between the response of prostatic epithelial cells to androgen ablation and metastatic progression. Caveolae are involved in calcium transport, storage, and potentially Ca^{++}-mediated signaling in various nonprostatic cells *(36)*. In the prostate, widespread apoptosis following androgen ablation in vivo is the result of increased intracellular Ca^{++} levels within prostatic glandular cells which drive Ca^{++}/Mg^{++}-dependent endonuclease activities *(18,26)*. This provides a conceptual framework for studies that attempt to reconcile coselection for metastasis and androgen resistance in prostate cancer based on the modulation of and/or response to Ca^{++}-mediated signal transduction by elevated caveolin-1/caveolae levels.

The association of caveolin-1 overexpression with drug resistance is also consistent with survival functions of caveolin-1/caveolae in malignancy. There are interesting functional similarities between caveolin-1 and well-established drug resistant genes such as P-glycoprotein. P-glycoprotein is a plasma membrane ATPase and energy-dependent drug efflux pump that can effectively reduce high intracellular concentration of cytotoxic molecules, leading to multidrug resistance and enhanced survival in P-glycoprotein-expressing cancer cells *(51)*. This mechanism of action can be compared to the molecular transport properties of caveolin-1 *(13)*. Caveolin-1/caveolae transports intracellular cholesterol to the cell surface for efflux from the cell *(8)*. Alternatively, many drugs such as taxol can activate a variety of signal transduction pathways that could be subverted or blocked by caveolin-1/caveolae. Caveolin-1/caveolae also regulate multiple signalling pathways including nitric oxide synthase, mitogen-activated kinases, and lipid-signaling molecules (reviewed in refs. *31,36*), and thereby provide potential overlapping downstream activities through which caveolin-1 could potentially modulate the effects of cytotoxic drugs such as taxol.

To reconcile the survival vs growth-suppressive functions of caveolin-1, and to further extend these concepts, it is interesting to consider the properties of the bcl-2 family of genes. Bcl-2 and other family members can block entry into the cell cycle, and thus inhibit growth but also provide well-defined survival functions *(50)*. During differentiation of myelomonocytic progenitor cells, bcl-2 appears to potentiate cell-cycle arrest and irreversible withdrawal into the nonproliferating (G0) state. Subsequent activities of differentiation inducers then allow for the cell to commit to the differentiation pathway. Functional maturation of these cells appears to downregulate bcl-2 levels and thus lead to apoptosis. However, during the maturation process, overexpression of bcl-2 can protect the cells from various apoptotic stimuli. A recent study also demonstrated that unlike low levels of bcl-2 protein, which exhibit antiapoptotic activities, high levels of bcl-2 can exhibit proapoptotic activities in human glioma cells *(37)*. Although analogies to human prostatic cell differentiation may be premature, the fully differentiated and secretory prostatic cell demonstrates low to undetectable levels of caveolin-1 *(54)*, and therefore may be poised to undergo apoptosis following a variety of stimuli, including withdrawal of androgenic steroids. Since bcl-2 also protects against cytotoxic drugs, it has been suggested that the properties of bcl-2 involved in blocking entry into the cell cycle, as well as its protective activities, could provide double protection against drugs—as both cell-cycle entry and response to apoptotic stimuli are required for effective induction of apoptosis by chemotherapeutic agents *(15)*.

The available information clearly points to a possible overlap among the metastatic, the androgen-resistant, and the drug resistant phenotypes through overexpression of caveolin-1. The conditional inhibitory effects of caveolin-1 on cell growth and the rapidly growing body of data that assign it antiapoptotic functions can be compared to the well-studied properties of the bcl-2 family of genes.

6. CONCLUSION

We have provided evidence indicating that caveolin-1 overexpression is associated with metastasis and the androgen-resistant phenotype in prostate cancer. Additionally, caveolin-1 overexpression occurs during the development of resistance to chemotherapeutic drugs in multiple human cancer cell lines. The possible overlap of relevant characteristics between the metastatic environment and that induced in prostate tissue by castration could provide the conceptual framework to explain coselection for metastasis and androgen resistance in prostate cancer cells. Metastatic prostate cancer cells lose appropriate cell–cell and cell–matrix interactions as they enter the vasculature, where they are exposed to significant alterations in the level of available androgens and polypeptide growth factors. Similar conditions are associated with the prostate environment following castration. Therefore, it is conceivable that during metastatic progression, prostate cancer cells are selected in part for survival in the metastatic environment based on properties that overlap with those necessary for survival in a castration environment. Extrapolation to drug resistance of this overlapping selection criteria concept for metastasis/androgen resistance is facilitated by consideration of the general properties of caveolin-1/caveolae. Based on the antiapoptotic properties and the potential to interact with signal transduction cascades that may intersect with those stimulated by chemotherapeutic drugs, caveolin-1 overexpression establishes a general paradigm of protection to both natural and cytotoxic drug-mediated barriers to malignant progression. Recent reports demonstrating that caveolin-1 can suppress growth under some conditions are not inconsistent with the antiapoptotic functions of caveolin-1, and with antiapoptotic genes in general. For example, under some conditions, bcl-2 gene-family members can block entry into the cell cycle, yet also protect against many apoptotic stimuli. Certainly, these concepts and speculations are untested, but they do provide a framework for relevant questions to be addressed in future studies. However, because of the rapid accumulation of information associating upregulation of caveolin-1 with metastasis and androgen and drug resistance, this area of investigation should be the focus of numerous studies that seek to understand the functional significance of caveolin-1 as a survival factor as well as the various levels of regulation that control its expression in prostate cancer.

REFERENCES

1. Bubendorf, L., J. Kononen, P. Koivisto, P. Schraml, H. Moch, T. C. Gasser, et al. 1999. Survey of gene amplifications during prostate cancer progression by high-throughput fluorescence in situ hybridization on tissue microarrays. *Cancer Res.* **59:** 803–806.
2. Buttyan, R., I. S. Sawczuk, M. C. Benson, J. D. Siegal, and C. A. Olsson. 1987. Enhanced expression of the c-myc protooncogene in high-grade human prostate cancers. *Prostate* **11:** 327–337.
3. Coffey, D. S. 1986. *Endocrine control of normal and abnormal growth of the prostate*, in *Urologic Endocrinology*, (Rajfer J., ed.), WB Saunders, Philadelphia, PA, pp. 170–195.
4. Egawa, S., D. Kadmon, G. J. Miller, P. T. Scardino, and T. C. Thompson. 1992. Alterations in mRNA levels for growth-related genes after transplantation into castrated hosts in oncogene-induced clonal mouse prostate carcinoma. *Mol. Carcinog.* **5:** 52–61.
5. Engelman, J. A., C. C. Wykoff, S. Yasuhara, K. S. Song, T. Okamoto, and M. P. Lisanti. 1997. Recombinant expression of caveolin-1 in oncogenically transformed cells abrogates anchorage-independent growth. *J. Biol. Chem.* **272:** 16,374–16,381.

6. Engelman, J. A., X. L. Zhang, F. Galbiati, and M. P. Lisanti. 1998. Chromosomal localization, genomic organization, and developmental expression of the murine caveolin gene family (Cav-1, -2, and -3). Cav- 1 and Cav-2 genes map to a known tumor suppressor locus (6-A2/7q31). *FEBS Lett.* **429:** 330–336.

7. Epstein, J., M. Carmichael, A. Partin, and P. Walsh. 1994. Small high grade adenocarcinoma of the prostate in radical prostatectomy specimens performed for nonpalpable disease: pathogenetic and clinical implications. *J. Urol.* **151:** 1587–1592.

8. Fielding, P. E. and C. J. Fielding. 1995. Plasma membrane caveolae mediate the efflux of cellular free cholesterol. *Biochemistry* **34:** 14,288–14,292.

9. Fleming, W. H., A. Hamel, R. MacDonald, E. Ramsey, N. M. Pettigrew, B. Johnston, et al. 1986. Expression of the c-myc protooncogene in human prostatic carcinoma and benign prostatic hyperplasia. *Cancer Res.* **46:** 1535–1538.

10. Galbiati, F., D. Volonte, J. A. Engelman, G. Watanabe, R. Burk, R. G. Pestell, et al. 1998. Targeted downregulation of caveolin-1 is sufficient to drive cell transformation and hyperactivate the p42/44 MAP kinase cascade. *EMBO J.* **17:** 6633–6648.

11. Gleason, D. 1997. *Histologic grading and clinical staging of prostatic carcinoma*, in *Urologic pathology: The Prostate*, (Tannenbaum M., ed.), Lea & Febiger, Philadelphia, pp. 171–197.

12. Hall, S. J. and T. C. Thompson. 1997. Spontaneous but not experimental metastatic activities differentiate primary tumor-derived vs metastasis-derived mouse prostate cancer cell lines. *Clin. Exp. Metastasis* **15:** 630–638.

13. Harder, T. and K. Simons. 1997. Caveolae, DIGs, and the dynamics of sphingolipid-cholesterol microdomains. *Curr. Opin. Cell Biol.* **9:** 534–542.

14. Hiramatsu, M., M. Kashimata, N. Minami, A. Sato, and M. Murayama. 1988. Androgenic regulation of epidermal growth factor in the mouse ventral prostate. *Biochem. Int.* **17:** 311–317.

15. Huang, D. C. S., L. A. O'Reilly, A. Strasser, and S. Cory. 1997. The anti-apoptosis function of Bcl-2 can be genetically separated from its inhibitory effect on cell cycle entry. *EMBO J.* **16:** 4628–4638.

16. Hurlstone, A. F., G. Reid, J. R. Reeves, J. Fraser, G. Strathdee, M. Rahilly, et al. 1999. Analysis of the CAVEOLIN-1 gene at human chromosome 7q31.1 in primary tumours and tumour-derived cell lines. *Oncogene* **18:** 1881–1890.

17. Jenkins, R. B., J. Qian, M. M. Lieber, and D. G. Bostwick. 1997. Detection of c-myc oncogene amplification and chromosomal anomalies in metastatic prostatic carcinoma by fluorescence *in situ* hybridization. *Cancer Res.* **57:** 524–531.

18. Kyprianou, N., H. F. English, and J. T. Isaacs. 1988. Activation of a Ca2+-Mg2+-dependent endonuclease as an early event in castration-induced prostatic cell death. *Prostate* **13:** 103–117.

19. Kyprianou, N. and J. T. Isaacs. 1987. Biological significance of measurable androgen levels in the rat ventral prostate following castration. *Prostate* **10:** 313–324.

20. Landis, S. H., T. Murray, S. Bolden, and P. A. Wingo. 1999. Cancer Statistics, 1999. *CA Cancer J. Clin.* **49:** 8–31.

21. Lavie, Y., G. Fiucci, and M. Liscovitch. 1998. Up-regulation of caveolae and caveolar constituents in multidrug-resistant cancer cells. *J. Biol. Chem.* **273:** 32,380–32,383.

22. Lee, S. W., C. L. Reimer, P. Oh, D. B. Campbell, and J. E. Schnitzer. 1998. Tumor cell growth inhibition by caveolin re-expression in human breast cancer cells. *Oncogene* **16:** 1391–1397.

23. Li, J., C. Yen, D. Liaw, K. Podsypanina, S. Bose, S. I. Wang, et al. 1997. PTEN, a putative protein tyrosine phosphatase gene mutated in human brain, breast, and prostate cancer. *Science* **275:** 1943–1947.

24. Lu-Yan, G., D. McLarren, J. Wasson, and J. Wennberg. 1993. An assessment of radical prostatectomy time trends, geographic variation and outcomes. The prostate patient outcomes research Team,. *JAMA* **269:** 2633–2636.

25. Maehama, T. and J. E. Dixon. 1998. The tumor suppressor, PTEN/MMAC1, dephosphory-lates the lipid second messenger, phosphatidylinositol 3,4,5-trisphosphate. *J. Biol. Chem.* **273:** 13,375–13,378.

26. Martikainen, P. and J. Isaacs. 1990. Role of calcium in the programmed death of rat prostatic glandular cells. *Prostate* **17:** 175–187.

27. McKeehan, W., M. Kan, J. Hou, F. Wang, P. Adams, and P. Mansson. 1991. *Heparin-binding (fibroblast) growth factor/receptor gene expression in the prostate*, in *Molecular and Cellular Biology of Prostate Cancer* (Karr, J., D. S. Coffey, R. G. Smith, and D. J. Tindall, eds.). Plenum Press, New York, pp. 115–126.

28. Nasu, Y., T. L. Timme, G. Yang, C. H. Bangma, L. Li, C. Ren, et al. 1998. Suppression of caveolin expression induces androgen sensitivity in metastatic androgen-insensitive mouse prostate cancer cells. *Nat. Med.* **4:** 1062–1064.

29. Nupponen, N. N., L. Kakkola, P. Koivisto, and T. Visakorpi. 1998. Genetic alterations in hormone-refractory recurrent prostate carcinomas. *Am. J. Pathol.* **153:** 141–148.

30. Ohori, M., J. R. Goad, T. M. Wheeler, J. A. Eastham, T. C. Thompson, and P. T. Scardino. 1994. Can radical prostatectomy alter the progression of poorly differentiated prostate cancer? *J. Urol.* **152:** 1843–1849.

31. Okamoto, T., A. Schlegel, P. E. Scherer, and M. P. Lisanti. 1998. Caveolins, a family of scaffolding proteins for organizing "preassembled signaling complexes" at the plasma membrane. *J. Biol. Chem.* **273:** 5419–5422.

32. Qian, J., D. G. Bostwick, S. Takahashi, T. J. Borell, J. F. Herath, M. M. Lieber, et al. 1995. Chromosomal anomalies in prostatic intraepithelial neoplasia and carcinoma detected by fluorescence *in situ* hybridization. *Cancer Res.* **55:** 5408–5414.

33. Sager, R., S. Sheng, A. Anisowicz, G. Sotiropoulou, Z. Zou, G. Stenman, et al. 1994. RNA genetics of breast cancer: maspin as paradigm. *Cold Sprg. Hrbr. Symp. Quant. Biol.* **59:** 537–546.

34. Sakr, W. A., J. A. Macoska, P. Benson, D. J. Grignon, S. R. Wolman, J. E. Pontes, et al. 1994. Allelic loss in locally metastatic, multisampled prostate cancer. *Cancer Res.* **54:** 3273–3277.

35. Shabsigh, A., D. T. Chang, D. F. Heitjan, A. Kiss, C. A. Olsson, P. J. Puchner, et al. 1998. Rapid reduction in blood flow to the rat ventral prostate gland after castration: preliminary evidence that androgens influence prostate size by regulating blood flow to the prostate gland and prostatic endothelial cell survival. *Prostate* **36:** 201–206.

36. Shaul, P. W. and R. G. Anderson. 1998. Role of plasmalemmal caveolae in signal trans-duction. *Am. J. Physiol.* **275:** L843–851.

37. Shinoura, N., Y. Yoshida, M. Nishimura, Y. Muramatsu, A. Asai, T. Kirino, et al. 1999. Expression level of Bcl-2 determines anti- or proapoptotic function. *Cancer Res.* **59:** 4119–4128.

38. Stambolic, V., A. Suzuki, J. L. de la Pompa, G. M. Brothers, C. Mirtsos, T. Sasaki, et al. 1998. Negative regulation of PKB/Akt-dependent cell survival by the tumor suppressor PTEN. *Cell* **95:** 29–39.

39. Stanford, J., R. Stephenson, L. Coyle, J. Cerhan, R. Correa, J. Eley, et al. 1999. *Prostate Cancer Trends 1973–1995, SEER Program*. National Cancer Institute. NIH Pub. No. 99-4543, Bethesda, MD.

40. Steck, P. A., M. A. Pershouse, S. A. Jasser, W. K. Yung, H. Lin, A. H. Ligon, et al. 1997. Identification of a candidate tumour suppressor gene, MMAC1, at chromosome 10q23.3 that is mutated in multiple advanced cancers. *Nat. Genet.* **15:** 356–362.

41. Suzuki, H., D. Freije, D. R. Nusskern, K. Okami, P. Cairns, D. Sidransky, et al. 1998. Interfocal heterogeneity of PTEN/MMAC1 gene alterations in multiple metastatic prostate cancer tissues. *Cancer Res.* **58:** 204–209.

42. Szallasi, Z. 1998. Bioinformatics. Gene expression patterns and cancer. *Nat. Biotechnol.* **16:** 1292–1293.

43. Tamura, M., J. Gu, K. Matsumoto, S. Aota, R. Parsons, and K. M. Yamada. 1998. Inhibition of cell migration, spreading, and focal adhesions by tumor suppressor PTEN. *Science* **280:** 1614–1617.
44. Tenniswood, M. P., M. L. Montpetit, and J. G. Leger. 1990. Epithelial-stromal interactions and cell death in the prostate, in *The prostate as an endocrine gland* (Farnsworth, W. E. and R. J. Ablin, eds.), CRC Press, Boca Raton, FL. pp. 187–204.
45. Thompson, T., T. Timme, L. Li, A. Goltsov, and G. Yang. 1999. Caveolin-1: a complex and provocative therapeutic target in prostate cancer and potentially other malignancies. *Emerging Therapeutic Targets* **3:** 337–346.
46. Thompson, T., T. Timme, and I. Sehgal. 1996. The role of p53 in prostate cancer progression, in *Accomplishments in cancer research, 1996* (Fortner, J. and P. Sharp, eds.), Lippincott-Raven Publishers, Philadelphia, pp. 280–289.
47. Thompson, T. C., S. H. Park, T. L. Timme, C. Ren, J. A. Eastham, L. A. Donehower, et al. 1995. Loss of p53 function leads to metastasis in ras+myc-initiated mouse prostate cancer. *Oncogene* **10:** 869–879.
48. Thompson, T. C., J. Southgate, G. Kitchener, and H. Land. 1989. Multistage carcinogenesis induced by ras and myc oncogenes in a reconstituted organ. *Cell* **56:** 917–930.
49. Thompson, T. C., T. L. Timme, and I. Sehgal. 1998. Oncogenes, growth factors, and hormones in prostate cancer, in *Hormones and growth factors in development and neoplasia*, (Dickson, R. B. and D. S. Salomon, eds.), Wiley-Liss, Inc., New York, pp. 327–359.
50. Vairo, G., K. M. Innes, and J. M. Adams. 1996. Bcl-2 has a cell cycle inhibitory function separable from its enhancement of cell survival. *Oncogene* **13:** 1511–1519.
51. van Veen, H. W. and W. N. Konings. 1997. Multidrug transporters from bacteria to man: similarities in structure and function. *Semin. Cancer Biol.* **8:** 183–191.
52. Whitmore, W. 1990. Natural history of low stage prostatic cancer and the impact of early detection. *Urol. Clin. N. Am.* **17:** 689–700.
53. Yang, C. P., F. Galbiati, D. Volonte, S. B. Horwitz, and M. P. Lisanti. 1998. Upregulation of caveolin-1 and caveolae organelles in Taxol-resistant A549 cells. *FEBS Lett.* **439:** 368–372.
54. Yang, G., L. D. Truong, T. L. Timme, C. Ren, T. M. Wheeler, S. H. Park, et al. 1998. Elevated expression of caveolin is associated with prostate and breast cancer. *Clin. Cancer Res.* **4:** 1873–1880.
55. Zeitman, A., R. Edelstein, J. Coen, R. Babayan, and R. Krane. 1994. Radical prostatectomy for adenocarcinoma of the prostate: the influence of preoperative and pathologic findings on biochemical disease-free outcome. *Urology* **43:** 828–833.
56. Zuck, B., C. Goepfert, A. Nedlin-Chittka, K. Sohrt, K. D. Voigt, and C. Knabbe. 1992. Regulation of fibroblast growth factor-like protein(s) in the androgen-responsive human prostate carcinoma cell line LNCaP. *J. Steroid Biochem. Mol. Biol.* **41:** 659–663.

17

Angiogenesis and Prostate Cancer

Ingrid B. J. K . Joseph, DVM, PhD and John T. Isaacs, PhD

1. INTRODUCTION

Prostate cancer is the most commonly diagnosed nonskin malignancy in American men, with an estimated 184,000 new cases projected for 2000 *(8)*. It will be responsible for more than 34,000 deaths this year, ranking it second only to lung cancer in cancer-related mortality *(8)*. Two features make prostate cancer relatively unique among neoplasms—its androgen sensitivity and its relatively low growth fraction. It has been known for almost 60 years that androgen deprivation through surgical or chemical castration results in significant tumor regression *(29,162,169)*. Recently, the mechanism for this regression has been demonstrated to be caused by induction of programmed cell death in the androgen responsive prostate cancer cells *(38)*. Unfortunately, this effect is transient, and inevitably selects for cell populations that can grow independent of androgens. It is believed that prostate cancer begins as a single androgen sensitive cell and expands clonally *(38)*. Over time, this clonal population develops genetic alterations, some of which lead to androgen independence. Thus, by the time of clinical detection, these cancers are composed of heterogeneous populations ranging from androgen dependent to androgen sensitive and independent cells. At this point, although androgen ablation can result in significant cell death of the androgen dependent cells, it eventually selects for androgen sensitive and independent cancer cells. In reference to the low-growth fraction, at any given time the vast majority of the prostate cancer cells are in a proliferatively quiescent (i.e., nondividing) state termed G_0, which makes them relatively resistant to many of the traditional chemotherapeutic agents that are targeted at dividing cells. Normal prostate glandular cells have an extremely low proliferation rate (approx 0.2%/d), which is balanced by the rate of death, and thus no net growth of the gland occurs *(17)*. In metastatic prostate cancer patients, the median proliferation rate of cancer cells within lymph nodes is 3.1%/d, and the median death rate is about 1.1%/d *(17)*. In the bone, the median proliferation rate of prostate cancer cells is low—about 2.2%/d, and the death rate is about 2.1% d *(17)*. These figures demonstrate that the proliferation rate for metastatic prostate cancer cells is remarkably low (<3%/d), and this explains why antiproliferative chemotherapy has had limited value against metastatic disease.

Based on the distinct characteristics that prostate cancer progresses to androgen independence and it has such a low growth fraction, the therapeutic challenge is to find

From: *Prostate Cancer: Biology, Genetics, and the New Therapeutics*
Edited by: L. W. K. Chung, W. B. Isaacs, and J. W. Simons © Humana Press Inc., Totowa, NJ

nonandrogen ablation approaches to induce death of androgen independent prostate cancer cells without requiring them to be proliferatively dividing. There are at least three targets for proliferation independent activation of programmed cell death in the prostate cancer cells. The first is to stimulate the host immune system to induce a cytotoxic antitumor response. Several laboratories around the country are currently exploring this approach. Recently, an autologous granulocyte macrophage-colony stimulating factor (GM-CSF) vaccine has been initiated for the treatment of androgen refractory prostate cancer in patients *(168)*. The second approach is to target the DNA synthesis independent intracellular pathways to activate the programmed-cell-death pathway within the cancer cells, since they still retain the machinery required to undergo programmed cell death despite becoming androgen independent. A number of drugs have been developed that interfere with the intracellular signaling pathways, and are at various stages of testing *(40,43,63)*. The third approach is to block tumor angiogenesis.

Since Dr. Judah Folkman first proposed the idea that tumor growth is dependent on angiogenesis in 1971, researchers around the world have analyzed the process and developed over 300 antiangiogenic compounds which are in various stages of testing *(122)*. If successful, these antiangiogenic therapies would offer the possibility of improved efficacy and reduce toxicity associated with current chemotherapeutic regimens. There are several advantages to targeting the endothelium over that of directly targeting tumor cells themselves with conventional therapies. The vascular endothelial cells are directly accessible to circulating antiangiogenic therapies, thus alleviating the need to penetrate deep into the tumor tissue *(147)*. Conventional chemotherapeutic agents must cross the endothelial lining of the tumor blood vessel to reach the extracellular space and travel through extracellular matrix (ECM) to arrive at the tumor *(184)*. Then they must travel to poorly vascularized hypoxic areas of the tumor. High interstitial pressure in the tumor and low microvessel pressure may offer resistance to extravasation into tumor tissue *(129,130)*. A single capillary supports a large number of tumor cells *(184)*. Thus, inhibition of a few capillaries should theoretically disrupt the exponential growth of a large number of tumor cells. Tumor cells are genetically unstable, have enhanced survivability, and are prone to acquiring drug resistance *(184)*. Endothelial cells are diploid nontransformed, genetically stable cells that are normally quiescent *(184)*. Therefore, with chronic treatment they are less likely to acquire drug resistance. This is exemplified by clinically successful chronic use of α-interferon for the treatment of hemangiomas *(202)*. Since the initial steps of the metastatic cascade of events are similar to angiogenesis, antiangiogenic agents should also prevent metastasis by preventing the access of tumor cells to the vasculature.

2. GENERAL OVERVIEW OF VASCULOGENESIS AND ANGIOGENESIS

Vascular development consists of two stages: an early stage termed vasculogenesis and a later stage termed angiogenesis. Vasculogenesis involves the *in situ* differentiation of endothelial cells from the mesodermally derived precursors and the assembly of these cells into discrete blood vessels, which then form a primitive vascular network *(152,153)*. This network is subsequently transformed into the mature vasculature through an angiogenic remodeling process that encompasses sprouting, branching,

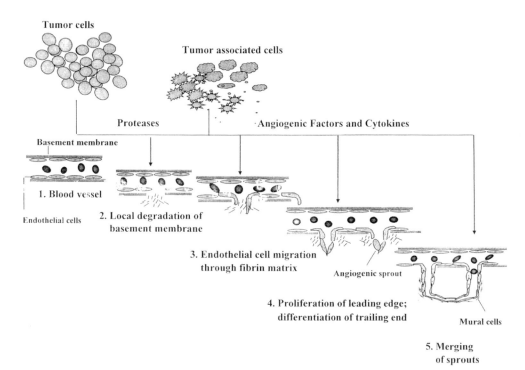

Fig. 1. Schematic representation of sequential steps in the angiogenic process. Under the influence of proteases, angiogenic factors, and cytokines, basement membrane degradation, endothelial cell migration, and proliferation takes place. Migrated endothelial cells differentiate to form a basement membrane around the newly formed vascular sprout. Sprouts formed from different parental vessels merge to form a vessel along which transport of blood occurs. Recruitment of mural cells leads to stabilization of the newly formed vascular bed.

pruning, differential growth of vessels, and the recruitment of supporting mural cells. Angiogenesis occurs both in embryogenesis and postnatal life. Angiogenesis that occurs in postnatal life—i.e. in the process of wound healing *(36)* and during the female reproductive cycle (e.g., during ovulation and gestation) *(155,201)*—is tightly regulated. The angiogenic process associated with normal tissue growth of the body is stopped after the tissue needs are met. In contrast, angiogenesis that occurs in pathological conditions such as diabetic retinopathy, macular degeneration, neovascular glaucoma, psoriasis, arthritis, and hemangiomas, and in malignancies, continues and thus results in aberrant tissue growth.

Angiogenesis, the formation of new blood vessels from preexisting vessels, is a multistep process involving more than just endothelial cell proliferation (Fig. 1) *(152)*. Under the influence of stimulatory angiogenic factors (Table 1), the quiescent endothelial cells degrade the underlying basement membrane and migrate through a provisional matrix formed by fibrin deposits that are formed by leaked fibrinogen from the vessels. Proliferation of endothelial cells occurs at the leading edge of what becomes a migrating column. Differentiation of migrated endothelial cells trails behind the advancing front to form a basal membrane around the newly formed vascular sprout. Sprouts formed from different parental vessels eventually merge to form a vessel along

Table 1
Endogenous Regulators of Angiogenesis

Stimulating factors	Inhibitory factors
Fibroblast growth factor [acidic (aFGF) and basic (bFGF)]	Angiostatin
Transforming growth factor-α (TGF-α)	Endostatin
Transforming growth factor-β (TGF-β)	Antithrombin
Tumor necrosis factor-α (TNF-α)	Interferon-α (INF-α)
Placental growth factor (PlGF)	Interferon-β (INF-β)
Platelet-derived growth factor (PDGF)	Interferon-γ (INF-γ)
Platelet-derived endothelial cell-growth factor (PD-ECGF)	Interferon-γ inducible
Granulocyte- and granulocyte-macrophage-	protein (IP-10)
colony-stimulating factor (G-CSF and GM-CSF)	Interleukin 1α and β
Vascular endothelial-growth factor/	Interleukin 12 (IL-12)
Vascular permeability factor (VEGF/VPF)	Platelet factor 4
Hepatocyte growth factor/scatter factor (HGF/SF)	Prolactin 16-kd fragment
Pleotropin (PTN)	
Proliferin	TGF-β
Prostaglandin E1, E2	TNF-α
Insulin-like growth factor 1 (IGF-1) (Somatomedin C)	Thrombospondin-1, -2
Interleukin 1 (IL-1)	Tissue inhibitor of
Interleukin 6 (IL-6)	metalloproteinase-1 and –2
Interleukin 8 (IL-8)	1,25-Dihydroxy-vitamin D3
Angiotropin	Retinoic acid
Angiopoietin-1	Plasminogen activator inhibitor
Angiotensin-converting enzyme (ACE)	types 1 and 2 (PAI-1, PAI-2)

which transport of blood can occur. Stabilization of the newly formed vascular bed is achieved by recruitment of mural cells.

3. ROLE OF MURAL CELLS IN ANGIOGENESIS

During the process of angiogenesis, a considerable amount of vascular remodeling occurs. This is the process through which the newly formed vascular tubes become a stable and mature vascular bed, and is mediated by the recruitment of mural cells—i.e., smooth muscle cells (SMCs) and pericytes to assume a perivascular position (Fig. 1) *(35)*. Studies by Alon et al. *(6)* have shown that during their development, vessels are dependent on exogenous survival factors such as vascular endothelial growth factor (VEGF) for a critical period. Subsequently, they reported that the association of newly forming vascular tubes with the mural cells marks the end of this critical period of growth factor dependence *(16)*. Thus, although VEGF is essential to sustain the newly formed vessels, this survival factor is dispensable for the mature vascular network *(6)*. Some of the molecular signals that can promote vascular maturation have been identified recently. Tie-1 and Tie-2 receptors are specifically expressed in developing vascular endothelial cells, and have distinct roles in blood vessel formation *(160)*. The former is important for vascular network formation, and the latter confers structural integrity to the vessel *(160)*. Tie-2 and its ligands, angiopoietin-1 (Ang1), and angiopoietin-2

(Ang2)—as well as the related orphan receptor Tie-1—have been shown to play important roles in the recruitment of mural cells *(37,67,119,175,176)*. Ang2 is the endogenous inhibitor of the Tie-2 receptor *(119)*. Ang2 expression is highest during the early stages of angiogenesis, perhaps minimizing Tie2 activity to allow newly forming vasculature to respond to angiogenic stimuli *(119)*. Subsequently, Ang2 expression is decreased and Ang1 expression is elevated, activating Tie2 and resulting in the stabilization and maturation of the neovessels *(119)*. Failure of the switch from Ang2 to Ang1 expression in atretic ovarian follicles has been thought to trigger vascular regression secondary to the absence of the maintenance signal provided by Tie2 activation *(67)*.

Platelet derived growth factor has been implicated in the proliferation and migration of pericytes *(34)*, while HB-EGF has been demonstrated to induce VEGF secretion by vascular SMCs *(2)*. It has also been documented that endothelial cells recruit mural-cell precursors through the secretion of PDGF-BB *(82,83)*, and that mice null for PDGF-B lack pericytes in some vascular beds *(116)*. More recent studies demonstrate that direct cell–cell contact between endothelial and mural cells results in activation of latent TGF-β, which leads to vessel stabilization at multiple steps, including inhibition of endothelial cell proliferation and migration as well as induction differentiation of mural cells *(11,82)*. TGF-β is also known to alter integrin profiles and stimulate basement membrane production and accumulation *(108)*. Earlier studies documenting that basement membrane is deposited only after endothelial-mural cell association has occurred lend credence to this idea *(30)*. Collectively, these studies demonstrate the involvement of a plethora of factors in a complex sequence of steps in vessel remodeling and maturation, once the initial events of angiogenesis leading to tube formation are complete. Many of these observations were made using genetically manipulated mice, and illustrate the importance of these factors in the development of vasculature via vasculogenesis and angiogenesis.

4. DIFFERENCES BETWEEN THE VASCULATURE OF TUMORS AND NORMAL TISSUES

There are fundamental anatomical, morphological, and behavioral differences between blood vessels in tumors and normal tissues *(24)*. A growing tumor recruits new blood vessels from the host vasculature to meet the nutritional requirements and to eliminate the metabolic waste products. These metabolites, catabolites, and other specific angiogenic factors act as stimulants for neoangiogenesis that subsequently takes place in the tumor *(164)*. Thus, the tumor vasculature is composed of two types of vessels: the existing vessels in the surrounding normal tissues into which the tumor has invaded, and the tumor microvessels arising from neovascularization. These vessels are highly irregular and tortuous, and have arterio-venous shunts, blind ends, or sinusoids with incomplete endothelial linings, and basement membranes with no smooth-muscle layer or inervation *(42,164)*. Recent studies have shown that well-established human tumors contain a significant fraction of immature blood vessels that are devoid of pericytes *(16)*. As a consequence of these characteristics of tumor blood vessels, blood flow is sluggish and highly irregular, and these vessels are usually hyperpermeable *(45,89)*. In some tumors, blood may flow even from one vein to another *(89)*. This type of chaotic arrangement of tumor vessels, together with the compression of tumor vessels by the tumor cells themselves, results in pockets of hypoxia and acidity in low-flow regions.

Tumor vasculature is constantly exposed to a microenvironment which is very high in growth factors that induce and sustain immature vessels in the relative absence of mural cells *(35)*. Benjamin et al. *(16)* have demonstrated that both xenografted tumors and primary human tumors contain a sizable fraction of immature blood vessels which have not yet recruited periendothelial cells, and that withdrawal of VEGF not only leads to an inhibition of the growth of these vessels, but also causes regression of them. More recent studies indicate that TGF-β1 secreted by primary gallbladder wall tumor inhibits vessel formation, leukocyte-endothelial cell interactions, and tumor growth at distant cranial sites *(68)*. Enhanced expression of Tie2 has been found in blood vessels of metastatic melanomas, breast tumors, and hemangioblastomas. Blockade of the Tie2 pathway using antiangiogenic gene therapy was found to inhibit tumor growth and metastasis *(114)*. These observations suggest that tumor vessel stabilization also results from a balance between stimulators such as VEGF and Tie2 and inhibitors such as TGF-β in the tumor microenvironment.

5. TUMOR ANGIOGENESIS

The development of solid tumors is demarcated by two phases *(140)*. The first is the prevascular phase that is characterized by limited tumor growth with few or no metastases. This phase can persist for up to several years before switching to a vascular phase. The second phase is the vascular phase (Fig. 1). Growth of primary carcinomas beyond 2–3 mm depends on a switch to the vascular phase during which the formation of new blood vessels occurs *(56,57)*. Many studies have suggested a strong correlation between the degree of tumor vascularization and the rate of metastasis or patient outcome *(202)*. Neoangiogenesis that occurs during the vascular phase is regulated by several factors produced endogenously—either by the tumor cells themselves or tumor-associated cells such as macrophages, endothelial cells, mast cells, and others. These factors include both angiogenesis activators and inhibitors, and the list of these factors is rapidly expanding (Table 1) *(55,107)*. The whole angiogenic process is orchestrated by the interaction of angiogenic growth factors and cytokines with their cognate receptors on the endothelium, and by the interaction of these cells with their surrounding matrix. Matrix-degrading proteases such as plasminogen activators (PAs), matrix metalloproteinases (MMPs), and adhesion molecules such as integrins regulate this.

The major angiogenic stimulators include acidic and basic fibroblast growth factor (aFGF and bFGF), VEGF, PDGF, platelet derived endothelial cell growth factor (PD-ECGF), hepatocyte growth factor (HGF) and tumor necrosis factor alpha (TNF-α). These growth factors bind to their cognate receptors, leading to signal trasduction followed by activation of resting vasculature. Some of the endogenous inhibitors of angiogenesis are thrombospondin-1 (TSP-1) and plasminogen activator inhibitor type-2 (PAI-2), angiostatin, and endostatin *(77,139)*. The progression of carcinomas *in situ* to the angiogenic phenotype results from an imbalance between the positive and negative regulators of angiogenesis, and is called the "angiogenic switch" *(77)*. Important inducers of this angiogenic switch are genetic mutations (i.e., activation of oncogenes or the inactivation of tumor suppressor genes) and/or tumor microenvironmental events such as hypoxia. This notion is supported by the following observations *(123,163)*. The endothelial-specific proangiogenic factor, VEGF, has been shown to be upregulated in cell lines expressing constitutively active oncogenic forms or *H-ras* and *K-ras* *(124,137)*. More recent studies have demonstrated that tumor-derived expression of VEGF is critical for *ras*-mediated tumorigenesis, and the loss of tumorigenic expression of VEGF causes dramatic decreases in vascular density and permeability and increases in tumor cell apoptosis *(72)*. VEGF has also been shown to be upregulated in human colon cancer cells possessing mutant p53 *(21,98)*. In human fibroblasts and mammary epithelial cells, loss of a wild-type allele of p53 tumor suppressor gene has been associated with downregulation of the expression of the potent angiogenic inhibitor TSP-1 *(77,189)*. Human renal carcinoma cells that either lacked endogenous wild-type von Hippel-Lindau tumor (VHL) suppressor gene or were transfected with an inactive mutant VHL showed deregulated expression of VEGF on the mRNA and protein level. This was reversed by introduction of wild-type VHL *(167)*. Further, blockade of epidermal growth factor and ErbB-2/neu receptor tyrosine kinases have also been shown to downregulate VEGF production by tumor cells in vitro and in vivo *(143)*. More recent studies have demonstrated that inactivation of the PTEN tumor suppressor gene is associated with increased angiogenesis in clinically localized prostate carcinoma *(64)*. However, this increase is angiogenesis was not attributed to downregulation of TSP-1 expression, as shown with glioblastomas *(64)*.

6. ROLE OF PROTEINASES IN ANGIOGENESIS

Degradation of basement membrane and ECM components is crucial for angiogenesis, invasion, and metastasis. Two families of proteases—the PAs and MMPs—are strongly implicated in the process of angiogenesis and matrix degradation *(151)*. The vast majority of epithelial-derived malignancies are known to express uPA and MMPs, and these are produced by the same cells that elaborate angiogenic factors *(10,198)*. Both uPA and MMPs are secreted in inactive proenzyme forms, and require activation via proteolytic cleavage. UPA is produced as pro uPA, which binds to the cell surface uPA receptor (uPAR). It is readily converted to two-chain active uPA by plasmin, kallikrein, and cathepsin B *(84,100)*. The activity of uPA is inhibited by plasminogen-activator inhibitors types 1 and 2 (PAI-1, -2) *(105)*. Enhanced expression of uPA has also been reported in a variety of human cancers, including breast, colon, lung, stomach, and prostate, as well as in gliomas, astrocytomas, and malignant melanomas. This has been correlated with tumor invasiveness. In rat prostate cancer sublines, the pattern of expression of plasminogen activator and MMPs were found to correlate with their metastatic behavior in vivo *(149)*. Expression of recombinant PAI-2 in HT1080 sarcoma cells inhibited their invasiveness *(111)*. Blockade of uPA receptor has been demonstrated to inhibit neovascularization and tumor growth in several types of cancers, including prostate cancer and B16 melanoma *(48,128)*. More recent studies have demonstrated that human prostate carcinoma cells (PC-3, Du-145 and LnCaP) express enzymatic activity that can convert plasminogen to the endogenous angiogenesis inhibitor angiostatin *(62)*.

The MMPs are a family of at least 17 endopeptidases, and based on their substrate specificity, they are classified into subgroups of collagenases (MMP-1, -2, -13) stromelysins (MMP-3, -7, -10, -11, -12), gelatinases (MMP-2, -9), membrane-type MMPs (MMP-14, to -17) and other MMPs (MMP-19, 20) *(198)*. Although the exact mechanism of activation of MMPs is unclear, it appears that the cell-surface proteolytic cascade is mediated at least in part via the uPA/uPAR system *(198)*. Tissue inhibitors of metalloproteinases (TIMPs) inhibit the activity of MMPs in the extracellular space. The TIMP family consists of four structurally related members: TIMP-1, -2, -3 and -4. TIMP-1, -2 and -4 are secreted, while TIMP-3 is associated with the ECM *(198)*. The proposed role of MMPs in angiogenesis and tumor invasion is based mainly on observations of high-level expression of distinct MMPs in invasive malignant tumors *(13,91)*, although some direct evidence for their role in angiogenesis is available. In vitro assays have demonstrated that the activity of collagenase-1 is required for the migration of epithelial cells through a type-1 collagen matrix *(144)*. Knockout studies have demonstrated that mice lacking MMP-7 showed reduction in intestinal tumorigenesis, while mice lacking MMP-2 showed reduced angiogenesis and tumor progression *(85,199)*. Increased expression of TIMPs by host or tumor cells has been found to result in reduced invasion and metastatic ability of transformed cells *(3,104)*. These studies demonstrate the critical role of PAs and MMPs in angiogenesis and tumorigenesis.

7. ROLE OF MACROPHAGES IN ANGIOGENESIS

Among the tumor infiltrating cells, tumor-associated macrophages play a key role in tumor angiogenesis *(145,174)*. When they become activated by appropriate stimuli such as GM-CSF or interferon (INF) γ, or platelet activating factor, they switch to an angiogenic phenotype and secrete a number of proteases, protease inhibitors, cytokines, and growth factors. They play important roles in each phase of the angiogenesis process, influencing endothelial cell proliferation, migration, and differentiation. These macrophages alter the components of the ECM and induce changes in endothelial-cell shape and morphology. They produce ECM components, but also degrade the ECM by elaborating proteases. In addition to producing angiogenic factors, macrophages also produce a number of factors that inhibit angiogenesis. These include TSP-1, PAI-2, and cytokines such as INF-α, macrophage endothelial-cell inhibitory factor (MECIF), interleukin (IL)-1, IL-6, TNF-α and TGF-β in appropriate concentrations *(145,174)*. It is well-known that the angiogenic switch during tumor development results from the tumor's loss of ability to produce inhibitors of angiogenesis. Recent studies have suggested that macrophages must also undergo a similar switch if they are to participate effectively in the timely growth and regression of capillaries in granulation tissues laid down during wound healing *(146)*. In this situation, macrophages switch from a proangiogenic to an angio-inhibitory phenotype, in contrast to the angiogenic switch that occurs in tumors *(146)*. Thus, it is conceivable that macrophages that fail to undergo this conversion may contribute to the unwarranted angiogenesis that occurs in tumors. This is substantiated by direct and indirect evidence suggesting that when macrophages fail to produce appropriate levels of the angio-inhibitory TSP-1, they can contribute to the persistent angiogenic activity seen in solid tumors. Thus, macrophage-derived factors have both positive and negative effects on tumor angiogenesis.

Table 2
VEGF, VEGF-Related Molecules and their Receptors

Members of VEGF Family	Isoforms	Receptor	Vascular target
VEGF	$VEGF_{121}$	VEGFR-1	Hematic endothelium
	$VEGF_{165}$	VEGFR-2	
	$VEGF_{189}$		
	$VEGF_{206}$		
	$VEGF_{145}$		
PlGF	PlGF-1	VEGFR-1	Hematic endothelium
	PlGF-2		
	PlGF-3		
VEGF-B	$VEGF-B_{167}$	VEGFR-1	Hematic endothelium
	$VEGF-B_{186}$		
VEGF-C	VEGF-C	VEGFR-2	Lymphatic endothelium
		VEGFR-3	Hematic endothelium
VEGF-D	VEGF-D	VEGFR-2	Lymphatic endothelium
		VEGFR-3	Hematic endothelium
VEGF-E	VEGF-E		

(Adapted from ref. *136*).

8. VASCULAR ENDOTHELIAL GROWTH FACTOR AND RELATED MOLECULES

Among the known angiogenic factors, the most potent and specific growth factor for endothelial cells is VEGF, produced by virtually all types of tumors *(51,52,92,93)*. VEGF can exist in five different isoforms ($VEGF_{121}$, $VEGF_{165}$, $VEGF_{189}$, and $VEGF_{206}$, $VEGF_{145}$) because of alternative splicing of a single VEGF gene (Table 2). $VEGF_{165}$ is the predominant form secreted by a variety of normal and malignant cells. $VEGF_{189}$ and $VEGF_{206}$ are more basic, bind heparin with a greater affinity than $VEGF_{165}$, and are sequestered in the ECM. $VEGF_{121}$ is a freely soluble protein that is acidic and does not bind heparin. Recently, at least six new molecules have been added to the VEGF family of growth factors. They include placenta growth factor (PlGF), VEGF-A, VEGF-B, VEGF-C, and VEGF-D, VEGF-E *(96)*. All of these contribute to endothelial cell proliferation and vasculogenesis during development *(154)*. As the name implies, PlGF expression is restricted to the placenta *(136)*. VEGF-B is present in a variety or normal organs, and is particularly abundant in heart and skeletal muscle *(96)*. VEGF-C is expressed during embryonal development in regions where lymphatics sprout from venous vessels. In the adult, it becomes largely restricted to the lymphatic endothelium and has been implicated in lymphangiogenesis. It has been reported that VEGF-B and VEGF-C are expressed in a variety of human tumors *(136)*. VEGF-C mRNA expression was found to be higher in lymph node positive prostatic carcinomas as compared with node-negative carcinoma, suggesting that VEGF-C may play a role in lymph node metastasis *(187)*. VEGF-C has been shown to stimulate migration of bovine capillary endothelial cells in collagen gels *(95)*. This observation suggests that its actions may extend beyond the lymphatic system. However, the major function of VEGF in tissues is to increase the perfusion of that tissue. This is accomplished through a number of mechanisms. First, VEGF increases the number of blood vessels in the tissues by inducing angiogenesis *(51)*. Second, it increases blood flow directly by nitric oxide-induced vasodilation *(106)* and thirdly, it may chronically decrease peripheral resistance by increasing microvascular radius *(14)*.

VEGF binds to three tyrosine kinase receptors—VEGF receptor (VEGFR)-1 (Flt-1), VEGFR-2 (KDR/Flk-1), and VEGFR-3 (Flt-4)—leading to receptor dimerization, autophosphorylation, and signal transduction *(51,134)*. However, transfection experiments have suggested that several angiogenic activities associated with VEGF, such as endothelial cell proliferation, chemotaxis, and changes in morphology, are mediated through VEGFR-2 rather than VEGFR-1 *(192)*. PlGF and VEGF-B also bind VEGFR-1, while VEGF-C and VEGF-D bind both VEGF-2 and VEGF-3 and induce tyrosine autophosphorylation *(95,136)*. PlGF and VEGF-B can form heterodimers with VEGF, and thus may reduce the bioavailability of VEGF. Some earlier studies have indicated that the expression of VEGFR-1 and VEGFR-2 are tightly restricted to endothelial cells and their progenitors *(142,150)*. However, other studies have reported their expression in other types of cells, including ovarian tumor cells and trophoblasts *(135)*. VEGFR-2 is found in the β-cell of the pancreatic islet, and VEGFR-1 has been reported in renal glomerular mesangial, melanoma cells and bovine retinal pericytes *(135,179,180)*.

Signaling pathways activated by VEGF have been described by Bates et al. *(15)*. Both VEGFR-1 and VEGFR-2 are tyrosine-phosphorylated, and dimerize in response to binding VEGF. Receptor autophosphorylation is followed by association with phospholipase C-γ (PLC-γ) and phosphorylation of phosphotidylinositol 3-kinase (PI3K), *ras* GTPas-activating protein, and Nek *(73)*. Activation of PLC-γ is accompanied by increases in inositol 1,4,5-triphosphate (IP3) and diacylglycerol (DAG) production, and increased IP3 activity. Production of DAG is known to activate PKC. An increase in the calcium-sensitive isoforms of PKC (α and β$_{II}$ and δ) in membrane fractions isolated from the retinas of eyes injected intravitrially with VEGF has been reported *(5)*. Other studies have demonstrated that VEGF-stimulated bovine aortic endothelial cells show an increase in PKC-α and -β$_{II}$ in their membrane fractions, and that the mitogenic response of these cells to VEGF can be blocked by β-selective PKC inhibitors *(5,200)*.

It has been reported that activation of PKC, through *raf* activation, leads to phosphorylation of a form of mitogen activated protein kinase (MAPK), the extracellular-regulated kinase (ERK1/2) and its translocation to the nucleus *(133)*. Activation of PLC-γ-PKC-ERK1/2 (MAPK) pathways have been demonstrated for both VEGFR-1 and VEGFR-2 *(161,181)*. Alternatively, ERK1/2 can be activated by VEGF receptor tyrosine kinase through the formation of a receptor Shc/Grb2/SOS complex with subsequent activation of the *ras/raf* cascade *(103)*.

VEGF is also known to stimulate phosphorylation of related adhesion-focal tyrosine kinase (RAFTK), focal adhesion kinase (FAK), and focal adhesion-associated protein paxillin, and promotes their association with focal adhesions *(1,133)*. RAFTK (PYK2) can be activated either by agents that increase intracellular calcium or independently through PKC. By feeding into the *ras/raf* pathway, RAFTKs can also cause ERK1/2 activation *(113)*. Activation of Rac by RAFTK can lead to signaling through the stress-activated protein kinase 2 (SAPK-2), leading to phosphorylation of c-jun. Mukhopadhyay et al. *(133)* have also reported that VEGF-stimulates activation of c-jun NH$_2$-terminal kinase (JNK). This is consistent with the previous observation. JNK has been reported to activate endothelial specific transcription factor Ets-1, which induces expression of matrix degrading proteins that enable growing vessels to migrate through interstitium *(87)*.

9. HYPOXIA-INDUCED ANGIOGENESIS

Hypoxia is an important promoter of tumor-induced angiogenesis *(50,157)*. It is believed that tumors become hypoxic when their growth rate exceeds the growth rate of new blood vessels or when their fragile, poorly organized vasculature partially collapses under interstitial pressure *(79)*. High oxygen and glucose consumption rates also lead to steep gradients of these metabolites in solid tumors *(177)*. Oxygen concentrations have been reported to gradually decrease from normoxic perivascular regions of proliferating cells across the hypoxic layers of resting cells, reaching anoxic conditions in the necrotic centers *(177)*. Tumor cells that do not adapt to severe oxygen and nutrient deprivation undergo apoptosis or necrosis. However, it has also been shown that hypoxia positively affects tumor growth by inducing cellular adaptations (i.e., anaerobic glycolysis) as well as local (i.e., angiogenesis) and genetic (e.g., p53 mutation) alterations. At the molecular level, this is accomplished by increased expression of Glut^3-1, glycolytic enzymes and VEGF *(20,196)*. Tumor cells harboring a mutant *p53* gene are more resistant to apoptosis induced by tissue hypoxia, implying that hypoxic stress can select for tumor cells that have diminished apoptotic potential *(71)*. Hypoxia has also been reported to induce wild-type p53 by a different pathway than DNA-damaging agents *(70)*. Further, p53 mutation has proangiogenic effects because wild-type p53 induces TSP-1, a potent angiogenesis inhibitor, and inhibits angiogenesis *(32,131)*. Available evidence indicates that heterodimeric transcription factor HIF-1 is a key mediator of oxygen homeostasis *(196)*. Recent studies show that hypoxic/anoxic p53 induction is HIF-1α dependent, and that HIF-1α can be coimmunoprecipitated together with p53, suggesting that HIF-1α: p53 interaction stabilizes p53 *(9)*. However, a subsequent study demonstrated that hypoxia can induce HIF-1α without concomitant p53 upregulation, suggesting that other anoxically driven mechanisms may be required for p53 induction *(197)*. An AP-1 transcription-factor-binding site has been known to cooperate with the HIF-1 site to potentiate hypoxia induction of VEGF gene by twofold, although this site on its own is unable to confer hypoxia responsiveness *(33)*. Other studies have reported that H-*ras* oncogene can enhance hypoxia induction of VEGF via the HIF-1 promoter element *(123)*. H-*ras* induction of VEGF appears to involve the phosphotidylinositol 3-kinase/Akt signaling pathway *(121,123,124)*. Hypoxia induction of human VEGF expression has been reported to involve activation of c-src *(132)*, although subsequent studies have argued against a regulatory role for src kinase in the induction of VEGF as well as other hypoxia-induced genes *(6)*.

It is known that transcriptional activation and mRNA stabilization both contribute to the hypoxic induction of VEGF mRNA *(69,171)*. In addition to hypoxia, growth factors and cytokines have also been shown to increase steady-state VEGF mRNA levels

(58). VEGF mRNA and protein levels have been induced by PDGF-BB *(59,186)*, bFGF *(186)*, IGF-1, *(194)*, TGF-β *(141)*, EGF *(186)*, TNF-α *(53)*, keratinocyte growth factor *(58)* IL-1β, and IL-6 *(28,53)* in a variety of cultured cells. Enhanced VEGF expression has been reported upon activation of protein kinase C by tumor-promoting phorbol esters *(59,61)*.

Although hypoxia, *ras* oncoprotein, and mutant p53 are potent inducers of VEGF mRNA, they do not increase VEGF-B or VEGF-C mRNA levels *(65)*. Serum and its components, PDGF, EGF, TGF-β and PMA, stimulate VEGF-C mRNA expression, but have no effect on VEGF-B expression *(47)*. Yet these growth factors and hypoxia downregulated Ang1, the ligand for Tie-2 receptor *(47)*. This is consistent with the fact that Ang1 has no role in immediate response to growth-factor-induced angiogenesis, but may play a role in stabilization of newly formed vessels. This notion is also supported by the observation that VEGF, bFGF, and hypoxia stimulate Ang2 mRNA levels in bovine microvascular endothelial cells *(120)*. Elevated Ang2 will counteract the vessel maturation and stabilization effect of Ang1 by binding to its receptor, Tie2. More recent studies have demonstrated that hypoxia and VEGF upregulate Tie1 in bovine aortic endothelial cells *(125)*. Using TSU-Pr1 human prostate cancer cells, we demonstrated that hypoxia upregulates VEGF secretion, but not bFGF secretion, with these cells *(93)*. It has been reported that hypoxia directly slows down endothelial cell proliferation, and suppresses endothelial cell bFGF expression *(165)*. However, subsequent studies show that hypoxia can induce growth of hypoxic endothelial cells, and this is caused by hypoxia-mediated induction of a/b FGF and PDGF in macrophages that in turn stimulate the endothelial cells in a paracrine manner *(109)*.

Hypoxia has been described as a mechanism of upregulating both Flt1 and KDR/Flk1 VEGF receptors *(188)*. Using cultured cerebral tissue slices, Kremer et al. *(102)* demonstrated that hypoxia induced VEGFR-2 expression through stimulation of VEGF in this tissue. Similarly, VEGF was also found to induce VEGFR-1 in HUVEC cells.

10. REGULATION OF ANGIOGENESIS IN NORMAL AND MALIGNANT PROSTATE TISSUES

It has been reported that the vast majority of latent prostate cancers detectable in autopsy material from men who died from prostate cancer have very low capillary density ratios compared to prostate cancers that produced clinical symptoms and metastasized *(60,190)*. Independent studies using immunohistochemical techniques have confirmed an increase in microvessel density in prostate cancer specimens compared with specimens of normal prostate cancer tissue and benign prostatic hyperplasia *(18,166)*. A stepwise increase in microvessel density toward the center of the prostate carcinomas has also been observed, suggesting that angiogenic promoters may have their highest activity in the center of the neoplasm *(166)*. Additional studies have demonstrated that microvessel density is an independent predictor of pathologic stage in prostate cancer patients, as well as a valuable prognostic indicator in patients with clinically localized prostate cancer treated with radiotherapy *(22,75,195)*. These observations suggest that the development and progression of prostate cancer as well as the prognosis of the disease are related to angiogenesis.

Although a great deal is known about factors regulating angiogenesis in other malignancies, the knowledge in this area in prostate cancer is sparse. Campbell et al. *(25)* have demonstrated that normal human prostate epithelial cells express a variety of cytokines that have been shown to have angiogenic properties in various systems. These include VEGF, bFGF, TGF-α, TGF-β, IL-8, TNF-α, GM-CSF, and G-CSF, with VEGF the most abundant. Several studies have demonstrated the widespread expression of VEGF in malignant and nonmalignant prostate tissue as well as in the seminal vesicles and testes *(23,53,88,92,93,117)*. Basic FGF expression has been detected in normal and malignant prostate tissues as well as in cell lines *(92,93,117)*. Both TGF-βs and their cognate receptors are expressed in developing and mature prostates, and have been reported to inhibit proliferation and induce apoptosis of prostate epithelial cells in vitro and in vivo *(182)*. TGF-β1 is known to be upregulated in prostate glandular epithelial cells during castration-induced programmed cell death *(31,110)*. However, TGF-β1 was found to be overexpressed in prostate cancer, and plasma levels of this cytokine have been reported to be significantly elevated in patients with invasive prostate cancer *(46,86,172)*. This has been attributed to the fact that prostate cancer cells acquire reduced sensitivity to the growth-inhibitory effects of TGF-β1 *(172)*. Elevated TGF-β1 levels promote angiogenesis and ECM formation and enhance metastatic potential *(178)*.

Recent studies have demonstrated that patients with metastatic prostate cancers have higher serum VEGF levels than patients with localized disease or healthy controls *(44)*. Other studies have documented that the mean level of PD-ECGF in prostatic adenocarcinomas is higher than that in neighboring normal prostatic tissues, and is localized to endothelial cells, macrophages, and lymphocytes *(173)*. It has been reported that bFGF is a potent angiogenic inducer and is expressed in malignant prostate tissues. In these prostate cancer patients, serum bFGF levels were significantly higher than in normal men *(126)*.

Recent studies have demonstrated that in addition to being expressed in vascular endothelial cells of prostate cancers, Flt1 and Flk1 receptors have also been found to be expressed in BPH tissue glandular epithelial cells and in the basal-cell layer, respectively *(54)*. These studies also reported the expression of Flt1 in DU145 and LnCaP prostate cancer cell lines, and suggest that in addition to playing a paracrine role in tumor angiogenesis, VEGF may also play an autocrine role in tumor-cell activation.

11. ANDROGEN REGULATION OF TUMOR ANGIOGENESIS

It is well known that androgens regulate both cell proliferation and cell death in normal and malignant prostate tissue *(39)*. We and others have reported that androgens also regulate blood flow to the normal rat ventral prostate as well as to Dunning tumors *(78,112)*. We have also demonstrated that castration induces a significant reduction of the weights and VEGF content in the rat ventral prostate glands, and that replacement of dihydrotestosterone (DHT) results in an increase in VEGF in these glands *(92)*. Two other groups of investigators have confirmed these observations both at mRNA and protein levels *(74,170)*. The latter investigators further demonstrated that Flk-1/KDR and Flt-1 receptor levels are unaffected by castration and testosterone treatment. Lissbrant et al. *(117)* reported that the effects of castration on the ventral prostate glands included reductions in endothelial cell proliferation rate, the total weights of vessel walls, blood vessel lumina, endothelial cells, glandular epithelial cells, and total organ weights. However, replacement of testosterone restored these parameters within 2 d, except total glandular epithelial weights and organ weights, which took two additional days.

We have demonstrated that androgen ablation-induced growth inhibition of androgen responsive PC-82, A-2 and LnCaP human prostate cancer xenografts and the Dunning G and H rodent prostate cancers involves direct activation of programmed (apoptotic) death of these cells. It also involves a reduction in tumor angiogenesis secondary to a reduction in tumor VEGF content *(92,93)*. We have also reported that castration led to a decrease in blood vessel density within the Dunning tumors as well as a reduction in blood flow to these tumors *(78)*. VEGF is known to increase the number of blood vessels in the tissues by inducing angiogenesis, and to increase blood flow directly by nitric oxide induced vasodilatation *(49)*. This is consistent with our observations. Using the androgen-dependent Shionogi mammary carcinoma model, Jain et al. *(90)* also showed that castration of tumor-bearing mice led to tumor regression with a concomitant reduction in VEGF expression. They also studied the sequence of events leading to tumor vessel regression, and reported that tumor endothelial cells undergo apoptosis before tumor cells, and rarefaction of tumor vessels precedes the decrease in tumor size.

Previous studies have suggested that the effects of DHT on prostate epithelial cells are mediated through stromal epithelial interactions *(41)*. However, using LnCaP prostate cancer cells, we have demonstrated that DHT can directly stimulate VEGF secretion by these cells in vitro *(92)*. Using a human immortalized prostate epithelial cell line, PNT1, Sordello et al. *(170)* have also confirmed this observation both at mRNA and secreted protein levels. Although androgen can directly regulate VEGF in these androgen responsive cells, following castration, androgen responsive tumors progress to become resistant to androgen ablation because of the heterogeneous presence of both androgen dependent and independent cells. Jain et al. *(90)* reported that 2 wk after castration, a second wave of angiogenesis and tumor growth begins with a concomitant increase in VEGF expression. We have demonstrated that androgen independent human prostate cancer cells—TSU-Pr1, DU-145, and PC-3—constitutively express high levels of VEGF, and in these cells, upregulation of VEGF occurs not with androgens but through cellular hypoxia *(92)*. Thus, patients may benefit if antiangiogenic therapy is administered as an adjuvant to androgen ablation. Using the androgen responsive PC-82 human xenograft model, we demonstrated that when androgen ablation was combined with the antiangiogenic agent Linomide, it potentiated the antiangiogenic and antitumor effects of castration *(93)*. We have also reported that treatment of Dunning H tumor-bearing rats with Linomide along with castration resulted in a prolonged inhibition of tumor growth over a period of 1 yr *(78)*. As long as Linomide was administered, the growth of these tumors remained supressed. However, when Linomide was withdrawn, the tumor began to regrow.

12. STRATEGIES FOR DEVELOPING ANTIANGIOGENIC THERAPIES

At least three different strategies have been developed to inhibit tumor angiogenesis. The first is to inhibit the release of angiogenic molecules by the tumor cells or tumor-associated cells. The second is to inhibit the activity of these angiogenic molecules, and the third is to inhibit the endothelial response to these angiogenic molecules. Several different approaches have been used to develop these antiangiogenic therapies. These include antibody therapies *(41,158)*, soluble growth-factor receptors *(115)*, antisense approaches *(36,193)*, ribozymes *(36,159)*, gene therapies *(101)*, and isolation and purification of endogenous inhibitors angiogenesis–i.e., angiostatin, endostatin, and small-molecule inhibitors *(138,147)*. Table 3 lists some of these approaches.

Experimental animal models have demonstrated that tumor growth can be inhibited by anti-VEGF antibodies *(51)*. A current clinical trial is presently evaluating the safety and efficacy of a humanized anti-VEGF antibody in cancer patients. *(148)*. An alternative to MAb is to use soluble VEGF receptor domains. Aiello et al. *(4)* have demonstrated that retinal neovascularization in vivo can be suppressed by inhibition of VEGF using soluble VEGF-receptor chimeric proteins.

13. ANTIANGIOGENESIS USING GENE THERAPY

Various proof-of-principle animal experiments have indicated that gene therapy may be an effective method to deliver antiangiogenic therapy to solid tumors *(99)*. One of the approaches has been to transfer antisense sequences or ribozymes that will deplete mRNA that code for angiogenic factors. Using an antisense construct for VEGF, Cheng et al. *(27)* demonstrated that calcium phosphate transfection of glioblastoma cells with this construct resulted in a decrease in VEGF mRNA and protein production. In addition, implantation of the antisense VEGF transfected cell to nude mice led to a decrease in tumorigenicity. A second approach is based on the concept that interference with the function of the receptors for angiogenic molecules should disrupt the angiogenic cascade. This was demonstrated by the construction of a dominant negative Flk-1 mutant VEGF receptor encoded by a retrovirus vector *(127)*. This mutant retains the extracellular and transmembrane domain but lacks the intracellular domain. Thus, although the receptor remains cell associated, it is dysfunctional. When endothelial cells are infected with a retrovirus vector coding for the mutant receptor, it dimerizes with the wild-type Flk-1 receptor on endothelial cells but does not induce signal transduction like the wild-type Flk-1 homodimers. When an ectopic packaging cell line producing a retrovirus vector coding for the mutant receptor was coimplanted with glioblastoma cells in nude mice; the tumor growth was suppressed compared to control mice *(127)*. Although gene therapy is still in its infancy, these examples demonstrate that it may be an effective means to deliver antiangiogenic therapies to solid tumors.

14. SMALL-MOLECULE INHIBITORS OF ANGIOGENESIS

Many small-molecule inhibitors of various mechanisms of actions are currently being evaluated for antiangiogenic activity *(76)*. These compounds are at various stages of testing. A small number of these are currently undergoing clinical trials for treatment of cancer (Table 3). These include thalidomide, TNP-470, fumagillin analog, carboxyamidotriazole (CAI), a calcium channel blocker, SU 5416, another inhibitor of the tyrosine kinase activity of the Flk-1 receptor, and batimastat (BB-94) and marimastat (BB-2516), two matrix metalloproteinase inhibitors.

Table 3
Strategies for Antiangiogenic Therapy

Mechanism	Antiangiogenic agent
Neutralization or sequestration of angiogenic molecule	Anti-VEGF MAb
	Ani-bFGF MAb
	Antiangiogenin MAb
	Chimeric soluble Flt-IgG heavy-chain protein
	Suramin[a]
	Sulfated polysaccharide-peptidoglycan complex (tecogalan; DS-4152)[a]
	Pentosan sulfate
Interference with the endothelial response to angiogenic molecules	Specific inhibitors of receptor kinases
	Specific inhibitors of Flk-1 receptor
	SU 5416[a]
	Chimeric soluble Flt-IgG heavy-chain protein
Inhibition of functions of basement and extracellular matrix	Anti-αvβ3 integrin MAb
	Batimastat (BB-94)[a] and Marimastat (BB-2516)[a]
	CGS 27023A
	AG-3340
	BAY-12-9566[a]
	Angiostatic steroids
Direct endothelial cell injury (vascular targeting)	VEGF-diphtheria toxin conjugates
	Antibody-directed vascular targeting of tissue factor to induce vascular thrombosis
Unknown mechanisms of actions on:	AGM-1470 (TNP-470)[a]
	Linomide
	Interferon α
	Interferon β
	Angiostatin
	Endostatin
	Angiostatin
	Interleukin 12[a]
	Carboxyaminotriazlole
	Recombinant platelet factor 4[a]
	Retinoids
	Tamoxifen
	D-penicillamine
	Nitric-oxide synthase inhibitor
	Thalidomide[a]

[a] Currently in clinical trial; adapted from ref. *101*.

15. FUTURE AREAS OF STUDY

Identification of factors that promote and inhibit the angiogenic process has led to the use of these naturally occurring or synthetic compounds for the treatment of various diseases that involve aberrant angiogenesis. Antiangiogenic proteins or small molecules are being used to inhibit neovascularization to curtail tumor growth and metastasis, and angiogenesis-stimulating agents are being used to promote new blood-vessel formation in ischemic diseases, in processes that stimulate the development of collateral arteries in peripheral or myocardial ischemia *(7)*. Recent phase I clinical studies have established that intramuscular gene transfer may be used to safely and successfully accomplish therapeutic angiogenesis in patients with critical limb ischemia *(118)*. Tio et al. *(185)* have demonstrated that in a porcine model of myocardial ischemia, direct intramyocardial gene therapy using a plasmid DNA-encoding $VEGF_{165}$ can achieve therapeutic angiogenesis. Phase I human trials with direct intramyocardial administration of an adenovirus vector expressing $VEGF_{121}$ cDNA to individuals with clinically significant severe coronary artery disease have demonstrated success. Improved patient symptoms and improved myocardial perfusion was demonstrated by single-photon emission computed tomography imaging and coronary angiography *(156)*. The angiogenic effects of VEGF are known to be mediated at least in part by stimulation of u-PA production by migrating endothelial cells and SMCs *(121)*. One of the fatal complications of acute myocardial infarction (AMI) is cardiac rupture. This is attributed to the dilatation and wall-thinning effect of u-PA and MMP-9 during matrix remodeling, which occurs after AMI *(81)*. Myocardium is known to contain more interstitial collagen than other tissues, and thus has a greater requirement for u-PA in the revascularization process *(26)*. Although temporary administration of PAI-1 and TIMP-1 completely protected against cardiac rupture, it impaired therapeutic angiogenesis and caused cardiac failure *(81)*. We and others have demonstrated that the antiangiogenic effect of Linomide is at least in part mediated through an increase in PAI-2 production by macrophages *(19,94)*. In a clinical trial involving multiple sclerosis patients, administration of Linomide resulted in AMIs in a small number of patients (unpublished observation). Recent studies have demonstrated that angiostatin can also bind to SMCs in the coronary artery and inhibit SMC proliferation and migration in vitro *(191)*.

Currently, antiangiogenic compounds are tested in preclinical animal models using young adults who have healthy coronary vessels. In these models, such cardiac toxicities will not be detected. Thus, appropriate animal models should be used to test for the cardiac toxicities of long-term use of antiangiogenic compounds. Until this issue is resolved, these observations warrant against prolonged use of antiangiogenic agents for patients with cancer or other inflammatory diseases. A more effective approach may be to use intermittent antiangiogenic therapy in combination with cytotoxic chemotherapies or radiation therapy. Preclinical animal model studies have demonstrated the beneficial effect of combining radiation therapy with antiangiogenic therapy in a cyclical fashion *(80,97,183)*. Using preclinical prostate cancer models, it has been demonstrated that when antiangiogenic therapy (i.e., Linomide) is given as an adjuvant to androgen ablation therapy, the combination holds the tumor growth in check for a longer period than either monotherapy *(78)*.

REFERENCES

1. Abedi, H. and I. Zachary. 1997. Vascular endothelial growth factor stimulates tyrosine phosphorylation and recruitment of new focal adhesions of focal adhesion kinase and paxillin in endothelial cells. *J. Biol. Chem.* **272:** 15,442–15,451.

2. Abramovitch, R., M. Neeman, R. Reich, I. Stein, E. Keshet, J. Abraham, et al. 1998. Intercellular communication between vascular smooth muscle and endothelial cells mediated by HB-EGF and VEGF. *FEBS Lett.* **425:** 4441–4447.

3. Ahonen, M., A. Baker, and V.-M. Kahari. 1998. Adenovirus-mediated gene delivery of tissue inhibitor of metalloproteinases-3 inhibits invasion and induces apoptosis in melanoma cells. *Cancer Res.* **58:** 2310–2315.

4. Aiello, L. P., E. Pierce, E. Foley, H. Takagi, H. Chen, L. Riddle, et al. 1995. Suppression of retinal neovascularization in vivo by inhibition of vascular endothelial growth factor receptor (VEGF) using soluble VEGF-receptor chimeric proteins. *Proc. Natl. Acad. Sci. USA* **92:** 10,457–10,461.

5. Aiello, L. P., S. Bursell, A. Clermont, E. Duh, H. Ishii, C. Takagi, et al. 1997. Vascular endothelial growth factor induced retinal permeability is mediated by protein kinase C in vivo and suppressed by orally effective beta-isoform-selective inhibitor. *Diabetes* **46:** 1473–1480.

6. Alon, T., I. Hemo, A. Itin, J. Pe'er, J. Stone, and E. Keshet. 1995. Vascular endothelial growth factor acts as a survival factor for newly formed retinal vessels and has implications for retinopathy of prematurity. *Nat. Med.* **1:** 1024–1028.

7. Amant, D., L. Berthou, and K. Walsh. 1999. Angiogenesis and gene therapy in man: dream or reality? *Drugs* **58:** 33–36.

8. Greenlee, R., T. Murrays, S. Bolden, P. A. Wingo. 2000. Cancer Statistics 2000. *Ca. G. Clin.* **50:** 7–11.

9. An, W. G., M. Kanekal, M. Somon, E. Maltepe, M. Blagosklonny, and L. Neckers. 1998. Stabilization of wild-type p53 by hypoxia-inducible factor 1 HIF-1. *Nature (Lond)* **392:** 405–408.

10. Andreasen, P. A., L. Kjoller, L. Christensen, and M. Duffy. 1997. The urokinase-type plasminogen activator system in cancer metastasis: a review. *Int. J. Cancer* **72:** 1–22.

11. Antonelli-Orlidge, A., K. Saunders, S. Smith, and P. D'Amore. 1989. An activated form of transforming growth factor beta is produced by coculture of endothelial cells and pericytes. *Proc. Natl. Acad. Sci. USA* **86:** 4544–4548.

12. Arbiser, J. L., M. Moses, C. Fernandez, N. Ghiso, Y. Cao, N. Klauber, et al. 1997. Oncogene H-ras stimulates tumor angiogenesis by two distinct pathways. *Proc. Natl. Acad. Sci. USA* **94:** 861–866.

13. Basset, P., A. Okada, M. Chenard, R. Kannan, I. Stoll, P. Anglard, et al. 1997. Matrix metalloproteinases as stromal effectors of human carcinoma progression: therapeutical implications. *Matrix Biol.* **15:** 535–541.

14. Bates, D. O. 1998. The chronic effects of vascular endothelial growth factor (VEGF) on individually perfused frog mesenteric microvessels. *J. Physiol.* **513:** 225–233.

15. Bates, D. O., D. Lodwick, and B. Williams. 1999. Vascular endothelial growth factor and microvascular permeability. *Microcirculation* **6:** 83–96.

16. Benjamin, L. E., D. Golijanin, A. Itin, D. Pode, and E. Keshet. 1999. Selective ablation of immature blood vessels in established tumors follows vascular endothelial growth factor withdrawal. *J. Clin. Investig.* **103:** 159–165.

17. Berges, R. R., J. Vukanovic, J. Epstein, M. Carmichael, L. Cisek, D. Johnson, et al. 1995. Implication of the cell kinetic changes during the progression of human prostatic cancer. *Clin. Cancer Res.* **1:** 473–480.

18. Bigler, S. A., R. Deering, and M. Brawer. 1993. Comparison of microscopic vascularity in benign and malignant prostate tissue. *Human Pathol.* **24:** 220–226.

19. Billstrom, A., B. Kinnby, I. Lecander, and B. Astedt. 1996. Production of plasminogen activator inhibitor type-2 in human peripheral blood monocytes upregulated in vitro by the quinoline-3-carboxamide, Linomide. *Fibrinolysis* **10:** 277–283.

20. Blancher, C. and A. Harris. 1998. The molecular basis of the hypoxia response pathway: Tumor hypoxia as a therapy target. *Cancer Metastasis Rev.* **17:** 187–194.

21. Bouvet, M., L. Ellis, M. Nishizaki, T. Fujiwara, W. Liu, C. Bucana, et al. 1998. Adeno-virus-mediated wild-type p53 gene transfer downregulates vascular endothelial growth factor expression and inhibits angiogenesis in human colon cancer. *Cancer Res.* **58:** 2288–2292.

22. Brawer, M. K., R. Deering, B. Marianne, D. Preston, and S. Bigler. 1994. Predictors of pathologic stage in prostatic carcinoma: the role of neovascularity. *Cancer* **73:** 678–687.

23. Brown, L. F., K. Yeo, B. Berse, A. Morgentaler, H. Dvorak, and S. Rosen. 1995. Vascular permeability factor/vascular endothelial growth factor is strongly expressed in normal male genital tract and is present in substantial quantities in semen. *J. Urol.* **154:** 576–579.

24. Brown, J. M. and A. Giaccia. 1998. The unique physiology of solid tumors: opportunities (and problems) for cancer therapy. *Cancer Res.* **58:** 1408–1416.

25. Campbell, C. L., D. Savarese, P. Quesenberry, and T. Savarese. 1999. Expression of mul-tiple angiogenic cytokines in cultured normal human prostate epithelial cells: predomi-nance of vascular endothelial growth factor. *Int. J. Cancer* **80:** 868–874.

26. Carmeliet, P. and D. Collen. 1998. Vascular development and disorders: molecular analy-sis and pathological insights. *Kidney Int.* **53:** 1519–1549.

27. Cheng, S. Y., H. Huang, M. Nagane, X. Jo, D. Wang, and C. Shih. 1996. Suppression of glioblastoma angiogenicity and tumorigenicity by inhibition of endogenous expression of vascular endothelial growth factor. *Proc. Natl. Acad. Sci. USA* **93:** 8502–8507.

28. Cohen, T., D. Nahari, L. Cerem, G. Neufeld, and B. Levi. 1996. Interleukin 6 induces the expression of vascular endothelial growth factor. *J. Biol. Chem.* **271:** 736–741.

29. Crawford, E. D., M. Eisenberger, D. McLeod, J. Spaulding, R. Benson, F. Dorr, et al. 1989. A control randomized trial of Leuprolide with and without flutamide in prostate cancer. *N. Engl. J. Med.* **321:** 419–424.

30. Croker, D. J., T. Murad, and J. Greer. 1970. Role of pericytes in wound healing: an ultra-structural study. *Exp. Mol. Pathol.* **13:** 5–65.

31. Culig, Z., A. Hobisch, M. Cronauer, C. Radmayr, A. Hittmair, J. Zhang, et al. 1996. Regulation of prostatic growth and function by peptide growth factors. *Prostate* **28:** 392–405.

32. Dameron, K. M., O. Volpert, M. Tainsky, and N. Bouck. 1994. Control of angiogenesis in fibroblasts by p53 regulation of thrombospondin-1. *Science* **265:** 1582–1584.

33. Damert, A., E. Ikeda, and W. Risau. 1997. Activator-protein-1 potentiates the hypoxia-inducible factor-1 mediated hypoxia-induced transcriptional activation of vascular endot-helial growth factor expression in C6 glioma cells. *Biochem J.* **327:** 419–423.

34. D'Amore, P. A. and S. Smith. 1993. Growth factor effects on cells of the vascular wall: a survey. *Growth Factors* **8:** 61–75.

35. Darland, D. C. and P. D'Amore. 1999. Blood vessel maturation: vascular development comes of age. *J. Clin. Investig.* **103:** 157,158.

36. Davidson, J. M. and S. Benn. 1996. Regulation of angiogenesis and wound repair. Interac-tive role of the matrix and growth factors, in *Cellular and Molecular Pathogenesis* (Sirica, A. E., ed.), Lippincott-Raven, Philadelphia, pp. 79–107.

37. Davis, S., T. Aldrich, P. Jones, A. Acheson, D. Compton, V. Jain, et al. 1996. Isolation of angiopoietin-1, a ligand for Tie- receptor, by secretion-trap expression cloning. *Cell* **87:** 1161–1169.

38. Denmeade, S. R., X. Lin, and J. Isaacs. 1996. Role of programmed (apoptotic) cell death during the progression and therapy for prostate cancer. *Prostate* **28:** 251–265.

39. Denmeade, S. R., D. McCloskey, I. Joseph, H. Hahm, J. Isaacs, and D. Davidson. 1997. Apoptosis in hormone responsive malignancies. *Adv. Pharmacol.* **41:** 553–583.

40. Denmeade, S. R. and J. Isaacs. 1998. Enzymatic activation of prodrugs by prostate-spe-cific antigen: targeted therapy for metastatic prostate cancer. *Cancer J. Sci. Am.* (**Suppl. 1**) **4:** S15–21.

41. Derbyshire, E. J. and P. Thorpe. 1997. Targeting the tumor endothelium using specific antibodies, in *Tumor Angiogenesis* (Bicknell, R. L. and E. Claire, eds.), Oxford University Press, Oxford, England, pp. 343–356.

42. Dewhirst, M. W., C. Tso, R. Oliver, C. Gustafson, T. Secomb, and J. Gross. 1989. Morphologic and hemodynamic comparison of tumor and healing normal tissue microvasculature. *Int. J. Radiat. Oncol. Biol. Phys.* **17:** 91–99.

43. Dionne, C. A., A. Camoratto, J. Jani, E. Emerson, N. Neff, J. Vaught, et al. 1998. Cell cycle-independent death of prostate adenocarcinoma is induced by the *trk* tyrosine kinase inhibitor CEP-751 (KT6587). *Clin. Cancer Res.* **4:** 1887–1898.

44. Duque, J. L., K. Loughlin, R. Adam, P. Kantoff, D. Zurakowski, and M. Freeman. 1999. Plasma levels of vascular endothelial growth factor are increased in patients with metastatic prostate cancer. *Urology* **54:** 523–527.

45. Dvorak, H. F., L. Brown, M. Detmar, and A. Dvorak. 1995. Vascular permeability factor/vascular endothelial growth factor, microvascular hyperpermeability. *Am. J. Pathol.* **146:** 1029–1039.

46. Eastham, J. A., L. Truong, E. Rogers, M. Kattan, K. Flanders, P. Scardino, et al. 1995. Transforming growth factor-beta 1: comparative immunohistochemical localization in human primary and metastatic prostate cancer. *Lab. Investig.* **73:** 628–635.

47. Enholm, B., K. Paavonen, A. Ristimaki, V. Kumar, Y. Gunji, U. Erikson, et al. 1997. Comparison of VEGF, VEGF-B, VEGF-C and Ang-1 mRNA regulation by serum, growth factors, oncoproteins and hypoxia. *Oncogene* **14:** 2475–2483.

48. Evans, C. P., F. Elfman, S. Parangi, M. Conn, G. Cunha, and M. Shuman. 1997. Inhibition of prostate cancer neovascularization and growth by urokinase plasminogen activator receptor blockade. *Cancer Res.* **57:** 3594–3599.

49. Ferrara, N., K. Houck, L. Jakeman, J. Winer, and D. Leung. 1991. The vascular endothelial growth factor family of polypeptides. *J. Cell Biochem.* **47:** 211–218.

50. Ferrara, N. and S. Buntings. 1996. Vascular endothelial growth factor. A specific regulator of angiogenesis. *Curr. Opin. Nephrol. Hypertens.* **5:** 35–44.

51. Ferrara, N. and T. Davis-Smyth. 1997. The biology of vascular endothelial growth factor. *Endocr. Rev.* **18:** 4–25.

52. Ferrara, N. 1999. Molecular and biological properties of vascular endothelial growth factor. *J. Mol. Med.* **77:** 527–543.

53. Ferrer, F. A., L. Miller, R. Andrawis, S. Kurtzman, P. Albertsen, V. Laudone, et al. 1997. Vascular endothelial growth factor (VEGF) expression in human prostate cancer: *in situ* and in vitro expression of VEGF by human prostate cancer cells. *J. Urol.* **157:** 2329–2333.

54. Ferrer, F. A., L. Miller, R. Lindquist, P. Kowalezyk, V. Laudone, P. Albertsen, et al. 1999. Expression of vascular endothelial growth factor receptors in human prostate cancer. *Urology* **54:** 567–572.

55. Fidler, I. J. and L. Ellis. 1994. The implications of angiogenesis for the biology and therapy of cancer metastasis. *Cell* **79:** 185–188.

56. Folkman, J. 1985. Tumor angiogenesis. *Adv. Cancer Res.* **43:** 175–203.

57. Folkman, J. and M. Klagsbrun. 1987. Angiogenic factors. *Science* **235:** 442–447.

58. Frank, S., G. Hubner, G. Breier, M. Longaker, D. Greenhalgh, and S. Werner. 1995. Regulation of vascular endothelial growth factor expression in cultured keratinocytes. Implications for normal and impaired wound healing. *J. Biol. Chem.* **270:** 12,607–12,613.

59. Frankenzeller, G., D. Marme, H. Weich, and H. Hug. 1992. Platelet derived growth factor-induced transcription of the vascular endothelial growth factor gene is mediated by protein kinase C. *Cancer Res.* **52:** 4821–4823.

60. Furusato, M., H. Wakui, H. Sasaki, and S. Ushigome. 1994. Tumor angiogenesis in latent prostate carcinoma. *Br. J. Cancer* **70:** 1244–1246.

61. Garrido, C., S. Saule, and D. Gospodarowicz. 1993. Transcriptional regulation of vascular endothelial growth factor gene expression in ovarian bovine granulosa cells. *Growth Factors* **8**: 109–117.

62. Gatley, S., P. Twardowski, M. Stack, M. Patrick, L. Boggio, D. Cundiff, et al. 1996. Human prostate carcinoma cells express enzymatic activity that converts human plasminogen to the angiogenesis inhibitor angiostatin. *Cancer Res.* **56**: 4887–4890.

63. George, D. J., C. Dionne, J. Jani, T. Angeles, C. Murakata, J. Lamb, et al. 1999. Sustained in vivo regression of Dunning H rat prostate cancers treated with combinations of androgen ablation and *Trk* tyrosine kinase inhibitors, CEP-751 (KT-6587) or CEP-701 (KT-5555). *Cancer Res.* **59**: 2395–2401.

64. Giri, D. and M. Ittmann. 1999. Inactivation of the PTEN tumor suppressor gene is associated with increased angiogenesis in clinically localized prostate carcinoma. *Hum. Pathol.* **30**: 419–424.

65. Gleadle, G. M., B. Ebert, D. Firth, and P. Rathcliffe. 1995. Regulation of angiogenic growth factor expression by hypoxia, transition metals, and chelating agents. *Am. J. Physiol.* **268**: C1362–C1368.

66. Gleadle, J. M. and P. Ratcliffe. 1997. Induction of hypoxia-inducible factor 1, erythropoietin, vascular endothelial growth factor, and glucose transporter-1 by hypoxia: evidence against a regulatory role for *src* kinases. *Blood* **89**: 503–509.

67. Goede, V., T. Schmidt, S. Kimmina, and H. Augustin. 1998. Analysis of blood vessel maturation processes during cyclic ovarian angiogenesis. *Lab. Investig.* **78**: 1385–1394.

68. Gohongi, T., D. Fukumura, Y. Boucher, C. Yun, G. Soff, C. Compton, et al. 1999. Tumor-host interactions in the gall bladder suppress distal angiogenesis and tumor growth: involvement of transforming growth factor 1. *Nat. Med.* **5**: 1203–1208.

69. Goldberg, M. A. and T. Schneider. 1994. Similarities between the oxygen-sensing mechanisms regulating the expression of vascular endothelial growth factor and erythropoietin. *J. Biol. Chem.* **269**: 4355–4359.

70. Graeber, T. G., J. Peterson, M. Tsai, K. Monica, A. Forance, and A. Giaccia. 1994. Hypoxia induces stimulation of p53 protein, but activation of a G1-phase checkpoint by low-oxygen condition is independent of p53 status. *Mol. Cell Biol.* **14**: 6264–6277.

71. Graeber, T. G., C. Osmanian, T. Jacks, D. Housman, C. Koch, S. Lowe, et al. 1996. Hypoxia-mediated selection of cells with diminished apoptotic potential in solid tumors. *Nature (Lond.)* **379**: 88–91.

72. Grunsein, J., W. Roberts, O. Mathieu-Costello, D. Hanahan, and R. Johnson. 1999. Tumor-derived expression of vascular endothelial growth factor is a critical factor in tumor expansion and vascular function. *Cancer Res.* **59**: 1592–1598.

73. Guo, D., Q. Jia, H. Song, R. Warren, and D. Donner. 1995. Vascular endothelial growth factor promotes tyrosine phosphorylation of mediators of signal transduction that contain SH2 domains. Association with endothelial cell proliferation. *J. Biol. Chem.* **270**: 6729–6733.

74. Haggstrom, S., I. Lissbrant, A. Bergh, and J. Damber. 1999. Testosterone induces vascular endothelial growth factor synthesis in the ventral prostate in castrated rats. *J. Urol.* **161**: 1620–1625.

75. Hall, M. C., P. Troncoso, A. Pollack, H. Zhau, G. Zagars, L. Chung, et al. 1994. Significance of tumor angiogenesis in clinically localized prostate carcinoma treated with external beam radiotherapy. *Urology* **44**: 869–875.

76. Hamby, J. M. and D. Hollis Showalter. 1999. Small molecule inhibitors of tumor-promoted angiogenesis, including protein tyrosine kinase inhibitors. *Pharmacol. Ther.* **82**: 169–193.

77. Hanahan, D. and J. Folkman. 1996. Patterns and emerging mechanisms of the angiogenic switch during tumorigenesis. *Cell* **86**: 353–363.

78. Hartley-Asp, B., J. Vukanovich, I. Joseph, K. Strandgarden, J. Polacek, and J. Isaacs. 1997. Anti-angiogenic treatment with Linomide as adjuvant to surgical castration in experimental prostate cancer. *J. Urol.* **158:** 902–907.

79. Helmlinger, G., P. Netti, H. Lichtenbeld, R. Melder, and R. Jain. 1997. Solid stress inhibits the growth of multicellular tumor spheroids. *Nat. Biotechnol.* **15:** 778–783.

80. Herbst, R. S., H. Takeuchi, and B. Teicher. 1998. Pacitaxel/carboplatin administration along with antiangiogenic therapy in non-small-cell lung and breast carcinoma models. *Cancer Chemother. Pharmacol.* **41:** 497–504.

81. Heymans, S., A. Luttun, D. Nuyens, G. Theilmeier, E. Creemers, L. Moons, et al. 1999. Inhibition of plasminogen activators or matrix metalloproteinases prevents cardiac rupture but impairs therapeutic angiogenesis and causes cardiac failure. *Nat. Med.* **5:** 1135–1142.

82. Hirschi, K. K., S. Rohovsky, and P. D'Amore. 1998. PDGF, TGF-beta, and heterotypic cell-cell interactions mediate the recruitment and differentiation of 10T1/2 cells to a smooth muscle cell fate. *J. Cell Biol.* **141:** 805–814.

83. Hirschi, K., S. Rohovsky, L. Beck, S. Smith, and P. D'Amore. 1999. Endothelial cells modulate the proliferation of mural cell precursors via platelet derived growth factor -BB and heterotypic cell contact. *Circ. Res.* **84:** 298–305.

84. Ichinose, A., K. Fugikawa, and T. Suyama. 1986. The activation of pro-urokinase by plasmin, kallikrein and its inactivation by thrombin. *J. Biol. Chem.* **261:** 3486–3489.

85. Itoh, T., M. Tanioka, H. Yoshida, T. Yoshioka, H. Nishimoto, and S. Itohara. 1998. Reduced angiogenesis and tumor progression in gelatinase-A deficient mice. *Cancer Res.* **58:** 1048–1051.

86. Ivanovic, V., A. Melman, B. Davis-Joseph, M. Valcic, and J. Geliebter. 1995. Elevated plasma levels of TGF-beta 1 in patients with invasive prostate cancer. *Nat. Med.* **1:** 282–284.

87. Iwasaka, C., K. Tanaka, M. Abe, and Y. Sato. 1996. Ets-1 regulates angiogenesis by inducing the expression of urokinase-type plasminogen activator and matrix metalloproteinase-1 and the migration of vascular endothelial cells. *J. Cell Physiol.* **169:** 522–531.

88. Jackson, M. W., J. Bentel, and W. Tilly. 1997. Vascular endothelial growth factor (VEGF) expression in prostate cancer and benign prostatic hyperplasia. *J. Urol.* **157:** 2323–2328.

89. Jain, R. K. 1988. Determinants of blood flow: a review. *Cancer Res.* **48:** 2641–2658.

90. Jain, R. K., N. Safabakhsh, A. Sckell, Y. Chen, P. Jiang, L. Benjamin, et al. 1998. Endothelial cell death, angiogenesis, and microvascular function after castration in an androgen-dependent tumor: role of vascular endothelial growth factor. *Proc. Natl. Acad. Sci. USA* **95:** 10,820–10,825.

91. Johnsen, M., L. Lund, J. Rohmer, K. Almholt, and K. Dano. 1988. Cancer invasion and tissue remodeling: common themes in proteolytic matrix degradation. *Curr. Opin. Cell Biol.* **10:** 667–671.

92. Joseph, I. B. J. K. and J. Isaacs. 1997. Potentiation of the antiangiogenic ability of Linomide by androgen ablation involves down-regulation of vascular endothelial growth factor in human androgen-responsive prostatic cancers. *Cancer Res.* **57:** 1054–1057.

93. Joseph, I. B. J. K., J. Nelson, S. Denmeade, and J. Isaacs. 1997. Androgens regulate vascular endothelial growth factor content in normal and malignant prostatic tissue. *Clin. Cancer Res.* **3:** 2507–2511.

94. Joseph I. B. J. K. and J. Isaacs. 1998. Macrophage role in the anti-prostate cancer response to one class of antiangiogenic agents. *J. Natl. Cancer Inst.* **90:** 1648–1653.

95. Joukov, V., K. Pajusola, A. Kaipainen, D. Chilov, I. Lahtinen, E. Kukk, et al. 1996. A novel vascular endothelial growth factor, VEGF-C, is a ligand for the Flt4 (VRGFR-3) and KDR (VEGFR-2) receptor kinases. *EMBO J.* **15:** 290–298.

96. Joukov, V., A. Kaipainen, M. Jeltsch, K. Pajusola, B. Olofsson, V. Kumar, et al. 1997. Vascular endothelial growth factors VEGF-B and VEGF-C. *J. Cell Physiol.* **173:** 211–215.

97. Kakeji, Y. and B. Teicher. 1997. Preclinical studies of the combination of angiogenic inhibitors with cytotoxic agents. *Investig. New Drugs* **15**: 39–48.

98. Kang, S.-M., K. Maeda, N. Onoda, Y. Chung, B. Nakata, Y. Nishiguchi, et al. 1997. Combined analysis of p53 and vascular endothelial growth factor expression in colorectal carcinoma for determination of tumor vascularity and liver metastasis. *Int. J. Cancer* **74**: 502–507.

99. Ke, L. D., J. Fueyo, X. Chen, P. Steck, Y. Shi, S. Im, et al. 1998. A novel approach to glioma gene therapy: down regulation of vascular endothelial growth factor in glioma cells using ribozymes. *Int. J. Cancer* **74**: 502–507.

100. Kobayashi, H., M. Schmitt, I. Goretzki, N. Chucholowski, J. Calvete, M. Kramer, et al. 1991. Cathepsin B efficiently activates the soluble and the tumor cell receptor bound form of proenzyme urokinase-type plasminogen activator (pro-uPA). *J. Biol. Chem.* **266**: 5147–5152.

101. Kong, H.-L. and R. Crystal. 1998. Gene therapy strategies for tumor antiangiogenesis. *J. Natl. Cancer Inst.* **90**: 273–286.

102. Kremer, C., G. Breier, W. Risau, and K. Plate. 1997. Up-regulation of flk-1/vascular endothelial growth factor receptor 2 by its ligand in a cerebral slice culture system. *Cancer Res.* **57**: 3852–3859.

103. Kroll, J. and J. Waltenberger. 1997. The vascular endothelial growth factor receptor KDR activates multiple signal transduction pathways in porcine aortic endothelial cells. *J. Biol. Chem.* **272**: 32,521–32,527.

104. Kruger, A., O. Sanchez Sweatmann, D. Maritn, J. Fata, A. Ho, F. Orr, et al. 1998. Host TIMP-1 overexpression confers resistance to experimental brain metastasis of a fibrosarcoma cell line. *Oncogene* **16**: 2419–2423.

105. Kruithof, E. K. O. 1988. Plasminogen activator inhibitors—a review. *Enzyme* **40**: 113–121.

106. Ku, D. D., J. Zaleski, S. Liu, and T. Brock. 1993. Vascular endothelial growth factor induces EDRF-dependent relaxation in coronary arteries. *Am. J. Physiol. Heart Circ. Physiol.* **265**: H586–H592.

107. Kuiper, R. A., J. Schellens, G. Blijham, J. Beijneen, and E. Voest. 1998. Clinical research on antiangiogenic therapy. *Pharmacol. Res.* **37**: 1–16.

108. Kumar, N. M., S. Sigurdson, D. Sheppard, and J. Lwebuga-Mukasa. 1995. Differential modulation of integrin receptors and extracellular matrix laminin by transforming growth factor-beta 1 in rat alveolar epithelial cells. *Exp. Cell Res.* **221**: 385–394.

109. Kuwabara, K., S. Ogawa, M. Matsumoto, S. Koga, M. Clauss, D. Pinsky, et al. 1995. Hypoxia-mediated induction of acidic/basic fibroblast growth factor and platelet-derived growth factor in mononuclear phagocytes stimulates growth of hypoxic endothelial cells. *Proc. Natl. Acad. Sci. USA* **92**: 4606–4610.

110. Kyprianou, N. and J. Isaacs. 1989. Expression of transforming growth factor-beta in the rat ventral prostate during castration-induced programmed cell death. *Mol. Endocrinol.* **3**: 1515–1522.

111. Laung, W. E., X. Cao, Y. Yu, H. Shimada, and E. Kruithof. 1993. Inhibition of invasion of HT1080 sarcoma cells expressing recombinant plasminogen activator inhibitor-2. *Cancer Res.* **53**: 6051–6057.

112. Lekas, E., M. Johansson, A. Wildmark, A. Bergh, and J. Damber. 1997. Decrement of blood flow precedes the involution of the ventral prostate in the rat after castration. *Urol. Res.* **25**: 309–314.

113. Lev, S., H. Moreno, R. Martinez, P. Canoll, I. Peles, J. Musacchio, et al. 1995. Protein kinase PYK2 involved in Ca (2+)-induced regulation of ion channel and MAP kinase functions. *Nature* **376**: 737–745.

114. Lin, P., J. Buxton, A. Acheson, et al. 1998. Antiangiogenic gene therapy targeting the endothelium-specific receptor tyrosine kinase Tie2. *Proc. Natl. Acad. Sci. USA* **95**: 8829–8834.

115. Lin, P., S. Sankar, S. Shan, M. Dewhirst, P. Polverini, T. Quin, et al. 1998. Inhibition of tumor growth by targeting tumor endothelium by using a soluble vascular endothelial growth factor receptor. *Cell Growth Differ.* **9:** 49–58.

116. Lindahl, P., B. Johansson, P. Leveen, and C. Betsholz. 1997. Pericyte loss and microaneurysm formation in PDGF-B-deficient mice. *Science* **277:** 242–245.

117. Lissbrant, I. F., S. Haggstrom, J. Damber, and A. Bergh. 1998. Testosterone stimulates angiogenesis and vascular regrowth in the ventral prostate in castrated adult rats. Endocrinology **139:** 251–256.

118. Losordo, D. W., P. Vale, and J. Isner. 1999. Gene therapy for myocardial angiogenesis. *Am. Heart J.* **138 (2 pt 2):** 132–141.

119. Maisonpierre, P. C., C. Suri, P. Jones, S. Bartunkova, S. Wiegand, C. Radziejewski, et al. 1997. Angiopoietin-2, a natural antagonist for Tie2 that disrupts in vivo angiogenesis. *Science* **277:** 55–60.

120. Mandriota, S. J., G. Seghezzi, J. Vassalli, N. Ferrara, S. Wasi, R. Mazzieri, et al. 1995. Vascular endothelial growth factor increases urokinase receptor expression in vascular endothelial cells. *J. Biol. Chem.* **270:** 9709–9716.

121. Mandriota, S. J. and Pepper, M. S. 1998. Regulation of angiopoietin-2 mRNA levels in bovine microvascular endothelial cells by cytokines and hypoxia. *Circ. Res.* **83:** 852–859.

122. Marshall, E. 1998. The power of the front page of *The New York Times. Science* **280:** 996,997.

123. Mazure, N. M., E. Chen P. Yeh, K. Laderoute, and A. Giaccia. 1996. Oncogenic transformation and hypoxia synergistically act to modulate vascular endothelial growth factor expression. *Cancer Res.* **56:** 3436–3440.

124. Mazure, N. M., E. Chen, P. Yeh, K. Laderoute, and A. Giaccia. 1997. Induction of vascular endothelial growth factor by hypoxia is modulated by a phosphotidylinositol 3-kinase/Akt signaling pathway in H-*ras* transformed cells through a hypoxia inducible element. *Blood* **90:** 3222–3331.

125. McCarthy, M. J., M. Crowther, P. Bell, and N. Brindle. 1998. The endothelial receptor tyrosine kinase tie-1 is upregulated by hypoxia and vascular endothelial growth factor. *FEBS Lett.* **423:** 334–338.

126. Meyer, G. E., E. Yu, A. Seigal, J. Petteway, N. Blumenstein, and M. Brawer. 1995. Serum basic fibroblast growth factor in men with and without prostate carcinoma. *Cancer* **76:** 2304–2311.

127. Millauer, B., L. Shawver, K. Plate, W. Risau, and A. Ullrich. 1994. Glioblastoma growth inhibited in vivo by a dominant-negative Flk-1 mutant. *Nature* **367:** 576–579.

128. Min, H.-Y., L. Doyle, C. Vitt, C. Zandonella, and J. Stratton-Thomas. 1996. Urokinase receptor antagonists inhibit angiogenesis and primary tumor growth in syngeneic mice. *Cancer Res.* **56:** 2428–2433.

129. Molema, G., L. de Leij, and D. Meijer. 1997. Tumor vascular endothelium: barrier or target in tumor directed drug delivery and immunotherapy. *Pharmacol. Res.* **14:** 2–10.

130. Molema, G., D. Meijer, and L. de Leij. 1998. Tumor vasculature targeted therapies. Getting the players organized. Biochem. *Pharmacol.* **55:** 1939–1945.

131. Mukhopadhyay, D., L. Tsiokas, and V. Sukhatme. 1995. Wild-type p53 and v-Src exert opposing influences on human vascular endothelial growth factor gene expression. *Cancer Res.* **55:** 6161–6165.

132. Mukhopadhyay, D., L. Tsiokas, X. Zhou, D. Foster, J. Brugge, and V. Sukhatme. 1995. Hypoxic induction of vascular endothelial growth factor expression through c-*src* activation. *Nature* **375:** 577–581.

133. Mukhopadhyay, D., J. Nagy, E. Manseau, and H. Dvorak. 1998. Vascular permeability factor/vascular endothelial growth factor-mediated signaling in mouse mesentry vascular endothelium. *Cancer Res.* **58:** 1278–1284.

134. Mustonen, T. and K. Alitalo. 1995. Endothelial receptor kinases involved in angiogenesis. *J. Cell Biol.* **129:** 895–898.

135. Neufeld, G., S. Tessler, H. Gitay-Goran, T. Cohen, and B. Levi. 1994. Vascular endothelial growth factor and its receptors. *Prog. Growth Factor Res.* **5:** 89–97.

136. Nicosia, R. F. 1998. What is the role of vascular endothelial growth factor-related molecules in tumor angiogeneis? *Am. J. Pathol.* **153:** 11–16.

137. Okada, F., J. Rak, B. Croix, B. Lieubeau, M. Kaya, L. Roncari, et al. 1998. Impact of oncogenes in tumor angiogenesis: mutant K-*ras* upregulation of vascular endothelial growth factor/vascular permeability factor is necessary, but not sufficient for tumorigenicity of human colorectal carcinoma cells. *Proc. Natl. Acad. Sci. USA* **95:** 3609–3614.

138. O'Reilly, M. S. 1997. Angiostatin: an endogenous inhibitor of angiogenesis and of tumor growth. *EXS* **79:** 273–294.

139. O'Reilly, M. S., T. Boehm, Y. Shing, N. Fukai, G. Vasios, W. Lane, et al. 1997. Endostatin: an endogenous inhibitor of angiogenesis and tumor growth. *Cell* **88:** 277–285.

140. Pepper, M. S., R. Montesano, S. Mandriota, L. Orci, and J. Vasalli. 1996. Angiogenesis: a paradigm for balanced extracellular proteolysis during cell migration and morphogenesis. *Enzyme Protein* **49:** 138–162.

141. Pertovaara, L., A. Kaipainen, T. Mustonen, A. Orpana, N. Ferrara, O. Saksela, et al. 1994. Vascular endothelial growth factor is induced in response to transforming growth factor-beta in fibroblastic and epithelial cells. *J. Biol. Chem.* **269:** 6271–6274.

142. Peters, K. G., C. De Vries, and L. Williams. 1993. Vascular endothelial growth factor expression during embryogenesis and tissue repair suggests a role in endothelial differentiation and blood vessel growth. *Proc. Natl. Acad. Sci. USA* **90:** 8915–8919.

143. Petit, A. M. V., J. Rak, M. Hung, P. Rockwell, N. Goldstein, B. Fendly, et al. 1997. Neutralizing antibodies against epidermal growth factor and ErbB/neu receptor tyrosine kinases have also been shown to down-regulate vascular endothelial growth factor production by tumor cells in vitro and in vivo: angiogenic implications for signal transduction therapy of solid tumors. *Am. J. Pathol.* **151:** 1523–1530.

144. Pilcher, B., J. Dumin, B. Sudbek, S. Krane, H. Welgus, and W. Parks. 1997. The activity of collagenase-1 is required for keratinocyte migration on type I collagen matrix. *J. Cell Biol.* **137:** 1445–1457.

145. Polverini, P. J. 1989. Macrophage induced angiogenesis: a review, in *Cytokine and Macrophage-Derived Cell Regulatory Factors* (Sorg, C., ed.), Karger Verlag, Basel, pp. 54–73.

146. Polverini, P. J. 1996. How the extracellular matrix and macrophages contribute to angiogenesis-dependent diseases. *Eur. J. Cancer* **32A:** 2430–2437.

147. Powell, D., J. Skotnicki, and J. Upeslacis. 1997. Angiogenesis inhibitors. *Ann. Rep. Med. Chem.* **32:** 161–170.

148. Presta, L. G., H. Chen, S. O'Connor, V. Chisholm, Y. Meng, L. Krummen, et al. 1997. Humanization of an anti-vascular endothelial growth factor monoclonal antibody for the therapy of solid tumors and other disorders. *Cancer Res.* **57:** 4593–4599.

149. Quax, P. H. A., A. de Bart, J. Schalken, and J. Verheijen. 1997. Plasminogen activator and matrix metalloproteinase production and extracellular matrix degradation by rat prostate cancer cells in vitro: correlation with metastatic behavior in vivo. *Prostate* **32:** 196–204.

150. Quinn, T. P., K. Peters, C. De Vries, and N. Ferrara. 1993. Fetal liver kinase 1 is a receptor for vascular endothelial growth factor and is selectively expressed in vascular endothelium. *Proc. Natl. Acad. Sci USA* **90:** 7533–7537.

151. Rabbani, S. A. 1998. Metalloproteases and urokinase in angiogenesis and tumor progression. *In Vivo* **12:** 135–142.

152. Risau, W. 1991 Vasculogenesis, angiogenesis and endothelial cell differentiation during embryonic development, in *The Development of the Vascular System* (Feinberg, R. N., Shere, G. K., and Auerbach, R., eds.), Karger, Basel, pp. 58–68.
153. Risau, W. 1995. Differentiation of endothelium. *FASEB J.* **9:** 926–933.
154. Risau, W. 1997. Mechanism of angiogenesis. *Nature* **386:** 671–674.
155. Reynolds, R. P. and D. Redmer. 1998. Expression of the angiogenic factors, basic fibroblast growth factor and vascular endothelial growth factor. *J. Anim. Sci.* **76:** 1671–1681.
156. Rosengart, T. K., L. Lee, S. Patel, T. Sanborn, M. Parikh, G. Bergman, et al. 1999. Angiogenesis gene therapy: phase I assessment of direct intramyocardial administration of an adenovirus vector expressing VEGF121 cDNA to individuals with clinically significant severe coronary artery disease. *Circulation* **100:** 468–474.
157. Royds, J. A., S. Dower, E. Qwarnstrom, and C. Lewis. 1998. Response of tumor cells to hypoxia: role of p53 and MFkB. *Mol. Pathol.* **51:** 55–61.
158. Saleh, M., S. Stacker, and A. Wilks. 1996. Inhibition of growth of C6 glioma cells in vivo by expression of antisense vascular endothelial growth factor sequence. *Cancer Res.* **56:** 393–401.
159. Sandberg, J. A., K. Bouhana, A. Gallegos, A. Agarwal, S. Grimm, F. Wincott, et al. 1999. Pharmacokinetics of an antiangiogenic ribozyme (angiozyme) in the mouse. *Antisense Nucleic Acid Drug Dev.* **9:** 271–277.
160. Sato, T. N., Y. Tozawa, U. Deutsch, K. Wolburg-Buchholz, Y. Fujiwara, M. Gendron-Maguire, et al. 1995. Distinct roles of the receptor tyrosine kinases Tie-1 and Tie-2 in blood vessel formation. *Nature* **376:** 70–74.
161. Sawano, A., T. Takahashi, S. Yamaguchi, and M. Shibuya. 1997. The phosphorylated 1169-tyrosine containing region of flt-1 kinase (VEGFR-1) is a major binding site for PLC gamma. *Biochem. Biophys. Res. Commun.* **238:** 487–491.
162. Scott, W. W., M. Menon, and P. Walsh. 1980. Hormonal therapy for prostatic cancer. *Cancer* **45:** 1929–1936.
163. Sekido, Y., K. Fong, and J. Minna. 1998. Progress in understanding the molecular pathogenesis in human lung cancer. *Biochim. Biophys. Acta* **1378:** F21–F59.
164. Shah-Yukich, A. A. and A. Nelson. 1988. Characterization of solid tumor microvasculature: a three-dimensional analysis using polymer casting technique. *Lab. Investig.* **58:** 236–244.
165. Shreeniwas, R., S. Ogawa, F. Cozzolino, G. Torcia, N. Braunstein, C. Butura, et al. 1991. Macrovascular and microvascular endothelium during long-term hypoxia: alterations in cell growth, monolayer permeability, and cell surface coagulant properties. *J. Cell Physiol.* **146:** 8–17.
166. Siegal, J. A., E. Yu, and M. Brawer. 1995. Topography of neovascularity in human prostate carcinoma. *Cancer* **75:** 2545–2551.
167. Siemeister, G., K. Weindel, K. Mohrs, B. Barleon, G. Martiny-Baron, and D. Marme. 1996. Reversion of deregulated expression of vascular endothelial growth factor in human renal carcinoma cells by von Hippel-Lindau tumor suppressor protein. *Cancer Res.* **56:** 2299–2301.
168. Simons, J. W., B. Mikhak, J. Chang, A. DeMarzo, M. Carducci, M. Lim, et al. 1999. Induction of immunity to prostate cancer antigens: results of a clinical trial of vaccination with irradiated autologous prostate tumor cells engineered to secrete granulocyte-macrophage colony-stimulating factor using ex vivo gene transfer. *Cancer Res.* **59:** 5160–5168.
169. Sinha, A. A., C. Blackard, and U. Seal. 1977. A critical analysis of tumor morphology and hormone treatment in the untreated and estrogen treated responsive and refractory human prostatic carcinomas. *Cancer* **40:** 5070–5075.
170. Sordello, S., N. Bertrand, and J. Plouet. 1998. Vascular endothelial growth factor is up-regulated in vitro and in vivo by androgens. *Biochem. Biophys. Res. Commun.* **25:** 287–290.

171. Stein, I., M. Neeman, D. Shweiki, A. Itin, and E. Keshet. 1995. Stabilization of vascular endothelial growth factor mRNA by hypoxia and hypoglycemia and coregulation with other ischemia-induced genes. *Mol. Cell Biol.* **15:** 5363–5368.

172. Steiner, M. S. 1995. Transforming growth factor-beta and prostate cancer. *World J. Urol.* **13:** 329–336.

173. Sugamoto, T., N. Tanji, S. Nishio, and M. Yokoyama. 1999. Expression of platelet-derived endothelial cell growth factor in prostatic adenocarcinoma. *Oncol. Rep.* **6:** 519–552.

174. Sunderkotter, C., K. Steinbrink, M. Goebeler, R. Bhardwaj, and C. Sorg. 1994. Macrophages and angiogenesis. *J. Leukoc. Biol.* **55:** 410–422.

175. Suri, C., P. Jones, S. Patan, S. Bartunkova, P. Maisonpierre, T. Sato, et al. 1996. Requisite role for angiopoietin-1 a ligand for the Tie-2 receptor, during embryonic angiogenesis. *Cell* **87:** 1171–1180.

176. Suri, C., J. McClain, G. Thurston, D. McDonald, H. Zhou, E. Oldmixon, et al. 1998. Increased vascularization in mice overexpressing angiopoietin-1. *Science* **282:** 468–471.

177. Sutherland, R. M. 1986. Importance of critical metabolites and cellular interactions in the biology of microregions of tumors. *Cancer* **58:** 1668–1680.

178. Taipale, J., J. Saharinen, and J. Keski-Oja. 1998. Extracellular matrix-associated transforming growth factor-beta: role in cancer cell growth and invasion. *Adv. Cancer Res.* **75:** 87–134.

179. Takagi, H., G. King, and L. Aiello. 1996. Identification and characterization of vascular endothelial growth factor receptor (Flt) in bovine retinal pericytes. *Diabetes* **45:** 1016–1023.

180. Takahashi, Y., Y. Kitadai, C. Bucana, K. Cleary, and L. Ellis. 1995. Expression of vascular endothelial growth factor and its receptor KDR correlates with vascularity, metastasis, and proliferation of human colon cancer. *Cancer Res.* **55:** 3364–3968.

181. Takahashi, T. and M. Shibuya. 1997. The 230 kDa mature form of KDR/Flk-1 (VEGF receptor-2) activates the PLC-gamma pathway and partially induces mitogenic signals in NIH3T3 fibroblasts. *Oncogene* **14:** 2079–2089.

182. Tang, B., K. de Castro, H. Barnes, W. Parks, L. Stewart, E. Bottinger, et al. 1998. Loss of responsiveness to transforming growth factor beta induces malignant transformation of nontumorigenic rat prostate epithelial cells. *Cancer Res.* **59:** 4834–4842.

183. Teicher, B. A., G. Ara, K. Menon, and R. Schaub. 1996. In vivo studies with interleukin-12 alone and in combination with monocyte colony-stimulating factor and/or fractionated radiation treatment. *Int. J. Cancer* **65:** 80–84.

184. Thorpe, P. E. and F. Burrows. 1995. Antibody-directed targeting of the vasculature of solid tumors. *Br. Cancer Res. Trt.* **36:** 237–251.

185. Tio, R. A., T. Tkebuchava, T. Scheuermann, C. Lebherz, M. Magner, M. Kearny, et al. 1998. Intramyocardial gene therapy with naked DNA encoding vascular endothelial growth factor improves collateral flow to ischemic myocardium. *Hum. Gene Ther.* **10:** 2953–2960.

186. Tsai, J. C., C. Goldman, and G. Gillespie. 1995. Vascular endothelial growth factor in human glioma cell lines: induced secretion by EGF, PDGF-BB and bFGF. *J. Neurosurg.* **82:** 864–873.

187. Tsurusaki, T., S. Kanda, H. Sakai, H. Kanetake, Y. Saito, K. Alitalo, et al. 1999. Vascular endothelial growth factor -C expression in human prostatic carcinoma and its relationship to lymph node metastasis. *Br. J. Cancer* **80:** 309–313.

188. Tuder, R. M., B. Flook, and N. Voelkel. 1995. Increased gene expression of VEGF and the VEGF receptors KDR/Flk and Flt in lungs exposed to acute or chronic hypoxia. *J. Clin. Investig.* **95:** 1798–1807.

189. Volpert, O. V., K. Dameron, and N. Bouck. 1997. Sequential development of an angiogenic phenotype by human fibroblasts progressing to tumorigenicity. *Oncogene* **14:** 1495–1502.

190. Wakui, S., M. Furusato, T. Itoh, H. Sasakt, A. Ariyama, I. Kinoshito, et al. 1992. Tumor angiogenesis in prostatic carcinoma with and without bone marrow metastasis: a morphometric study. *J. Pathol.* **168:** 257–262.

191. Walter, J. J. and D. Sane. 1999. Angiostatin binds smooth muscle cells in the coronary artery and inhibits smooth muscle cell proliferation and migration in vitro. Arterioscler. *Throm. Vasc. Biol.* **19:** 2041–2048.

192. Walttenberger, J., L. Claesson, A. Siegbahn, M. Shibuya, and C. Heldin. 1994. Different signal transduction properties of KDR and Flt1 two receptors for vascular endothelial growth factor. *J. Biol. Chem.* **269:** 26,988–26,995.

193. Wang, Y. and D. Becker. 1997. Antisense targeting of basic fibroblast growth factor and fibroblast growth factor receptor -1 in human melanomas blocks intratumoral angiogenesis and tumor growth. *Nat. Med.* **3:** 887–893.

194. Warren, R. S., H. Yuan, M. Matli, N. Ferrara, and D. Donner. 1996. Induction of vascular endothelial growth factor by insulin-like growth factor 1 in colorectal carcinoma. *J. Biol. Chem.* **271:** 29,483–29,488.

195. Weidner, N. 1993. Tumor angiogenesis correlates with metastasis in invasive prostate carcinoma. *Am. J. Pathol.* **143:** 401–409.

196. Wenger, R. H. and M. Gassmann. 1997. Oxygen(es) and hypoxia-inducible factor-1. *Biol. Chem.* **378:** 609–616.

197. Wenger, R. H., G. Camenisch, I. Desbaillets, D. Chilov, and M. Gassmann. 1998. Up-regulation of hypoxia-inducible factor 1- HIF-1 is not sufficient for hypoxia/anoxic p53 induction. *Cancer Res.* **58:** 5678–5680.

198. Wetermarck, J. and V. Kahari. 1999. Regulation of matrix metalloproteinase expression in tumor invasion. *FASEB J.* **13:** 781–792.

199. Wilson, C., K. Heppner, P. Labosky, B. Hogan, and L. Matrisian. 1997. Intestinal tumorigenesis is suppressed in mice lacking the metalloproteinase matrilysin. *Proc. Natl. Acad. Sci. USA* **94:** 1402–1407.

200. Xia, P., L. Aiello, H. Ishii, Z. Jiang, D. Park, and G. Robinson. 1996. Characterization of vascular endothelial growth factor's effect on the activation of protein kinase C its isoforms and endothelial cell growth. *J. Clin. Investig.* **98:** 2018–2026.

201. Yamamoto, S., I. Konishi, Y. Tsurura, K. Nanbu, M. Mandai, H. Kuroda, et al. 1997. Expression of vascular endothelial growth factor (VEGF) during folliculogenesis and corpus luteum formation in the human ovary. *Gynecol. Endocrinol.* **11:** 371–381.

202. Zetter, B. R. 1998. Angiogenesis and tumor metastasis. *Ann. Rev. Med.* **49:** 407–424.

18

Prostate Specific Membrane Antigen

Denise S. O'Keefe, PhD, Dean J. Bacich, PhD, and Warren D. W. Heston, PhD

1. INTRODUCTION

The molecular basis of prostate carcinoma has always been less understood than that of other cancers, despite its high incidence in the population. One of the reasons for this is that the molecular pathways leading to prostate cancer do not seem to parallel that of other cancers, and until recently there have been few markers for this tumor. One of the most exciting recent findings in prostate cancer was the discovery of prostate specific membrane antigen (PSMA). PSMA is a glutamate carboxypeptidase that switches from a cytosolically located protein in the normal prostate to a membrane-bound protein in prostatic carcinoma. The majority of PSMA expression appears to be restricted to the prostate, with some expression seen in the brain, salivary glands, and small intestine. Intriguingly, our group recently found that PSMA is expressed in the endothelial cells of the neovasculature of nearly all solid tumors examined. The membrane-bound nature of this protein—and the limited sites of expression as well as expression in tumor-associated neovasculature—makes PSMA an ideal marker and therapeutic target for clinical studies and treatment of not only prostate cancer, but of other solid tumors as we progress into the 21st century.

2. THE DISCOVERY OF PSMA

The antigen itself was discovered by Horoszewicz et al. *(28)*, who isolated LNCaP cell membranes and immunized mice with the mixture, producing the antibody known as 7E11C5.3. The LNCaP cell line is derived from a Lymph Node metastasis from a Carcinoma of the Prostate, and is considered the most relevant of the few prostatic cell lines available, because it retains expression of prostate specific antigen (PSA), prostatic acid phosphatase (PAP) and the androgen receptor, among other characteristics typical of human prostate cancers in vivo *(23,25,29,30)*. Characterization of the antibody revealed that it specifically bound epithelial cells of normal prostate, benign prostatic hypertrophy (BPH), and prostatic carcinoma specimens, making PSMA an attractive prostate-specific marker *(28)*. The rights to the 7E11C5.3 antibody were then bought by a biotechnology company called Cytogen Corporation (Princeton, NJ).

Cytogen modified the antibody so that it could be labeled with [111]Indium while retaining its specificity, and renamed it Cyt-356. The radiolabeled antibody was then

From: *Prostate Cancer: Biology, Genetics, and the New Therapeutics*
Edited by: L. W. K. Chung, W. B. Isaacs, and J. W. Simons © Humana Press Inc., Totowa, NJ

administered to nude mice carrying tumors established from the LNCaP cell line. After 3 d, 30% of the injected dose had localized to the LNCaP xenograft, with no significant amounts found in other tissues *(42)*. This occurred despite the fact that the same investigators had noted that immunohistochemical staining using this modified antibody against normal human tissues showed weak reactivity with cardiac muscle, proximal kidney tubules, and sweat glands. There was also strong binding to a subset of skeletal muscle cells. A phase I clinical study using radiolabeled Cyt-356 as an imaging agent for metastatic deposits was then carried out in patients with prostate cancer and known distant metastases *(78)*. No adverse affects of the agent were noted in the patients, and the results showed promise for use of the immunoconjugate as an imaging agent. At this stage it was clear that a deeper understanding of the molecular basis and function of PSMA expression in prostate cancer was needed.

3. CLONING AND EXPRESSION PATTERN OF PSMA

The complementary DNA (cDNA) sequence encoding PSMA was cloned in 1993 using a classic textbook approach *(33)*. The monoclonal antibody Cyt-356 was used to immunoprecipitate PSMA from LNCaP cell membranes, and the protein was then electrophoresed on and isolated from a polyacrylamide gel. PSMA was then subjected to proteolytic digestion and the subsequent peptide fragments were microsequenced to determine their amino acid composition. Based on the amino acid sequence, degenerate oligonucleotide primers were designed that could theoretically amplify the PSMA cDNA sequence from LNCaP reverse-transcribed mRNA. The resulting PCR product was cloned and used to probe a LNCaP cDNA library and isolate the full-length PSMA transcript of 2653 nucleotides (the sequence can be found in Genbank under the accession number M99487).

Translation of the cDNA sequence predicted that the protein consists of 750 amino acids with a molecular wt of 84 kDa before posttranslational modifications *(33)*. It was later shown that in vitro translation of the PSMA cDNA sequence with and without dog pancreatic microsomal membranes (which permit glycosylation of proteins to occur in vitro) produces proteins of 100 and 84 kDa, respectively. This is consistent with the 100 kDa molecular wt of PSMA seen in LNCaP cells *(32)*. PSMA is a Type II integral membrane protein, and as such the short N-terminal of the protein is located on the cytoplasmic side of the membrane, with the majority of the protein located on the extracellular side of the membrane, making it available for clinical and therapeutic targeting *(33)*. Northern analyses using the PSMA cDNA probe and ribonuclease protection assays using a probe corresponding to nucleotides 242–588 of the PSMA cDNA sequence showed no expression of PSMA mRNA in the prostatic cell lines PC-3 and DU145, and no expression in normal tissues from kidney, liver, lung, mammary gland, pancreas, placenta, skeletal muscle, spleen, and testis. However, there was high expression in normal prostate and prostatic carcinomas, and barely detectable expression in salivary gland, whole brain, and small intestine. Expression of PSMA mRNA in BPH specimens was either reduced relative to that of normal prostate, or absent altogether *(32)*, which is most likely an indication of the major cell type that constitues BPH (stromal cells that do not express PSMA), rather than a biologic phenomenon. Interestingly, our group and others recently found that PSMA is expressed in the endothelial cells of neovasculature associated with almost all solid tumors, but not in normal vasculature *(40,61)*. Immunohistochemistry using five different antibodies against PSMA has confirmed this, as have *in situ* hybridization and RT-PCR results *(8,9)*. In fact, the only tumor which does not seem to consistently express PSMA in the associated vasculature is that of the prostate (2/12 prostate cancer specimens expressed PSMA in the vasculature), perhaps providing a clue to the function of PSMA in these cells *(9)*.

As PSA expression is modulated by androgens, Israeli et al. examined the effect of various steroids on PSMA expression in LNCaP cells *(32)*. In contrast to PSA expression, PSMA is downregulated in the presence of androgens, with the highest amount of PSMA expressed in LNCaP cells grown in charcoal-stripped (and therefore steroid-reduced) media. This finding was later supported both in vitro in LNCaP cells, and in vivo by Wright et al., *(76)*, who found that in 55% (11 of 20) and 100% (4 of 4) primary and metastatic tumor specimens, PSMA expression was significantly upregulated in patients who had undergone some form of hormonal deprivation, relative to matched specimens from the patients before treatment. These findings are particularly significant, because of the implication that PSMA can be a highly useful clinical and therapeutic target for patients with recurrent disease.

4. REGULATION OF PSMA EXPRESSION: CLONING OF THE PSMA PROMOTER AND ENHANCER

To obtain more information about the genetic regulation of PSMA expression, we set out to determine the complete sequence of the gene. A bacteriophage P1 library containing fragments of DNA from normal human lymphocytes approx 60–80 kb in size was screened using PCR. Two sets of oligonucleotide primers were used—one set corresponding to the 5′ end of the PSMA cDNA sequence, and one set corresponding to the 3′ end of the sequence. The advantage of this method of screening was that the gene spanned more than 60 kb of DNA, and two P1 clones that overlapped by about 5.6 kb had to be analyzed to acquire the entire sequence *(50)*.

Comparison of the genomic and cDNA sequences of the PSMA gene revealed 19 exons ranging in size from 64 to 379 nucleotides, and 18 introns from 300 to 7363 base pairs (Fig. 1). The entire genomic sequence of the gene can be found in Genbank, under accession number AF007544. One of the most striking features of the genomic sequence was the presence of a CpG island at the 5′ end of the gene. From nucelotides 2661–2990 of the genomic sequence—which extends from exon 1 into the first intron of the gene—the observed/expected ratio of the CpG dinucleotide was 1.85, which is significantly greater than the ratio for bulk human DNA (0.25)*(1,50)*. CpG islands are substrates for DNA methyltransferase, and the presence of a CpG island in the 5′ region of the PSMA gene suggests a role for DNA methylation in the regulation of PSMA expression.

Once we had the genomic sequence of the 5′ portion of the gene, we were able to clone the promoter controlling transcription of PSMA mRNA. To confirm the transcription start site indicated by the initial PSMA cDNA sequence *(33)*, we carried out 5′ Rapid Amplification of cDNA Ends (5′ RACE). 5′ RACE is a form of PCR that uses one primer based in the known cDNA sequence of the gene, and one primer that binds to 5′ ends of all mRNA transcripts. Thus, only one primer is specific to the gene of

```
   1  ctcaaaaggg gccggatttc cttctcctgg aggcagatgt tgcctctctc tctcgctcgg attggttcag tgcactctag aaacactgct

  91  gtggtggaga aactggaccc caggtctgga gcgaattcca gcctgcaggg ctgataagcg aggcattagt gagattgaga gagactttac

 181  cccgccgtgg tggttggagg gcgcgcagta gagcagcagc acaggcgcgg gtcccgggag gccggctctg ctcgcgccga gATGTGGAAT

 271  CTCCTTCACG AAACCGACTC GGCTGTGGCC ACCGCGCGCC GCCCGCGCTG GCTGTGCGCT GGGGCGCTGG TGCTGGCGGG TGGCTTCTTT
                    ▼ INTRON 1- 2130 BP

 361  CTCCTCGGCT TCCTCTTCGG GTGGTTTATA AAATCCTCCA ATGAAGCTAC TAACATTACT CCAAAGCATA ATATGAAAGC ATTTTTGGAT
                              ▼ INTRON 2 - 5626 BP

 451  GAATTGAAAG CTGAGAACAT CAAGAAGTTC TTATATAATT TTACACAGAT ACCACATTTA GCAGGAACAG AACAAAACTT TCAGCTTGCA

 541  AAGCAAATTC AATCCCAGTG GAAAGAATTT GGCCTGGATT CTGTTGAGCT AGCACATTAT GATGTCCTGT TGTCCTACCC AAATAAGACT
                              ▼ INTRON 3 - 7363 BP

 631  CATCCCAACT ACATCTCAAT AATTAATGAA GATGGAAATG AGATTTTCAA CACATCATTA TTTGAACCAC CTCCTCCAGG ATATGAAAAT
                              INTRON 4 - 6023 BP ▼

 721  GTTTCGGATA TTGTACCACC TTTCAGTGCT TTCTCTCCTC AAGGAATGCC AGAGGGCGAT CTAGTGTATG TTAACTATGC ACGAACTGAA
                                                                                  INTRON 5 - 788 BP ▼

 811  GACTTCTTTA AATTGGAACG GGACATGAAA ATCAATTGCT CTGGGAAAAT TGTAATTGCC AGATATGGGA AAGTTTTCAG AGGAAATAAG

 901  GTTAAAAATG CCCAGCTGGC AGGGGCCAAA GGAGTCATTC TCTACTCCGA CCCTGCTGAC TACTTTGCTC CTGGGGTGAA GTCCTATCCA

 991  GATGGTTGGA ATCTTCCTGG AGGTGGTGTC CAGCGTGGAA ATATCCTAAA TCTGAATGGT GCAGGAGACC CTCTCACACC AGGTTACCCA
            ▼ INTRON 6 - 2426 BP

1081  GCAAATGAAT ATGCTTATAG GCGTGGAATT GCAGAGGCTG TTGGTCTTCC AAGTATTCCT GTTCATCCAA TTGGATACTA TGATGCACAG
            ▼ INTRON 7 - 7195 BP

1171  AAGCTCCTAG AAAAAATGGG TGGCTCAGCA CCACCAGATA GCAGCTGGAG AGGAAGTCTC AAAGTGCCCT ACAATGTTGG ACCTGGCTTT
                              ▼ INTRON 8 - 881 BP

1261  ACTGGAAACT TTTCTACACA AAAAGTCAAG ATGCACATCC ACTCTACCAA TGAAGTGACA AGAATTTACA ATGTGATAGG TACTCTCAGA
            ▼ INTRON 9 - 1415 BP

1351  GGAGCAGTGG AACCAGACAG ATATGTCATT CTGGGAGGTC ACCGGGACTC ATGGGTGTTT GGTGGTATTG ACCCTCAGAG TGGAGCAGCT
                                        ▼ INTRON 10 - 2079 BP

1441  GTTGTTCATG AAATTGTGAG GAGCTTTGGA ACACTGAAAA AGGAAGGGTG GAGACCTAGA AGAACAATTT TGTTTGCAAG CTGGGATGCA
                              ▼ INTRON 11 - 1932 BP

1531  GAAGAATTTG GTCTTCTTGG TTCTACTGAG TGGGCAGAGG AGAATTCAAG ACTCCTTCAA GAGCGTGGCG TGGCTTATAT TAATGCTGAC
            ▼ INTRON 12 - 4426 BP                                                       ▼ INTRON 13 - 6659 BP

1621  TCATCTATAG AAGGAAACTA CACTCTGAGA GTTGATTGTA CACCGCTGAT GTACAGCTTG GTACACAACC TAACAAAAGA GCTGAAAAGC
                                                                            INTRON 14 - 1144 BP ▼

1711  CCTGATGAAG GCTTTGAAGG CAAATCTCTT TATGAAAGTT GGACTAAAAA AAGTCCTTCC CCAGAGTTCA GTGGCATGCC CAGGATAAGC
                                                            INTRON 15 - 2206 BP ▼

1801  AAATTGGGAT CTGGAAATGA TTTTGAGGTG TTCTTCCAAC GACTTGGAAT TGCTTCAGGC AGAGCACGGT ATACTAAAAA TTGGGAAACA

1891  AACAAATTCA GCGGCTATCC ACTGTATCAC AGTGTCTATG AAACATATGA GTTGGTGGAA AAGTTTTATG ATCCAATGTT TAAATATCAC

1981  CTCACTGTGG CCCAGGTTCG AGGAGGGATG GTGTTTGAGC TAGCCAATTC CATAGTGCTC CCTTTTGATT GTCGAGATTA TGCTGTAGTT
                                                                      INTRON 16- 300 BP ▼

2071  TTAAGAAAGT ATGCTGACAA AATCTACAGT ATTTCTATGA AACATCCACA GGAAATGAAG ACATACAGTG TATCATTTGA TTCACTTTTT
                                                            ▼ INTRON 17 - 5115 BP

2161  TCTGCAGTAA AGAATTTTAC AGAAATTGCT TCCAAGTTCA GTGAGAGACT CCAGGACTTT GACAAAAGCA ACCCAATAGT ATTAAGAATG
                                                                            ▼ INTRON 18 - 1693 BP

2251  ATGAATGATC AACTCATGTT TCTGGAAAGA GCATTTATTG ATCCATTAGG GTTACCAGAC AGGCCTTTTT ATAGGCATGT CATCTATGCT

2341  CCAAGCAGCC ACAACAAGTA TGCAGGGGAG TCATTCCCAG GAATTTATGA TGCTCTGTTT GATATTGAAA GCAAAGTGGA CCCTTCCAAG

2431  GCCTGGGGAG AAGTGAAGAG ACAGATTTAT GTTGCAGCCT TCACAGTGCA GGCAGCTGCA GAGACTTTGA GTGAAGTAGC CTAAgaggat

2521  tctttagaga atccgtattg aatttgtgtg gtatgtcact cagaaagaat cgtaatgggt atattgataa attttaaaat tggtatattt

2611  gaaataaagt tgaatattat atataaaaaa aaaaaaaaaa aaa
```

Fig. 1. The cDNA sequence of the human PSMA gene. The 5′ and 3′ untranslated regions are shown in lower case; the coding region is in upper case. The start and stop codons are underlined, and intron positions and sizes are indicated by the arrowhead.

interest, but by using this method it is possible to determine the exact start sites of transcription and therefore predict the sequence encompassing the promoter region of the gene. Our 5′ RACE experiments confirmed the original start site (+1 of the cDNA sequence), but also showed other start sites within this region, at −195 and −235, in addition to the original start site at −262 relative to the translation initiation codon of the gene. Such heterogeneity of transcription start sites is not uncommon in genes where the promoter lacks a TATA box. Consistent with this finding, the DNA sequence upstream of these start sites has no typical TATA boxes (50). We next cloned the 1244 base pair region of genomic DNA spanning the start sites, and approx 1 kb of the region 5′, into a reporter vector to test whether the region was capable of driving transcription of the firefly luciferase gene. To our surprise, not only did this region of the gene have significant activity/mg of cell protein relative to the strong SV-40 viral promoter/enhancer in LNCaP cells, but it also appeared to be prostate specific, in that we could not detect significant levels of luciferase in the DU145 and MCF-7 cell lines (prostate and breast carcinoma lines). These cell lines do not express PSMA, and therefore presumably do not contain the appropriate trancription factors for activation of the PSMA promoter.

Interestingly, we did see luciferase expression driven by the PSMA promoter in PC-3 cells—another prostatic cell line that does not express PSMA—at levels corresponding to about 10% of that of the control SV-40 promoter/enhancer *(50)*. This led us to examine the genomic region of PC-3 DNA containing the CpG island for hypermethylation by Southern analysis with methylation sensitive restriction enzymes. We were able to demonstrate that while DNA from normal male lymphocytes and the LNCaP cell line was not hypermethylated, DNA from PC-3 cells was at least partially hypermethylated in this region. We next treated PC-3 cells with the demethylating agent 5-azacytidine, but were unable to detect expression of PSMA after treatment with the drug (O'Keefe et al., unpublished data), and we are still investigating this phenomenon.

In further experiments to delineate the minimal promoter region of the gene, we discovered that our original estimation of the strength of the PSMA promoter was somewhat high. We had calculated the strength of the PSMA promoter relative to that of the usually strong SV-40 promoter/enhancer in the luciferase-reporter experiments. However, when we transfected various cell lines with the SV-40 promoter alone—and after adjusting for transfection efficiency compared these transfections to those with the SV-40 promoter/enhancer combination—we were surprised to find that in LNCaP cells, addition of the SV-40 enhancer to the basal SV-40 promoter did not enhance reporter gene transcription and in some cases repressed it. In contrast, in other cell lines such as PC-3, the SV-40 promoter/enhancer combination significantly increases reporter gene transcription (O'Keefe et al., unpublished data). Other laboratories have reported similar findings in LNCaP cells when combining the SV-40 enhancer with other basal promoters such as the PSA minimal promoter (Peter Molloy, personal communication) although the reason for this remains unclear.

Deletion constructs of the promoter region allowed us to localize the minimal promoter to between bases 461–1097. The original promoter construct had contained an *Alu* repeat sequence, and we also found that once this region was deleted, reporter gene expression increased (Horiguchi et al., unpublished data). Although PSMA expression is regulated by androgens *(32,76)*, there are no typical androgen-response elements in the promoter region or in the entire PSMA genomic sequence. However, because there might be novel androgen response elements, we tested the deletion constructs and the original promoter construct for androgen responsiveness in LNCaP cells.

Although the minimal PSMA promoter described here appeared to exhibit prostate-specificity, it could only promote basal levels of reporter gene expression *(75)*. Watt et al. *(75)* cloned the PSMA enhancer region (PSME) using an "enhancer trap" system. The enhancer trap library was created by partial digestion of the P1 bacteriophage clones containing the PSMA genomic sequence, and subcloning the resultant fragments into a vector containing the PSMA promoter-driving expression of the Green Fluorescent Protein (GFP) gene. Screening of the library for DNA fragments able to increase GFP expression over that seen by the promoter alone was carried out in LNCaP cells and a number of other non-PSMA expressing cell lines. Using this method, a fragment of DNA that was able to increase transcription from the PSMA promoter by 250-fold was identified. When the enhancer was linked to other stronger basal promoters instead of the PSMA promoter, transcription levels were increased by at least 10-fold; in the most impressive experiment, the PSME was linked to the herpes virus thymidine kinase (TK) promoter and transcription was nearly threefold that of the Rous-Sarcoma Virus promoter/enhancer, which in itself is a strong viral promoter. The PSME retains prostate-specificity even when linked to the TK promoter—which is not prostate restricted in expression—and the PSME also shows repression by androgens *(75)*. As such, the PSME shows excellent promise for use in gene therapy approaches targeting prostate cancer in the near future.

5. ALTERNATIVE SPLICING OF THE PSMA GENE

Using RT-PCR of normal prostate tissue, Su et al. *(64)* discovered the first reported mRNA splice-variant of the PSMA gene. The variant, PSM′ (PSM-prime), transcribes from the regular PSMA promoter and uses an alternative 5′ splice donor site within exon one of the gene, deleting bases 114–379, which includes the translation start codon for PSMA. Initiation of translation of the PSM′ protein begins at nucleotide 427, producing a glycoprotein of about 95 kDa that lacks the intracellular and transmembrane domains of PSMA. As such, PSM′ is located within the cytoplasm, but still retains the enzymatic activity of PSMA *(21)*. RNase protection assays differentiating PSMA from PSM′ mRNA transcripts revealed that in normal prostate PSM′ is the dominant isoform, whereas in prostate tumors and the LNCaP cell line PSMA is more prevalent *(36,64)*. Compilation of the data to form a "tumor index" comparing the ratio of PSMA:PSM′ resulted in a score of 9–11 for LNCaP cells, 3–6 for prostate carcinoma, 0.75–1.6 for BPH, and 0.075–0.45 for the normal prostate. Unfortunately, further analysis of the ratio of PSMA:PSM′ in clinical specimens has not been reported, so it remains unclear whether or not this tumor index could have a clinical impact.

Another alternative splice form of PSMA that was isolated from the human brain, prostate, and liver deletes amino acids 657–688 of the protein *(5)*, and creates an amino acid substitution (Asn→Lys). These amino acids correspond to the entire 18th exon of the gene, so the splicing event probably occurs by "exon skipping." We have also seen this splice form in cDNA derived from a colon tumor. Further investigation of this variant is required to determine whether it retains the activity of the full length PSMA protein, and whether it exists in significant levels relative to PSMA and PSM′.

Finally, when we implemented 5′ RACE of the PSMA gene using LNCaP cells, we discovered a number of novel transcripts. The first, which we have called PSM-C, begins transcription at the same nucleotides as the PSMA and PSM′ transcripts, then uses the same splice donor site as PSM′ (nt 114), but uses an alternative splice acceptor site located within intron one. Nucleotides 3270–3402 of the genomic PSMA sequence are transcribed, followed by exon 2 and exon 3. Translation of this variant containing a previously unidentified exon, which we have termed exon 1b, would result in a protein identical to PSM′. Another variant, PSM-D, again uses the same splice donor site as PSM′, and a unique splice acceptor site in intron one, including another novel exon (exon 1c) which is from nucleotides 4289–4389 of the genomic PSMA sequence. The putative translation of this protein reveals a new translation-initiation start site located in exon 1c, followed by 42 novel amino acids and the rest of the PSMA protein in-frame. Interestingly, a motif in the novel region consisting of the peptide Ala-Ala-Tyr-Ala-Cys-Thr-Gly-Cys-Leu-Ala is similar to that seen in the growth-factor cys-knot family of proteins. Using RT-PCR, we were able to demonstrate the existence of this variant in normal prostate and LNCaP cells; however, we were unable to demon-strate significant amounts of this mRNA splice variant via RNase protection assays on these tissues.

At least one other group has also found splice variants arising from novel exons in intron one of the gene; one exon continuing on from the 3′ end of exon 1 for 68 nucle-otides, and another extending for 97 nucleotides. All three variants include exon 1 (nt 1–379), and thus would be predicted to translate into a protein with a transmem-brane domain. One of the variants contains both new exons aligned in tandem, and the three variants are expected to produce proteins between 40 and 805 amino acids in length *(53)*. Novel variants such as those described here have not been proven to con-tribute to or be functionally involved in prostate cancer. Therefore, their clinical sig-nificance remains uncertain.

6. MAPPING OF THE PSMA GENE AND IDENTIFICATION OF THE PSMA-LIKE GENE

Chromosomal localization of the PSMA gene has proven to be controversial. Initial mapping by two independent research groups using Fluorescent In Situ Hybridization (FISH) and the full-length cDNA sequence as a probe indicated two regions for the gene—11p11-12, and 11q14 *(38,56)*. To identify the true location of the PSMA gene, Leek et al. *(38)* used PCR of somatic cell hybrids containing various regions of chro-mosome 11, assigned the gene to 11p, and suggested that the 11q14 locus represented a PSMA pseudogene. Rinker-Schaeffer et al. used two P1 clones containing approx 120 kb of the PSMA gene and surrounding sequence to repeat the FISH experiment, and under conditions of high stringency, assigned the gene to 11q14 *(56)*. Later, it became apparent that FISH can be subject to artifact under conditions of high strin-gency when one of the regions involved is close to a centromere, which in this case is the 11p11 locus. We therefore mapped the gene again, using a number of sets of oligo-nucleotide primers designed to bind both intronic and exonic sequences of the gene, and PCR against a panel of somatic cell hybrids containing various regions of chromo-some 11. We found that the PSMA gene does map to 11p11, approx 7 Mb from D11S1350. We also established that the "PSMA pseudogene" sequence reported on Genbank as mapping to 11q14 (accession number HSU93599) did not exist, but instead a gene that is highly homologous to the PSMA gene resides on 11q14.3 *(50)*. Further analysis of the gene at the 11q14 locus (which we have termed the "PSMA-like" gene, Genbank accession number AF261715), revealed that exons 2–19 of the PSMA gene are duplicated on the long arm of chromosome 11, along with their corresponding introns. We have been unable to detect duplication of the promoter region, or of exon

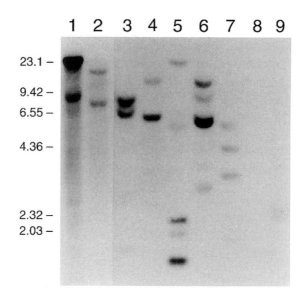

Fig. 2. Zoo-Blot using PSMA cDNA as a probe. Genes homologous to PSMA exist in many other species, including yeast. Lanes 1–9 are hybridized with genomic DNA from: (1) human, (2) monkey, (3) rat, (4) mouse, (5) dog, (6) bovine, (7) rabbit, (8) chicken, and (9) yeast.

one *(50)*. This would suggest a different mechanism of regulation, and therefore a different tissue expression pattern of the PSMA-like gene. The exonic sequences of the two genes are highly conserved (97% identical), and we have determined that the PSMA-like gene is transcribed and expressed in kidney and liver tissue, but not in prostate samples (O'Keefe et al., unpublished data). Complete characterization of the PSMA-like gene is needed. Thus, clinical and therapeutic strategies targeting PSMA can be designed to avoid PSMA-like expressing tissues or targets, and subsequently limit lack of specificity and unecessary toxicity.

7. MOLECULAR EVOLUTION OF THE PSMA FAMILY OF PROTEINS

Comparison of the intronic sequence differences of the PSMA and PSMA-like genes allowed us to calculate that evolutionary period in which the original gene duplicated was 22 million years ago *(50)*. This data is consistent with the report that the tyrosinase gene, which is closely linked to the PSMA-like gene on chromosome 11q14, was subject to duplication to 11p 24 million years ago *(17)*. It would therefore seem that the locus at 11q14 contained the original gene, and that a little more than 20 million years ago—after the divergence of man and rodent, but before the separation of man and chimp—this locus was duplicated on 11p11. Both genes then evolved further, with the PSMA gene gaining expression in the prostate. Southern blot analysis has shown that PSMA homologs exist in many species, and this is supported by the finding of homologs as far back in evolution as yeast and *C. Elegans* (Fig. 2; Heston et al., unpublished; *[55]*). Similarly, it is interesting to note that although PSMA homologs have been cloned in several of these species, there are no reports of PSMA expression in the prostate *(2,5,22)*. Instead, these PSMA homologs seem to be primarily expressed in the

Table 1
Homology Between Human PSMA and Selected Homologs and Paralogs

Species	Protein	Size (aa)	AA/NT homology to PSMA	Folate Hyd. activity	DPP IV activity	NAALA-Dase activity	GenBank accession number	Reference
Human	PSMA	750	100/100%	+	+	+	M99487	(8)
	NAALADase II	740	67/74%	nt	+	+	AJ012370	(30)
	NAALADase L	740	35/ns%	nt	+	–	AJ012371	(30)
	PGCP	542	27/ns%	nt	nt	+	AF119386	(29)
	DPP IV	766	29/ns%	nt	+	nt	M80536	(33)
	Transferin Receptor.	760	31/ns%	–	–	–	M11507	(34)
Mouse	MoPSM (PSMA homolog)	752	86/85%	+	nt	+	AF026380	(2)
Rat	NAALADase (PSMA homolog)	752	86/85%	+[a]	nt	+	U75973	(21)
	I100[b]	746	41/ns%	nt	+	–	AF009921	(35)
Pig	Folypoly-γ-glutamate Carboxypeptidase (PSMA homolog)	751	91/88%	+	nt	+	AF050502	(27)

[a] Bacich et al. unpublished observations;

[b] rat homolog of NAALADase L protein; The amino acid (AA) and nucleotide (NT) homologies to PSMA are shown; NT homologies were determined by a BLAST 2 sequences alignment using standard parameters. "ns" refers to a nonsignificant alignment (BLOSUM 62). "nt" refers to enzymatic activities that have not been tested.

small intestine, brain, and kidney of other species. In the species which is most often used as an experimental model resembling man—the mouse—there is clearly no prostatic expression of the murine homolog of PSMA (termed MoPSM), as determined by northern analysis and RT-PCR (2). Furthermore, there is only one gene in the mouse, and the MoPSM gene maps to mouse chromosome 7D1-2, which is syntenic with human 11q14 (2). Considering these facts, it is tempting to suggest that the PSMA-like gene contributes to the extraprostatic expression currently attributed to PSMA, and that expression of PSMA in the prostate may somehow put the prostate at high risk for developing mutations and subsequent carcinogenesis.

8. ENZYMATIC ACTIVITY OF PSMA AND RELATED GENES

Recently, PSMA homologs have been cloned from mouse (2), rat (5), and pig (22), in addition to the cloning of more distantly related paralogs of PSMA in humans (18,51). The cloning and comparison of these homologs and paralogs has shed considerable light on some of the activities of PSMA, and provided some insight into which amino acid sequences appear to be crucial in these activities. PSMA has three known activities: a folate poly γ glutamyl carboxypeptidase (folate hydrolase) (54), a NAALADase (7) and a dipeptidyl peptidase IV (51). A comparison of these three activities in the PSMA homologs and paralogs is summarized in Table 1.

The folate hydrolase activity of PSMA describes the sequential removal of γ-linked glutamates from conjugated folates and folate analogs such as methotrexate γ-glutamate and pteroylpentaglutamate, as shown in Fig. 3A *(54)*. The folate hydrolase activity of PSMA is maintained in the presence of sulfhydryl reducing agents and *p*-hydroxy-mercuribenzonate, in contrast to an unrelated folate hydrolase enzyme that is located in lysosomes.

PSMA also possesses NAALADase activity, because it is able to hydrolyze the neuropeptide N-acetyl-L-aspartyl-L-glutamate (NAAG) to form *N*-acetyl-L-aspartate and glutamate. This is hydrolysis of the aspartyl α linkage, as shown in Fig. 3B. This activity was first reported by Robinson et al. *(57)* in 1986 in the rat brain, and was demonstrated to be inhibited by quisqualate. NAALADase and its neuropeptide substrate NAAG have been implicated in the regulation of excitatory signaling in the nervous system *(14,77)*. Altered activity of NAALADase has been associated with various neurolgical disorders, including schizophrenia *(11,73)*, Alzheimer's disease, and Huntington's disease *(52)*. In addition, increased levels of NAALADase have been observed in animal models for epilepsy *(45–47,52)* and amylotrophic lateral sclerosis *(58,72,74)*.

Carter et al. *(7)* used antisera to purified rat NAALADase to screen a rat-brain expression library, resulting in the isolation of a partial 1428 nt cDNA clone that had 86% homology to part of the human PSMA cDNA sequence. The entire rat PSMA/ NAALADase sequence was subsequently cloned by *(5)*, and when transiently transfected into PC-3 cells (which are NAALADase-negative), they gained NAALADase activity that could be inhibited by quisqualic acid. Human PSMA was also demonstrated to have NAALADase activity *(7)*. Further characterization by Luthi-Carter et al. demonstrated that the human brain NAALADase could be immunoprecipitated with the MAb 7E11-C5 *(44)*. As this antibody binds to residues not conserved in PSMA-like (O'Keefe et al., unpublished), it suggests that human NAALADase and PSMA are derived from the same gene. In addition, Luthi-Carter amplified RNA by RT-PCR, a sequence identical to the LNCaP-derived PSMA sequence, from human cerebellum, indicating that this RNA is present, but in itself not proving that all of the NAALADase activity found in the brain is from PSMA.

Recently, it was shown that PSMA also has dipeptidyl peptidase IV activity, which refers to the ability to hydrolyze Glycine-Proline-7-amido-4-methylcoumarin *(51)*. This amino dipeptidyl peptidase IV activity cleaves the bond between the proline residue and amido methylcoumarin molecule, as shown in Fig. 3C. It was first reported that PSMA possesses this activity when Pangalos et al. *(51)* transiently transfected COS cells with PSMA cDNA and assayed for the dipeptidyl peptidase IV activity. Although the mock-transfected COS cells had dipeptidyl peptidase IV activity, the PSMA-transfected COS cells had significantly more activity. The physiolgical role of the dipeptidyl peptidase IV activity of PSMA is unclear; however, it may play a role in the regulation of various biologically active peptides, including collagen, neuropeptide Y, and growth hormone releasing factor *(51)*. As such, it would appear that PSMA is a multifunctional enzyme, possessing both amino and carboxy-peptidase activities as a mono and dipeptidase.

Rawlings and Barrett predicted the secondary structure of PSMA using a number of protein prediction and protein alignment programs, modifying the results so that the potential zinc ligand binding sites and other blocks of secondary structures were aligned

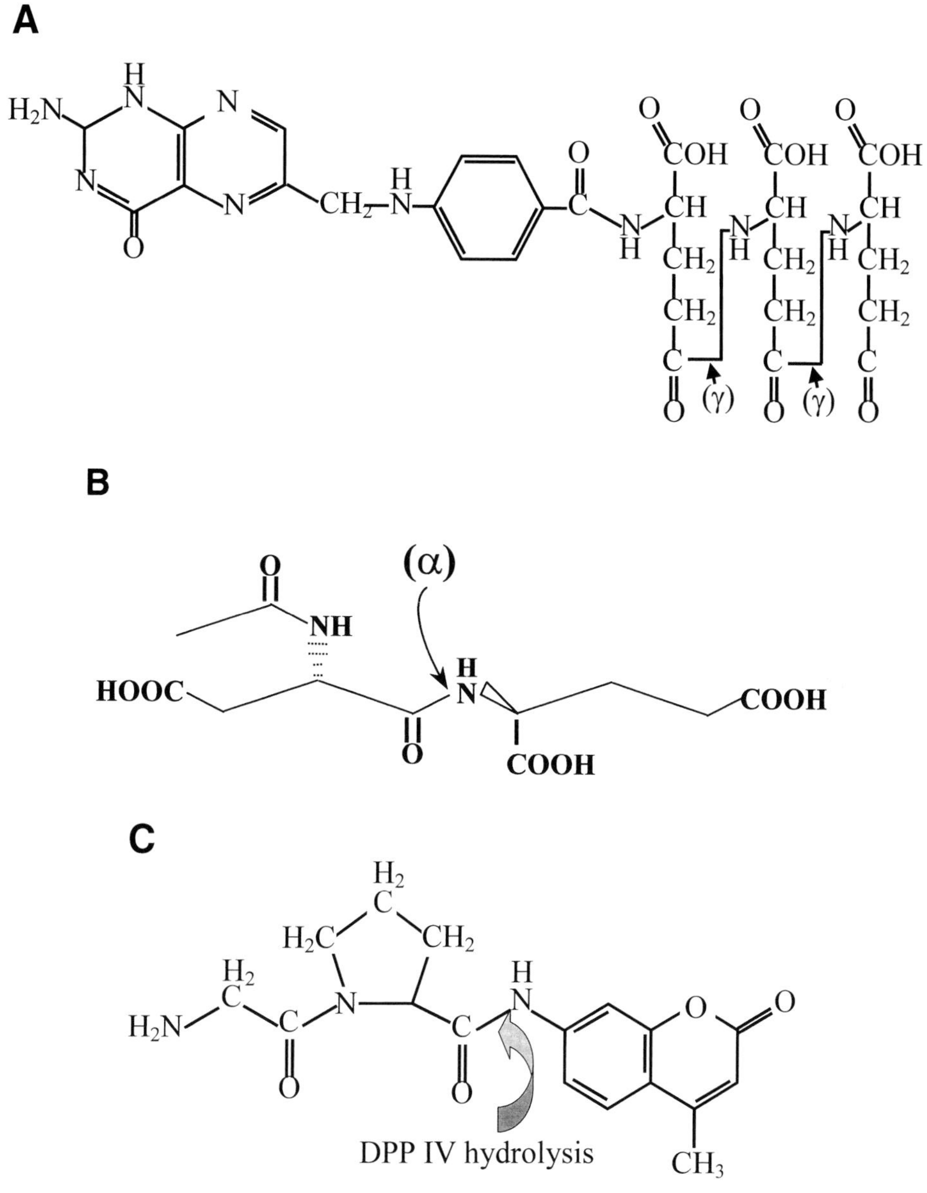

A

B

C

DPP IV hydrolysis

Fig. 3. PSMA substrates. **(A)** folic-acid polyglutamate, **(B)** *N*-acetyl-aspartylglutamate (NAAG), and **(C)** glycine-proline-7-amido-4-methylcoumarin. Arrows indicate the bond that is hydrolyzed by PSMA.

(55). They predicted that PSMA is made up of six organizational domains, with domain E (a.a. 273–587) responsible for the catalytic activity. They were then able to assign this catalytic domain to the M28 peptidase family, and predicted that Asp[377], Asp[387], Glu[425], Asp[453] and His[553] are ligands for two atoms of zinc required for catalytic activity *(55)*. Speno et al. performed site-directed mutagenesis experiments alter-

ing these residues resulting in severely reduced NAALADase activity, and were also able to demonstrate that substitution of some amino acids near the putative zinc ligands has a major impact on enzyme structure and/or function *(63)*.

9. THE ROLE OF PSMA IN PROSTATE CARCINOGENESIS AND PROGRESSION

PSMA is believed to be involved both in glutamatergic signaling and folate metabolism. Although there is no evidence that the PSMA substrate NAAG is present in the prostate, our laboratory has demonstrated the existence of Glu 2/3 and Glu 4 glutamate receptors using immunohistochemistry *(26)*. This would suggest that when PSMA is expressed on the surface of the prostate epithelial cell—and particularly when the membrane-bound form of PSMA is upregulated in cancer—sufficient quantities of glutamate could be released to stimulate these receptors, leading to oxidative stress and subsequent cell and DNA damage *(12)*, and further enhancing the ability of the cell to mutate and the cancer to progress.

Another possible function of PSMA was recently reported by Liu et al. *(41)*, who observed a di-leucine motif in the amino terminal of the protein, indicating a possible role in internalization of ligands via PSMA. Incubation of LNCaP cells with antibodies against PSMA followed by laser scanning confocal microscopy revealed that the antibodies were internalized and remained in endosomes within the cell. The endocytosis occurred via clathrin-coated pits and was shown to occur constitutively, although it was enhanced by the presence of antibodies, suggesting a role for PSMA in the internalization of as yet undefined ligand(s) *(41)*.

Our most favored theory is based on the folate hydrolase activity of PSMA and PSM', which releases the terminal gamma-linked glutamates from folates. To appreciate how the folate hydrolase activity of PSMA might be involved in carcinogenesis and the progression of prostate cancer, it is first necessary to understand the role of folate in this tissue. Dietary folates are generally polygammaglutamated. However, folate can only enter the cell by passive diffusion if it has been deglutamated (although most extracellular folate is monoglutamated). Within the cell, folate is polyglutamated so that it cannot diffuse out of the cell. The presence of PSM' in the cell would lead to deglutamation of the polyglutamated folate, and subsequent loss of folate from the cell. In the prostate, there is an increased need for folate relative to that of other tissues *(24)*. Folate hydrolase would be expected to deglutamate folate, and allow it to be in a form that could easily diffuse out of the cell—thus placing the cell at risk of becoming folate deficient *(54)*. Folate deficiency is associated with DNA damage and carcinogenesis *(13,34)*.

Folic-acid deficiency can lead to DNA damage via increased uracil incoporation, resulting in single-stranded DNA breaks and decondensation of chromosomes *(4,37)*. Folate deficiency may also lead to carcinogenesis by reducing DNA methylation, which in turn has been proven to lead to the overexpression of certain genes, including a number of oncogenes *(3,16,35)*. Folate is integral to a number of basic metabolic processes in the cell, including DNA synthesis, DNA methylation, and the formation of methionine and polyamines. The prostate is the major organ responsible for polyamines, producing between eightfold and 100-fold greater amounts than other polyamine-producing tissues *(24)*. This high production of polyamines places stress on the folate-methionine pathway, and as a result the prostate is at greater risk of DNA damage induced by a low-folate environment.

Therefore it is our hypothesis that PSM′, the cytosolic version of PSMA expressed in normal prostate epithelial cells, would be a "catalyst" of DNA damage, and subsequently carcinogenesis, by depleting the prostate of intracellular folate. PSMA, the membrane-bound isoform highly expressed in the tumor and metastatic deposits, could also be expected to hydrolyze poly-γ-glutamated folates, allowing them to diffuse into cells in the local microenvironment. Although poly-γ-glutamated folates are not typically considered extracellular substances, there are a large number of dead or dying cells that can liberate these polyglutamated folates within an environment such as a prostate tumor. Therefore, cells expressing a membrane folate hydrolase such as PSMA would have a growth and survival advantage over nonexpressing cells, especially if the levels of PSM′ decreased in the PSMA-expressing cells. A possible extension of this hypothesis might explain why the neovasculature of most solid tumors express PSMA, tumors which characteristically have an inadequate blood supply may be able to sequester folate from dead cells if they can induce the endothelial cells of the vasculature to express such a folate hydrolase.

After the switch of mRNA splicing to predominantly form PSMA—the membrane-bound isoform of the protein—folate uptake by the cell would be enhanced. This in turn would lead to a greater proliferation rate for the cell, and could possibly also lead to enhanced mutation rates via glutamate receptors and oxidative stress on the cell. In this case, increased expression of PSMA could assist in evolution of the tumor and tumor growth, and progression of the cancer.

To assess this theory in the laboratory, we are currently using the transgenic mouse model. This is significantly assisted by the fact that the murine prostate does not express the homolog of PSMA, MoPSM. We have created transgenic mice expressing human PSMA and/or PSM′ under the control of a prostate-specific promoter, and are examining the effect of folate deficiency on the rate of DNA damage in the presence of the PSMA isoforms (Bacich et al., unpublished).

10. CLINICAL UTILITY OF PROSTATE SPECIFIC MEMBRANE ANTIGEN

The potential of PSMA as a marker of clinical progression was first noted during characterization of the 7E11C5.3 antibody *(28)*. Sera from 20 of 43 patients with prostate cancer appeared to carry molecules reactive with the 7E11C5.3 antibody. However, none of the 30 normal blood donors or seven patients with BPH exhibited such reactivity. The authors also reported that prostate cancer patients who tested positive were more likely to be in progression ($p < 0.05$) *(28)*, although other groups have been unable to detect PSMA in the serum of any patients with metastatic disease *(69)*. The possibility that PSMA could be used as a marker of circulating prostate cancer cells was quickly examined by a number of groups. Israeli et al. *(31)* developed a highly sensitive technique using reverse-transcriptase PCR with nested primer sets to amplify PSMA sequences from patient blood samples. Using similar nested, "enhanced," or radioactive PCR-based methods, the consensus appears to be that there is no correlation between PSMA-positive results and clinical stage, pathological stage, or tumor grade *(6,49,62)*. There are other reports of PSMA-mRNA expression in normal lymphocytes, urine, and bone marrow (including specimens from female controls), as the result of "illegitimate transcription"—insignificant numbers of PSMA transcripts produced to have any functional effect, but that are able to be detected by sensitive PCR techniques *(10,15,39,80)*.

As with all PCR-based methods to detect circulating cancer cells, the technique needs to be standardized between laboratories. It is clear from the literature that in the hands of different researchers, significant variation is found in test results. Furthermore, the presence of circulating cells does not appear to be directly related to metastatic potential of the primary tumor. For example, Loric et al. *(43)* have shown that patients with inflamed prostates also exhibit circulating prostate cells. However, new technologies currently available may be able to solve these problems. The advent of "Real-Time" PCR, which allows sensitive quantitation of PCR products and the expanding access to custom-designed "Gene Chips" should make it easier to quantitate one or a number of prostate specific transcripts. It has already been shown that a combination of RT-PCR methods for PSMA and PSA-expressing cells is more accurate than either technique alone *(20,79)*. In addition to combining several different markers for analysis, it might also be worthwhile to examine relative amounts of the PSMA mRNA splice variants—particularly PSM' vs PSMA.

PSMA RT-PCR—in combination with PSA RT-PCR—has also been used to determine the "molecular surgical margins" at radical prostatectomy, by examining five biopsy specimens from the prostatic fossa *(65)*. The results, although preliminary, are promising. The authors found a perfect correlation between a positive PCR result and histopathological determination of positive margins or extracapsular extension. Furthermore, control biopsy specimens taken from men undergoing radical cysto-prostatectomy for bladder cancer or abdominoperineal resection for rectal cancer were all negative for the test. Interestingly, in four of 16 cases with histopathologically negative surgical margins, the molecular margins were positive *(65)*. Validation of this unique method requires larger, longer, and multi-institutional studies.

At the present time, clinical imaging using PSMA-directed immunoconjugates utilize the Cyt-356 antibody, commercially known as the "Prostascint Scan™". While the results are promising, the test is probably not optimally designed. In studies localizing the target epitope of Cyt-356, Troyer et al. *(71)* found that the antibody binds to the short cytoplasmic domain of the protein. As such, Cyt-356 binds efficiently to dead cells, and not viable cells *(40,70,71)*. The ability of Cyt-356 to image metastatic deposits is most likely caused by necrotic cells in the tumors, and therefore the sensitivity of imaging would be expected to be enhanced through the use of antibodies directed against the external domain of PSMA. A number of groups have developed such "second generation" antibodies *(40,48)*, and are currently carrying out phase I trials using the antibodies as both imaging agents and therapeutic vectors.

11. THE FUTURE OF CLINICAL AND THERAPEUTIC STRATEGIES UTILIZING PSMA

In an immunotherapeutic approach, Tjoa et al. *(66)* showed that T-cell proliferation could be induced in vitro by autologous dendritic cells pulsed with peptides from the PSMA amino acid sequence. Dendritic cells are professional antigen-presenting cells that can induce T-cell proliferation and cytotoxicity against specific antigens. This study was followed by Phase I and II clinical trials, which showed positive results, with partial responders identified in groups of patients with both metastatic and suspected local recurrent disease. Follow-up of the responsive patients nearly 300 d later revealed that more than 50% of the subjects were still responding *(59,60,67,68)*. While these results indicate a promising future for immunotherapeutic strategies against prostate cancer, there are several intrinisic problems. The therapy described here is restricted to patients of major histocompatibility antigen type A2 (HLA-A2) tissue type. Furthermore, HLA antigens are downregulated by tumor cells, and thus would not be available for immuno-targeting.

Using an innovative approach to avoid these restrictions, Gong et al. *(19)* devised an immunotherapeutic method that completely circumvents the need for MHC-mediated presentation of peptides. An artificial T-cell receptor was generated by cloning the DNA sequence responsible for recognition of PSMA by the J-591 antibody described here *(40)*, followed by a linker region and the zeta chain receptor, into a retroviral vector *(19)*. T-cells (CD4+ and CD8+) from prostate cancer patients were then transduced with the vector, and their response to cells expressing PSMA was examined. The transduced cells efficiently and specifically lysed PSMA-expressing cells, and also released cytokines in response to PSMA, suggesting that a prolonged response might be feasible *(19)*. If these results are as impressive in vivo as they are in vitro, such an approach should be able to target both the primary tumor and metastatic deposits, as well as the neovasculature of other solid tumors.

Other therapeutic approaches targeting PSMA currently being investigated by our and other laboratories include the use of prodrug strategies and gene therapy. To investigate prodrug strategies against prostate cancer, NIH3T3+/– PSMA and PC-3+/– PSMA-transfected cells and LNCaP cells were grown in the presence of methotrexate triglutamate *(27)* and Heston et al. (unpublished). In the cells expressing PSMA, the drug was converted into its cytotoxic derivative methotrexate, and cell growth was inhibited. However, in the non-PSMA-expressing cells, the drug was nontoxic. While these results show promise, we are currently using the LNCaP xenograft model to determine whether toxicity is specifically targeted to the tumor, or affects other cells expressing the murine homologs of the genes described in Table 1.

Cloning of the PSMA promoter, and more particularly the enhancer, has made the use of gene therapy constructs carrying either therapeutic or cytotoxic genes a viable alternative to those described here *(50a)*. In this approach, cytotoxic genes such as the cytosine deaminase (CD) or herpes virus TK genes are linked to the PSME and a compatible promoter, and the patient is treated with cytotoxic prodrugs such as 5-fluorocytosine or gancyclovir. However, the first challenge is to demonstrate prostate-specificity of the PSME in the transgenic mouse model, and we are currently evaluating this process (Bacich et al., unpublished).

12. INTO THE 21ST CENTURY

The PSMA story has yielded several unexpected surprises so far, but we still do not know whether expression of this gene influences the development or progression of prostate cancer and if so, how. The possible role of PSMA in the angiogenic pathway of tumors is intriguing, but it also suggests that we have much to learn about this fascinating protein. The expression of PSMA in tumor-associated vasculature, as well as its high expression in virtually all prostate tumors and metastases, and particularly in hormone refractory disease for which there is currently no efficient treatment, indicates that targeting of PSMA may be highly valuable as a treatment for not only prostate cancer, but several types of solid tumors.

ACKNOWLEDGMENT

This work was supported in part by a grant from the AFUD/AUA Research Scholar Program and the CR Bard Foundation (D.S. O'Keefe) AFUD/AUA and the Yamanouchi Foundation (D. J. Bacich), as well as grants PC990017 (D.S. O'Keefe), and DAMD17-00-1-0043, DAMD17-99-1-9523 (W.D.W. Heston) from the US Army Medical Research Acquisition Activity, Ft. Detrick, MD; and NIH grants CA29502-16 (D.J. Bacich) and DK/CA47650 (W.D.W. Heston). The information contained within this manuscript does not necessarily reflect the position or policy of the US government.

REFERENCES

1. Antequera, F. and A. Bird. 1995. Number of CpG islands and genes in human and mouse. *Proc. Natl. Acad. Sci. USA* **90:** 11,995–11,999.
2. Bacich, D. J., J. T. Tong, W. P. Heston, and J. T. Pinto. Cloning, expression, genomic localization and glutamyl carboxypeptidase activities of the murine homologue of prostate-specific membrane antigen / NAALADase. *Mammalian Genome* (in press).
3. Bestor, T. H. and B. Tycko. 1996. Creation of genomic methylation patterns. *Nat. Genet.* **12:** 363–367.
4. Blount, B. C. and B. N. Ames. 1994. Analysis of uracil in DNA by gas chromatography-mass spectrometry. *Anal. Biochem.* **219:** 195–200.
5. Bzdega, T., T. Turi, B. Wroblewska, D. She, H. S. Chung, H. Kim, et al. 1997. Molecular cloning of a peptidase against N-acetylaspartylglutamate from a rat hippocampal cDNA library. *J. Neurochem.* **69:** 2270–2277.
6. Cama, C., C. A. Olsson, A. J. Raffo, H. Perlman, R. Buttyan, K. O'Toole, et al. 1995. Molecular staging of prostate cancer. II. A comparison of the application of an enhanced reverse transcriptase polymerase chain reaction assay for prostate specific antigen versus prostate specific membrane antigen. *J. Urol.* **153:** 1373–1378.
7. Carter, R. E., A. R. Feldman, and J. T. Coyle. 1996. Prostate-specific membrane antigen is a hydrolase with substrate and pharmacologic characteristics of a neuropeptidase. *Proc. Natl. Acad. Sci. USA* **93:** 749–753.
8. Chang, S. S., D. S. O'Keefe, D. J. Bacich, W. D. W. Heston, V. E. Reuter, and P. B. Gaudin. 1999. prostate-specific membrane antigen (PSMA) is produced in tumor-associated neovasculature. *Clin. Cancer Res.* **5:** 2674–2681.
9. Chang, S. S., V. E. Reuter, W. D. W. Heston, N. H. Bander, L. S. Grauer, and P. B. Gaudin. 1999. Five different anti-prostate-specific membrane antigen (PSMA) antibodies confirm PSMA expression in tumor-associated neovasculature. *Cancer Res.* **59:** 3192–3198.
10. Clements, J. A., P. Rohde, V. Allen, V. J. Hyland, M. L. Samaratunga, W. D. Tilley, et al. 1999. Molecular detection of prostate cells in ejaculate and urethral washings in men with suspected prostate cancer. *J. Urol.* **161:** 1337–1343.
11. Coyle, J. T. 1997. *Neurobiological Disorders* **4:** 231–238.
12. Coyle, J. T. and P. Puttfarcken. 1993. Oxidative stress, glutamate and neurodegenerative disorders. *Science* **262:** 689–695.
13. Eto, I. and C. L. Krumdiek. 1986. Role of vitamin B12 and folate deficiencies in carcinogenesis. *Adv. Exp. Med. Biol.* **206:** 313–330.

14. Fuhrman, S., M. Palkovits, M. Cassidy, and J. H. Neale. 1994. The regional distribution of N-acetylaspartylglutamate (NAAG) and peptidase activity against NAAG in the rat nervous system. *J. Neurochem.* **62:** 275–281.

15. Gala, J. L., M. Heusterspreute, S. Loric, F. Hanon, B. Tombal, P. Van Cangh, et al. 1998. Expression of prostate-specific antigen and prostate-specific membrane antigen transcripts in blood cells: implications for the detection of hematogenous prostate cells and standardization. *Clin. Chem.* **44:** 472–481.

16. Ghoshal, A. K. and E. Farber. 1984. The induction of liver cancer by dietary dificiency of choline and methionine without added carcinogens. *Carcinogenesis* **5:** 1367–1370.

17. Giebel, L. B., K. M. Strunk, and R. A. Spritz. 1991. Organization and nucleotide sequences of the human tyrosinase gene and a truncated tyrosinase-related segment. *Genomics* **9:** 435–445.

18. Gingras, R., C. Richard, M. El-Alfy, C. R. Morales, M. Potier, and A. V. Pshezhetsky. 1999. Purification, cDNA cloning, and expression of a new human blood plasma glutamate carboxypeptidase homologous to N-acetyl-aspartyl-alpha-glutamate carboxypeptidase/prostate-specific membrane antigen. *J. Biol. Chem.* **274:** 11,742–11,750.

19. Gong, M. C., J. B. Latouche, A. Krause, W. D. W. Heston, N. H. Bander, and M. Sadelain. 1999. Cancer patient T cells genetically targeted to prostate-specific membrane antigen specifically lyse prostate cancer cells and release cytokines in response to prostate-specific membrane antigen. *Neoplasia* **1:** 123–127.

20. Grasso, Y. Z., M. K. Gupta, H. S. Levin, C. D. Zippe, and E. A. Klein. 1998. Combined nested RT-PCR assay for prostate-specific antigen and prostate-specific membrane antigen in prostate cancer patients: correlation with pathological stage. *Cancer Res.* **58:** 1456–1459.

21. Grauer, L. S., K. D. Lawler, J. L. Marignac, A. Kumar, A. S. Goel, and R. L. Wolfert. 1998. Identification, purification, and subcellular localization of prostate-specific membrane antigen PSM' protein in the LNCaP prostatic carcinoma cell line. *Cancer Res.* **58:** 4787–4789.

22. Halsted, C. H., E. H. Ling, R. Luthi-Carter, J. A. Villanueva, J. M. Gardner, and J. T. Coyle. 1998. Folylpoly-gamma-glutamate carboxypeptidase from pig jejunum. Molecular characterization and relation to glutamate carboxypeptidase II. *J. Biol. Chem.* **273:** 20,417–20,424.

23. Hasenson, M., B. Lundh, R. Stege, K. Carlstrom, and A. Pousette. 1989. PAP and PSA in prostatic carcinoma cell lines and aspiration biopsies: relation to hormone sensitivity and to cytological grading. *Prostate* **14:** 83–90.

24. Heston, W. D. W. 1991. Prostatic polyamines and polyamine targeting as a new approach to therapy of prostate cancer, in *Prostate Cancer Cell and Molecular Mechanisms in Diagnosis and Treatment* (Isaacs, J. T., ed.), Cold Spring Harbor Laboratory Press, Cold spring Harbor, NY.

25. Heston, W. D. W. 1997. Biologic implications for prostatic function following identification of prostate-specific membrane antigen as a novel folate hydrolase/neurocarboxypeptidase, in *Prostate: Basic and Clinical Aspects* (Naz, R. K., ed.), CRC Press: pp. 267–298.

26. Heston, W. D. W., D. A. Silver, I. Pellicer, W. R. Fair, C. Cordon-Cardo. 1996. Ionotropic glutamate receptor distribution in prostate tissue. *J. Urol.* **155:** 513A.

27. Heston, W. D. W., W-P. Tong, and J. T. Pinto. 1997. Prostate-specific membrane antigen: a unique folate hydrolase: potential target for prodrug therapy. *Mol. Urol.* **1:** 215–219.

28. Horoszewicz, J. S., E. Kawinski, and G. P. Murphy. 1987. Monoclonal antibodies to a new antigenic marker in epithelial prostatic cells and serum of prostatic cancer patients. *Anticancer Res.* **7:** 927–935.

29. Horoszewicz, J. S., S. S. Leong, T. M. Chu, Z. L. Wajsman, M. Friedman, L. Papsidero, et al. 1980. The LNCaP cell line—a new model for studies on human prostatic carcinoma. *Prog. Clin. Biol. Res.* **37:** 115–132.

30. Horoszewicz, J. S., S. S. Leong, E. Kawinski, J. P. Karr, H. Rosenthal, T. M. Chu, et al. 1983. LNCaP model of human prostatic carcinoma. *Cancer Res.* **43:** 1809–1818.

31. Israeli, R. S., W. H. Miller, Jr., S. L. Su, C. T. Powell, W. R. Fair, D. S. Samadi, et al. 1994. Sensitive nested reverse transcription polymerase chain reaction detection of circulating prostatic tumor cells: comparison of prostate-specific membrane antigen and prostate-specific antigen-based assays. *Cancer Res.* **54:** 6306–6310.

32. Israeli, R. S., C. T. Powell, J. G. Corr, W. R. Fair, and W. D. W. Heston. 1994. Expression of the prostate-specific membrane antigen. *Cancer Res.* **54:** 1807–1811.

33. Israeli, R. S., C. T. Powell, W. R. Fair, and W. D. Heston. 1993. Molecular cloning of a complementary DNA encoding a prostate-specific membrane antigen. *Cancer Res.* **53:** 227–230.

34. Jennings, E. 1995. Folic acid as a cancer-preventing agent. *Med. Hypotheses* **45:** 297–303.

35. Jones, P. A. and J. D. Buckley. 1990. The role of methylation in cancer. *Adv. Cancer Res.* **54:** 1–23.

36. Kawakami, M. and J. Nakayama. 1997. Enhanced expression of prostate-specific membrane antigen gene in prostate cancer as revealed by *in situ* hybridization. *Cancer Res.* **57:** 2321–2324.

37. Krumdiek, C. L. and P. N. Howard-Peebles. 1983. On the nature of folic acid-sensitive fragile sites in human chromosomes: an hypothesis. *Am. J. Med. Genet.* **16:** 23–28.

38. Leek, J., N. Lench, B. Maraj, A. Bailey, I. M. Carr, S. Andersen, et al. 1995. Prostate-specific membrane antigen: evidence for the existence of a second related human gene. *Br. J. Cancer* **72:** 583–588.

39. Lintula, S. and U. H. Stenman. 1997. The expression of prostate-specific membrane antigen in peripheral blood leukocytes. *J. Urol.* **157:** 1969–1972.

40. Liu, H., P. Moy, S. Kim, Y. Xia, A. Rajasekaran, V. Navarro, et al. 1997. Monoclonal antibodies to the extracellular domain of prostate-specific membrane antigen also react with tumor vascular endothelium. *Cancer Res.* **57:** 3629–3634.

41. Liu, H., A. K. Rajasekaran, P. Moy, Y. Xia, S. Kim, V. Navarro, et al. 1998. Constitutive and antibody-induced internalization of prostate-specific membrane antigen. *Cancer Res.* **58:** 4055–4060.

42. Lopes, A. D., W. L. Davis, M. J. Rosenstraus, A. J. Uveges, and S. C. Gilman. 1990. Immunohistochemical and pharmacokinetic characterization of the site-specific immuno-conjugate CYT-356 derived from antiprostate monoclonal antibody 7E11-C5. *Cancer Res.* **50:** 6423–6429.

43. Loric, S., F. Dumas, P. Eschwege, P. Blanchet, G. Benoit, A. Jardin, et al. 1995. Enhanced detection of hematogenous circulating prostatic cells in patients with prostate adenocarci-noma by using nested reverse transcription polymerase chain reaction assay based on pros-tate-specific membrane antigen. *Clin. Chem.* **41:** 1698–1704.

44. Luthi-Carter, R., A. K. Barczak, H. Speno, and J. T. Coyle. 1998. Molecular characteriza-tion of human brain N-acetylated alpha-linked acidic dipeptidase (NAALADase). *J. Pharmacol. Exp. Ther.* **286:** 1020–1025.

45. Meyerhoff, J. L., R. E. Carter, D. L. Yourick, B. S. Slusher, and J. T. Coyle. 1992. Activity of a NAAG-hydrolyzing enzyme in brain may affect seizure susceptibility in genetically epilepsy-prone rats. *Epilepsy Res. Suppl.* **9:** 163–172.

46. Meyerhoff, J. L., R. E. Carter, D. L. Yourick, B. S. Slusher, and J. T. Coyle. 1992. Geneti-cally epilepsy-prone rats have increased brain regional activity of an enzyme which liber-ates glutamate from N-acetyl-aspartyl-glutamate. *Brain Res.* **593:** 140–143.

47. Meyerhoff, J. L., M. B. Robinson, M. A. Bixler, S. S. Richards, and J. T. Coyle. 1989. Seizures decrease regional enzymatic hydrolysis of N-acetyl-aspartylglutamate in rat brain. *Brain Res.* **505:** 130–134.

48. Murphy, G. P., T. G. Greene, W. T. Tino, A. L. Boynton, and E. H. Holmes. 1998. Isola-tion and characterization of monoclonal antibodies specific for the extracellular domain of prostate specific membrane antigen. *J. Urol.* **160:** 2396–2401.

49. Noguchi, M., J. Miyajima, K. Itoh, and S. Noda. 1997. Detection of circulating tumor cells in patients with prostate cancer using prostate specific membrane-derived primers in the polymerase chain reaction. *Int. J. Urol.* **4:** 374–379.

50. O'Keefe, D. S., S. L. Su, D. J. Bacich, Y. Horiguchi, Y. Luo, C. T. Powell, et al. 1998. Mapping, genomic organization and promoter analysis of the human prostate-specific membrane antigen gene. *Biochim. Biophys. Acta* **1443:** 113–127.

50a. O'Keefe, D. S., A. Uchida, D. J. Bacich, F. B. Watt, A. Matorana et al. 2000. Prostate-specific suicide gene therapy using the prostate specific membrane antigen promoter and enhancer. *Prostate* (in press).

51. Pangalos, M. N., J. M. Neefs, M. Somers, P. Verhasselt, M. Bekkers, L. van der Helm, et al. 1999. Isolation and expression of novel human glutamate carboxypeptidases with N-acetylated alpha-linked acidic dipeptidase and dipeptidyl peptidase IV activity. *J. Biol. Chem.* **274:** 8470–8483.

52. Passani, L. A., J. P. Vonsattel, R. E. Carter, and J. T. Coyle. 1997. N-acetylaspartylglutamate, N-acetylaspartate, and N-acetylated alpha-linked acidic dipeptidase in human brain and their alterations in Huntington and Alzheimer's diseases. *Mol. Chem. Neuropathol.* **31:** 97–118.

53. Peace, D. J. Z., Y. Holt, G. Ferrer, et al. 1999. Identification of three novel splice variants of prostate-specific membrane antigen in prostate cancer cells. American Association for Cancer Research 90th Annual Meeting, April 10–14, 1999, Philadelphia, PA.

54. Pinto, J. T., B. P. Suffoletto, T. M. Berzin, C. H. Qiao, S. Lin, W. P. Tong, et al. 1996. Prostate-specific membrane antigen: a novel folate hydrolase in human prostatic carcinoma cells. *Clin. Cancer Res.* **2:** 1445–1451.

55. Rawlings, N. D. and A. J. Barrett. 1997. Structure of membrane glutamate carboxypeptidase. *Biochim. Biophys. Acta* **1339:** 247–252.

56. Rinker-Schaeffer, C. W., A. L. Hawkins, S. L. Su, R. S. Israeli, C. A. Griffin, J. T. Isaacs, et al. 1995. Localization and physical mapping of the prostate-specific membrane antigen (PSM) gene to human chromosome 11. *Genomics* **30:** 105–108.

57. Robinson, M. B., R. D. Blakely, R. Couto, and J. T. Coyle. 1987. *J. Biol. Chem.* **262:** 14,498–14,506.

58. Rothstein, J. D., G. Tsai, R. W. Kuncl, L. Clawson, D. R. Cornblath, D. B. Drachman, et al. 1990. Abnormal excitatory amino acid metabolism in amyotrophic lateral sclerosis. *Ann. Neurol.* **28:** 18–25.

59. Salgaller, M. L., P. A. Lodge, J. G. McLean, B. A. Tjoa, D. J. Loftus, H. Ragde, et al. 1998. Report of immune monitoring of prostate cancer patients undergoing T-cell therapy using dendritic cells pulsed with HLA-A2-specific peptides from prostate-specific membrane antigen (PSMA). *Prostate* **35:** 144–151.

60. Salgaller, M. L., B. A. Tjoa, P. A. Lodge, H. Ragde, G. Kenny, A. Boynton, et al. 1998. Dendritic cell-based immunotherapy of prostate cancer. *Crit. Rev. Immunol.* **18:** 109–119.

61. Silver, D. A., I. Pellicer, W. R. Fair, W. D. W. Heston, and C. Cordon-Cardo. 1997. Prostate-specific membrane antigen expression in normal and malignant human tissues. *Clin. Cancer Res.* **3:** 81–85.

62. Sokoloff, M. H., C. L. Tso, R. Kaboo, S. Nelson, J. Ko, F. Dorey, et al. 1996. Quantitative polymerase chain reaction does not improve preoperative prostate cancer staging: a clinicopathological molecular analysis of 121 patients. *J. Urol.* **156:** 1560–1566.

63. Speno, H. S., R. Luthi-Carter, W. L. Macias, S. L. Valentine, A. R. Joshi, and J. T. Coyle. 1999. Site-directed mutagenesis of predicted active site residues in glutamate carboxypeptidase II. *Mol. Pharmacol.* **55:** 179–185.

64. Su, S. L., I. P. Huang, W. R. Fair, C. T. Powell, and W. D. W. Heston. 1995. Alternatively spliced variants of prostate-specific membrane antigen RNA: ratio of expression as a potential measurement of progression. *Cancer Res.* **55:** 1441–1443.

65. Theodorescu, D., H. F. Frierson, Jr., and R. A. Sikes. 1999. Molecular determination of surgical margins using fossa biopsies at radical prostatectomy. *J. Urol.* **161:** 1442–1448.
66. Tjoa, B., A. Boynton, G. Kenny, H. Ragde, S. L. Misrock, and G. Murphy. 1996. Presentation of prostate tumor antigens by dendritic cells stimulates T-cell proliferation and cytotoxicity. *Prostate* **28:** 65–69.
67. Tjoa, B. A., S. J. Erickson, V. A. Bowes, H. Ragde, G. M. Kenny, O. E. Cobb, et al. 1997. Follow-up evaluation of prostate cancer patients infused with autologous dendritic cells pulsed with PSMA peptides. *Prostate* **32:** 272–278.
68. Tjoa, B. A., S. J. Simmons, A. Elgamal, M. Rogers, H. Ragde, G. M. Kenny, et al. 1999. Follow-up evaluation of a phase II prostate cancer vaccine trial. *Prostate* **40:** 125–129.
69. Troyer, J. K., M. L. Beckett, and G. L. Wright, Jr. 1995. Detection and characterization of the prostate-specific membrane antigen (PSMA) in tissue extracts and body fluids. *Int. J. Cancer* **62:** 552–558.
70. Troyer, J. K., M. L. Beckett, and G. L. Wright, Jr. 1997. Location of prostate-specific membrane antigen in the LNCaP prostate carcinoma cell line. *Prostate* **30:** 232–242.
71. Troyer, J. K., Q. Feng, M. L. Beckett and G. L. Wright Jr. 1995. Biochemical characterization and mapping of the 7E11C5.3 epitope of the prostate-specific membrane antigen. *Urologic Oncology* **1:** 29–37.
72. Tsai, G., L. C. Cork, B. S. Slusher, D. Price, and J. T. Coyle. 1993. Abnormal acidic amino acids and N-acetylaspartylglutamate in hereditary canine motoneuron disease. *Brain Res.* **629:** 305–309.
73. Tsai, G., L. A. Passani, B. S. Slusher, R. Carter, L. Baer, J. E. Kleinman, et al. 1995. Abnormal excitatory neurotransmitter metabolism in schizophrenic brains. *Arch. Gen. Psychiatry* **52:** 829–836.
74. Tsai, G. C., B. Stauch-Slusher, L. Sim, J. C. Hedreen, J. D. Rothstein, R. Kuncl, et al. 1991. Reductions in acidic amino acids and N-acetylaspartylglutamate in amyotrophic lateral sclerosis CNS. *Brain Res.* **556:** 151–156.
75. Watt, F. B., D. E. Ho, T. Martorana, A. Kingsley, E. O'Keefe, D. S. Russell, et al. 2000. A Tissue-specific enhancer of the prostate-specific membrane antigen gene. *Genomics* (in press).
76. Wright, G. L., Jr., B. M. Grob, C. Haley, K. Grossman, K. Newhall, D. Petrylak, et al. 1996. Upregulation of prostate-specific membrane antigen after androgen- deprivation therapy. *Urology* **48:** 326–334.
77. Wroblewska, B., M. R. Santi, and J. H. Neale. 1998. N-acetylaspartylglutamate activates cyclic AMP-coupled metabotropic glutamate receptors in cerebellar astrocytes. *Glia* **24:** 172–179.
78. Wynant, G. E., G. P. Murphy, J. S. Horoszewicz, C. E. Neal, B. D. Collier, E. Mitchell, et al. 1991. Immunoscintigraphy of prostatic cancer: preliminary results with 111In-labeled monoclonal antibody 7E11-C5.3 (CYT-356). *Prostate* **18:** 229–241.
79. Zhang, Y., C. D. Zippe, F. Van Lente, E. A. Klein, and M. K. Gupta. 1997. Combined nested reverse transcription-PCR assay for prostate-specific antigen and prostate-specific membrane antigen in detecting circulating prostatic cells. *Clin. Cancer Res.* **3:** 1215–1220.
80. Zippelius, A., P. Kufer, G. Honold, M. W. Kollermann, R. Oberneder, G. Schlimok, et al. 1997. Limitations of reverse-transcriptase polymerase chain reaction analyses for detection of micrometastatic epithelial cancer cells in bone marrow. *J. Clin. Oncol.* **15:** 2701–2708.

19

Targeting Antiapoptotic Genes Upregulated by Androgen Withdrawal Using Antisense Oligodeoxynucleotides to Enhance Androgen- and Chemo-Sensitivity in Prostate Cancer

Martin E. Gleave, MD, Hideaki Miyake, MD, PhD, Colleen Nelson, PhD, Paul Rennie, PhD, and Simon Leung, MB

1. INTRODUCTION

Androgen withdrawal is the only effective form of systemic therapy for men with advanced disease, producing symptomatic and/or objective response in 80% of patients. Unfortunately, androgen independent (AI) progression and death occurs within a few years in the majority of these cases *(6)*. Prostate cancer is highly chemoresistant, with objective response rates of 10% and no demonstrated survival benefit *(28)*. Hormone refractory prostate cancer (HRPC) is therefore the main obstacle to improving the survival and quality of life in patients with advanced disease, and novel therapeutic strategies that target the molecular basis of androgen and chemo-resistance are required.

In this chapter we summarize the progress we have made in utilizing antisense oligodeoxynucleotides (AS-ODN) to therapeutically target genes that appear to play functionally relevant roles in the progression to androgen independence. Progression to androgen independence is a complex process involving variable combinations of clonal selection *(14)*, adaptive upregulation of antiapoptotic survival genes *(2,20,22,)*, androgen receptor transactivation in the absence of androgen from mutations or increased levels of coactivators *(4,33)* and alternative growth factor pathways *(4,26)*. Characterization of changes in gene expression during AI progression identifies potential targets that can be manipulated therapeutically. Identification of genes expressed during AI progression must be followed by an investigation of their functional significance in this process. Genes with a causative role in hormone independence can then be targeted for therapeutic intervention. Reproducible tumor models and efficient high-throughput technologies are required to accomplish these objectives. Once proof of principle is demonstrated in preclinical model systems, appropriate phase I and II studies can be initiated in men with prostate cancer.

From: *Prostate Cancer: Biology, Genetics, and the New Therapeutics*
Edited by: L. W. K. Chung, W. B. Isaacs, and J. W. Simons © Humana Press Inc., Totowa, NJ

2. RELIABLE MODEL SYSTEMS OF AI PROGRESSION

Because prostate cancer is highly heterogeneous and varies widely in its biological aggressiveness, androgen sensitivity, and histologic appearance, it is unrealistic to expect that a singular model will perfectly mimic the diverse human condition. However, insights and understanding into the nature of human prostate cancer will come from developing useful concepts through careful extrapolation from appropriate types of tumor models *(8)*. The Shionogi tumor model is a mouse androgen-dependent (AD) mammary carcinoma that, like human prostate cancer, regresses after castration and later recurs as AI tumors *(8)*. Although the Shionogi tumor model is of mouse-mammary origin, it shares a number of features characteristic of human prostate cancer—it is androgen dependent, has a functional androgen receptor, and undergoes extensive castration-induced apoptosis following androgen withdrawal with subsequent AI tumor recurrence after 1 mo. At the molecular level, the Shionogi tumor model shares a number of characteristics with human prostate cancers *(2,20,22,26)*.

The human LNCaP cell line is androgen responsive, prostate specific antigen (PSA)-secreting, and immortalized in vitro *(13)*. Like clinical prostate cancer, serum PSA levels in the LNCaP tumor model are initially regulated by androgen, are directly proportional to tumor vol, and increase after prolonged periods of growth after castration to signal progression and androgen independence *(9)*. Apoptotic tumor regression does not consistently occur after castration, but tumor growth stabilizes, and serum and tumor cell PSA levels decrease by 80% for several wk after castration, after which LNCaP tumor growth rates and PSA expression increase above precastration levels.

3. IDENTIFICATION OF POTENTIAL THERAPEUTIC TARGETS

Comparative hybridization of high density cDNA array is one method to rapidly and efficiently characterize changes in gene expression after androgen withdrawal and during AI progression of androgen dependent tumors in both LNCaP and Shionogi model systems. Computer-assisted subtractive analysis of arrays highlights increases or decreases in gene expression at various points in time during AI progression. Northern analysis is then used to confirm the array data. In general, androgen withdrawal results in a programmatic drift in gene expression, with upregulation of at least 20 genes in the Shionogi or LNCaP tumor models (Fig. 1). Many genes become upregulated early (within days) of androgen withdrawal associated with tumor cell apoptosis (e.g., TRPM-2, cathepsins, Bcl-2, Bcl-xL, IGFBP-2, and IGFBP-5). Expression levels of several genes are increased later in AI recurrent tumors (e.g., vimentin, c-*fos*, c-*myc*, and TGF-β). Some genes initially dependent on androgens for expression, such as PSA, decrease in the early postcastration period but become constitutively expressed in AI recurrent tumors. Finally, a few genes (e.g., Nm22, IGFBP3) are downregulated after androgen withdrawal.

4. ANTISENSE STRATEGIES TO TARGET RELEVANT GENES

Targeting cell survival genes upregulated by androgen withdrawal may enhance castration-induced apoptosis and thereby prolong time to overt recurrence. Antisense oligodeoxynucleotide (AS-ODN) therapy is one strategy to specifically target functionally relevant genes. AS-ODNs are chemically modified stretches of single-stranded

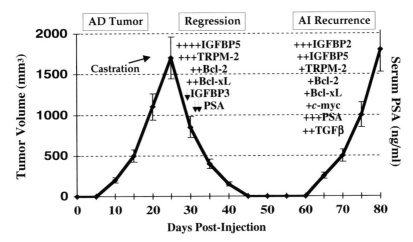

Fig. 1. Schematic drawing summarizing changes in tumor volume and serum PSA in the androgen-dependent Shionogi and LNCaP tumor model systems, respectively. Shionogi tumors undergo complete regression following castration, but recur as rapidly growing AI tumors 1 mo later. LNCaP tumor growth stabilizes and serum PSA decrease by 80% after castration before increasing 4–6 wk later. The expression of antiapoptotic genes TRPM-2, Bcl-2 and Bcl-xL increase beginning 4 d after castration, and remain overexpressed in AI tumors.

DNA complementary to mRNA regions of a target gene that inhibit translation by forming RNA/DNA duplexes, thereby reducing mRNA and protein levels of the target gene *(5)*. Antisense ODN strategy is based on the understanding that cellular ribosomal machinery translates mRNA into proteins. Amounts of specific proteins can be reduced by blocking this translation, and subsequent cascades of protein–protein signaling control of cellular proliferation, differentiation, homeostasis, and apoptosis can altered. The specificity and efficacy of antisense ODNs rely on precise targeting afforded by strand hybridization, where only a perfect match between the target sequence and the antisense ODN will lead to hybridization and inhibition of translation (Fig. 2). Phosphorothioate AS-ODNs are water-soluble, stable agents manufactured to resist nuclease digestion through substitution of a nonbridging phosphoryl oxygen of DNA with sulfur, which become associated with high-capacity, low-affinity serum binding proteins after parental administration *(31)*. AS-ODNs targeting several oncogenes have been reported to specifically inhibit expression of these genes and delay progression in several types of tumors *(5,15,23,31,38)*.

To date, new nonhormonal therapies have been traditionally evaluated late in HRPC and when used in this end-stage setting, most are ineffective *(28)*. A more rational treatment strategy would involve adjuvant therapy that targets the adaptive changes in gene expression precipitated by androgen withdrawal in order to enhance castration-induced apoptosis and delay emergence of the AI phenotype. After maximal apoptotic regression has occurred, additional targeting of proliferation-associated genes may further delay emergence of resistant tumors. Integration and appropriate timing of combination therapies, based on biological mechanism of progression and castration-induced changes in gene expression, may provide means to delay AI progression in a major way.

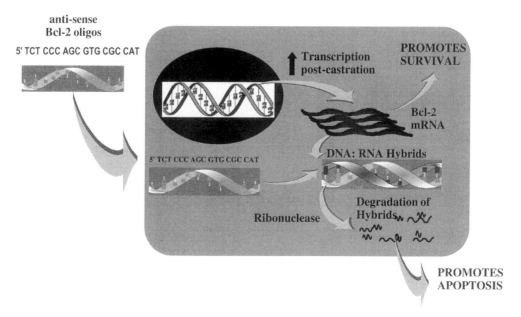

Fig. 2. Schematic drawing and illustrating mechanism of action of antisense oligonucleotides.

5. BCL-2

Bcl-2 has emerged as a critical regulator of apoptosis in numerous tissues as part of a growing family of apoptosis regulatory gene products, which function as either death antagonists (e.g., Bcl-2, Bcl-xL) or death agonists (Bax, Bcl-Xs, Bad) *(3,19,29,32,36)*. The ratio of death antagonists to death agonists determines how a cell responds to an apoptotic signal. In the prostate gland, Bcl-2 is expressed in the less differentiated basal cell layer of prostatic acini, but not in benign differentiated luminal cells or AD prostate cancer cells. In prostate cancer cells, Bcl-2 is upregulated within mo after androgen withdrawal *(27)* and remains increased in AI tumors *(3,29)*. Bcl-2 upregulation after androgen withdrawal may be an adaptive mechanism that helps some prostate cancer cells survive castration-induced apoptosis and subsequently progress to androgen independence. Induction of apoptotic cell death after androgen ablation or chemotherapy may be enhanced through functional inhibition of Bcl-2. Indeed, recent reports indicate that Bcl-2 AS-ODNs induce apoptosis and enhance chemosensitivity in various types of malignant cell lines, including small cell lung cancer *(38)*, melanoma *(15)*, and lymphoma *(35)*.

5.1. Enhancing Castration-Induced Apoptosis Using Bcl-2 AS-ODN

In both the LNCaP and Shionogi tumor models, Bcl-2 gene expression increases severalfold after castration and during AI progression. In both cell lines, Bcl-2 AS-ODN treatment reduced Bcl-2 mRNA and protein levels by >90% in a sequence-specific and dose-dependent manner (Fig. 3). In vivo treatment of athymic male mice bearing SQ LNCaP tumors with human Bcl-2 AS-ODN stabilized LNCaP tumor growth after castration. Serum PSA levels and LNCaP tumor vol increased 5–10 times faster in control MM-ODN treated mice compared to mice treated with Bcl-2 AS-ODN *(10)*. Treatment of mice bearing Shionogi tumors with mouse antisense Bcl-2 ODN begin-

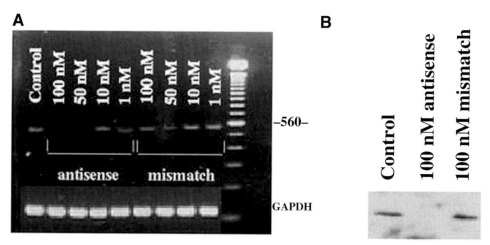

Fig. 3. (A) Antisense Bcl-2 ODN treatment of LNCaP cells in vitro results in sequence-specific and dose-dependent decreases in Bcl-2 mRNA levels within 24 h. No effect on Bcl-2 mRNA levels was observed after treatment with a 2-base mismatch-control ODN (5′ tct ccc agc atg tgc cat). Lane 1: serum-free control + 10 μL lipofectin; Lanes 2–5: 100, 50, 10, and 1 n*M* antisense bcl-2 ODN plus 10 μL lipofectin. Lanes 6–9: 100, 50, 10, and 1 n*M* mismatch bcl-2 ODN plus 10 μL lipofectin. **(B)** Western blot analysis of bcl-2 protein in LNCaP cells after treatment with 100 n*M* antisense and mismatch ODNs. Cells were treated for 6-h incubations with 100 n*M* antisense or mismatch ODN every 24 h for 5 d. Control cells were incubated in medium plus 10 mL lipofectin alone.

ning 1 d postcastration resulted in a 70% reduction in Bcl-2 mRNA levels, earlier onset of apoptosis, a more rapid regression of tumors, and a significant delay of emergence of androgen independent recurrent tumors *(4)* (Fig. 4).

5.2. Enhancing Chemosensitivity Using Bcl-2 AS-ODN

Bcl-2 also blocks proapoptotic signals by a variety of chemotherapy agents, conferring a multidrug resistant phenotype which may be operative in AI prostate cancer. This evidence raises the possibility that bcl-2 overexpression in AI prostate cancer helps mediated intrinsic chemoresistance, and suggests that modulation of bcl-2 levels may enhance chemosensitivity. Indeed, the IC_{50} of taxol and mitoxanthrone is reduced by a factor of 1 log in both LNCaP and Shionogi tumor models when Bcl-2 AS-ODNs are combined with either agent in vitro *(21)*. Characteristic apoptotic DNA laddering and cleavage of PARP were demonstrated only after combined treatment. Taxanes are known to phosphorylate and inactivate Bcl-2 *(11)*. Although Bcl-2 expression levels were not changed by paclitaxel treatment, paclitaxel treatment induced Bcl-2 phosphorylation and consequently inhibited the formation of Bcl-2/Bax heterodimer formation in a dose-dependent manner. Adjuvant in vivo administration of Bcl-2 AS-ODN and taxol following castration resulted in significant delay in the emergence of AI recurrent tumors compared to administration of either agent alone. Furthermore, regression of established AI Shionogi tumors was significantly greater with combined Bcl-2 AS-ODN plus taxol compared to treatment with either agent alone (Fig. 5A). Synergistic activity

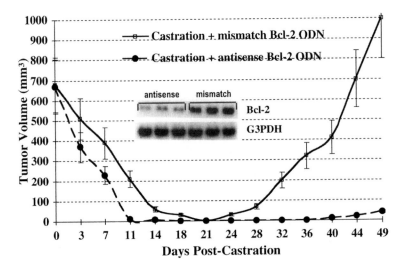

Fig. 4. Male mice bearing Shionogi tumors 1–2 cm in diameter were castrated and randomized for treatment with antisense Bcl-2 vs mismatch-control ODN. Antisense Bcl-2 ODN treatment resulted in a 70% decrease in Bcl-2 mRNA levels in Shionogi tumors (*inset*), faster and earlier complete tumor regression, and significant delay in recurrence of AI tumors compared to mismatch-control ODN treatment.

between AS-ODN and taxanes results from AS-ODN induced decreases in Bcl-2 mRNA and protein levels and taxol induced Bcl-2 phosphorylation (Fig. 5B). These findings suggest that downregulation of Bcl-2 by antisense ODN chemosensitizes AI tumors to paclitaxel over and above the effects of paclitaxel-induced phosphorylation of Bcl-2. Clinical studies using Bcl-2 AS-ODNs either alone or in combination with chemotherapy in prostate cancer are now underway at several institutions.

6. TRPM-2

Testosterone repressed prostate message-2 (*TRPM-2*), also known as *clusterin* or *sulfated glycoprotein-2*, was first isolated from ram rete testes fluid, and has been implicated in tissue remodeling, lipid transport, reproduction, complement regulation, and apoptotic cell death *(30)*. Since TRPM-2 expression is induced or highly enhanced in various normal and malignant tissues undergoing apoptosis, TRPM-2 has been regarded as a marker for cell death and possible mediator of apoptosis. Although TRPM-2 was initially reported as an androgen repressed gene in prostate tissue *(24)*, the functional role of TRPM-2 in apoptosis remains undefined. Overexpression of TRPM-2 in LNCaP cells enhances resistance to apoptosis induced by TNF-α *(34)*. However, other reports illustrate possible dichotomous roles for TRPM-2 following apoptosis induced by various types of stimuli *(12)*.

In Shionogi tumors, TRPM-2 expression is upregulated more than 10-fold within 4 d after castration and maintained at eightfold higher levels in AI tumors compared to AD tumors before castration. TRPM-2/clusterin staining also dramatically increases in prostate cancer cells after neoadjuvant hormone therapy compared to those without any treatment. Changes in TRPM-2 expression pattern after castration are similar to

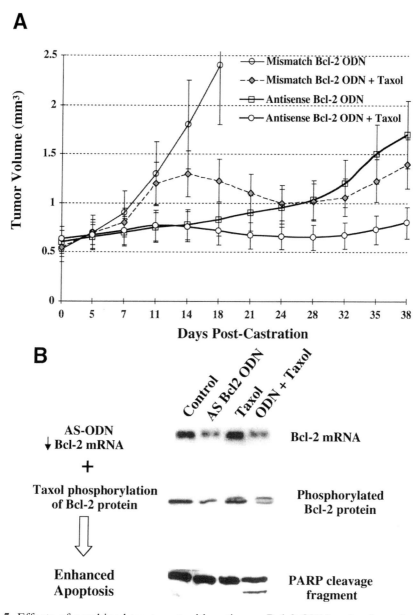

Fig. 5. Effects of combined treatment with antisense Bcl-2 ODN and polymeric micellar taxol on AI Shionogi tumor growth. (**A**) Male mice bearing AI Shionogi tumors between 1 and 2 cm in diameter were randomly selected for treatment with either antisense Bcl-2 ODN alone, antisense Bcl-2 ODN plus taxol, mismatch-control ODN plus taxol, or mismatch-control ODN alone. 12.5 mg/kg antisense Bcl-2 or mismatch-control ODN were injected intraperitoneally once daily for 14 d. Beginning d 10 postcastration, 0.5 mg polymeric micellar taxol was administered intravenously once daily for 5 d. Combined treatment with antisense Bcl-2 ODN plus taxol resulted in the most significant delay in recurrence. (**B**) After completion of treatment as described in (**A**), poly A⁺ RNA was extracted from AI Shionogi tumors, and Bcl-2 and mRNA levels were analyzed by Northern blotting *(top)*, by Western blotting with an anti-Bcl-2 antibody *(middle)*, or Western blotting with an anti poly PARP *(bottom)*. Apoptosis, as measured by PARP cleavage, was detected in only AI tumors treated with antisense Bcl-2 ODN and micellar taxol.

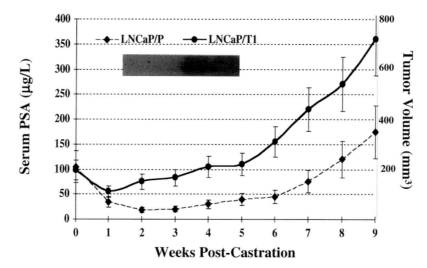

Fig. 6. Overexpression of TRPM-2 accelerates time to AI progression in the LNCaP tumor model. LNCaP cells were transfected with TRPM-2 cDNA expression vector pRC-CMV/TRPM-2 or the pRC-CMV vector alone as a control. As shown in insert, abundant levels of TRPM-2 mRNA were detected in TRPM-2-transfected clones (LNCaP/T), while the parental LNCaP (LNCaP/P) or control vector-transfected cell line (LNCaP/C) did not express detectable TRPM-2 mRNA levels. One million LNCaP/C and LNCaP/T1 and LNCaP/T2 were inoculated subcutaneously in intact male nude mice. After castration, LNCaP/T tumor vol and serum PSA levels continued to increase after castration, increasing threefold faster than in controls.

previously reported findings in the rat prostate *(24)* and human prostate cancer xenografts *(18)*.

To investigate the functional significance of TRPM-2 upregulation after androgen withdrawal, the effects of TRPM-2 overexpression on time to AI progression after androgen ablation was evaluated by stably transfecting LNCaP cells with *TRPM-2* cDNA expression vector. Tumor volume and serum PSA levels increased fourfold faster after castration in TRPM-2 overexpressing LNCaP tumors compared to control tumors (Fig. 6). Furthermore, overexpressing TRPM-2 LNCaP tumors were more resistant to taxol chemotherapy than the control tumors. Collectively, these experiments illustrate that TRPM-2 expression helps to confer both an androgen and a chemoresistant phenotype. The upregulation of TRPM-2 in human prostate cancer tissues after castration and the accumulating findings implicating TRPM-2 in protection of apoptosis suggests that targeting TRPM-2 upregulation precipitated by androgen ablation may enhance castration-induced apoptosis and delay AI progression.

6.1. Enhancing Apoptosis Using TRPM-2 AS-ODN

TRPM-2 AS-ODN corresponding to the TRPM-2 translation initiation site reduced TRPM-2 RNA levels in a dose-dependent and sequence-specific manner (Fig. 7). Adjuvant treatment with TRPM-2 AS-ODN after castration of mice bearing Shionogi tumors decreased TRPM-2 mRNA levels by 70% and resulted in earlier onset and more rapid apoptotic tumor regression, with significant delay in recurrence of AI

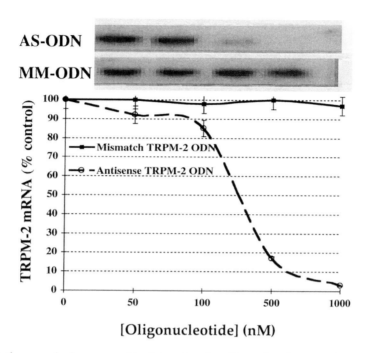

Fig 7. Northern analysis was used to determine the effect of antisense (5′-GCACAGCAGG AGAAT-CTTCAT-3′) vs a 2-base mismatch (5′-GCACAGCAGGAGGATATT-CAT-3′) TRPM-2 ODN on TRPM-2 mRNA expression. Daily treatment of Shionogi tumor cells with antisense TRPM-2 ODN (50, 100, 500 or 1000 n*M*) for 2 d reduced TRPM-2 mRNA levels by 2, 15, 81, or 98%, respectively. Mismatch ODN did not alter TRPM-2 mRNA levels.

tumors. After an observation period of 50 d after castration, mean tumor vol in the mismatch-ODN control group was six times greater than that of the TRPM-2 AS-ODN group. These experiments illustrate that TRPM-2 AS-ODN enhance castration-induced apoptosis. Furthermore, as shown in Fig. 8, TRPM-2 AS-ODN increased the cytotoxic effects of mitoxanthrone and paclitaxel in vitro, reducing the IC-50 by 75–90%. Synergy between TRPM-2 AS-ODN and chemotherapy also occurs in vivo. The recurrence of AI tumors is delayed longest with combined antisense TRPM-2 and paclitaxel compared to either agent alone. Although TRPM-2 AS-ODN had no effect on the growth of established AI tumors, TRPM-2 AS-ODN enhanced paclitaxel-induced tumor regression producing tumor vol 50–70% lower than paclitaxel alone. Collectively, these findings illustrate that TRPM-2 is an antiapoptotic rather than an androgen-repressed gene that confers resistance to androgen ablation and chemotherapy.

6.2. Systemic Effects of AS-ODN

The adverse effects of AS-ODN targeted against a specific cellular regulatory molecule, such as TRPM-2 or Bcl-2, on normal organs remains undefined. Because TRPM-2 and Bc-2 are expressed in many normal organs, including brain, kidney, spleen, and prostate, the effects of AS-ODN on the expression levels and function in these organs must be carefully evaluated. This is especially important in the context of combination therapy with cytotoxic chemotherapy, where inhibiting an anitapoptotic gene may

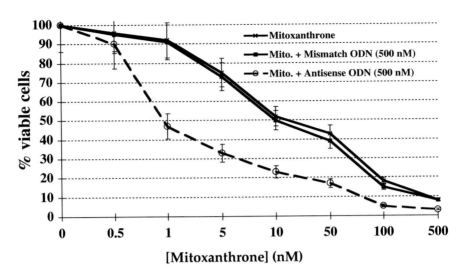

Fig. 8. To determine whether treatment with antisense TRPM-2 ODN enhances chemosensitivity, Shionogi tumor cells were treated with various concentration of antisense TRPM-2 or mismatch control ODN once daily for 2 d and then incubated with various concentrations of mitoxanthrone for 2 d. The MTT assay was then performed to determine cell viability. Antisense TRPM-2 ODN increased the cytotoxic effects of mitoxanthrone in vitro, shifting the dose-response curve to the left, and reduced the IC_{50} by 90% compared to a mismatch-control ODN.

worsen myelosuppression, nephrotoxicity, or GI toxicity. However, despite significant decreases in Bcl-2 or TRPM-2 expression after respective AS-ODN treatment in prostate and tumor tissues that undergo apoptosis after castration, target-gene expression was not altered by AS-ODN in the remaining normal organs examined *(20,22)*. Indeed, dose-dependent studies did not reveal any obvious toxicity in mice treated with up to 50 mg/kg of TRPM-2 AS-ODN. These results suggest that tissues undergoing apoptosis may be more sensitive to TRPM-2 AS-ODN treatment relative to intact organs, and that tumor tissues might be more sensitive to phosphorothioate ODN treatment compared to normal organs. One can speculate that preferential uptake of ODN in tumor tissues occurs because of differences in biodistribution or increased membrane permeability. Monia et al. reported reduced C-*raf* mRNA levels in mouse tissues following iv administration of antisense C-*raf* mRNA ODN, but observed no significant toxicity from these effects *(23)*. A phase I dose-escalation trial using antisense Bcl-2 ODN in nine patients with lymphoma reported objective and subjective responses with no significant toxicity *(37)*. These findings suggest that therapeutic doses of systemic phosphorothioate antisense ODN targeted against important cellular proteins do not cause significant toxicity in normal tissues.

7. OTHER POTENTIAL TARGETS

Many other genes are upregulated after androgen withdrawal and may be associated with either tumor-cell apoptosis or proliferation (e.g., Bcl-xL, IGFBP-5, c-*myc*). For example, we recently reported >100-fold upregulation of IGFBP-5 after castration and during AI progression in the Shionogi tumor model *(26)*. Accumulating evidence implicates insulin-like growth factor (IGF)-I in the pathophysiology of prostatic disease. The biological response of cells to IGFs, a potent mitogen for prostate cells, is regulated by various factors in the microenvironment, including the IGF-binding proteins (IGFBPs) *(16)*. Several IGFBPs are produced by normal prostate epithelial and/or stromal cells, and function to modulate IGF activity through high-affinity interactions *(16,26)*. After castration, the expression levels of certain IGFBPs change rapidly in the rat ventral prostate *(25)*. Differences in expression of various IGFBPs in benign and malignant prostatic epithelial cells have also been reported, with increases in IGFBP-2 and IGFBP-5, and decreases in IGFBP-3 in malignant vs benign cells *(7)*. Increased IFGBP-5 levels after castration has been shown to be an adaptive cell survival response that helps potentiate the antiapoptotic and mitogenic effects of IGF-1, thereby accelerating AI progression (*see* ref. *22a*). Other therapeutic approaches to targeting the IGF axis are utilizing AS-ODN against the IGF-1 receptor, or anti-IGF-1 receptor antibodies.

As discussed above, the *bcl-2* family plays key roles in the regulation of apoptotic cell death induced by a wide variety of stimuli. One gene in this family is *bcl-x*, which encodes two proteins—a long form (Bcl-xL) and a short form (Bcl-xS)—through alternative splicing mechanisms. Bcl-xL blocks apoptosis, whereas Bcl-xS, lacking 63 amino acids contained within Bcl-xL, is a dominant inhibitor of Bcl-2 activity *(1)*. Increased expression of Bcl-xL has been reported in prostate cancer, suggesting that Bcl-xL, like Bcl-2, may help facilitate progression to androgen-independence through the inhibition of apoptotic cell death *(17)*. Indeed, Bcl-xL is upregulated in the Shionogi tumor model after castration, and experiments using Bcl-xL AS-ODN are underway to try to enhance castration-induced apoptosis and chemotherapy in combination with other AS-ODN targets.

8. INTEGRATED COMBINATORIAL MOLECULAR THERAPIES

Since numerous genes and cellular pathways control the rate of tumor progression, inhibition of a single target gene will likely be insufficient to adequately suppress tumor progression. Exploration of additive or synergistic effects of combination antisense targeting in preclinical models will help guide further clinical protocols. For example, an additional combination of antisense TRPM-2 ODN with antisense Bcl-2 ODN and paclitaxel further enhanced the cytotoxic effects of paclitaxel, illustrating that combination targeting of other antiapoptotic genes may produce additive benefits (Fig. 9). Many additional novel biologic strategies are being developed to target various facets of this complex process, and include inhibitors of signal transduction pathways, angiogenesis, autocrine or paracrine growth factor pathways, or cell-cell communication. Inhibition of biologic activity can be accomplished using specific enzyme inhibitors, receptor antagonists, antisense ODNs, differentiation agents, and cell-cycle inhibitors. To achieve the additive benefits of integrated androgen ablation and combination therapy, stratagems that evaluate optimal timing, in vivo delivery and efficacy of these therapies are required. Once target mechanisms and proof-of-principle for novel agents are established in preclinical model systems, then significant methodological challenges confront clinicians, industry, and regulatory agencies to transfer testing to the clinical arena. Trial design for drug approval has traditionally required survival as an endpoint, but when the natural history is lengthy even in advanced disease, such an endpoint proves difficult and very expensive. It is critical that novel agents targeting biologic mechanisms be tested at appropriate times in the

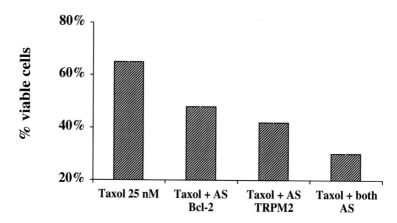

Fig. 9. To determine whether combined treatment of Bcl-2 and TRPM-2 AS-ODNs have additive effects in enhancing chemosensitivity, Shionogi tumor cells were treated with various concentration of Bcl-2 and/or TRPM-2 antisense or mismatch control ODN once daily for 2 d and then incubated with various concentration of paclitaxel for 2 d. The MTT assay was then performed to determine cell viability. Combined targeting of both antiapoptotic genes increased the cytotoxic effects of 25 n*M* paclitaxel beyond the effects of either AS-ODN alone.

natural history of the disease. This requires earlier, adjuvant administration with androgen ablation to take maximal advantage of castration-induced cell death, adaptive changes in gene expression, and smaller tumor burden. The challenges inherent to successful translation of an integrated and combinatorial systemic therapy for prostate cancer will require close communication and collaboration among bench scientists, clinicians, industry, and regulatory agencies.

ACKNOWLEDGMENTS

Supported in part by a Grant 009002 from the National Cancer Institute of Canada. We thank Mary Bowden and Virginia Yago for their excellent technical assistance.

REFERENCES

1. Boise, L., M. Gonzalez-Garcia, C. Postema, L. Ding, T. Lindsten, L. Turka, et al. 1993. bcl-x, a bcl-2-related gene that functions as a dominant regulator of apoptotic cell death. *Cell* **74:** 597–608.
2. Bruchovsky N., P. S. Rennie, A. J. Coldman, S. L. Goldenberg, M. To, and D. Lawson. 1990. Effects of androgen withdrawal on the stem cell composition of the Shionogi carcinoma. *Cancer Res.* **50:** 2275–2282.
3. Colombel, M., F. Symmans, S. Gil, K. M. O'Toole, D. Choplin, and M. Benson. 1993. Detection of the apoptosis-suppressing oncoprotein Bcl-2 in hormone-refractory human prostate cancers. *Am. J. Pathol.* **143:** 390–400.
4. Craft, N., Y. Shostak, M. Carey, and C. Sawyers. 1999. A mechanism for hormone-independent prostate cancer through modulation of androgen receptor signaling by the HER-2/neu tyrosine kinase. *Nat. Med.* **5:** 280–285.
5. Crooke, S. T. 1993. Therapeutic applications of oligonucleotides. *Annu. Rev. Pharmacol. Toxicol.* **32:** 329–376.

6. Denis, L. and G. P. Murphy. 1993. Overview of phase III trials on combined androgen treatment in patients with metastatic prostate cancer. *Cancer* **72:** 3888–3895.

7. Figueroa, J. A., S. De Raad, L. Tadlock, V. O. Speights, and J. J. Rinehart. 1998. Differential expression of insulin-like growth factor binding proteins in high versus low Gleason score prostate cancer. *J. Urol.* **159:** 1379–1383.

8. Gleave, M. E. and J. T. Hsieh. 1997. Animal models in prostate cancer, in *The Principles and Practice of Genitourinary Oncology* (Raghavan, D., H. Scher, S. Leibel, and P. H. Lange, eds.), Philadelphia: J B Lippincott Co., Philadelphia, pp. 367–378.

9. Gleave, M. E., J. T. Hsieh, H.-C. Wu, and L. W. K. Chung. 1992. Serum PSA levels in mice bearing human prostate LNCaP tumor are determined by tumor volume and endocrine and growth factors. *Cancer Res.* **52:** 1598–1605.

10. Gleave, M. E., A. Tolcher, H. Miyake, E. Beraldi, and J. Goldie. 1999. Antisense Bcl-2 oligos delay progression to androgen-independence after castration in the LNCaP prostate tumor model. *Clinical Cancer Research* **5:** 2891–2898.

11. Halder, S., A. Basu, and C. M. Croce. 1997. Bcl2 is the guardian of microtubule integrity. *Cancer Res.* **57:** 229–233.

12. Ho, S-H. 1998. Lack of association between enhanced TRPM-2/clusterin expression and increased apoptotic activity in sex-hormone-induced prostatic dysplasia of the noble rat. *Am. J. Pathol.* **153:** 131–139.

13. Horoszewicz, J., S. Leong, T. Chu, Z. Wajsman, M. Friedman, L. Papsidero, et al. 1980. The LNCaP cell line—a new model for studies on human prostatic carcinoma. *Prog. Clin. Biol. Res.* **37:** 115–132.

14. Isaacs, J. T., N. Wake, D. S. Coffey, and A. A. Sandberg. 1982. Genetic instability coupled to clonal selection as a mechanism for progression in prostatic cancer. *Cancer Res.* **42:** 2353.

15. Jansen, B., H. Schlagbauer-Wadl, B. D. Brown, R. N. Bryan, A. van Elsas, and M. Muller. 1998. bcl-2 antisense therapy chemosensitizes human melanoma in SCID mice. *Nat. Med.* **4:** 232–234.

16. Jones, J. I. and D. R. Clemmons. 1995. Insulin-like growth factors and their binding proteins: biological actions. *Endocr. Rev.* **16:** 3–34.

17. Krajewska, M., S. Krajewski, J. I. Epstein, A. Shabaik, J. Sauvageot, K. Song, S. Kitada, and J. C. Reed. 1996. Immunohistochemical analysis of bcl-2, bax, bcl-x, and mcl-1 expression in prostate cancer. *Am. J. Pathol.* **148:** 1567–1576.

18. Kyprianou, N., H. F. English, and J. T. Isaacs. 1990. Programmed cell death during regression of PC-82 human prostate cancer following androgen ablation. *Cancer Res.* **50:** 3748–3753.

19. McDonnell, T. J., P. Troncoso, S. M. Brisby, C. L. Logothetis, L. W. K. Chung, and J. T. Hsieh. 1992. Expression of the protooncogene Bcl-2 in the prostate and its association with emergence of androgen-independent prostate cancer. *Cancer Res.* **52:** 6940–6944.

20. Miyake, H., A. Tolcher, and M. E. Gleave. 1999. Antisense Bcl-2 oligodeoxynucleotides delay progression to androgen-independence after castration in the androgen dependent Shionogi tumor model. *Cancer Res.* **59:** 4030–4034.

21. Miyaki, H., A. Tolcher, and M. E. Gleave. 2000. Antisense Bcl-2 oligodeoxynucleotides enhance taxol chemosensitivity and synergistically delays progression to androgen-independence after castration in the androgen dependent Shionogi tumor model. *JNCI* **92:** 34–41.

22. Miyake, H., P. Rennie, C. Nelson, and M. E. Gleave. 2000. TRPM/2 clusterin is an antiapoptotic protein that helps mediate hormone independence in prostate cancer. *Cancer Res.* **60:** 170–176.

22a. Miyake, H., C. Nelson, P. Rennie, M. Gleave. 2000. Overexpression of IGFBP-5 helps accelerate progression to androgen independence in the human prostate LNCaP tumor model through activation of P13K pathway. *Endocrinology* **141:** 2257–2265.

23. Monia, B. P., J. F. Johnston, T. Geiger, M. Muller, and D. Fabbro. 1996. Antitumor activity of a phosphorothioate antisense oligodeoxynucleotide targeted against C-raf kinase. *Nat. Med.* **2:** 668–675.

24. Montpetit, M. L., K. R. Lawless, and M. Tenniswood. 1986. Androgen-repressed messages in the rat ventral prostate. *Prostate* **8:** 25–36.

25. Nickerson, T., M. Pollak, and H. Huynh. 1998. Castration-induced apoptosis in rat ventral prostate is associated with increased expression of genes encoding insulin-like growth factor binding proteins 2, 3, 4 and 5. *Endocrinology* **139:** 807–810.

26. Nickerson, T., H. Miyake, M. E. Gleave, and M. Pollak. 1999. Castration-induced apoptosis of androgen-dependent Shionogi carcinoma is associated with increased expression of genes encoding insulin-like growth factor binding proteins. *Cancer Res.* **59:** 3392–3395.

27. Patterson, R., M. Gleave, E. Jones, J. Zubovits, S. L. Goldenberg, and L. D. Sullivan. 1999. Immunohistochemical analysis of radical prostatectomy specimens after 8 months of neoadjuvant hormone therapy. *Mol. Urol.* **3:** 277–286.

28. Oh, W. K. and P. W. Kantoff. 1998. Management of hormone refractory prostate cancer: current standards and future prospects. *J. Urol.* **160:** 1220–1229.

29. Raffo, A. J., H. Periman, M. W. Chen, J. S. Streitman, and R. Buttyan. 1995. Overexpression of bcl-2 protects prostate cancer cells from apoptosis in vitro and confers resistance to androgen depletion in vivo. *Cancer Res.* **55:** 4438–4445.

30. Rosenberg, M. E. and J. Silkensen. 1995. Clusterin. Physiologic and pathophysiologic considerations. *Int. J. Biochem. Cell. Biol.* **27:** 633–645.

31. Saijo, Y., L. Perlaky, H. Wang, and H. Busch. 1994. Pharmacokinetics, tissue distribution, and stability of antisense oligodeoxynucleotide phosphorothioate ISIS 3466 in mice. *Oncol. Res.* **6:** 243–249.

32. Sato, T., M. Hanada, S. Bodnig, S. Ine, N. Iwana, L. H. Boise, et al. 1994. Interactions among members of the bcl-2 protein family analysed with a yeast two-hybrid systems. *Proc. Nat. Acad. Sci. USA* **91:** 9238–9242.

33. Sato, N., M. D. Sadar, N. Bruchovsky, F. Saatcioglu, P. S. Rennie, S. Sato, et al. 1997. Androgenic induction of prostate-specific antigen gene is repressed by protein-protein interaction between androgen receptor and AP-1c-Jun in the human prostate cancer cell line LNCaP. *J. Biol. Chem.* **272:** 17,485–17,494.

34. Sensibar, J. A. 1995. Prevention of cell death induced by tumor necrosis factor in α LNCaP cells by overexpression of sulfated glycoprotein-2 (clusterin). *Cancer Res.* **55:** 2431–2437.

35. Smith, M. R., Y. Abubakr, R. Mohammad, T. Xie, M. Hamdan, and A. al-Katib. 1995. Antisense oligodeoxyribonucleotide down-regulation of bcl-2 gene expression inhibits growth of the low-grade non-Hodgkin's lymphoma cell line WSU-FSCCL. *Cancer Gene Ther.* **2:** 207–212.

36. Tsujimoto, Y. and C. M. Croce. 1986. Analysis of the structure, transcripts, and protein products of bcl-2, the gene involved in human follicular lymphoma. *Proc. Nat. Acad. Sci. USA* **83:** 5214–5218.

37. Webb, A. 1997. BCL-2 antisense therapy in patients with non-Hodgkin lymphoma. *Lancet* **349:** 1137–1141.

38. Zieger, A., G. H. Luedke, D. Fabbro, K.-H. Altman, R. A. Stahel, and U. Zangemeister-Wittke. 1997. Induction of apoptosis in small-cell lung cancer cells by an antisense oligodeoxynucleotide targeting the Bcl-2 coding sequence. *JNCI* **89:** 1027–1036.

20

Stromal-Epithelial Interaction

From Bench to Bedside

Leland W. K. Chung, PhD and Haiyen E. Zhau, PhD

1. INTRODUCTION

Even as we hail the arrival of the 21st century, we must realize that prostate cancer and prostate cancer metastasis will soon threaten a greater percentage of the US population than ever before *(43)*. Prostate cancer and all its associated costs will be on the rise in the next decades, impacting the health industry and the productivity of the general economy as the baby boomers of World War II add to the general trends of the aging population. Faced with this uncertain future, the NIH and Congress have increased funding for prostate cancer research in recent years in the expectation that researchers will conduct translational research from bench to bedside. The opportunity exists to reduce the incidence of prostatic diseases through innovative prevention trials, to delay disease progression, and to treat men with hormone refractory, recurrent, and metastatic lymph node or bone diseases by specific hormonal, radiation, and chemotherapeutic strategies with clearly defined molecular targets. Future endeavors to identify additional critical molecular targets and develop therapeutic approaches exploiting these targets and processes have begun. Our intentions here are to review and summarize:

1. Our past research developing a molecular understanding of stromal and epithelial interaction in prostate growth and development.
2. The establishment of human prostate cancer progression models addressing the reciprocal roles of stromal and epithelial interaction and the expression by tumor epithelium of androgen independent and metastatic characteristics in host animals.
3. The use of human prostate cancer models to screen for therapeutic agents that can block local tumor growth and its distant metastases.
4. The dissection of genetic and phenotypic changes of prostate cancer cells during disease progression, and the categorization and validation of novel biomarkers to predict clinical prostate cancer development and disease progression, and
5. The designing of Phase I clinical trials, based on preclinical animal studies, to translate the findings from bench to the bedside for therapeutic targeting of men who have hormone-refractory primary prostate cancer and metastases to lymph nodes and skeleton.

From: *Prostate Cancer: Biology, Genetics, and the New Therapeutics*
Edited by: L. W. K. Chung, W. B. Isaacs, and J. W. Simons © Humana Press Inc., Totowa, NJ

2. STROMAL-EPITHELIAL INTERACTION IN PROSTATE DEVELOPMENT AND PROSTATE CANCER PROGRESSION

Reciprocal cellular interactions between stroma and epithelium are involved in fetal prostate development, postnatal prostate growth and maturation, maintenance of differentiation status, hormonal responsiveness, and the aging and senescence of the prostate gland in adulthood *(16,21)*. During neoplastic progression, stromal-epithelial interactions have been shown to accelerate local tumor growth *(11,15)* and distant metastasis *(67)*, and increase the genetic instability of the tumor epithelium *(70)* and its subsequent androgen independent progression *(28,66,67)*. The intricate intercellular communication between stromal and epithelial cells involves cell-cell, cell-insoluble extracellular matrices (ECMs), cell-soluble factors, and cell-androgen receptor-mediated processes—all of which are the subject of intensive investigation. To understand the molecular pathways that may affect intercellular communication and subsequent intracellular signaling, we must first identify key cell types, soluble factors, and insoluble ECMs participating in these communication processes between tumor epithelium and stroma. The next step involves identifying key metabolic and signaling pathways that may mediate the functions of regulatory molecules in tumor epithelium in a rate-limiting manner. Obviously, these are complex, interactive, and often redundant pathways whose regulation is highly cell-background and cell-microenvironment interaction dependent. The challenge is to determine how the cells mediate, integrate, interpret, and organize intercellular communications, and how the signals ultimately dictate the structure, function, and behavior of the cells. The reciprocal nature of the stromal-epithelial interaction can be clearly seen in pathologic specimens obtained from primary prostate tumors and in prostate tumors metastasized to bone (Fig. 1: *arrows* represent areas of stromal-epithelial interaction).

Three important features of stromal-epithelial interactions are noteworthy. First, whereas androgen receptor (AR), a key nuclear transcription factor in the stromal cells, is responsible for regulating *fetal* prostate development *(19,22)*, AR in the epithelium could assume the regulatory role and determine the ultimate growth and differentiation potential of the adult normal and tumor epithelium *(17,37)*. Experimental evidence using cocultured human BPH-derived stromal and epithelial cells indicates that the expression of AR, PSA and 5α-reductase in the epithelial cells relies on the inductive influence of neighboring stromal cells *(6,32)*. Similarly, in cocultured rat prostate epithelial and fibroblast cells, the androgen responsiveness of prostate epithelial cells can be conferred by the presence of fibroblastic cells *(12)*. However, studies using transplantable PC-82 human prostate cancer xenografts in athymic mice clearly indicated that once prostate cancer cells acquire the ability to grow autonomously (as exhibited by their ability to be passaged and grown in competent hosts), AR in the epithelium rather than the stroma is responsible for controlling the androgen responsiveness of prostate tumors in vivo *(25)*.

Second, genetic changes in the tumor epithelium are required, but are not sufficient in themselves to drive the metastatic cascade. Using a human prostate cancer epithelial cell line, LNCaP as a model, we demonstrated that despite its extensive chromosomal changes, this cell line remains nontumorigenic and nonmetastatic in castrated hosts *(67)*. By interacting in vivo with prostate or bone fibroblasts followed by in vitro cell cul-

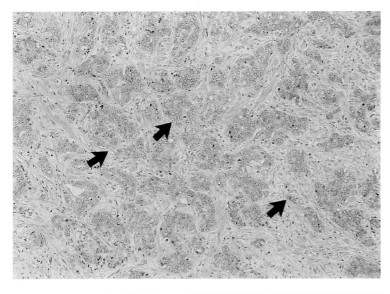

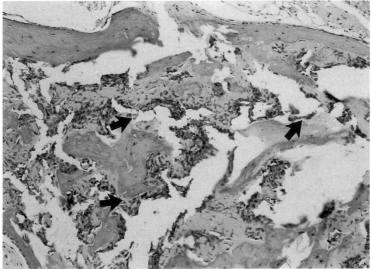

Fig. 1. Histopathology of primary human prostate cancer and its skeletal metastasis. In both of these specimens, stromal-epithelial interaction is apparent, as indicated by *arrows*.

tures, we observed that LNCaP cells acquired tumorigenic and metastatic potential in castrated hosts *(28,67)*. These observations demonstrated the importance of cell-cell contacts and soluble and insoluble molecules in the microenvironment, which together could be inductive and permanently alter the genotypes and the behavior of tumor epithelial cells.

Third, to gain access to distant anatomical sites, metastatic prostate cancer cells must fulfill a number of conditions: local cell proliferation, invasion through the basement membranes, attachment to the basolateral surfaces of the endothelial cells, migration and invasion through the intercellular space between the endothelium or the lining cells in the lymphatic channels, intravasation through the intercellular space of the

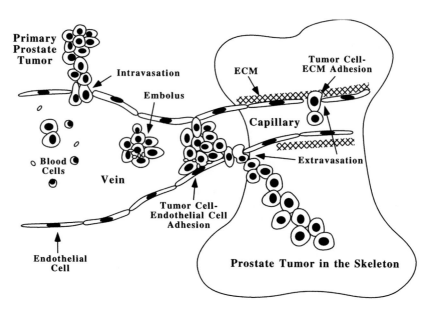

Fig. 2. Prostate tumor metastasis from primary to lymph node and bone. Multi-step processes of prostate cancer metastasis from primary to lymph node and bone involve cell proliferation at the primary site, intravasation into the blood or lymphatic circulation, attachment and adhesion to endothelial cells, extravasation to distant organs including the skeleton, and reciprocal cellular interaction with osteoblasts in the skeleton and the resulting increased cell proliferation of both prostate cancer and osteoblasts (osteoblastic reaction).

endothelium to the blood circulation to form circulating tumor emboli, attachment to endothelial cells, and finally, invasion, migration, and extravasation at the metastatic site (such as lymph node or skeleton). Once tumor cells arrive at the metastatic site, they will reestablish their proliferative and enhance their potential, induce local stromal growth (such as the eliciting of osteoblastic reactions in bone), and further invade, migrate, and metastasize to other body compartments, the so-called metastasis metastases (*see* Fig. 2). This general scheme of metastatic cascade is shared by many different forms of cancer, including prostate, breast, lung and skin, and should be further explored for potential new strategies for the prevention and therapy of prostate tumors.

In a series of early studies, we provided experimental evidence that chimeric prostate tumors comprised of tumor epithelial cells and prostate or bone fibroblasts can be grown in immune-compromised athymic or SCID mice *(28,77,78)*. We observed that once PSA is produced by tumors, the removal of testicular androgens (for example, by surgical castration) promotes androgen independent disease progression, which is manifested by the continued production of PSA by tumor cells in the absence of testicular androgens *(18,27,28,67)*. Taking advantage of these behavioral changes of tumor cells in vivo in response to androgen deprivation, we have cloned androgen independent and metastatic LNCaP sublines, designated as C4, C4-2, C4-2B sublines, that have been genetically and phenotypically altered from the parental LNCaP cells *(66,67,77)*. Notably, C4-2 and C4-2B cells, when administered either subcutaneously or orthotopically to either intact or castrated mice, metastasized to lymph node and skeleton. The latency periods varied from 2–10 mo, with tumor cell metastasis to bone more

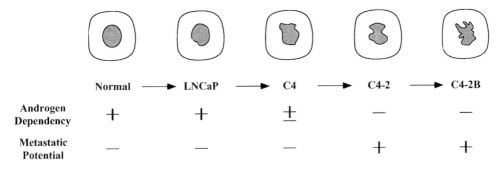

Fig. 3. A cell model of prostate cancer progression. A series of lineage-related cell lines derived from a human prostate cancer parental cell line, LNCaP, was developed in our laboratory. These cell lines have altered androgen dependency and metastatic potential when evaluated in vivo. In comparison to normal prostatic epithelial cells, the parental LNCaP cells have already undergone genetic and phenotypic changes, although they remain nontumorigenic in castrated hosts. The derivative LNCaP sublines C4, C4-2, and C4-2B have acquired decreased androgen dependency and increased metastatic potential.

frequently observed in castrated animals *(67)*. Prostate tumor cells appearing in the bone produced dramatic osteoblastic reactions, with animals developing gross paraplegia followed shortly by death at an incidence between 12.5-25% at the term of the study *(67)*. Figure 3 summarizes the androgen independent progression of prostate cancer cells under the influence of prostate or bone stromal cells. The development of *lineage-related LNCaP sublined through in vivo cell-cell interaction* is valuable for the following reasons:

1. These cell lines have been used by us *(13,35)* and others *(14,20a,23a)* to identify genes and evaluate pathways that may be associated with prostate cancer progression. Specifically, novel genes have been cloned through the use of these models, and results have been confirmed and validated in clinical prostate cancer specimens *(13* and Zhou et al., unpublished results).
2. These cell lines are also valuable for establishing models to study drug *(23a,63)* and gene *(26,30,31,40)* therapies for the treatment of prostate cancer metastasis. For example, we have used these models to study the effectiveness of antibodies (Law et al, unpublished results) and antiangiogenic drugs *(63)* on the growth and androgen independent progression of prostate cancer cells.
3. These cell lines are useful for defining mechanisms regulating cell growth, differentiation, and survival under various growth conditions *(14,15,17,18)*. Yeung et al. (unpublished results) in our laboratory have used this model to dissect the molecular mechanisms of prostate-specific antigen regulation in androgen-independent prostate cancer cell lines.

Using these cell lines as tools to explore cell-ECM interaction, we have observed additional behavioral changes of these cells with respect to their attachment, migration, and invasion through bone-matrix proteins such as osteopontin, vitronectin, and laminin. We observed that integrin utilization as a result of integrin switching in LNCaP sublines may be the key determinant in signaling external stimuli to the inside of the cells that alters the growth, survival, and differentiation of the tumor epithelial cells (Edlund, Miyamoto et al., unpublished observations). Some salient features of the LNCaP progression model deserve further comment:

1. Induction of solid tumor formation, promotion of androgen independent progression, and associated acquisition of increased invasion and metastatic potentials of prostate-tumor cells in vivo can be accomplished through cellular interaction with organ specific stroma *(28,57,67)*. Although extracellular matrices (such as Matrigel) and growth factors (such as basic FGF, EGF, HGF/SF) can also induce tumor formation in vivo, derivative cell lines from such induction by soluble and matrix-associated molecules failed to acquire increased metastatic potential in vivo (unpublished results). These results suggest that a host of factors expressed in a coordinated manner may be the key determinants underlying tumor-stroma interaction.

2. These observations are significant in view of the existing animal models, where a few growth factors or transforming oncogenes are overexpressed, or a single gene is knocked out in mice with well-defined genetic backgrounds, rarely resulting in metastasis *(8,32a,52a,54,61)*. Although a few of these models have been reported to exhibit metastatic potential, none have demonstrated metastasis from primary sites to lymph node and bone with clearly discernible osteoblastic reactions and paralysis of the hind legs of the animal subsequent to tumor cell metastasis to the spine. Figure 4 demonstrates at the histopathologic level how LNCaP and LNCaP sublines have the propensity to induce osteoblastic reactions in the spine.

3. The LNCaP progression model is a convenient way to pinpoint certain specific chromosome regions that can be considered "hot" spots *(35)*. Once these regions are identified, a confirmatory study can be performed in human prostate cancer specimens to validate the changes observed in the cell lines *(65)*. This model is also useful for identifying the expression of genes that may be altered during androgen independent progression. Using this LNCaP progression model, we have identified specific chromosomal regions *(35)* and proteins that may be altered during prostate cancer progression *(13)*.

In addition to the LNCaP progression model, we have also established an ARCaP model, a human prostate cancer cell line isolated from the ascites fluid of a patient with metastatic prostate cancer, which appears to be highly virulent and metastatic when administered orthotopically to test animals *(83)*. ARCaP cells have unique properties in their negative response to androgen and estrogen-induced proliferation. That is, the growth of ARCaP cells in vitro and tumors in vivo is suppressed by androgen and estrogen. ARCaP cells appear to have upregulated erb-B family growth factor receptor genes such as erb-B1 (EGF receptor), erb-B2/neu, erb-B3, and erb-B4 cell-surface receptors *(83)*. It is conceivable that this cell line may acquire growth and invasive advantages over other prostate epithelial cells through cellular interaction with soluble growth factors secreted by the surrounding tumor epithelium and stroma.

Based on the cell models of prostate cancer progression, we propose that androgen dependent tumors can progress to androgen independence. Within the androgen independent tumors, there are at least three different phenotypes: androgen responsive (AI-1), androgen insensitive (AI-2), and androgen suppressed (AI-3). In any given prostate tumor mass, it is possible that tumor cells with these variant phenotypes exist in different ratios (e.g., androgen dependent and the progressive AI type 1, 2, and 3 tumors). Upon disease progression and treatment, the ratios of these variant phenotypes may be altered, and consequently the behaviors of the tumors could be changed. For example, hormonal therapy could result in the dominance of androgen independent cells exhibiting C4-2 and ARCaP phenotypes. Relative ratios of AI type 1, 2, and 3 prostate cancer cells within the tumor are dependent upon the durations for which prostate cancer cells are exposed to androgen-deprived growth conditions. Several lines of evidence in the literature suggest that prostate cancer cells, when maintained in

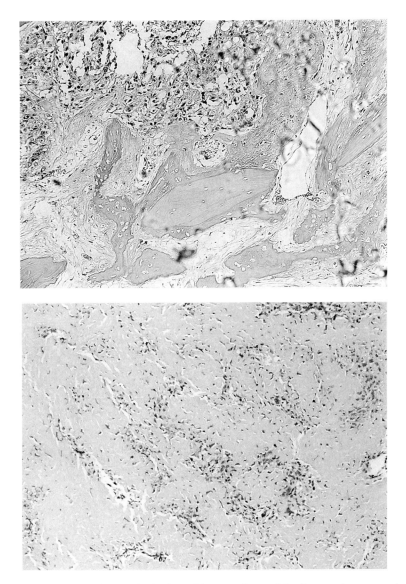

Fig. 4. Representative histopathologic evidence of osteoblastic reactions seen in athymic mice inoculated either subcutaneously or orthotopically with metastatic LNCaP sublines C4-2 or C4-2B. We demonstrated that osteoblastic reactions, which can be clearly seen in the skeleton, harbor metastatic human prostate tumors.

castrated hosts for longer duration, develop more aggressive phenotypes. Depending on the ultimate ratios of these cell populations in the tumor, responsiveness to chemotherapy, radiation therapy, or additional hormonal therapy might vary. The tumors may manifest varying degrees of androgen independence, aggressiveness, and differentiation, and an increased expression of invasive phenotype (e.g., increased expression of neuroendocrine and poorly differentiated fibroblastic phenotypes with decreased PSA expression) could be predicted through the analysis of cell models of human prostate cancer. The graph in Fig. 5 depicts the progression of prostate cancer cell models

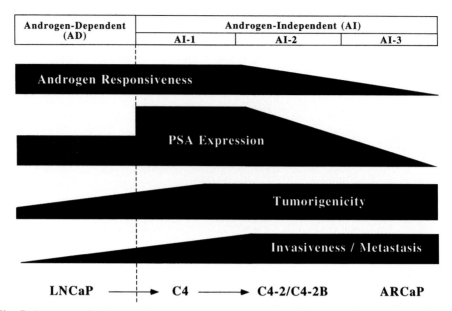

Fig. 5. A proposed schema of prostate cancer progression from an androgen dependent (AD) to androgen independent (AI) state. Based on cell models of prostate carcinogenesis (the LNCaP and ARCaP models), we propose that AI human prostate tumors can be derived from originally AD human prostate tumors. In this diagram, we depicted that among AI states, there are three progressive stages; androgen independent stage 1 (AI-1), androgen independent stage 2 (AI-2) and androgen independent stage 3 (AI-3). In clinical settings, we believe that most patients—when categorized as androgen-independent—most frequently belong to AI-1 and AI-2 stages. Thus, these patients are responsive to androgen blockade therapy. However, as disease progresses, some patients may progress to AI-3. AI-3 tumors are highly aggressive and invasive, but have depressed expression of PSA and become progressively negatively regulated by androgen or estrogen. These tumors may benefit from intermittent androgen suppression or flutamide withdrawal treatment.

from the androgen dependent to the androgen independent state with associated changes in PSA expression and metastatic potential. Figure 6 illustrates a hypothetical model predicting altered secondary hormonal responsiveness and tumor behavioral changes following hormonal therapy. For example, a short-term castration results in the elimination of androgen-dependent prostate cells and the retention of progressive AI type 1, 2, and 3 cells. Upon long-term castration, a shift in the proportion of AI type 1, 2, and 3 cells may occur within prostate tumors. For example, patients with phenotype A may respond favorably to antiandrogen therapy, whereas patients exhibiting phenotype C may respond favorably to intermittent androgen suppression and flutamide withdrawal therapy. This altered tumor cell ratio may affect tumor treatment, response, and recurrence. The implications of these progression schemes are:

1. In the androgen independent state, androgen insensitivity (such as in C4-2) and androgen repression (as in ARCaP) may be central to tumor progression and the expression of malignant phenotypes. A tumor cell expressing androgen insensitive phenotypes (defined as capable of growing in castrated hosts) can still respond positively to a pharmacologic dose of androgen with enhanced growth and PSA expression. Aggressive human prostate cancer may exhibit an increased reliance on growth-factor receptor and ECM signaling,

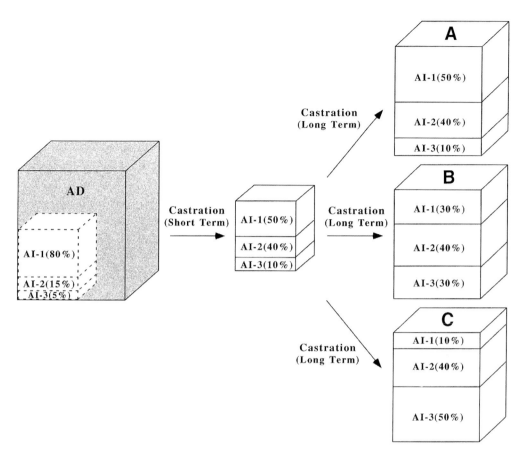

Fig. 6. A hypothetical model to illustrate the kinetics of androgen independent progression. Upon short-term castration the AI-1 cell population may decrease in proportion and in actual cell numbers, whereas AI-2 and AI-3 may expand in proportion and cell numbers when compared to the original population of AI cells in tumors before castration. Upon longer term of castration, relative ratios of AI-1, AI-2, and AI-3 cells may vary depending on the genetic and host microenvironment interaction. For example, a patient may have virtually unchanged AI-1, AI-2, and AI-3 cells in tumors following long-term castration (phenotype A). On the other hand, long-term castration could alter the phenotype of tumors to phenotype B and C with expansion of proportions of AI-2 and AI-3 cells at the expense of AI-1 cells. Consequently, patients with phenotype A may benefit from continued androgen withdrawal or blockade, whereas patients with phenotype C may benefit from intermittent androgen suppression, flutamide withdrawal, or combinations of these approaches in a sequential manner. Hypothetically, it is possible to employ intermittent androgen suppression or flutamide withdrawal to eliminate AI-3 cells, followed by the return of complete androgen blockade to eliminate AI-1 cells; AI-2 cells may be eliminated by treatment with other non-hormonal modalities.

which determines the growth, survival, and differentiation of the tumor epithelium. The expression of these phenotypes may be facilitated through stromal-epithelial interaction in hosts deprived of testicular androgen.

2. The fact that the growth of ARCaP cells in vitro and tumors in vivo is suppressed by androgen and estrogen suggests that under certain conditions, pharmacological levels of androgen and estrogen can suppress tumor growth directly—possibly mediated by the

nuclear receptors and their intracellular interaction with other cognate factors. The significance of this suppression is presently unknown. It is conceivable that the suppression of prostate tumor growth by androgen or estrogen could partly explain the clinical observations of prostate tumor responsiveness to secondary hormone treatment such as intermittent androgen suppression *(2,10)* and flutamide withdrawal *(59,60)*, where the rebound of testicular androgen at the off-period of hormonal therapy may be responsible for the suppression of tumor growth in selected patients.

3. The low levels of PSA expression detected in the aggressive ARCaP model pose the possibility that men with aggressive forms of prostate cancer may express low levels of PSA despite disease progression. It may be important to define the genotypic and phenotypic traits of ARCaP cells and tumors, which together could provide insight into the possibility of differentiating the indolent from the virulent forms of human prostate cancer.

The metastatic models of human prostate cancer were developed through the dedicated efforts of many of our talented colleagues: Ploutarchos Anezinis, Shi-Ming Chang, Bao-Qi Chen, Rodney Davis, Michal Chen, Martin Gleave, Jer-Tsong Hsieh, Andy Law, Chang-Ling Li, Sen Pathak, Hong-Woo Rhee, Robert Sikes, Mitchell Sokoloff, George Thalmann, Steve Wu, Tony Wu, Fan Yeung, and Jian-Guang Zhou. The molecular basis of androgen and estrogen action in these cells is currently under investigation by Bekir Cinar and Qinong Ye.

3. MOLECULAR TARGETING OF PROSTATE CANCER GROWTH THROUGH INTERRUPTION OF STROMAL-EPITHELIAL COMMUNICATION

Figure 7 illustrates our current view of stromal-epithelial interaction in localized and disseminated prostate cancers. At least five potential levels of molecular targeting can be achieved through the design of specific targeting molecules.

3.1. Extracellular Matrix Cell Surface Integrin Receptor Signaling

This can be accomplished through the use of integrin-specific antibodies *(9,24)*, cell-surface peptides *(3,52)*, or designed small molecules *(3,52,58,82)* that recognize or block the function of cell-surface receptors, including integrins, nonintegrins, and their interactive molecules. An increasing number of new cell-surface targets and ligands that recognize such targets are being identified through cDNA microarray and proteomics technologies, and by such techniques as chemical synthesis of small ligands based on the 3-dimensional structures of receptor molecules analyzed by X-ray crystallography or phage-display, to identify small peptides that may recognize specific epitopes on cell-surface receptors with either known or unknown structures *(76)*. Once the cell-surface receptor and the ligand interaction can be clearly defined, the target molecules can be either radiolabeled or conjugated to toxins or therapeutic viruses for efficient targeting at tumor cell and stromal-cell surfaces *(47,55a)*.

3.2. Growth Factor-Growth Factor Receptor Signaling

This pathway can be targeted through the use of receptor-specific antibodies and conjugation of these antibodies to radiolabeled molecules, toxins, and other therapeutic molecules *(5)*. In addition, both matrix and growth-factor-receptor initiated signaling pathways can be blocked successfully by the use of dominant negative or antisense strategies to interrupt outside-in and inside-out signaling mediated by the critical inter- and intracellular communication network *(46)*.

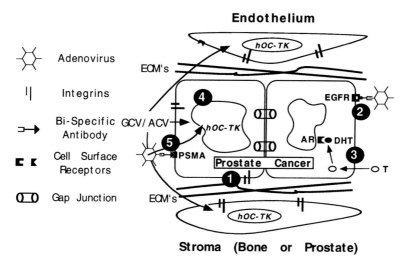

Fig. 7. Stromal-epithelial interaction as therapeutic target. Prostate cancer cells maintain close gap junctional communication as well as autocrine, paracrine, and cell-matrix interaction loops with adjacent stroma (bone or prostate) and endothelial cells. We propose that there are at least five levels of molecular targeting that can be implemented in affecting stromal-epithelial interaction in primary and metastatic prostate cancers. Interference in stromal-epithelial interaction can be achieved at: (**1**) extracellular matrix-cell surface integrin receptor signaling, (**2**) growth factor/growth-factor-receptor signaling, (**3**) nuclear androgen receptor signaling pathways, (**4**) by targeting specific cell structure and organelles such as nuclear matrix, and (**5**) gene therapeutic targeting to increase tumor cell death and decrease its proliferating potential. These strategies could prove to be valuable in preventing prostate cancer development, progression, and its subsequent evolution to express increasing malignant potential.

3.3. Nuclear Androgen Receptor Signaling Pathway

The androgen receptor mechanism in the stroma may be critical for the growth, differentiation, and early development and morphogenesis of the prostate gland, whereas the androgen receptor in the epithelium may be required to maintain the functional integrity of the adult and aging prostate glandular epithelium *(16,21)* and could function autonomously in prostate cancer and the relapse to androgen independence, without influence from adjacent stroma *(37)*. Androgen receptor gene amplification *(73)* and mutations (occurring most frequently at the steroid hormone binding domain *(69,74)* have been reported in clinical specimens obtained from men with androgen independent disease progression, suggesting that the aberrant function of the androgen receptor may be fundamental to the acquisition of androgen independence and metastatic potential by prostate tumor cells. Androgen receptor-mediated signaling pathways can be targeted through the use of androgen receptor antagonists, 5α-reductase inhibitors, or drugs that interfere with androgen receptor posttranscriptional modifications—such as phosphorylation—or interruption of androgen receptor function through the use of dominant negative or antisense strategies *(38)*.

3.4. Specific Cell Structures and Organelles

The nuclear matrix structure discovered by Donald S. Coffey and colleagues *(4,7)* has been employed as an attractive diagnostic *(55)* and therapeutic *(53,71)* target.

Microtubule structure and assembly proved susceptible to the drug estramustine *(50)*. In addition, various ion channels, cell-membrane pores, and transport-associated organelles have been used as targets for the discoveries of novel therapeutic agents *(80)*.

3.5. Gene Therapy Targeting

Therapeutic toxic genes or tumor suppressors have been delivered successfully to prostate-tumor cells with a high degree of efficiency using infectious adenoviral (Ad) vectors *(33,62,64)*. The goal of this approach is to severely interrupt the basal cellular metabolism so that the targeted tumor epithelium will be destroyed. Fractions of tumor cell-kill can be enhanced through the use of replication-competent adenoviruses *(45,81)*, the prolongation of gene expression through the use of the third generation of the gutless version of the Ad vectors which markedly decrease the host antiviral immunity *(20)*, and the use of locoregional perfusion techniques to concentrate the viruses in tumors locally. Specificity of targeting can be achieved through the use of tissue-specific promoters *(20,30,36)*, controlled activation of *cis*-acting DNA-responsive elements in the promoters with small inducing molecules *(1,79)*, or retargeting tumor metastasis by the use of specific antibodies or their conjugates to prevent damage to normal organs *(29)*.

In our laboratory, through the dedicated effort of many talented collaborators (including Jun Cheon, Thomas Gardner, Akinobu Gotoh, Chia-Ling Hsieh, Chinghai Kao, Se Joong Kim, Author Ko, Kenneth Koeneman, Yen-Chuan Ou, Toshiro Shirakawa, Yoshitaka Wada, and Ms. Fan Yeung), we have developed novel targeting strategies that use tissue-specific and tumor-restrictive promoters, such as PSA, osteocalcin, bone sialoprotein, and osteonectin, to drive the expression of therapeutic genes in prostate cancer epithelium, its supporting stroma, or both cellular compartments. These strategies should allow us to promote tumor destruction by eliminating the growth of tumor cells and by altering possible metabolic cooperation between tumor epithelium and its supporting stroma and interrupting intercellular communication between these two cellular components.

4. STROMAL-EPITHELIAL INTERACTION: POSSIBLE TARGETS FOR GENE THERAPY

Gene therapy holds promise for the treatment of metabolic diseases and cancer. However, this form of therapy is still limited by inefficient gene delivery to target cells, by the difficulty of expressing therapeutic gene specifically at tumor sites without damaging the normal organs, and by elicited host immune responses that prevent repeated and long-term applications of therapeutic viruses to hosts with an intact immune system. In a series of studies in our laboratory *(26,40,49)*, we have developed strategies for delivering therapeutic genes to prostate cancer epithelium and its supporting stoma through the use of tissue-specific and tumor-restrictive promoters that are capable of driving the expression of therapeutic genes in calcified tumor cells and supporting prostate stromal cells and osteoblasts. Bone matrix proteins are known to function in the bone remodeling involved in bone growth, differentiation, and maturation *(56)*. Experimental evidence from our laboratory *(42,78)* and others *(23,75)* supports the concept that prostate cancer cells, after they become metastatic with the propensity of homing to the skeleton, acquire osteomimetic and calcification properties, including the synthesis, secretion, and deposition of bone matrix proteins such as osteopontin, osteocalcin, bone sialoprotein, and osteonectin *(23,42,44,68,75)*. In a series of studies, we observed that osteocalcin (OC) promoter-driven therapeutic genes can effectively target the growth of osteosarcoma, brain tumors, prostate cancer, and chimeric tumors comprised of human prostate cancer cells and bone stromal cells *(26,39–41)*. The viral vector chosen for our studies was adenovirus (Ad) because of its high infectivity, its capability of infecting both proliferating and quiescent cells, high titers of Ad vector preparation that allow increased efficiency of infection, its stability and ability to accommodate relatively large DNA insert sizes, and broad-range cell specificity which permits the infection of both epithelial and stromal cells *(34)*. The therapeutic toxic gene used in these studies is the herpes simplex virus-Thymidine Kinase (hsv-TK), which can convert a pro-drug Acyclovir (ACV) or Ganciclovir (GCV) to its phospho-rylated form, and upon incorporation into cellular DNA blocks its elongation and thus stops cell replication. We have obtained promising preclinical data to suggest that Ad-OC-TK/ACV markedly inhibited the growth of previously established prostate tumors, grown either subcutaneously, orthotopically, or intraosseously *(26,41)*. In a series of animal toxicology studies, we noted that Ad-OC-TK/ACV was safe and did not cause any mortality or damage to normal organs as evaluated by gross morphology and histo-pathology. In sharp contrast, we observed that the Ad vector bearing the hsv-TK gene driven by a universal cytomegalovirus (CMV) promoter, when administered with ACV, killed 90% of the animals and induced severe liver toxicities in host animals. Despite the significant differential of toxicity observed between Ad-OC-TK/ACV and Ad-CMV-TK/ACV, both of these Ad vectors exhibited strong antitumor effects when adminis-tered in vivo (Wada et al., unpublished results). These promising preclinical results prompted our effort to seek a Phase I clinical trial testing the effect of Ad-OC-TK plus an oral form of ACV, valacyclovir (Val), in men with hormone-refractory and recur-rent prostate cancer and metastatic prostate cancer to lymph node and bone.

We evaluated OC protein expression in pathologic specimens obtained from men with either primary or metastatic prostate cancers. Figure 8 shows representative human prostate cancer specimens from primary, lymph node, and bone sites, stained by an OC-specific antibody. We concluded that OC protein is prevalently expressed by pros-tate cancer cells, prostate stromal component and osteoblasts (see arrows indicating positive immunostaining). OC immunostaining was found in 85% of the primary pros-tate cancer (23/27), and 100% of the prostate cancer metastasis to lymph node (12/12) and bone (10/10); low or absent levels of OC immunostaining were found in normal pros-tate cells. This series of preclinical studies clearly illustrated that Ad-OC-TK/ACV is safe and could potentially be beneficial to patients with metastatic prostate cancer.

5. IMPLEMENTATION OF A PHASE I CLINICAL TRIAL FOR MEN WITH HORMONE REFRACTORY RECURRENT PROSTATE CANCER AND PROSTATE CANCER METASTASES

Through the clinical effort and expertise provided by Thomas Gardner, Kenneth Koeneman, Jay Gillenwater, and David Kallmes, we have completed a dose escalation Phase I safety trial of Ad-OC-TK/Val in men with hormone-refractory, recurrent pri-

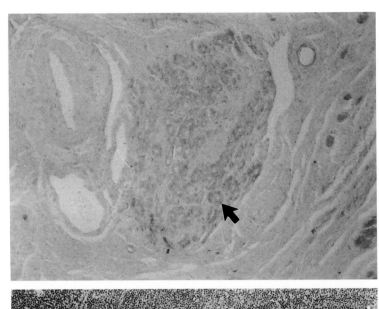

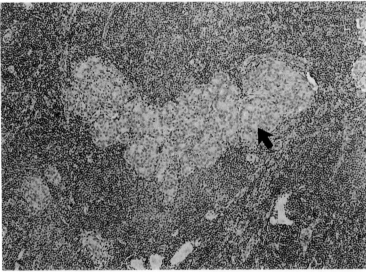

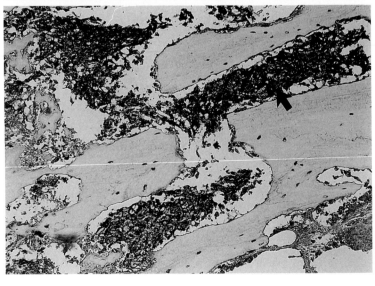

mary prostate cancer, and metastatic prostate cancer to lymph node and bone. A total of 11 patients were recruited. Each patient received two injections of Ad vectors, from 2.5×10^8 to 2.5×10^{10} PFU per injection, with a 7-d interval between the first and second dosing of the Ad-OC-TK. All patients were treated with a 21-d course of oral Val. Patients were monitored and evaluated subjectively by physical examination of symptomology and pain, and objectively by serum PSA and blood chemistry, including blood-cell count, liver and kidney function tests, blood coagulopathy, and viral titers in blood and urine samples. The status of tumors before, during, and after treatment was also monitored by chest X-ray, bone scan, transrectal ultrasound, CT and/or MRI-scan where indicated. In selected patients, positron emission tomography was also conducted. These imaging modalities can be used to evaluate the efficacy of gene therapy because all patients enrolled have bidimensionally measured index lesions. We are presently conducting laboratory correlative studies to determine if biomarkers associated with cell proliferation, differentiation, apoptosis, and local and systemic immune responses have predictive values for clinical responses. The conclusion of this study, as expected from the preclinical data, was that Ad-OC-TK/Val is safe at the highest dose of Ad vector administered. This finding is significant in relation to other similar gene therapy trials where the highest dose of Ad-CMV- or RSV-TK—when administered intratumorally to the localized prostate cancer lesions resulted in significant liver toxicity to selected patients *(62)*. Our trial, which involved administering Ad-OC-TK directly to the tumor lesions in the bone (the equivalent of iv administration) did not induce liver toxicity. This finding suggests the importance and advantage of employing tissue-specific and tumor-restrictive promoter, OC, as a vehicle to deliver therapeutic genes to tumor cells. In this trial, we noted in a dose-unrelated manner a transient elevation of activated prothromboplastin time (aPTT) in approx 50% of the patients. None of the treated patients, with or without aPTT elevation, experienced clinical coagulopathy or thrombolic episodes. A preliminary report of this study will appear in the *World Journal of Urology (41)*.

6. CONCLUSION AND FUTURE DIRECTIONS

Prostate cancer, in its progression from an androgen-dependent to an androgen-independent state with increasing metastatic potential, represents a serious threat to the health of the aging population. Clearly, we must find a cure for prostate cancer. Strategies to find such a cure are numerous. We have chosen to focus on intercellular communication between prostate cancer and its microenvironment, with special emphasis on prostate development, neoplastic progression, and the development of metastatic models of prostate cancer mimicking the disease process found in humans. Notably, we have created and characterized two mouse models of human prostate cancer

---

Fig. 8. *(facing page)* Immunohistochemical staining of osteocalcin in normal human prostate gland. Primary human prostate cancer, prostate cancer metastasis to lymph nodes, and prostate cancer metastasized to bone specimens. As clearly illustrated in these representative photomicrographs, OC expression is prevalent in primary and metastatic human prostate cancers. OC is either not expressed in normal prostate tissues, or is expressed in very low levels in the stromal compartment of some tissue specimens (data not shown).

metastases—the LNCaP progression and the ARCaP model—in which tumor cells acquired the ability to home to bone and induced osteoblastic and osteolytic reactions with gross paraplegia and death in experimental animals, more closely mimicking the human condition. We provided evidence to suggest that tumor progression toward androgen independence and acquisition of metastatic potential can be facilitated through cell-cell interaction. These cell models of human prostate cancer metastasis have proven to be valuable tools for conveniently and reliably assessing the genotypic and phenotypic changes of cells during disease progression. Some of these changes have been validated by clinical specimens. Drawing from the models and the molecular information generated by the study of prostate cancer progression, we developed a gene therapy program targeting both the tumor epithelium and its supporting stroma using a tissue-specific and tumor-restrictive promoter, OC, to direct the expression of the therapeutic gene hsv-TK in both the epithelial and stromal compartments. This strategy has been shown to be extremely effective in inhibiting the growth of tumors in preclinical models of prostate tumors, osteosarcoma, and brain tumors. Based upon these encouraging preclinical results, we conducted and completed a Phase I clinical trial of Ad-OC-TK/Val therapy in men with metastatic prostate cancer. The results of this trial indicate that Ad-OC-TK/Val is safe and can be further developed to increase its effectiveness for the treatment of localized and metastatic prostate cancers.

Future efforts in developing an understanding of the molecular biology of prostate cancer and devising potential therapies targeting the growth of localized and disseminated prostate cancer at the level of stromal-epithelial interactions may take the following directions:

1. Tumor cell heterogeneity has been appreciated by tumor biologists for years. Manipulating the tumor cell microenvironment, via tumor-associated stroma and tumor angiogenesis, could reduce the frequency of emergence of heterogenous and invasive clones of tumor cells. Tumor stroma could influence the growth, differentiation, invasiveness, survival, and senescence of tumor epithelium through secreted soluble and insoluble factor-mediated signaling cascades, and confer the overall genetic instability of the tumor cells. Angiogenic components in tumor stroma could be responsible not only for supporting the growth of tumors, but also for their ability to attach, migrate, and invade through basement membranes.

2. The tumor-stroma interaction may determine the sensitivity of tumor cells to hormonal therapy, chemotherapy, and radiation therapy. Understanding the molecular mechanisms underlying this interaction should help with the design of more effective preventive and therapeutic agents for treating prostate cancer metastasis.

3. New knowledge must be developed on the basic level as to how stroma react to tumor epithelium (e.g., the molecular basis of desmoplastic reaction), the biochemistry and molecular biology of normal and disease-associated stroma, and the possible regulatory role of stroma in the genetic stability of tumor epithelium. Such basic knowledge would help our future efforts to create genetic and genetic-microenvironment interaction models with transgenes expressed conditionally in different cell populations in mice, and to study the progression of prostate cancer in host animals under various experimental permutations.

4. The tumor-stroma interaction provides a rational basis for therapeutic targeting. The efficiency and specificity of such targeting may dictate the future success of the effort to eradicate tumor growth at metastatic sites. One theoretical advantage of targeting tumor-associated stroma is that it is normal and thus genetically stable in comparison to tumor epithelium. Thus, its therapeutic responses are predictable.

5. Although Ad vectors are highly efficient for the delivery of therapeutic genes to normal and tumor tissues, their inherent immunogenicity and potential fatal hepatic toxicity when injected intravenously must be addressed and fully understood to successfully advance this approach. In addition, novel imaging techniques need to be developed to visualize gene transduction to tumor cells and/or their surrounding stroma and levels of transgene expression, in order to determine therapeutic responses in a time-dependent manner directly and rapidly.

An era of combination therapy using multiple modalities is rapidly approaching for the treatment of prostate cancer metastasis. Very likely, genetic information on the tumor cells and their phenotypic expression (subject to stromal or host humoral-factor regulation, defined and validated in clinical samples) could guide future therapy. It is highly probable that individually designed therapies based on highly-specific phenotypic data obtained from each patient will ultimately yield the best clinical responses.

ACKNOWLEDGMENT

The authors are indebted to Mr. Gary Mawyer, MFA, for his outstanding editorial assistance and organizational skills. The authors are also grateful for the typing and proofreading of this chapter by Ms. Angela Sherman, and the artwork created by Arthur Ko (MD, PhD). This work is supported in part by the Kluge, CaP CURE, and Mellon Foundations, NASA NCC8-171, NIH CA76620 and NIH CA63341.

REFERENCES

1. Abruzzese, R. V., D. Godin, M. Burcin, V. Mehta, M. French, Y. Li, et al. 1999. Ligand-dependent regulation of plasmid-based transgene expression in vivo. *Human Gene Therapy* **10:** 1499–1507.
2. Akakura, K., N. Bruchovsky, S. L. Goldenberg, P. S. Rennie, A. R. Buckley, and L. D. Sullivan. 1993. Effect of intermittent androgen suppression on androgen-dependent tumors: apoptosis and serum prostate-specific antigen. *Cancer* **71:** 2782.
3. Arap, W., R. Pasqualini, and E. Ruoslahti. 1998. Cancer treatment by targeting drug delivery to tumor vasculature in a mouse model. *Science* **279:** 377–380.
4. Barrack, E. R. and D. S. Coffey. 1982. Biologic properties of the nuclear matrix: steroid hormone binding. *Recent Prog. Horm. Res.* **38:** 133–195.
5. Baselga, J., L. Norton, J. Albanell, Y. M. Kim, and J. Mendelsohn. 1998. Recombinant humanized anti-HER2 antibody (Herceptin) enhances the antitumor activity of paclitaxel and doxorubicin against HER2/neu overexpressing human breast cancer xenografts. *Cancer Res.* **58:** 2825–2831.
6. Bayne, C. W., F. Donnelly, K. Chapman, P. Bollina, A. C. Buck, P. Bollina, et al. 1998. A novel co-culture model for benign prostatic hyperplasia expressing both isoforms of 5-reductase. *J. Clin. Endocrinol. Metab.* **83:** 206–213.
7. Berezney, R. and D. S. Coffey. 1975. Nuclear protein matrix: association with newly synthesized DNA. *Science* **189:** 291–293.
8. Bhatia-Gaur R., A. A. Donjacour, P. J. Sciavolino, M. Kim, N. Desai, P. Young, et al. 1999. Roles for Nkx3.1 in prostate development and cancer. *Genes Dev.* **13:** 966–977.
9. Brooks, P. C., A. M. P. Montgomery, M. Rosenfeld, et al. 1994. Integrin $\alpha v \beta 3$ antagonists promote tumor regression by inducing apoptosis of angiogenic blood vessels. *Cell* **79:** 1157–1164.
10. Bruchovsky N., R. Snoek, P. S. Rennie, K. Akakura, S. L. Goldenberg, and M. Gleave. 1996. Control of tumor progression by maintenance of apoptosis. *Prostate Suppl.* **6:** 13–21.

11. Camps, J. L., S. M. Chang, T. C. Hsu, M. R. Freeman, S. J. Hong, H. Y. E. Zhau, et al. 1990. Fibroblast-mediated acceleration of human epithelial tumor growth in vivo. *Proc. Natl. Acad. Sci. USA* **87(1):** 75–79.

12. Chang, S.-M. and L. W. K. Chung. 1989. Interaction between prostatic fibroblast and epithelial cells in culture: role of androgen. *Endocrinology* **125(5):** 2719–2727.

13. Chen, M. E., S. H. Lin, L. W. K. Chung, and R. A. Sikes. 1998. Isolation and characterization of PAGE-1 and GAGE-7. *J. Biol. Chem.* **273:** 17,618–17,625.

14. Chen, T., R. W. Cho, P. J. Stork, and M. J. Weber. 1999. Elevation of cyclic adenosine 3′,5′—monophosphate potentiates activation of mitogen-activated protein kinase by growth factors in LNCaP prostate cancer cells. *Cancer Res.* **59:** 213–218.

15. Chung, L. W. K. and R. Davis. 1996. Prostate epithelial differentiation is dictated by its surrounding stroma. *Mol. Biol. Rep.* **23:** 13–19.

16. Chung, L. W. K., M. E. Gleave, J. T. Hsieh, et al. 1991. Reciprocal mesenchyme-epithelial interaction affecting prostate tumor growth and hormonal responsiveness. *Cancer Surv.* **11:** 91–121.

17. Chung, L. W. K. 1993. Implications of stromal-epithelial interaction in human prostate cancer growth, progression and differentiation. *Semin. Cancer Biol.* **4:** 183–192.

18. Chung, L. W. K., H. Y. E. Zhau, and T. T. Wu. 1997. Development of human prostate cancer models for chemoprevention and experimental therapeutics studies. *J. Cell. Biochem.* (**Suppl. 28/29):** 174–181.

19. Chung, L. W. K., N. G. Anderson, B. L. Neubauer, G. R. Cunha, T. C. Thompson, and A. K. Rocco. 1981. Tissue interactions in prostate development: roles of sex steroids, in *Prostatic Cells: Structure and Function*, Alan R. Liss, New York, 177–203.

20. Clemens, P. R., S. Kochanek, Y. Sunada, S. Chan, H. H. Chen, K. P. Campbell, et al. 1996. In vitro muscle gene transfer of full length dystrophies with an adenoviral vector that lacks all viral genes. *Gene Ther.* **3:** 965–972.

20a. Cox, M. E., P. D. Deeble, S. Lakhani, and S. J. Parsons. 1999. Acquisition of neuroendocrine characteristics by prostate tumor cells is reversible: implications for prostate cancer progression. *Cancer Res.* **59:** 3821–3830.

21. Cunha, G. R., L. W. K. Chung, J. M. Shannon, O. Taguchi, and H. Fujii. 1983. Hormone-induced morphogenesis and growth: role of mesenchymal-epithelial interactions. *Recent Prog. Horm. Res.* **39:** 559–598.

22. Cunha, G. R. and L. W. K. Chung. 1981. Stromal-epithelial interactions. I. Introduction of prostatic phenotype of urothelium of testicular feminized (Tfm/y) mice. *J. Steroid Biochem.* **14:** 1317–1321.

23. Curatolo, C., G. M. Ludovico, M. Correal, A. Pagliovolo, I. Abbate, M. E. Cirrilo, et al. 1992. Advanced prostate follow-up with PSA, PAP, osteocalcin and bone alkaline phosphatase. *Eur. Urol.* **1:** 105–107.

23a. El Etreby, U. F., Y. Liang, M. H. Johnson, and R. W. Lewis. 2000. Antitumor activity of mifepristone in the human LNCaP, LNCap-C4 and LNCap-C4-2 prostate cancer models in nude mice. *Prostate* **42:** 99–106.

24. Eliceiri, B. P. and D. A. Cheresh. 1999. The role of αv integrins during angiogenesis: insights into potential mechanism of action and clinical development. *J. Clin. Investig.* **103:** 1227–1230.

25. Gao, J. and J. T. Isaacs. 1998. Development of an androgen receptor-null model for identifying the initiation site for androgen stimulation of proliferation and suppression of programmed (apoptotic death) death of PC-82 human prostate cancer cells. *Cancer Res.* **58:** 3299–3306.

26. Gardner, T. A., S. C. Ko, C. Kao, T. Shirakawa, J. Cheon, A. Gotoh, et al. 1998. Exploiting stromal-epithelial interaction for model development and new strategies of gene therapy for prostate cancer and osteosarcoma metastases. *Gene Ther. Mol. Biol.* **2:** 41–58.

27. Gleave, M. E. and L. W. K. Chung. 1995. Stromal-epithelial interaction affecting prostatic tumour growth and humoral responsiveness. *Endocrine-Related Cancer* **2:** 243–265.

28. Gleave, M. E., J. T. Hsieh, A. C. von Eschenbach, and L. W. K. Chung. 1992. Prostate and bone fibroblasts induce human prostate cancer growth in vivo: Implications for bidirectional tumor-stromal cell interaction in prostate carcinoma growth and metastasis. *J. Urol.* **147:** 1151–1159.

29. Goldman, C. K., B. E. Rogers, J. T. Douglas, B. A. Sosnowski, W. Ying, G. P. Siegal, et al. 1997. Targeted gene delivery to Kaposi's sarcoma cells via the fibroblast growth factor receptor. *Cancer Res.* **57:** 1447–1451.

30. Gotoh, A., S. C. Ko, T. Shirakawa, J. Cheon, C. Kao, T. Miyamoto, et al. 1998. Development of prostate-specific antigen promoter-based gene therapy for androgen independent human prostate cancer. *J. Urol.* **160:** 220–229.

31. Gotoh, A., C. Kao, S. C. Ko, K. Hamada, T. J. Liu, and L. W. K. Chung. 1997. Cytotoxic effects of recombinant adenovirus p53 and cell-cycle regulator genes (p21$^{WAF1/ciP1}$ and p16^{INK4}) in human prostate cancers. *J. Urol.* **158:** 636–641.

32. Grant, E. S., K. W. Batchelor, and F. K. Habib. 1996. Androgen-independence of primary epithelial cell cultures of the prostate is associated with a down-regulation of androgen receptor gene expression. *Prostate* **29:** 339–349.

32a. Greenberg, N. M., F. J. DeMayo, M. J. Finegold, D. Medina, et al. 1995. Prostate cancer in a transgenic mouse. *Proc. Natl. Acad. Sci.* **92:** 3439–3443.

33. Herman, J. R., H. L. Adler, E. Aguilar-Cordova, A. Rojas-Martinez, S. Woo, T. L. Timme, et al. 1999. *In situ* gene therapy for adenocarcinoma of the prostate: a phase 1 clinical trial. *Human Gene Therapy* **10:** 1239–1249.

34. Hitt, M. M., R. J. Parks, and F. L. Graham. 1999. Structure and genetic organization of adenovirus vectors, in *The Development of Human Gene Therapy*, Cold Spring Harbor Laboratory, NY, pp. 61–86.

35. Hyytinen, E.-R., G. N. Thalmann, H. Y. E. Zhau, R. Karhu, O.-P. Kallioniemi, L. W. K. Chung, et al. 1997. Genetic changes associated with the acquisition of androgen independent growth, tumorigenicity and metastatic potential in a prostate cancer model. *Br. J. Cancer* **75:** 190–195.

36. Ido, A., et al. 1995. Gene therapy for hepatoma cells using a retrovirus vector carrying herpes simplex virus thymidine kinase gene under the control of human alpha-fetoprotein gene promoter. *Cancer Res.* **55:** 105–109.

37. Isaacs, J. T. 1999. The biology of hormone refractory prostate cancer. *Urol. Clin. N. Am.* **26:** 263–273.

38. Knudsen, K. E., W. K. Cavenee, and K. C. Arden. 1999. D-type cyclins complex with androgen receptor and inhibit its transcriptional transactivation ability. *Cancer Res.* **59:** 2297–2301.

39. Ko, S.-C., A. Tord, S.-J. Kim, T. A. Gardner, A. Kwon, H. K. Kim, et al. 2000. The treatment of malignant meningiomas using osteocalcin promoter based gene therapy in experimental models. *Neurosurgery* (submitted).

40. Ko, S.-C., J. Cheon, C. Kao, A. Gotoh, T. Shirakawa, R. A. Sikes, et al. 1996. Osteocalcin promoter-based toxic gene therapy for the treatment of osteosarcoma in experimental models. *Cancer Res.* **56:** 4614–4619.

41. Koeneman, K. S., C. Kao, S. C. Ko, L. Yang, Y. Wada, D. A. Kallmes, et al. 1999. Osteocalcin directed gene therapy for prostate cancer bone metastasis. *World J. Urol.* (in press).

42. Koeneman, K. S., F. Yeung, and L. W. K. Chung. 1999. Osteomimetic properties of prostate cancer cells: a hypothesis supporting the predilection of prostate cancer metastasis and growth in the bone environment. *Prostate* **39:** 246–261.

43. Landis, S. H., T. Murray, S. Bolden, and P. A. Wingo. 1999. Cancer Statistics. *Cancer J. Clin.* **49:** 8–31.
44. Levy, R. J., C. Gundberg, and R. Scheinman. 1983. The identification of the vitamin K-dependent bone protein osteocalcin as one of the α-carboxyglutamic acid containing proteins present in calcified atherosclerotic plaque and mineralized heart valves. *Atherosclerosis* **46:** 49–56.
45. McCormick, F. 1999. Cancer therapy based on p53. *Cancer J. Scientif. Am.* **5:** 139–144.
46. Miyake, H., A. Tolcher, and M. Gleave. 1999. Anti-sense bcl2 oligodeoxynucleotides inhibit progression to androgen-independence after castration in a Shionogi tumor model. *Cancer Res.* **59:** 4030–4034.
47. Nagy, A., et al. 1998. Synthesis and biologic evaluation of cytotoxic analogs of somatostatin. *Pro. Natl. Acad. Sci. USA* **95:** 1794–1799.
48. Newton, S. A., E. J. Reeves, H. Gralnick, S. Mohla, et al. 1995. Inhibition of experimental metastasis of human breast carcinoma cells in athymic nude mice by anti-α5β1 fibronectin receptor integrin antibodies. *Int. J. Oncol.* **6:** 1063–1070.
49. Ou, Y., T. A. Gardner, S. C. Ko, H. Y. E. Zhau, C. Kao, and L. W. K. Chung. 1999. Expression of osteocalcin in canine metastatic prostate cancer: an ideal prostate cancer animal model for osteocalcin promoter-based toxic gene therapy (*AUA 94th Annual Meeting, Dallas, TX*), p. 131.
50. Panda, D., H. P. Miller, K. Islam, and L. Wilson. 1997. Stabilization of microtubule dynamics by estramustine by binding to novel site in tubulin: a possible mechanistic basis for its anti-tumor action. *Proc. Natl. Acad. Sci. USA* **94:** 10,560–10,564.
51. Pang, S., S. Taneja, K. Dardashti, P. Cohan, R. Kaboo, M. Sokoloff, et al. 1995. Prostate tissue specificity of the prostate-specific antigen promoter isolated from a patient with prostate cancer. *Human Gene Ther.* **6:** 1417.
52. Pasqualini, R., E. Koivunen, and E. Ruoslahti. 1997. αv integrins as receptors for tumor targeting by circulating ligands. *Nat. Biotechnol.* **15:** 542–546.
52a. Perez-Stable, C., N. H. Altman, P. P. Mehta, L. J. Deftos, and B. A. Roos. 1997. Prostate cancer progression, metastasis, and gene expression in transgenic mice. *Cancer Res.* **57:** 900–906.
53. Pienta, K. J. and D. C. Smith. 1997. Paclitaxel, estramustine, and etoposide in the treatment of hormone-refractory prostate cancer. *Semin. Oncol.* **24(Suppl.15):** S-15–S-77.
54. Podsypanina, K., L. H. Ellenson, A. Nemes, J. Gu, M. Tamura, K. M. Yamada, et al. 1999. Mutations of Pten/Mmac1 in mice causes neoplasia in multiple organ systems. *Proc. Natl. Acad. Sci. USA* **96:** 1563–1568.
55. Replogle-Schwab, R., K. J. Pienta, and R. H. Getzenberg. 1996. The utilization of nuclear matrix proteins for cancer diagnosis. *Crit. Rev. in Eukaryot. Gene Expr.* **6:** 103–113.
55a. Robertson, C. N., K. M. Roberson, A. Pinero, J. M. Jaynes, and D. F. Paulson. 1998. Peptidyl membrane-interactive molecules are cytotoxic to prostate cancer cells in vitro. *World J. Urol.* **16:** 405–409.
56. Ross, F. P., J. Chappel, J. I. Alvarez, D. Sander, W. T. Butler, M. C. Farach-Carson, et al. 1993. Interactions between the bone matrix proteins OPN and BSP and the osteoclast integrin αvβ3 potentiate bone resorption. *J. Biochem. (Tokyo)* **268:** 9901–9907.
57. Rowley, D. R. 1999. What might a stromal response mean to prostate cancer progression? *Cancer Metast. Rev.* **17:** 411–419.
58. Saunder, J. and C. M. Tarby. 1999. Opportunities for novel therapeutic agents acting at chemokine receptors. *Drug Discovery Today* **4:** 80–92.
59. Scher, H. I., Z. F. Zhang, L. Cohen, and W. K. Kelly. 1995. Hormonally relapsed prostate cancer: lessons from the flutamide withdrawal syndrome. *Advances in Urol.* **8:** 61–95.
60. Scher, H. I. and L. W. K. Chung. 1994. Bone metastases: Improving the Therapeutic Index, in *Seminars in Oncology on Prostate Cancer* **21:** 630–656.

61. Schreiber-Aqus, N., Y. Meng, T. Hoang, H. Hou, K. Chen, R. Greenberg, et al. 1998. Role of Mxi-1 in aging organ systems and the regulation of normal and neoplastic growth. *Nature* **393**: 483–487.

62. Simons, J. W. and F. F. Marshall. 1998. The future of gene therapy in the treatment of urologic malignancies. *Urol. Clin. N. Am.* **25**: 23:28.

63. Sokoloff, M. H. and L. W. K. Chung. 1999. Targeting angiogenic pathways involving tumor-stromal interaction to treat advanced human prostate cancer. *Cancer Metastasis* **17**: 307–315.

64. Steiner, M. S. and J. R. Gingrich. 2000. Gene therapy for prostate cancer: where are we now? *J. Urol.* (in press)

65. Thalmann, G. N., R. A. Sikes, R. E. Devoll, J. A. Kiefer, R. Markwalder, I. Klima, et al. 1999. Osteopontin: possible role in prostate cancer progression. *Clin. Cancer Res.* **5**: 2271–2277.

66. Thalmann, G. N., R. A. Sikes, T. T. Wu, A. DeGeorges, S.-M. Chang, M. Ozen, et al. 2000. The LNCaP progression model of human prostate cancer: Androgen-independence and osseous metastasis. *The Prostate* **44**: 91–103.

67. Thalmann, G., P. Anezinis, S.-M. Chang, H. Y. E. Zhau, C. Hall, S. Pathak, et al. 1994. The LNCaP mouse model of human prostate cancer: androgen independent cancer progression and osseous metastasis. *Cancer Res.* **54**: 2577–2581.

68. Thalmann, G. N., P. Anezinis, R. Devoll, C. Farach-Carson, and L. W. K. Chung. 1997. Experimental approaches to skeletal metastasis of human prostate cancer, in *Principles and Practice of Genitourinary Oncology*, pp. 409–416, Lippincott and Raven, PA.

69. Tilley, W. D., G. Buchanan, T. E. Hickey, and J. M. Bentel. 1996. Mutations in the androgen receptor gene are associated with progression of human prostate cancer to androgen independence. *Clin. Cancer Res.* **2**: 277–285.

70. Tlsty, T. D. 1998. Cell-adhesion dependent influences on genomic instability and carcinogenesis. *Curr. Opin. Cell Biol.* **10**: 647–653.

71. Valkov, N. I., J. L. Gump, and D. M. Sullivan. 1997. Quantitative immunofluorescence and immunoelectron microscopy of the topoismerage II—associated with nuclear matrices from wild-type drug-resistant Chinese hamster ovary cell lines. *J. Cell. Biochem.* **67**: 112–130.

72. Vile, R. G. and I. R. Hart. 1993. Use of tissue-specific expression of the herpes simplex virus thymidine kinase gene to inhibit growth of established murine melanomas following direct intratumoral injection of DNA. *Cancer Res.* **53**: 3860–3864.

73. Visakorpi, T., E. Hyytinen, P. Koivisto, M. Tanner, R. Keinanen, C. Palmberg, et al. 1995. *In vivo* amplification of the androgen receptor gene and progression of human prostate cancer. *Nat. Genet.* **9**: 401–406.

74. Vldscholte, J., C. Ris-Stalpers, G. G. J. M. Kuiper, et al. 1990. A mutation in the ligand binding domain of the androgen receptor of human LNCaP cells affects steroid binding characteristics and response to antiandrogens. *BBRC* **175**: 534–543.

75. Waltregny, D., A. Bellaheene, I. V. Riet, L. W. Fisher, M. Young, P. Feunandez, et al. 1998. Prognostic value of bone sialoprotein expression in clinically localized human prostate cancer. *J. Natl. Cancer Inst.* **90**: 1000–1007.

76. Wood, D. W., W. Wu, G. Belfort, et al. 1999. A genetic system yields self-cleaving integrins for bioseparations. *Nat. Biotech.* **17**: 889–892.

77. Wu, H. S., J. T. Hsieh, M. E. Gleave, N. M. Brown, S. Pathak, and L. W. K. Chung. 1994. Derivation of androgen independent human LNCaP prostatic cancer cell sublines: role of bone stromal cells. *Int. J. Cancer* **57**: 406–412.

78. Wu, T. T., R. A. Sikes, Q. Cui, G. N. Thalmann, C. Kao, C. F. Murphy, et al. 1998. Establishing human prostate cancer cell xenografts in bone: induction of osteoblastic reaction by prostate-specific antigen-producing tumors in athymic and SCID/bg mice using LNCaP and lineage-derived metastatic sublines. *Int. J. Cancer* **77**: 887–894.

79. Yoshida, Y. and H. Hamada. 1997. Adenovirus-mediated inducible gene expression through tetracycline-controllable transactivator with nuclear localization signal. *Biochem. Biophys. Res. Commun.* **230:** 426–430.
80. Young, K., et al. 1998. Identification of a calcium channel modulator using a high-throughput yeast two-hybrid screen. *Nat. Biotechnol.* **16:** 946–950.
81. Yu, D. C., Y. Chen, M. Seng, J. Dilley, and D. R. Henderson. 1999. The addition of adenovirus type 5 region E3 enables calydon virus 787 to eliminate distant prostate tumor xenografts. *Cancer Res.* **59:** 4200–4203.
82. Zhao, M., H. K. Kleinman, M. Mokotoff. 1994. Synthetic laminin-like peptides and pseudopeptides as potential anti-metastatic agents. *J. Med. Chem.* **37:** 3383–3388.
83. Zhau, H. Y. E., S. M. Chang, B. Q. Chen, Y. Wang, H. Zhang, C. Kao, et al. 1996. Androgen-repressed phenotype in human prostate cancer. *Proc. Natl. Acad. Sci. USA* **93:** 15,152–15,157.

PART IV

CANCER THERAPEUTICS

21

Chemoprevention of Prostate Cancer

James D. Brooks, MD, William G. Nelson, MD, PhD

1. INTRODUCTION

During the twentieth century, approx 20 yr were added to the life expectancy of men and women in the United States (65). With this increased life expectancy, neoplastic diseases have emerged as major killers. Cancer has moved from a relatively infrequent killer in 1900—far behind tuberculosis, pneumonia, enteritis, and accidents—to the second leading cause of death in recent decades. Certainly, some of the gains in life expectancy are the result of improvements in medical technology such as the development of antibiotics for infectious disease and medical and surgical innovations in the management of cardiovascular disease. However, the largest improvements have arisen from public health efforts directed at disease prevention. Improvements in sanitation, vaccinations, and other public health efforts have dramatically reduced deaths from infectious disease, while accidental deaths have decreased substantially as a public health hazard with heightened regulation of workplace safety. Changes in diet and exercise habits and recent decreases in cigarette smoking have all lowered the cardiovascular death rate. Further decreases in cardiovascular deaths can be attributed to identification of important risk factors in the development of atherosclerotic disease, such as hypertension and elevated cholesterol, and the use of interventions targeted at ameliorating these conditions. In the 21st century, reduction in deaths from neoplasia, including prostate cancer, will also be targeted with prevention strategies. To achieve this goal, significant research efforts will be required to identify the risk factors for development of cancer, to devise nontoxic intervention strategies based on an understanding of the causes of cancer, and to develop biomarkers to assess the efficacy of these preventive interventions.

2. THE NEED FOR PROSTATE CANCER PREVENTION

For men in the United States, prostate cancer has the ignoble distinction of being the leading cancer diagnosis and the second leading cause of cancer death (12). African-American males are particularly devastated by this disease, with some of the highest incidence and mortality rates for prostate cancer in the world (39,49). Men with a family history of prostate cancer appear to be at increased risk for prostate cancer, and hereditary prostate cancer may account for as many as 10% of all cases diagnosed in the United States (11). Although the genes responsible for hereditary prostate cancer

From: *Prostate Cancer: Biology, Genetics, and the New Therapeutics*
Edited by: L. W. K. Chung, W. B. Isaacs, and J. W. Simons © Humana Press Inc., Totowa, NJ

have not been identified, prostate cancer development in high-risk prostate cancer families has been linked to genetic markers on chromosome 1 and on the X chromosome *(58,70)*. An increased risk of prostate cancer has been associated with polymorphisms in gene encoding for the androgen receptor *(23)*. The explosion of DNA-sequence information from the Human Genome Project will undoubtedly provide a number of other molecular markers for prostate cancer risk *(14)*. With the anticipated increase in the use of genetic information for the assignment of prostate cancer risk, it is incumbent on physicians to develop effective screening and prevention strategies for men considered at high risk for life-threatening prostate cancer development.

Prostate cancer prevention strategies will probably come from an improved understanding of the causes of prostate cancer and the discovery of nontoxic interventions that can be targeted at these underlying mechanisms of prostate carcinogenesis. Although the exact causes of prostate cancer have not yet been established, several recent epidemiologic and basic molecular studies have provided some clues to some of the underlying factors in prostate carcinogenesis *(5)*. As the factors that lead to prostate cancer are identified, rationally designed prevention strategies may become feasible. Such strategies are likely to involve elimination or avoidance of exogenous factors that contribute to prostate cancer development, buttressing of prostate cellular defenses against endogenous factors that cannot be avoided, or a combination of both approaches.

3. THE CURRENT STATUS OF PROSTATE CANCER PREVENTION

Androgens play a central role in the development of prostate cancer. Men who are castrated at an early age cannot develop prostate cancer. Androgen withdrawal has become a mainstay in the treatment of men with locally advanced and metastatic prostate cancer since the mid-twentieth century. Can antagonists of androgen action prevent the development of life-threatening prostate cancer? Recent progress in attempts to prevent breast cancer has brought this question into the forefront of prostate cancer prevention research. Estrogens have long been known to play an important role in the development of breast cancer in women *(46)*. Furthermore, tamoxifen—an antiestrogen— has been demonstrated to reduce breast cancer risk in a large ($n = 13,388$) randomized prospective trial *(19)*. The positive findings of this study emphasize the promise of preventive strategies targeted at the androgen axis in prostate cancer.

Oral antiandrogens have been available for a number of years. Thus far, these agents have not been widely considered for prostate cancer prevention largely because of undesirable side effects including erectile dysfunction, development of breast tissue, deranged liver function, and osteoporosis associated with their use. Several years ago, finasteride, a 5-alpha reductase with a more acceptable side-effect profile, was proposed as a prostate cancer preventive agent *(3)*. As a 5-alpha reductase inhibitor, finasteride blocks the conversion of testosterone to dihydrotestosterone, thereby muting the effects of androgen in the prostate. A prospective, randomized trial—the Prostate Cancer Prevention Trial (PCPT), involving some 18,000 men—is currently underway in the United States to test whether finasteride will prevent the development of clinically significant prostate cancer *(61)*. Study subjects had prostate biopsy at enrollment in the study, and exit biopsies are planned after 8 yr at the conclusion of the study period. Will finasteride prove effective at preventing prostate cancer? 5-alpha reductase inhibitors have demonstrated preclinical preventive efficacy in rat models for prostate and prostate/seminal vesicle cancer *(3,31,63)*. Yet some preliminary reports suggest that finasteride may not be effective in preventing human prostate cancer *(1)*. In a randomized trial of finasteride vs placebo for benign prostatic hyperplasia ($n = 3040$), 4.7% of men treated with finasteride and 5.1% of men treated with placebo were diagnosed with prostate cancer ($p = 0.7$), *(1)*. In a second smaller trial ($n = 52$), men with an elevated prostate specific antigen (PSA) and negative prostate biopsies were randomized to treatment with finasteride, or to no treatment, for 12 mo *(15)*. Repeat biopsies at the end of the study disclosed prostate cancer in 30% of men treated with finasteride compared with 4% of men left untreated ($p = 0.25$). Among the men in the trial found to have high-grade prostatic intraepithelial neoplasia (PIN) on the initial biopsy, finasteride appeared to have no effect on the PIN lesions. Furthermore, prostate cancer appeared after 12 mo of finasteride treatment in 6 of 8 men—vs 0 of 5 untreated men—with high-grade PIN ($p = 0.21$) *(15)*. The outcome of the PCPT, which targets a more general population of men, will hopefully provide definitive evidence of the presence or absence of efficacy of finasteride in the prevention of prostate cancer. In addition, data collected via the PCPT is also likely to shed significant light on the natural history of prostate cancer and benign prostatic hyperplasia.

Androgens are not the sole determinants of prostate cancer development. Abundant evidence suggests that other factors contribute to prostate carcinogenesis. One of the striking features of human prostate cancer epidemiology is the tremendous geographic variation in incidence and mortality rates. Unlike the United States and Western Europe, prostate cancer is rarely diagnosed, and contributes little to cancer mortality, in Asia *(5,12,72)* Several carefully conducted epidemiologic studies have failed to demonstrate differences in serum androgen levels or androgen metabolism between men in areas of low and high incidence *(47)*. Migration studies have suggested that lifestyle and/or environment are important determinants of prostate cancer pathogenesis *(16,25,56,69)*. Migrants from Asia to the United States acquire a higher clinical incidence of prostate cancer, and subsequent generations of American-born Asian men have a prostate cancer risk approaching that of Caucasian Americans. Although the exact environmental factors are unknown, diet has emerged as an important candidate risk modifier for prostate cancer development. A number of large studies have suggested that diets high in saturated fat (Western diets) may be associated with an increased risk of prostate cancer incidence and mortality *(22,38,54,68)*. Such findings have led some to propose that drastic reductions in fat consumption may attenuate prostate cancer progression. Possible mechanisms through which fat may act to increase the risk of prostate cancer are unknown, but such studies open the possibility that factors other than androgen are important in the development of prostate cancer.

4. A NEW HYPOTHESIS

In 1994, we described a somatic molecular genetic lesion that may provide some insight into the genesis of prostate cancer and suggest a possible rational strategy for its prevention. Virtually all human prostate cancers lose expression of the enzyme glutathione S-transferase-π (GSTP1) *(41)*. GSTP1 is one of a large family of glutathione transferases that act in concert with other Phase 2 detoxification enzymes to defend cells against damage *(27)*. Phase 2 enzymes protect cells against a barrage of exogenous and endogenous oxidant and electrophilic species that can damage DNA and cause cellular transformation. In prostate cancer, loss of GSTP1 expression may be the result of methylation of regulatory DNA sequences in a "CpG island' region encompassing the promoter and first intron of the GSTP1 gene *(40)*. This somatic genome alteration appears to be relatively unique to carcinoma of the prostate among genitourinary cancers, and is not found in any normal human tissue.

It is somewhat surprising that loss of any single member of the GST family could be associated with the development of cancer. However, mice carrying disrupted π-class GST genes manifest an earlier onset and an increased number of skin tumors after treatment with the carcinogen 7, 12-dimethylbenz anthracene (DMBA) *(30)*. As for *homo sapiens*, 40% of the Caucasian population in the United States carry null alleles for a member of the mu-class GST (GSTM1) and have only one phenotypic manifestation: increased risk of development of cancer *(2,4,26,35,37,55,62)*. This increased risk has been reported for several cancers, including lung, colon, and bladder cancer. Early molecular epidemiology studies have tentatively identified an increased risk for breast cancer and for prostate cancer associated with carrying polymorphic low activity GSTP1 alleles *(26,29,59)*. Taken together, these studies provide compelling evidence that loss of a single carcinogen defense enzyme can have profound affects on the development of cancer. Thus, we can speculate that the early loss of GSTP1 plays an important role in prostate carcinogenesis.

5. HOW CAN LOSS OF GSTP1 EFFECT PROSTATE CANCER DEVELOPMENT?

While all GSTs are effective at reduction of DNA-damaging electrophiles, GSTP1 may be more active at quenching oxygen-free-radical damage, perhaps by scavenging lipid peroxides. We hypothesize that prostate cancer initiation and progression may be the result of oxidant stress in the face of compromised oxidative defenses. In agreement with this hypothesis, loss of GSTP1 expression appears to occur early during prostate carcinogenesis: the lack of GSTP1 expression and *GSTP1* promoter methylation have both been found in prostatic intraepithelial neoplasia (PIN) lesions—putative precursors to prostate carcinomas *(8)*.

Several lines of evidence point to the important role that oxidative damage plays in prostate carcinogenesis. The prostate is replete with metabolic pathways, such as prostaglandin synthetic pathways, that generate abundant oxygen free radicals. Diets rich in saturated fats have been shown to increase oxidative stress and to produce potentially mutagenic DNA adducts in the kidneys and livers of laboratory animals *(42,43)*. Malins et al. have reported progressive alterations in DNA structure between normal, BPH, and cancerous prostatic tissues, which are the probable result of oxidative damage to the DNA template by the hydroxyl free radical *(45)*. Intriguingly, Ripple et al. have found that treatment of the prostate cancer cell line LNCaP with androgen resulted in a burst of an oxidative stress with a generation of reactive oxygen species, increased lipid peroxidation depletion of intracellular glutathione stores, and activation of transcription factors such as AP-1 and NF-κB *(52,53)*. As a whole, these data suggest that prostate cancer may occur as the result of significant oxidative stress in the face of compromised oxidant defenses. If this hypothesis is true, prostate cancer prevention may be accomplished through reduction of oxidative stress in the prostate or through strengthening the innate defenses of the prostate against oxidative damage.

6. PREVENTING PROSTATE CANCER THROUGH ATTENUATION OF OXIDATIVE DAMAGE

Since our initial report—which suggested that compromised prostate cell defenses against carcinogens, resulting from somatic inactivation of *GSTP1*, may play a critical role in the pathogenesis of prostate cancer—a number of additional observations have underscored the importance of oxidative damage in prostatic carcinogenesis. Several recent reports have identified dietary-derived antioxidants as protective agents against prostate cancer. The most striking of these, conducted by Giovannucci et al., revealed that men in the Health Professionals Follow-up Study (HPFS) who consumed large quantities of tomatoes had a substantially reduced risk (*RR* = 0.65, with a 95% confidence interval of 0.44–0.95 for a consumption frequency of greater than 10 vs less than 1.5 servings per wk) of developing prostate cancer, leading to the hypothesis that the antioxidant lycopene, present in tomatoes, might be responsible for this protective effect *(21)*. A recent pooled analysis of a number of epidemiologic studies confirmed the possible protective effect of lycopene for prostate cancer *(20)*. The ATBC intervention trial was designed to evaluate the possible protective roles of vitamin E, beta-carotene, or a combination of the two in Finnish smokers at high risk for the development of lung cancer. The beta-carotene arms of the study were closed prematurely because of the disappointing finding of increased risk of lung cancer in both beta-carotene treated groups compared to placebo *(60)*. Although no reduction in lung-cancer risk was observed for the groups treated with vitamin E, a possible benefit of vitamin E treatment in reducing prostate cancer risk was also detected. After a mean of 5 yr of follow-up, a 30% decrease in prostate cancer diagnosis and a 40% decrease in prostate cancer deaths were noted in the groups of men on vitamin E *(28)*. Although this finding may be relevant only to men who smoke, it again highlights the point that a free-radical-quenching agent—in this case, vitamin E—can reduce the risk of prostate cancer.

Selenium has recently gained considerable attention as a potential prostate cancer preventive agent. In 1996, Clark et al. reported a placebo-controlled trial directed at preventing skin cancer in high-risk individuals *(13)*. After 8 yr of follow-up of 1312 men and women, no differences were noted in the rates of skin cancer of any type. However, overall death rates from cancer were reduced by 50% in the group on 200 µg of selenized yeast compared to controls. Furthermore, prostate cancer diagnoses were decreased by two-thirds in the treated group. While the prostate cancer findings of the study have been criticized because the development of prostate cancer was a secondary endpoint of the study, the results have fueled great interest in selenium as a prostate cancer preventive agent. Since this report, a case-control study of men from the HPFS has substantiated the importance of selenium in prostate cancer development. Individuals in the lowest quintile of selenium measured in toenail clippings (a reflection of the total body selenium pool) had a twofold higher risk for the development of prostate cancer *(71)*. We have recently analyzed serum selenium values in a nested case-control study of men enrolled in the Baltimore Longitudinal Study of Aging. Our findings replicate those of the HPFS in that men with very low serum selenium levels manifested the highest risk for prostate cancer *(6)*. Intriguingly, in both studies, there appeared to be a threshold effect—that once a certain level of selenium was attained, no further reduction in risk occurred.

Selenium, an essential trace element, is incorporated into a small number of proteins in the form of selenocysteine. Selenoproteins include glutathione peroxidase, an enzyme which plays a critical role in defending against oxidative damage and is particularly effective at reducing lipid peroxides. In the past, GSTs have been suspected to function as "selenium-independent" glutathione peroxidases. It is tempting to speculate that selenium may attenuate prostatic carcinogenesis by compensating for the somatic inactivation of GSTP1 through increasing total glutathione peroxidase activity in prostatic cells.

A number of other compounds have been proposed as candidates for prostate cancer preventative agents. Soy products—particularly the isoflavone genistein—are regarded by many researchers as having prostate cancer protective effects *(18,33)*. Epigallocatechin gallate (EGCG), found in Asian green tea, has received considerable attention as a potential prostate cancer preventive *(24,44)*. The potential prostate cancer prevention activities of both agents are supported principally by the epidemiological observations that both are abundant in the diet among Asian populations, where prostate cancer incidence and mortality rates are relatively low. Both agents are known to be potent antioxidants, and thus remain intriguing candidates for prostate cancer prevention.

7. PROSTATE CANCER PREVENTION: A NEW PARADIGM

Both molecular genetic and epidimeologic evidence suggest that prostate cancer may arise from significant oxidative stress in the face of crippled defenses. Indeed, micronutrients thus far demonstrating promise as prostate cancer prevention agents all appear to share the capacity to quench free-radical damage. We speculate that modulation of the oxidative environment of the prostate may offer the best avenue for new, effective prostate cancer prevention strategies.

Our finding of universal somatic *GSTP1* inactivation in human prostate cancer suggests another mechanism-based prostate cancer prevention strategy. Since human prostate cancer cells and PIN cells appear to have a selective deficit in expression of the Phase 2 enzyme GSTP1, a rational prevention maneuver may be to compensate for GSTP1 loss by global induction of the broad array of Phase 2 enzymes, including other GSTs, within the prostate. A large body of evidence dating back to the 1950s suggests that induction of enzymes of carcinogen metabolism (Phase 2 enzymes), and in particular GSTs, may be an effective means of preventing neoplastic transformation or attenuating tumor promotion *(36,66,67,73)*. Indeed, several putative cancer preventive dietary micronutrients have been identified by their ability to induce Phase 2 enzyme activity *(59)*. Biomodulation of Phase 2 enzymes through orally administered agents has been documented to prevent carcinomas in a number of animal model systems. Clinical trials utilizing such Phase 2 enzyme inducing chemopreventive agents are currently in progress for several tumor types *(34,48,66)*. Since human prostate cancer is characterized by a defect in carcinogen defenses, therapeutic augmentation of Phase 2 enzymes through dietary means may act to prevent the development of prostate cancer or to attenuate prostate cancer progression.

We are currently developing therapeutic, global Phase 2 enzyme induction as a potential prostate cancer prevention strategy. In preliminary studies, we have screened a number of candidate carcinogen detoxification enzyme-inducer compounds for their ability to increase expression of Phase 2 enzymes in vitro *(9)*. Several candidate prostate cancer preventive agents have been identified in this screen. We are currently evaluating change in expression of a battery of Phase 2 enzymes with the intent of identifying a candidate gene or genes that could serve as a biomarkers of response in clinical trials. Induction of Phase 2 enzymes in the prostate depends on a number of factors, which cannot be evaluated in vitro, such as absorption of the compound from the gut, first-pass metabolism in the liver, penetration into prostatic tissues, and metabolism to active compounds within the prostate. Species differences in pharmacokinetics and susceptibility to prostate cancer make it difficult or impossible to assess putative Phase 2 inducing agents in a preclinical setting *(17,50,57,64)*. Identification of molecular biomarkers will allow assessment of efficacy in short-term strategic clinical trials. Dietary-derived candidate inducer compounds could be given in the window prior to radical prostatectomy. Thus, in short-term small clinical trials, effective inducer agents could be identified which may be suitable for larger clinical trials.

8. PROSTATE CANCER PREVENTION IN THE TWENTY-FIRST CENTURY

Over the next few years, our understanding of prostate cancer will be improved with the fostering of dedicated research efforts in areas such as molecular pathology, molecular genetics, genetic epidemiology, and genetic toxicology. Undoubtedly, research in these fields will provide fascinating new leads for prostate cancer prevention based on a more complete understanding of the mechanisms by which prostate cancer develops and evolves. New research technologies will play a critical role in all aspects of prostate cancer prevention research. Progressively, the mechanistic pathways by which candidate preventive agents act will be elucidated by the application of new technologies such as cDNA gene expression arrays and proteomics *(10,32)*. These new technologies will also provide new molecular biomarkers for cancer risk and for treatment effects *(7)*. New genomics technologies offer the potential for identification of men at high risk for prostate cancer development or at high risk for the development of other life-threatening diseases, and will allow for tailoring of specific preventive interventions to the appropriate specific diseases. Ultimately, the promise of prostate cancer prevention will be to offer hope that future generations of men will be free of any threat of morbidity or mortality from prostate cancer.

REFERENCES

1. Andriole, G. L., H. A. Guess, J. I. Epstein, H. Wise, D. Kadmon, E. Crawford, et al. 1998. Treatment with finasteride preserves usefulness of prostate specific antigen in the detection of prostate cancer: results of a randomized, double-blind, placebo-controlled clinical trial. PLESS Study Group. Proscar Long-Term Efficacy and Safety Study. *Urology* **52:** 195–201; 201–202 (discussion).

2. Anwar, W. A., S. Z. Abdel-Rahman, R. A. El-Zein, H. M. Mostafa, and W. W Au. 1996. Genetic polymorphism of GSTM1, CYP2E1 and CYP2D6 in Egyptian bladder cancer patients. *Carcinogenesis* **17:** 1923–1929.

3. Aquilina, J. W., J. J. Lipsky, and D. G. Bostwick. 1997. Androgen deprivation as a strategy for prostate cancer chemoprevention. *J. Natl. Cancer Inst.* **89:** 689–696.

4. Brockmoller, J., R. Kerb, N. Drakoulis, B. Staffeldt, and I. Roots. 1994. Glutathione S-transferase M1 and its variants A and B as host factors of bladder cancer susceptibility: a case-control study. *Cancer Res.* **54:** 4103–4111.

5. Brooks, J. D., W.-H. Lee, and W. G. Nelson. 1996a. Epidemiological and molecular features of prostatic carcinogenesis as clues for new prostate cancer prevention strategies. *Canadian J. Urol.* **(Suppl) 3:** 20–26.

6. Brooks, J. D., E. J. Metter, D. W. Chan, L. J. Sokoll, P. Landis, W. G. Nelson, et al. 1999. Prediagnostic serum selenium levels and the risk of prostate cancer development *J. Urol.* **261 (Suppl):** 69A (Abstract).

7. Brooks, J. D., and V. Paton. 1999. Potent Induction of Carcinogen Defense Enzymes with Sulforaphane, a Putative Prostate Cancer Chemopreventive Agent. *Prostate Cancer and Prostatic Diseases* **2 (3 Suppl):** 58.

8. Brooks, J. D., M. Weinstein, X. Lin, Y. Sun, S. S. Pin, G. S. Bova, et al. 1998. CG island methylation changes near the GSTP1 gene in prostatic intraepithelial neoplasia. *Cancer Epidemiol. Biomark. Prev.* **7:** 531–536.

9. Brooks, J. D., D. Wu, and W. G. Nelson. 1996b. Identification of prostate cancer chemopreventative agents through induction of phase II enzymes. *J. Urol.* **155:** 529A.

10. Brown, P. O. and D. Botstein. 1999. Exploring the new world of the genome with DNA microarrays. *Nat. Genet.* **21(1 Suppl):** 33–37.

11. Carter, B. S., T. H. Beaty, G. D. Steinberg, B. Childs, and P. C. Walsh. 1992. Mendelian inheritance of familial prostate cancer. *Proc. Natl. Acad. Sci. USA* **89:** 3367–3371.

12. Carter, B. S., H. B. Carter, and J. T. Isaacs. 1990. Epidemiologic evidence regarding predisposing factors to prostate cancer. *Prostate* **16:** 187–197.

13. Clark, L. C., G. F. Combs, Jr., B. W. Turnbull, E. H. Slate, D. K. Chalker, J. Chow, et al. 1996. Effects of selenium supplementation for cancer prevention in patients with carcinoma of the skin. A randomized controlled trial. Nutritional Prevention of Cancer Study Group. *JAMA* **276:** 1957–1963.

14. Collins, F. S. 1999. Shattuck lecture—medical and societal consequences of the Human Genome Project. *N. Engl. J. Med.* **341:** 28–37.

15. Cote, R. J., E. C. Skinner, C. E. Salem, S. J. Mertes, F. Z. Stanczyk, B. E. Henderson, et al. 1998. The effect of finasteride on the prostate gland in men with elevated serum prostate-specific antigen levels. *Br. J. Cancer* **78:** 413–418.

16. Danley, K. L., J. L. Richardson, L. Bernstein, B. Langholz, and R. K. Ross. 1995. Prostate cancer: trends in mortality and stage-specific incidence rates by racial/ethnic group in Los Angeles County, California (United States). *Cancer Causes Control* **6:** 492–498.

17. De Long, M. J., H. J. Prochaska, and P. Talalay. 1985. Tissue-specific induction patterns of cancer-protective enzymes in mice by tert-butyl-4-hydroxyanisole and related substituted phenols. *Cancer Res.* **45:** 546–551.

18. Fair, W. R., N. E. Fleshner, and W. Heston. 1997. Cancer of the prostate: a nutritional disease? *Urology* **50:** 840–848.

19. Fisher, B., J. P. Costantino, D. L. Wickerham, C. K. Redmond, M. Kavanah, W. M. Cronin, et al. 1998. Tamoxifen for prevention of breast cancer: report of the National Surgical Adjuvant Breast and Bowel Project P-1 Study. *J. Natl. Cancer Inst.* **90:** 1371–1388.

20. Giovannucci, E. 1999. Tomatoes, tomato-based products, lycopene, and cancer: review of the epidemiologic literature. *J. Natl. Cancer Inst.* **91:** 317–331.

21. Giovannucci, E., A. Ascherio, E. B. Rimm, M. J. Stampfer, G. A. Colditz, and W. C. Willett. 1995. Intake of carotenoids and retinol in relation to risk of prostate cancer. *J. Natl. Cancer Inst.* **87:** 1767–1776.

22. Giovannucci, E., E. B. Rimm, G. A. Colditz, M. J. Stampfer, A. Ascherio, C. C. Chute, et al. 1993. A prospective study of dietary fat and risk of prostate cancer. *J. Natl. Cancer Inst.* **85:** 1571–1579.

23. Giovannucci, E., M. J. Stampfer, K. Krithivas, M. Brown, A. Brufsky, J. Talcott, et al. 1997. The CAG repeat within the androgen receptor gene and its relationship to prostate cancer. *Proc. Natl. Acad. Sci. USA* **94:** 3320–3323.

24. Gupta, S., N. Ahmad, R. R. Mohan, M. M. Husain, and H. Mukhtar. 1999. Prostate cancer chemoprevention by green tea: in vitro and in vivo inhibition of testosterone-mediated induction of ornithine decarboxylase. *Cancer Res.* **59:** 2115–2120.

25. Haenzel, W. and M. Kurihara. 1968. Studies of Japanese migrants. I. Mortality from cancer and other diseases among Japanese men in the United States. *J. Natl. Cancer Inst.* **40:** 43–68.

26. Harries, L. W., M. J. Stubbins, D. Forman, G. C. Howard, and C. R. Wolf. 1997. Identification of genetic polymorphisms at the glutathione S- transferase Pi locus and association with susceptibility to bladder, testicular and prostate cancer. *Carcinogenesis* **18:** 641–644.

27. Hayes, J. D. and D. J. Pulford. 1995. The glutathione S-transferase supergene family: regulation of GST and the contribution of the isoenzymes to cancer chemoprotection and drug resistance. *Crit. Rev. Biochem. Mol. Biol.* **30:** 445–600.

28. Heinonen, O. P., D. Albanes, J. Virtamo, P. R. Taylor, J. K. Huttunen, A. M. Hartman, et al. 1998. Prostate cancer and supplementation with alpha-tocopherol and beta-carotene: incidence and mortality in a controlled trial. *J. Natl. Cancer Inst.* **90:** 440–446.

29. Helzlsouer, K. J., O. Selmin, H. Y. Huang, P. T. Strickland, S. Hoffman, A. J. Alberg, et al. 1998. Association between glutathione S-transferase M1, P1, and T1 genetic polymorphisms and development of breast cancer. *J. Natl. Cancer Inst.* **90:** 512–518.

30. Henderson, C. J., A. G. Smith, J. Ure, K. Brown, E. J. Bacon, and C. R. Wolf. 1998. Increased skin tumorigenesis in mice lacking pi class glutathione S- transferases. *Proc. Natl. Acad. Sci. USA* **95:** 5275–5280.

31. Homma, Y., M. Kaneko, Y. Kondo, K. Kawabe, and T. Kakizoe. 1997. Inhibition of rat prostate carcinogenesis by a 5alpha-reductase inhibitor, FK143. *J. Natl. Cancer Inst.* **89:** 803–807.

32. Iyer, V. R., M. B. Eisen, D. T. Ross, G. Schuler, T. Moore, J. C. F. Lee, et al. 1999. The transcriptional program in the response of human fibroblasts to serum. *Science* **283:** 83–87.

33. Jacobsen, B. K., S. F. Knutsen, and G. E. Fraser. 1998. Does high soy milk intake reduce prostate cancer incidence? The Adventist Health Study (United States). *Cancer Causes Control* **9:** 553–557.

34. Jacobson, L. P., B. C. Zhang, Y. R. Zhu, J. B. Wang, Y. Wu, Q. N. Zhang, et al. 1997. Oltipraz chemoprevention trial in Qidong, People's Republic of China: study design and clinical outcomes. *Cancer Epidemiol. Biomark. Prev.* **6:** 257–265.

35. Kelsey, K. T., M. R. Spitz, Z. F. Zuo, and J. K. Wiencke. 1997. Polymorphisms in the glutathione S-transferase class mu and theta genes interact and increase susceptibility to lung cancer in minority populations (Texas, United States). *Cancer Causes Control* **8:** 554–559.

36. Kensler, T. W., N. E. Davidson, J. D. Groopman, B. D. Roebuck, H. J. Prochaska, and P. Talalay. 1993. Chemoprotection by inducers of electrophile detoxication enzymes. *Basic Life Sci.* **61:** 127–136.

37. Kihara, M., M. Kihara, A. Kubota, M. Furukawa, and H. Kimura. 1997. GSTM1 gene polymorphism as a possible marker for susceptibility to head and neck cancers among Japanese smokers. *Cancer Lett.* **112:** 257–262.

38. Kolonel, L. N., C. N. Yoshizawa, and J. H. Hankin. 1988. Diet and prostatic cancer: a case-control study in Hawaii. *Am. J. Epidemiol.* **127:** 999–1012.

39. Landis, S. H., T. Murray, S. Bolden, and P. A. Wingo. 1999. Cancer statistics. 1999. *CA Cancer J. Clin.* **49:** 8–31.

40. Lee, W.-H., W. B. Isaacs, G. S. Bova, and W. G. Nelson. 1997. CG island methylation changes near the GSTP1 gene in prostatic carcinoma cells detected using the polymerase chain reaction: a new prostatic biomarker. *Cancer Epidemiol. Biomark. Prev.* **6:** 443–450.

41. Lee, W. H., R. A. Morton, J. I. Epstein, J. D. Brooks, P. A. Campbell, G. S. Bova, et al. 1994. Cytidine methylation of regulatory sequences near the pi-class glutathione S-transferase gene accompanies human prostatic carcinogenesis. *Proc. Natl. Acad. Sci. USA* **91:** 11,733–11,737.

42. Li, D. and K. Randerath. 1992. Modulation of DNA modification (I-compound) levels in rat liver and kidney by dietary carbohydrate, protein, fat, vitamin, and mineral content. *Mutat. Res.* **275:** 47–56.

43. Li, D. H. and K. Randerath. 1990. Association between diet and age-related DNA modifications (I- compounds) in rat liver and kidney. *Cancer Res.* **50:** 3991–3996.

44. Liao, S., Y. Umekita, J. Guo, J. M. Kokontis, and R. A. Hiipakka. 1995. Growth inhibition and regression of human prostate and breast tumors in athymic mice by tea epigallocatechin gallate. *Cancer Lett.* **96:** 239–243.

45. Malins, D. C., N. L. Polissar, and S. J. Gunselman. 1997. Models of DNA structure achieve almost perfect discrimination between normal prostate, benign prostatic hyperplasia (BPH), and adenocarcinoma and have a high potential for predicting BPH and prostate cancer. *Proc. Natl. Acad. Sci. USA* **94:** 259–264.

46. Nayfield, S. G., J. E. Karp, L. G. Ford, F. A. Dorr, and B. S. Kramer. 1991. Potential role of tamoxifen in prevention of breast cancer. *J. Natl. Cancer Inst.* **83:** 1450–1459.

47. Nomura, A. M., G. N. Stemmermann, P. H. Chyou, B. E. Henderson, and F. Z. Stanczyk. 1996. Serum androgens and prostate cancer. *Cancer Epidemiol. Biomark. Prev.* **5:** 621–625.

48. O'Dwyer, P. J., C. E. Szarka, K. S. Yao, T. C. Halbherr, G. R. Pfeiffer, F. Green, et al. 1996. Modulation of gene expression in subjects at risk for colorectal cancer by the chemopreventive dithiolethione oltipraz. *J. Clin. Invest.* **98:** 1210–1217.

49. Powell, I. J. 1997. Prostate cancer and African-American men. *Oncology* **11:** 599–605.

50. Raza, H. and H. Mukhtar. 1993. Differences in inducibility of cytochrome P-4501A1, monooxygenases and glutathione S-transferase in cutaneous and extracutaneous tissues after topical and parenteral administration of beta-naphthoflavone to rats. *Int. J. Biochem.* **25:** 1511–1516.

51. Rebbeck, T. R., A. H. Walker, J. M. Jaffe, D. L. White, A. J. Wein, and S. B. Malkowicz. 1999. Glutathione S-transferase-mu (GSTM1) and -theta (GSTT1) genotypes in the etiology of prostate cancer. *Cancer Epidemiol. Biomark. Prev.* **8:** 283–287.

52. Ripple, M. O., W. F. Henry, R. P. Rago, and G. Wilding. 1997. Prooxidant-antioxidant shift induced by androgen treatment of human prostate carcinoma cells. *J. Natl. Cancer Inst.* **89:** 40–48.

53. Ripple, M. O., W. F. Henry, S. R. Schwarze, G. Wilding, and R. Weindruch. 1999. Effect of antioxidants on androgen-induced AP-1 and NF-kappaB DNA- binding activity in prostate carcinoma cells. *J. Natl. Cancer Inst.* **91:** 1227–1232.

54. Ross, R. K., H. Shimizu, A. Paganini-Hill, G. Honda, and B. E. Henderson. 1987. Case-control studies of prostate cancer in blacks and whites in southern California. *J. Natl. Cancer Inst.* **78:** 869–874.

55. Ryberg, D., V. Skaug, A. Hewer, D. H. Phillips, L. W. Harries, C. R. Wolf, et al. 1997. Genotypes of glutathione transferase M1 and P1 and their significance for lung DNA adduct levels and cancer risk. *Carcinogenesis* **18:** 1285–1289.

56. Shimizu, H., R. K. Ross, L. Bernstein, R. Yatani, B. E. Henderson, and M. Mack. 1991. Cancers of the prostate and breast among Japanese and white immigrants in Los Angeles County. *Br. J. Cancer* **63:** 963–966.

57. Sisk, S. C. and W. R. Pearson. 1993. Differences in induction by xenobiotics in murine tissues and the Hepa1c1c7 cell line of mRNAs encoding glutathione transferase, quinone reductase, and CYP1A P450s. *Pharmacogenetics* **3:** 167–181.

58. Smith, J. R., D. Freije, J. D. Carpten, H. Gronberg, J. Xu, S. D. Isaacs, et al. 1996. Major susceptibility locus for prostate cancer on chromosome 1 suggested by a genome-wide search. *Science* **274:** 1371–1374.

59. Talalay, P., J. W. Fahey, W. D. Holtzclaw, T. Prestera, and Y. Zhang. 1995. Chemo-protection against cancer by phase 2 enzyme induction. *Toxicol. Lett.* **82:** 173–179.

60. The Alpha-Tocopherol, Beta Carotene Cancer Prevention Study Group. 1994. The effect of vitamin E and beta carotene on the incidence of lung cancer and other cancers in male smokers. *N. Engl. J. Med.* **330:** 1029–1035.

61. Thompson, I. M., C. A. Coltman, Jr., and J. Crowley. 1997. Chemoprevention of prostate cancer: the Prostate Cancer Prevention Trial. *Prostate* **33:** 217–221.

62. Tsuchida, S. and K. Sato. 1992. Glutathione transferases and cancer. *Crit. Rev. Biochem. Mol. Biol.* **27:** 337–384.

63. Tsukamoto, S., H. Akaza, M. Onozawa, T. Shirai, and Y. Ideyama. 1998. A five-alpha reductase inhibitor or an antiandrogen prevents the progression of microscopic prostate carcinoma to macroscopic carcinoma in rats. *Cancer* **82:** 531–537.

64. van Lieshout, E. M., D. M. Tiemessen, W. H. Peters, and J. B. Jansen. 1997. Effects of nonsteroidal anti-inflammatory drugs on glutathione S- transferases of the rat digestive tract. *Carcinogenesis* **18:** 485–490.

65. Famighetti, R., ed. 1998. Vital Statistics, in *The World Almanac and Book of Facts. 1999.* Primedia Reference Inc., Mahwah, NJ.

66. Wang, J. S., X. Shen, X. He, Y. R. Zhu, B. C. Zhang, J. B. Wang, et al. 1999. Protective alterations in phase 1 and 2 metabolism of aflatoxin B1 by oltipraz in residents of Qidong, People's Republic of China. *J. Natl. Cancer Inst.* **91:** 347–354.

67. Wattenberg, L. W. 1992. Inhibition of carcinogenesis by minor dietary constituents. *Cancer Res.* **52(7 Suppl.):** 2085S–2091S.

68. West, D. W., M. L. Slattery, L. M. Robison, T. K. French, and A. W. Mahoney. 1991. Adult dietary intake and prostate cancer risk in Utah: a case-control study with special emphasis on aggressive tumors. *Cancer Causes Control* **2:** 85–94.

69. Whittemore, A. S., L. N. Kolonel, A. H. Wu, E. M. John, R. P. Gallagher, G. R. Howe, et al. 1995. Prostate cancer in relation to diet, physical activity, and body size in blacks, whites, and Asians in the United States and Canada. *J. Natl. Cancer Inst.* **87:** 652–661.

70. Xu, J., D. Meyers, D. Freije, A. Isaacs, K. Wiley, D. Nusskern, et al. 1998. Evidence for a prostate cancer susceptibility locus on the X chromosome. *Nat. Genet.* **20:** 175–179.

71. Yoshizawa, K., W. C. Willett, S. J. Morris, M. J. Stampfer, D. Spiegelman, E B. Rimm, et al. 1998. Study of prediagnostic selenium level in toenails and the risk of advanced prostate cancer. *J. Natl. Cancer Inst.* **90:** 1219–1224.

72. Yu, H., R. E. Harris, Y. T. Gao, R. Gao, and E. L. Wynder. 1991. Comparative epidemiology of cancers of the colon, rectum, prostate and breast in Shanghai, China versus the United States. *Int. J. Epidemiol.* **20:** 76–81.

73. Zhang, Y., T. W. Kensler, C. G. Cho, G. H. Posner, and P. Talalay. 1994. Anticarcinogenic activities of sulforaphane and structurally related synthetic norbornyl isothiocyanates. *Proc. Natl. Acad. Sci. USA* **91:** 3147–3150.

22

Anatomic Radical Retropubic Prostatectomy for Prostate Cancer

Misop Han, MD and Alan W. Partin, MD, PhD

1. INTRODUCTION

In 1905, Hugh Hampton Young first described radical surgery for the treatment of prostate cancer in his report on radical perineal prostatectomy (RPP) *(11)*. In 1947, Millin described the radical retropubic prostatectomy (RRP), but complications such as bleeding, incontinence, and impotence prevented widespread early use of this operation. During the past two decades, many discoveries have been made, which have permitted surgeons to perform an anatomical dissection and reduce perioperative morbidity. Understanding of the anatomy of the dorsal vein complex has allowed precise dissection of the prostate in a relatively bloodless field *(8)*. Also, the identification of the anatomy of the pelvic nerve plexus and an improved understanding of the striated urethral sphincter have allowed better preservation of sexual function and urinary continence, respectively, in many men *(10)*. The goals of radical prostatectomy are cancer control, preservation of urinary control, and preservation of sexual function. In this chapter, we review the long-term results of radical retropubic prostatectomy on cancer control—the most important goal of this operation—based on extensive studies reported from centers within the United States.

2. CANCER CONTROL

A number of select academic centers in the United States have published their extended experiences in radical prostatectomy on cancer control: the Baylor College of Medicine, the Johns Hopkins Medical Institutions, the Mayo Clinic, UCLA (University of California, Los Angeles), and Washington University.

Follow-up among these centers was composed of routine serum prostate specific antigen (PSA) assays, digital rectal examinations, and radiological studies, when indicated. Disease recurrence was defined in three steps. First, a postoperative detectable serum PSA level was defined as a biochemical recurrence. Secondly, palpable induration at the operative site, with or without a positive biopsy and no radiographic evidence of distant disease, was defined as a local recurrence. And finally, a positive bone scan or other radiographic evidence of retroperitoneal adenopathy was defined as a distal recurrence. A few patients from the Washington University series were found with local or distant recurrence without biochemical evidence of recurrence *(1,2)*.

From: *Prostate Cancer: Biology, Genetics, and the New Therapeutics*
Edited by: L. W. K. Chung, W. B. Isaacs, and J. W. Simons © Humana Press Inc., Totowa, NJ

3. OVERALL PROGRESSION AND SURVIVAL

Mean ages of patients from different studies ranged from 59–65 yr. All studies had a mean follow-up of more than 28 mo, while a longer follow-up of more than 60 mo was reported by the Johns Hopkins and the Mayo Clinic series. The distribution of clinical stage T1 vs T2 patients was similar in all studies, except in the Mayo Clinic series, which was more heavily weighted to T2 patients. Also, there was a shift toward more patients presenting with T1 disease in more recent series from Johns Hopkins and Washington University (2,7). This shift can be explained by an increasing proportion of patients presenting with T1c stage resulting from a wide use of PSA screening testing and a subsequent early diagnosis of prostate cancer. Table 1 summarizes the patient demographics from various institutional series.

There were different patient exclusion criteria based on neoadjuvant/adjuvant hormonal/ radiation therapy from these series. For example, the patients who received post-operative adjuvant therapy prior to demonstration of cancer recurrence were excluded from the Johns Hopkins series (6), while the patients who received preoperative radio-therapy or adjuvant hormonal therapy were excluded from the Baylor College series (4). Patients who received neoadjuvant radiation or hormonal therapy were excluded from the UCLA study (9), while postoperative adjuvant radiation and/or hormonal therapy was used in 26% of patients in the Mayo Clinic series (12).

The patterns of tumor recurrence steps after RRP from three centers are summarized in Table 2. Overall recurrence rate after RRP ranged from 12–20%. Biochemical recurrence usually comprised the largest share of overall recurrence. Table 3 compares actuarial PSA progression-free survival, actuarial cause-specific survival, and actuarial metastasis-free survival rates from the different series. There were variations in PSA progression-free survival between institutions. For example, the 10-yr PSA progression-free survival rate from the Johns Hopkins, Washington University, and Baylor College series was higher than 65%, but the rate from the UCLA and Mayo Clinic series was lower than 52%. The ten-yr-actuarial cause-specific survival rate was higher than 90% in all three institutions that reported this data. When patients were grouped according to their tumor grade and stage, there was a significant decrease in the actuarial cause-specific survival with advancing histologic grade and pathologic stage (6,12). A metastasis-free survival rate was available only from the Johns Hopkins and the Mayo Clinic series (7,12). When compared with conservative therapy, the actuarial rate of development of metastasis for men after RRP was considerably lower (6,7).

4. CLINICAL STAGE AND PROGRESSION

Table 4 summarizes the actuarial recurrence-free rate based on clinical tumor stage after radical prostatectomy from the Johns Hopkins, Washington University, and Mayo Clinic series. As expected, clinical stage of the tumor was significantly associated with cancer recurrence. Palpable tumors in advanced clinical stages were more likely to recur following surgery from all series.

5. PREOPERATIVE PSA AND PROGRESSION

In the Johns Hopkins series, patients were placed into four groups based on pre-operative PSA levels. The Kaplan-Meier survival analysis was performed based on

Table 1
Demographics of Patients[a]

Institution	Primary author	Number of patients	Years of RRP	Mean age (y) (range)	Months, follow-up, mean (range)	% T1	% T2
Johns Hopkins	Pound (6)	1623	1982–1995	59 ± (34–76)	60.4 (12–156)	31	66
Johns Hopkins	Pound (7)	1997	1982–1997	59 ± 6	64 (6–180)	38	60
Washington University	Catalona (1)	925	1983–1993	63 ± 7 (41–79)	28 (0–123)	21	79
Washington University	Catalona (2)	1778[a]	1983–1997	63 ± 7 (38–79)	48	38	60
Baylor College	Ohori (4)	500	1983–1993	63 (43–79)	36 (1–114)	22	78
UCLA	Trapasso (9)	601	1972–1992	64 (44–80)	34[b] (12–237)	27	73
The Mayo Clinic	Zincke (12)	3170[c]	1966–1991	65 ± 4 (31–81)	60	7	93

[a] 4% of patients received postoperative adjuvant radiation therapy.
[b] Median.
[c] 26% of patients received postoperative adjuvant radiation and/or hormonal therapy.
[d] Modified from ref. 6.

379

Table 2
Recurrence Pattern After RRP[c]

Institution (ref.)	Overall (%)	Biochemical (%)	Local (%)	Distant (%)
Johns Hopkins (6)	17	7.9	2.5	5.4
Johns Hopkins (7)	15	N/A[b]	N/A[b]	5.2
Washington University (1)	12	8.4	3.2[a]	[a]
Washington University (2)	19	14.6	4.4[a]	[a]
UCLA (9)	20	8	7.2	5.3

[a] Local and distant metastasis.
[b] N/A : Not available.
[c] Modified from ref. 6.

Table 3
Progression[c]

Institution (ref.)	Actuarial PSA progression-free survival		Actuarial cause-specific survival			Actuarial metastasis-free survival	
	5-yr	10-yr	5-yr	10-yr	15-yr	10-yr	15-yr
Johns Hopkins (6,7)	80	68	99	94	91	87	82
Washington University (1,2)	78	65	97[a]	N/A[b]	N/A[b]	N/A[b]	N/A[b]
Baylor College (4)	76	73	N/A[b]	N/A[b]	N/A[b]	N/A[b]	N/A[b]
UCLA (9)	69	47	98	94	N/A[b]	N/A[b]	N/A[b]
The Mayo Clinic (12)	70	52	N/A[b]	90	82	82	76

[a] At 7 yr.
[b] N/A : not available.
[c] Modified from ref. 6.

these levels, and found that there was a statistically significant difference between progression-free probability of men in all PSA groups (6). In the Washington University series, patients were categorized into three groups based on preoperative PSA levels. Survival analysis showed that a higher preoperative PSA level (greater than 10 ng/mL) was also significantly associated with cancer recurrence (2). The summary of results is shown in Table 5.

6. PREOPERATIVE GLEASON SCORE AND PROGRESSION

The actuarial recurrence-free rate was significantly associated with preoperative Gleason score of patients. The Johns Hopkins and Baylor group showed a statistically significant difference in progression-free rate between men with Gleason score 6, 7, and 8–10 (4,6). When patients were divided into three groups by tumor grade, the Washington University group also observed statistically significant differences in survival function (1). The results are summarized in Table 6.

Table 4
Clinical Stage and Progression

Variable	Actuarial Recurrence-Free Rate (95% CI)					
Time	5-yr	5-yr	7-yr	10-yr	10-yr	15-yr
Institution	Johns Hopkins (6)	Washington U. (1)	Washington U. (2)	Johns Hopkins (6)	Mayo Clinic (12)	Mayo Clinic (12)
TNM						
T1a	100	90 (84–97)	79 (73–86)	100	70	62
T1b	89 (81–94)			89 (81–94)		
T1c	86 (75–93)	97 (93–100)		86 (75–93)		
T2a	85 (81–88)	74 (69–79)	66 (62–69)	68 (61–75)	56	43
T2b	69 (63–75)	N/A[c]		57 (48–65)	47	37
T2c	63 (51–73)	N/A[c]		53 (38–66)		
T3a	61 (42–75)		44 (22–67)[a]	52 (28–71)[b]	N/A[c]	N/A[c]

[a] All T3.
[b] 8-yr data.
[c] N/A : not available.

Table 5
Preoperative PSA and Progression

	Actuarial Recurrence Free-Rate (95% CI)			
Time	5-yr	5-yr	7-yr	10-yr
Institution	Johns Hopkins *(6)*	Washington U. *(1)*	Washington U. *(2)*	Johns Hopkins *(6)*
Serum PSA (ng/mL)				
0–4	94 (91–96)	95 (90–100)	*a*	87 (74–94)
4.1–10	82 (76–86)	93 (89–97)	76 (71–83)	75 (67–81)
10.1–20	72 (63–79) ⎤	71 (62–80) ⎤	49 (42–56)	30 (3–62)
>20	54 (39–66) ⎦	⎦		28 (9–51)

[a]93% for PSA <2.6 (86–99), 88% for PSA >2.6, <4.1(79–97).

7. PATHOLOGIC STAGE, GLEASON SCORE, AND SURGICAL MARGINS IN RELATION TO PROGRESSION

In the Johns Hopkins series, optimal stratification of actuarial progression-free probability was obtained by grouping patients based on a combination of pathologic stage, Gleason score, and surgical margin status *(3)*. For example, the 10-yr recurrence-free rate for patients with capsular penetration with Gleason grade 2–6 disease was 89% for patients with a positive surgical margin and 72% for patients with a negative margin. Patients with capsular penetration, Gleason grade 2–6 disease, and the absence of positive surgical margin had a recurrence rate similar to that of men with organ-confined disease. In patients with capsular penetration with Gleason 7 or higher disease, the presence of a positive surgical margin had a significant effect on actuarial progression-free rates, and the progression-free rates in these patients were similar to the progression-free rates of patients with the seminal vesicle invasion *(6)* (*see* Fig. 1).

The Washington University group reported that pathological tumor stage was significantly associated with cancer recurrence. The 5-yr and 7-yr recurrence rates for patients with seminal vesicle invasion and lymph node metastasis were higher compared to recurrence rate for patients with organ-confined disease *(1,2)*.

In the Baylor College of Medicine series, men who had tumors with positive surgical margins had a higher progression rate than patients whose tumors had negative surgical margins among the entire patient population. For example, the 5-yr progression-free rates for patients with tumors with and without positive surgical margins were 64% and 83%, respectively. The Baylor series also showed that the progression rate was strongly associated with tumor grade if the tumor extended outside of the prostate *(5)*.

In the UCLA series, the 5-yr biochemical recurrence-free rate was significantly different in individual pathological groups as well. When the patients who received RRP after 1987 were included in the analysis, the 5-yr biochemical recurrence-free rate for individual pathologic groups improved *(9)*. The results of recurrence-free rate according to pathologic stage from the Washington University, Baylor, and UCLA series are summarized in Table 7.

Table 6
Preoperative Gleason Score and Progression

	Actuarial Recurrence-Free Rate (95% CI)						
Time Institution Gleason Score	5-yr Johns Hopkins (6)	5-yr Washington U. (1)	5-yr Baylor College (4)	7-yr Washington U. (2)	10-yr Johns Hopkins (6)	10-yr Mayo Clinic (12)	15-yr Mayo Clinic (12)
2–4	100	89 (84–94)	N/A[c]	84 (79–89)	94 (62–99)	[a]	[a]
5	97 (94–99)		N/A[c]		91 (84–95)	53[a]	40[a]
6	92 (88–95)	78 (72–84)	90	68 (64–73)	78 (66–86)	[a]	[a]
7	66 (61–71)		64		46 (34–56)	35	25
8–10	41 (32–50)	51 (36–67)	28[b]	48 (39–57)	23 (13–35)		

[a] For Gleason 4–6.
[b] After 4 yr.
[c] N/A : not available.

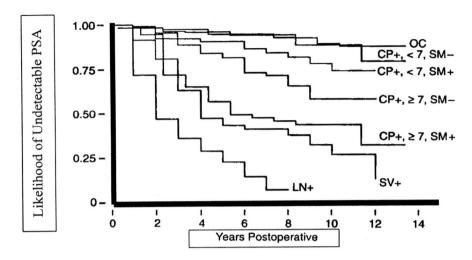

Fig. 1. Kaplan-Meier actuarial likelihood of PSA recurrence by a combination of pathologic stage, Gleason score, and surgical margin status from the Johns Hopkins series *(6)*. OC = organ-confined; CP+, <7, SM– = capsular penetration, Gleason score less than 7, and negative surgical margins; CP+, ≥ 7, SM+ = capsular penetration, Gleason score ≥ 7, and positive surgical margins; SV+ positive seminal vesicle with negative lymph nodes; LN+ = positive lymph nodes. (Reprinted with permission from ref. *6*).

8. TIMING OF PSA RECURRENCE, GLEASON SCORE, AND PATHOLOGIC STAGE AND DEVELOPMENT OF PROGRESSION

In the Johns Hopkins series, Pound et al. concluded that the timing of PSA recurrence, Gleason score greater than 7, and positive seminal vesicle or pelvic lymph nodes were the variables that best distinguished between local vs distant recurrences. For example, patients with PSA recurrence less than 2 yr after RRP or surgical pathology results with seminal vesicle or lymph node involvement were generally more likely to demonstrate distant metastases *(6)*.

In the subsequent series of 1,997 men undergoing radical prostatectomy for clinically localized prostate cancer, Pound et al. reported that 34% of 304 men with biochemical recurrence developed distant metastases with a median follow-up of 5.3 yr. After biochemical recurrence following RRP, the median time to develop distant metastasis was 8 yr, and the 5-yr metastasis-free rate was 63%. The actuarial median time from development of metastasis to death from prostate cancer was approx 5 yr. The only variable that reliably predicted the time to death resulting from prostate cancer was the time interval from surgery to development of metastatic disease. Pound et al. also found that PSA doubling time, in addition to the timing of PSA recurrence and Gleason score, was predictive of the probability and time to the development of metastatic disease *(7)*. This finding is consistent with the UCLA study, which reported a statistically significant difference in the median PSA doubling times from the patients with distal recurrence (4.3 mo) and from those with local or biochemical recurrence (11.7 mo) *(9)*.

9. POTENCY IN RELATION TO PROGRESSION

In the Johns Hopkins series, Pound et al. reported no difference in the actuarial recurrence-free rate between men who were potent and impotent postoperatively when

Table 7
Pathologic Stage and Progression

	Actuarial Recurrence-Free Rate (95% CI)						
Time	5-yr	5-yr	5-yr	5-yr[a]	7-yr	10-yr
Institution	Washington U. (1)	Baylor (4)	UCLA (9)	UCLA (9)	Washington U. (2)	Baylor (4)
Pathologic stage						
Organ-confined	91	94	87	92[a]	81	90
Capsular penetration	74		64	74[a]	[c]	
Involvement of seminal vesicle	32	61[b]	40	56[a]	26	59[b]
Metastasis to pelvic lymph nodes	N/A[d]		N/A	N/A	19	

[a] Only patients who received RRP after 1987.
[b] Nonorgan-confined.
[c] 57% for positive margins, 76% for negative margins.
[d] N/A : not available.

they were grouped by tumor stage. These groups of men had similar age distribution, Gleason score, and pathologic stage. There was no difference in actuarial biochemical recurrence rate between potent and impotent men with capsular penetration and positive surgical margins. Therefore, preservation of potency using anatomic RRP did not adversely influence cancer control *(6)*.

10. CONCLUSION

The studies in this chapter confirm that radical retropubic prostatectomy achieves excellent cancer control in men with clinically localized prostate cancer, although there are some differences in tumor progression after surgery from different institutions. Radical retropubic prostatectomy serves as an attractive treatment option for men with clinically localized prostate cancer who are otherwise healthy and have a life expectancy greater than 15-yr. With a better selection of surgical candidates using PSA screening and the incorporation of the anatomic radical retropubic prostatectomy, prostate cancer is being detected at an earlier stage, and the prognosis for patients with the disease will continue to improve.

REFERENCES

1. Catalona, W. J. and D. S. Smith. 1994. 5-year tumor recurrence rates after anatomical radical retropubic prostatectomy for prostate cancer. *J. Urol.* **152:** 1837–1842.
2. Catalona, W. J. and D. S. Smith. 1998. Cancer recurrence and survival rates after anatomic radical retropubic prostatectomy for prostate cancer: intermediate-term results. *J. Urol.* **160:** 2428–2434.
3. Epstein, J. I., et al. 1996. Prediction of progression following radical prostatectomy. A multivariate analysis of 721 men with long-term follow-up. *Am. J. Surg. Pathol.* **20:** 286–292.
4. Ohori, M. et al. 1994. Can radical prostatectomy alter the progression of poorly differentiated prostate cancer? *J. Urol.* **152:** 1843–1849.
5. Ohori, M., et al. 1995. Prognostic significance of positive surgical margins in radical prostatectomy specimens. *J. Urol.* **154:** 1818–1824.
6. Pound, C. R., et al. 1997. Prostate-specific antigen after anatomic radical retropubic prostatectomy. Patterns of recurrence and cancer control. *Urol. Clin. N. Am.* **24:** 395–406.
7. Pound, C. R., et al. 1999. Natural history of progression after PSA elevation following radical prostatectomy. *JAMA* **281:** 1591–1597.
8. Reiner, W. G. and P. C. Walsh. 1979. An anatomical approach to the surgical management of the dorsal vein and Santorini's plexus during radical retropubic surgery. *J. Urol.* **121:** 198–200.
9. Trapasso, J. G., et al. 1994. The incidence and significance of detectable levels of serum prostate specific antigen after radical prostatectomy. *J. Urol.* **152:** 1821–1825.
10. Walsh, P. C. and P. J. Donker. 1982. Impotence following radical prostatectomy: insight into etiology and prevention. *J. Urol.* **128:** 492–497.
11. Young, H. H. 1905. The early diagnosis and radical cure of carcinoma of the prostate. *Johns Hopkins Hop. Bull.* **16:** 315–321.
12. Zincke, H., et al. 1994. Long-term (15 years) results after radical prostatectomy for clinically localized (stage T2c or lower) prostate cancer. *J. Urol.* **152,**(5 Pt 2), 1850–1857.

23

Radiation Therapy as Applied to Prostate Cancer

Clinical, Technical, and Biologic Considerations

Naren R. Ramakrishna, MD, PhD
and Theodore L. DeWeese, MD

1. INTRODUCTION

Radiation has been used in the treatment of prostate cancer for nearly a century. Following Roentgen's discovery of the X-ray in 1895 *(96)*, and the isolation of radium by Pierre and Marie Curie in 1898 *(21)*, several physicians began treating prostate disorders, including prostate cancer, with radiation. In 1910, Paschkis and Tittinger inserted radium into the prostatic urethra with a cystoscope in what appears to be the first documented use of radiation for prostate cancer. Not long after, Hugh Young from Johns Hopkins reported a relatively large usage of treating prostate cancer patients with urethral and rectal radium "applicators" *(127)*. These early studies revealed that radiation applied in this crude fashion could improve a patient's local symptoms and eliminate prostate cancer, but was difficult to perform and uncomfortable for the patient. In 1928, Barringer was one of the first to report on the use of externally-delivered low-energy kilovoltage radiation for prostate cancer *(5)*. Dosimetric considerations were not well understood, and patients were treated until their skin turned red. These types of low-energy radiation machines were used until cobalt machines became available and provided the first opportunity to treat more deeply seated tumors in the body. The first reported series of prostate cancer patients treated with cobalt-60 therapy, by George et al. in 1965, focused on patients with unresectable disease *(40)*. It was not until the development of the megavoltage linear accelerator at Stanford University in the late 1950s *(62)* and the pioneering work of Bagshaw, Kaplan, Del Ragato, and others, that the modern era of radiation therapy for prostate cancer began revealing the possibility of radiation curability in this disease *(4,26)*. Drawing from these beginnings, we now use three-dimensional conformal plans to drive high-energy accelerators with sophisticated dynamic shielding in order to treat the prostate with a high dose of radiation while sparing the surrounding normal tissues.

The 20th century was what we term the "technical era" in radiation oncology, driven in large part by important contributions in physics to the understanding and application of radiation to the human body. We will surely continue to see refinements in technol-

From: *Prostate Cancer: Biology, Genetics, and the New Therapeutics*
Edited by: L. W. K. Chung, W. B. Isaacs, and J. W. Simons © Humana Press Inc., Totowa, NJ

ogy which will provide real benefit to the patient. However, we believe the next century will be the "molecular era" in radiation oncology, seizing upon the rapid advancements in genetics and molecular biology. These advances will allow the physician to more readily diagnose a patient's cancer and define certain tumor and patient-specific factors. These factors will suggest the appropriate dose and dose rate of radiation to use, and will also determine the class of radiation response modifier, which can be added to specifically increase tumor elimination while sparing normal cells in a particular patient. This chapter outlines the research and therapies being performed today which are setting the stage for the use of radiation therapy in the 21st century.

2. THE TECHNICAL ERA

2.1. Computer-Based Treatment Planning

Some of the most significant advances which have occurred in the delivery of radiation have been driven by the application of advanced computer technologies. This computer hardware and software development has allowed rapid advancement in the areas of imaging, treatment planning, treatment delivery, and verification. Slow and labor-intensive hand calculations are no longer needed to determine appropriate dosing parameters. The computer has fostered a revolution in approaches to treatment planning. Generally, the physician first decides what radiation field(s) to treat, and then allows the computer to calculate and display the resulting radiation dose distribution from that particular configuration. This procedure itself has evolved with the advent of highly sophisticated computer software and the speed of computers now available. In the future, physicians will decide the dose limits for the tumor and surrounding structures, and then allow the computer to determine the best field arrangement and radiation-beam parameters required to achieve the desired radiation dose within the prescribed limits. The computer can perform these calculations iteratively thousands of times, producing the treatment parameters required to meet the desired dose limitations. Today, the typical treatment-planning computers and algorithms cannot hope to complete this type of process in a reasonable amount of time. The result of this so-called inverse treatment planning is the best treatment plan, which provides very high doses of radiation to the tumor while minimizing radiation treatment to surrounding normal tissues.

2.2. Conformal External Beam Therapies

The ability to deliver high doses of radiation to the tumor while exposing the normal tissue surrounding the tumor to relatively small doses of radiation remains one of the most important goals in radiation oncology. Evidence has been presented by several authors which establishes the importance of local control to the long-term outcome of patients *(38,114)*. These authors have reviewed large-scale series revealing that improved local tumor control results in a diminished risk of metastatic disease and increased survival rates. In prostate cancer, higher radiation doses have been associated with increased tumor control in some stages of the disease *(50)*. However, higher doses to the prostate are also associated with higher doses to the rectum, with a consequent elevation in the risk of rectal injury *(128)*. Therefore, techniques that increase the conformation of the radiation dose to the shape of the prostate and that limit treatment of the anterior rectum result in an enhanced therapeutic ratio.

Several highly important technologies are employed in order to achieve the desired conformation of radiation dose. The first technology involves some form of imaging, usually computed tomography (CT), but also can include magnetic resonance imaging (MRI) and ultrasound. These technologies, combined with advanced computer software, allow for localization of the prostate in a three-dimensional space within the confines of a patient's particular anatomy. They also allow for discrimination of other important dose-limiting structures. Once the anatomic localization process is completed, the data is used to produce a three-dimensional image of the pelvis so that an optimal geometric placement of the radiation beams can be performed based on a determination of the amount of radiation to be received by the prostate with respect to the surrounding normal tissue.

Given the precise nature of conformal radiation therapy, successful delivery is highly dependent on patient immobilization. A variety of techniques to immobilize the patient can be used. One commonly used method involves producing a mold of the patient's pelvis and lower extremities on the day of treatment planning, cast in the exact position in which the patient will be treated. The patient can then be repositioned in the same way each day, and is also prevented from easily moving once in position.

This type of three-dimensional therapy has resulted in excellent disease-free survival. For patients with early stage (T1C-T2A), low-moderate grade (Gleason ≤6) and low pretreatment PSA (≤10 ng/mL) prostate cancer, treatment by conformal radiation therapy results in 85% of patients remaining free of disease 5 yr following this type of therapy *(49)*.

Several other exciting techniques currently under investigation provide an even more conformal delivery of radiation. These include intensity-modulated radiation therapy (IMRT) and proton beam therapy. IMRT is a technique designed to deliver a highly conformal dose of radiation, achieved by modulation of the X-ray beam intensity during the time the X-ray beam is on. For any particular radiation port being treated, part of that field may be blocked during a portion of the treatment time and may be unblocked for the remainder of the treatment time, with a resultant gradient of dose over that treatment field. This modulation of beam intensity allows for a much higher degree of spatial distribution of radiation dose, particularly for tumors with areas of concavity *(112)*. Sophisticated treatment planning, like inverse treatment planning, is usually required to provide the data used to achieve this modulated beam intensity. Computer model comparisons of a beam with a nonuniform intensity reveal better dosimetric coverage than those using standard beams with uniform intensity *(112)*. If this beam-intensity modulation is performed over multiple treatment fields, the end result is a highly conformal dose of radiation to the prostate and a considerably reduced relative dose of radiation to the rectum and bladder. Ideally, this will provide an improved method of dose escalation without a significant increase in rectal injury, and therefore result in an improved therapeutic ratio *(120)*. As yet, there have been no large trials reporting on the treatment of prostate cancer with IMRT, but several institutions are actively treating patients and results will soon follow.

Proton beam therapy and the conformation of dose it provides are primarily dependent on the physical characteristics of the proton and its interaction with human tissue. Regular photons (X-rays) have no mass and no charge. Protons possess mass and carry a positive charge. These characteristics can be exploited to deposit a dose of protons very precisely at any desired point, with very little dose beyond that point. The precision of the proton beam has been used successfully for some time in the treatment of tumors around the spinal cord and at the base of skull, where precision is exceedingly important *(81)*. Historically, its application to prostate cancer has been mixed *(104)*, but may be explained in part by patient selection factors. More recently, Slater et al. have reported their early experience in the treatment of prostate cancer with protons, and have found that they can deliver this therapy safely in a large number of patients *(106)*. Follow-up is still short, but early results suggest at least similar disease-free survival at 5 yr (5-yr actuarial bNED = 88%) when compared to more conventional photon (X-ray) three-dimensional therapy. These data will require longer follow-up, and ideally, confirmation by other sites. Until then, proton therapy for prostate cancer must be considered nonstandard, although promising. One particularly limiting factor in the widespread use of protons for cancer therapy—including prostate cancer—is the extreme expense incurred in the construction, staffing, and maintenance of a proton facility. Yet several modern, clinical proton beam facilities have been constructed worldwide and more are planned.

The use of neutrons in the treatment of prostate cancer also has a mixed history, but more recently has been improved by the incorporation of three-dimensional treatment planning and the ability to accurately shape the beam. Compared to photons (X-rays) or protons, neutrons have a significantly different biologic effect on human cells. Dose for dose, neutrons generally kill significantly more cells than either photons or protons. High-energy neutrons do not have a charge, and therefore can penetrate deeply compared to charged particles. They have a relatively large mass, which—given certain fundamental features of neutron interactions with water (the most abundant substance in the body)—increases the probability that a neutron will interact with the cell and its DNA, resulting in cell death. The relative biologic effect of neutrons can vary with cell type, but averages about 1.5–3 times greater than the effects of photons (X-rays) *(34,75)*. This improved biologic effect is considered to be greatest in cells with a low S-phase fraction such as prostate cancer *(6)*. The cytotoxic effects of neutrons are also less dependent on tumor oxygenation than photons (X-rays), providing another theoretic advantage for neutron therapy in overcoming tumor radioresistance. Unfortunately, the same properties which give neutrons their enhanced tumor killing potential also result in increased normal tissue damage and side effects. The clinical experience treating prostate cancer to date has been mixed. There are intriguing results in patients with locally-advanced prostate cancer treated with neutrons alone or with mixed neutrons and photons. Two randomized trials have been completed comparing neutron irradiation to photon irradiation for patients, with high-risk localized prostate cancer (T2, N0-N1, Gleason ≥8 or T3-T4, N0-N1, any grade) *(68,97)*. Both studies showed an increase in clinical local control, and one also revealed an increase in overall survival at 5 yr and 10 yr in patients receiving neutron irradiation. Unfortunately, these series also found that patients treated with neutrons had an increase in significant long-term side effects, including pelvic nerve damage and bowel injury. Investigators at Wayne State University have completed several trials of neutron beam irradiation for prostate cancer, including a comparison of mixed neutron irradiation to hyperfractionated photon irradiation in prostate cancer patients with high-risk local or locally advanced prostate disease *(35,36)*. Overall, these series have found that neutron irradiation delivered with sophisticated beam shaping results in excellent biochemical disease-free survival. As in the earlier neutron series, these investigators also found an increase in long-term side effects, including dose-limiting toxicity to muscle, resulting in hip stiffness *(16)*. The elevated risk of significant long-term side effects, as well as the expense and difficulty of building and maintaining a neutron facility, will limit its widespread application. If, however, the second randomized series confirms the overall survival advantage of neutron therapy found in the RTOG series, and, if modulation of some of the significant late side effects can be achieved through new dosing schemes and/or by incorporation of radiation-response modifiers, enthusiasm for neutron-based therapy may increase.

2.3. Interstitial Radiation Therapies

Recently, brachytherapy, using permanently implanted radioactive sources (seed implants), has become a much more common modality in the treatment of prostate cancer. Its evolution from a difficult-to-perform open procedure with poor results *(128)* to a more sophisticated transrectal ultrasound-guided transperineal approach *(56)* has dramatically increased its use and potential in the treatment of low-risk prostate cancer. Most contemporary published brachytherapy series report on the treatment of patients with early stage, low to moderate-grade, low-PSA prostate cancer. As an example, one recently published series of patients with early-stage (T1-T2 [1992 AJCC staging]) cancer revealed that 71% of patients had no evidence of disease 5 yr following treatment with iodine-125 brachytherapy *(94)*. These data and others reveal that patient selection is critical to the potential success of prostate brachytherapy. This selection is based on a combination of prognostic factors including stage, grade, and pretreatment PSA *(87)* which help to predict the likelihood of organ-confined disease. The importance of appropriate patient selection was also illustrated by D'Amico, et al. These authors showed that brachytherapy was inferior to either radical retropubic prostatectomy or external beam radiation therapy in patients whose prostate cancer was ≥ stage T2B, those with a Gleason score ≥7, or patients with pretreatment PSA ≥10 ng/mL *(23)*.

Brachytherapy can also been combined with external beam radiation therapy in an attempt to improve the outcome of patients treated with either modality separately. Suitable patients may first undergo treatment by an implant with ^{125}I at a reduced dose followed by a reduced dose of external beam radiation. This sequence of an implant followed by external beam radiation provides treatment with concomitant radiation to the prostate by two modalities, one at low dose rate (implant) and one at a high dose rate (external beam radiation). This has the potential to increase the killing of tumor cells, but may also result in increased side effects. To date, there is one series with an adequate length of follow-up to support this approach in early stage prostate cancer patients *(17)*. Specifically, patients with early stage, low to moderate grade prostate cancer, who were known to be pathologically node-negative underwent interstitial implantation with ^{125}I and then 3–6 wk later were treated with external beam radiation to the pelvis. Disease-free survival results from this single institution series are excellent with 79% and 72% of patients achieving a PSA ≤0.5 ng/mL at 5 yr and 10 yr respectively. Importantly, the side-effect profile from this therapy seems to be higher than either external beam radiation or brachytherapy individually *(18)*. It is also possible to treat patients in the reverse sequence—i.e., external beam radiation followed by an prostate implant. Theoretically, this approach may result in less tumor killing because the two radiation modalities are not given concomitantly, but this sequence may also have a preferable side-effect profile *(24)*.

Prostate brachytherapy also includes the use of temporary, high dose-rate interstitial implants either alone, or more frequently as a boost to external beam radiation. Ideally, this high dose-rate brachytherapy boost is meant to deliver a very high, localized dose of radiation to the prostate in 1–3 brief sessions (a few minutes each session) which is believed to achieve greater cell death than standard doses and dose rates of radiation *(47)*. A shortened course of standard external beam radiation is also performed to continue treatment of the prostate and to treat extraprostatic sites. Only a few investigators have reported results, and none have long-term follow-up. The early results suggests that this form of therapy provides an outcome similar to conformal radiation therapy alone, and the side-effect profile has varied between series *(30,113)*. Therefore, this therapy has not gained widespread acceptance.

2.4. Androgen Suppression and Radiation

As early as the 1960s, hormonal therapy was being added to radiation therapy in an attempt to modify the outcome of patients with stage C (T3) prostate cancer *(25)*. The rationale for the treatment of these patients was based on the knowledge that these patients had an inferior outcome compared to patients with earlier-stage prostate cancer treated with radiation therapy. These T3 tumors were also quite large, and it was believed that a course of cytoreductive therapy might provide a more favorable geometry for external irradiation and reduce the tumor burden *(44)*.

Over the years, a number of studies have been conducted involving the use of androgen suppression (AS) and radiation. These early series provided the necessary toxicity and efficacy data to allow the RTOG to begin the 86-10 study *(91)*. This was a randomized Phase III trial of radiation alone (standard treatment arm) vs neoadjuvant and concomitant total androgen suppression (TAS) and radiation (experimental treatment arm). Eligible patients were those with bulky, locally advanced tumors ($>25 \text{ cm}^2$), stage T2B-T4, N0-N1, M0. Those patients randomized to receive TAS were treated with goserelin acetate and flutamide for 2 mo before the start of radiation and during radiation therapy. A total of 471 patients were enrolled and randomized to one of the two treatment arms. Analysis of this series revealed that those patients treated with TAS and radiation had a statistically significant improvement in local control at 5 yr compared to those patients treated with radiation only ($p < 0.001$). A recent update of this trial with a median follow-up time of 6 yr continues to show a statistically significant difference in the 5-yr probability of local failure (22% vs 35%, $p < 0.004$) as well as a decreased incidence of distant metastasis (29 vs 39%, $p < 0.04$) in favor of the experimental arm *(92)*. To date, there is no difference in the overall survival of the two groups of patients. However, it is important to note that this study was limited because it did not routinely collect serum PSA on all patients prior to entry—a parameter that is now recognized to be an extremely important prognostic factor and indicator of disease extension. Therefore, there probably were a large number of patients with elevated serum PSAs in the range frequently associated with a high risk of micrometastatic disease. The study also included patients with node-positive disease—also recognized as a poor risk factor and one in which the value of any treatment modality to overall survival can be debated. Nonetheless, this important study, performed in a rigorous fashion, reveals important and measurable benefits with the addition of AS to radiation therapy for this high-risk group of patients.

The study by Laverdiere et al. *(69)* also provided important information. In this study, patients were randomized to receive either radiation alone, 3 mo of neoadjuvant TAS (LHRH-agonist plus flutamide) followed by radiation, or 3 mo of TAS followed by TAS plus radiation followed by 6 mo of adjuvant TAS. Patients with stage T2A-T4 were eligible. Interestingly, the addition of 3 mo of TAS prior to radiation reduced the 2-yr positive prostate biopsy rate from 65% (radiation only) to 28%. Those patients receiving neoadjuvant, concomitant, and adjuvant TAS and radiation had only a 5% positive prostate biopsy rate. While impressive, the length of follow-up was too short to determine whether the addition of TAS to radiation has made any significant impact on other meaningful endpoints such as biochemical no-evidence-of-disease survival (bNED), disease-free survival (DFS), or overall survival.

Finally, Bolla et al. recently published an analysis of the EORTC 22863 trial *(9)*. This was a Phase III trial which enrolled 415 patients with stage T3-T4, any grade, or stage T1-T2, WHO grade 3 prostate cancer with no evidence of nodal or metastatic disease. Patients were randomized to receive either radiation therapy alone (control arm) or AS plus radiation (experimental arm). Androgen suppression consisted of oral cyproterone acetate for 4 wk prior to radiation and an LHRH-agonist started on the first day of radiation and continued each mo for 3 yr. A total of 401 patients were analyzed with a median follow-up of 45 mo. The local recurrence-free survival rate was 97% in the experimental arm vs 77% in the control arm, ($p < 0.001$). The relapse-free survival rate was reported to be 85% in the experimental arm vs 48% in the control arm ($p < 0.001$). Most significantly, this study was the first to report an overall survival advantage with the addition of AS to radiation, with an estimated 5 yr overall survival of 79% in the experimental arm vs 62% in the control arm ($p = 0.001$). Whether this estimated difference will be maintained has not been determined—particularly since the median survival had not been reached for either group at the time of the analysis. In addition, at least 27% of the patients in the experimental arm were still receiving AS therapy at the time of the analysis. Nonetheless, this is a critically important study confirming the results of previous trials, and at least suggesting that androgen deprivation and radiation given in this protracted fashion to this group of patients can increase overall survival rates.

Human prostate cancer cells vary in their in vitro sensitivity to both acute radiation (like that delivered as external beam radiation) and low dose rate radiation (i.e., like that used in prostate brachytherapy) *(29)*. The radiosensitivity does not appear to be dependent on *P53* status or the ability of the cell to initiate a G_1 cell-cycle checkpoint—both previously considered to be important to radiation response. These studies also do not reveal dependence on androgen responsiveness *(29)*. Androgen-responsive prostate cells undergo programmed cell death (apoptosis) when deprived of androgens *(39)*. Like radiation, this death does not seem to be p53-dependent *(39)*. Several authors have performed in vivo analyses of radiation combined with androgen deprivation on androgen-responsive tumors of both prostate and nonprostate origin *(61,132)*. None of these studies have conclusively demonstrated synergy between radiation and androgen deprivation, but they do suggest that the timing of androgen deprivation may be critical. In one study of androgen withdrawal in the Shionogi breast tumor model, Zietman et al. found that a lower dose of radiation was required to control 50% of the tumors if androgens were used in combination with radiation. Specifically, animals treated with radiation following maximal androgen withdrawal-mediated tumor regression required 42.1 Gy of radiation to control 50% of the tumors, as compared to 89.0 Gy in animals treated with radiation only. The most direct interpretation of these data is that following androgen withdrawal, there is a smaller number of tumor clonogens for the radiation to eradicate. However, these data do not rule out direct biologic interactions between radiation and androgen suppressive therapies which are "more than additive." These data also do not rule out other potentially significant benefits of tumor-burden reduction, such as changes in the hypoxic cell fraction within the tumor or alterations in the number of cells able to undergo accelerated repopulation—both of which are associated with relatively radioresistant tumors.

The combination of AS and radiation for the treatment of locally advanced prostate cancer results in an apparent increase in local control and disease-free survival, as supported by several prospective, randomized trials *(9,69,91)*. There is conflicting data from such trials as to the benefit in overall survival *(9)*. It may also be true that other groups of patients who are at "high risk" for biochemical, local, and distant failure—but who do not fit the classic definition of having locally-advanced prostate cancer—might similarly benefit by treatment with this combined modality approach.

2.5. Conclusion

The latter half of the 20th century witnessed the accumulated knowledge of the first 50 yrs in physics and radiation biology applied safely and efficaciously to the treatment of prostate cancer. The last 10–15 yr of the 20th century provided the capacity to identify and localize the prostate with sophisticated noninvasive techniques, and to precisely deliver high doses of radiation heretofore not safely administered. We have also witnessed improved patient stratification based on an increasing knowledge of the clinical features of prostate cancer. This stratification allows for a matching of patients to the most appropriate therapy. This same understanding of high-risk clinical features has allowed the identification of patients who benefit from combined modality therapies, including androgen suppression and radiation. The 21st century will see a continued refinement of technology, which will provide improvement in the therapeutic ratio and an increase in the numbers of patients cured of prostate cancer. It will be critically important to develop these technologies in a way that will make them easily obtainable and useable worldwide.

3. THE MOLECULAR ERA: RADIATION THERAPY WITH A BIOLOGICAL PERSPECTIVE

Diverse genetic and epigenetic changes have been observed in prostate cancer—including mutations, or altered expression of tumor suppressors, oncogenes, growth factors, and electrophile detoxification proteins *(59,64)*. A central challenge of the molecular era will be to clearly define the relationship between these lesions and the heterogenous clinical behavior and response to radiotherapy of prostate cancer. As noted earlier, screening of molecular lesions may allow the prediction of disease radiosensitivity, invasiveness, metastatic potential, and overall prognosis. Large prospective clinical trials—made more feasible by advances in molecular screening—will be essential to clarify the association of these lesions to clinical endpoints. This will permit a new dimension to risk stratification, building upon the algorithms to assess likelihood of organ-confined disease developed during the technical era.

The major therapeutic advances of the technical era—dose escalation, the use of high LET particles such as neutrons, optimization of dose conformality, and the use of sequential or concurrent androgen suppression—are ultimately limited in their potential to address the biological diversity of prostate cancer. Emerging insights into the mechanistic basis of prostate cancer tumorigenesis and radioresistance should facilitate direct targeting of the molecular lesions central to radiation treatment response and overall outcome. Rapid progress in mechanism-based drug development and gene therapy should provide a vast new armamentarium of pharmacological and genetic tools. New classes of radiosensitizers, radioprotectors, molecular markers, and novel combined modality treatments may augment or eventually supersede current treatment schema.

3.1. Prostate Cancer Cell Radioresistance: Overview

The principal target of therapeutic radiation is DNA *(93)*. Irradiation of the cell results in the formation of free radical species which may induce DNA damage, including strand breaks, mutations, and crosslinking (Fig. 1). Tumor hypoxia may inhibit the capacity of free radical species to effect DNA damage. Following radiation-induced DNA damage, DNA damage-sensing and repair mechanisms are normally activated, and may trigger cell-cycle arrest. This arrest is believed to be a mechanism which allows repair of radiation damage prior to DNA synthesis or mitosis. In the case of repairable DNA damage, it is thought that cells reenter the cell cycle and then proceed normally with proliferation. When damage exceeds repair capacity, cells may undergo apoptosis, thereby limiting the proliferation of mutant cells. In cancer cells, defects in DNA damage sensing and repair systems can abrogate the normal induction of cell-cycle arrest and elimination of cells with accumulated DNA damage through apoptosis. Mutations of genes involved in cell-cycle arrest such as p53, Rb, and p21 are another means by which transformed cells may escape from cell-cycle arrest and potential apoptotic death. A wide range of signals modulate apoptosis itself. Radiation may induce the generation of the lipid second messenger ceramide in cells, which may activate apoptosis. Oncogenes such as *ras* and bcl-2 may inhibit the entry of cells into the apoptotic pathway. When cell death occurs following radiation, it may be through both apoptotic and nonapoptotic pathways. The fact that radiosensitivity varies widely, even between tumors of the same type, is likely a result of the diverse physicochemical and biological factors which govern cellular radiation response.

Radiosensitizers are used to improve therapeutic ratio by potentiating the effect of radiation in tumor cells to a greater extent than in normal cells. The premise that a radiosensitizer may improve tumor control is based upon the dose-response profiles of

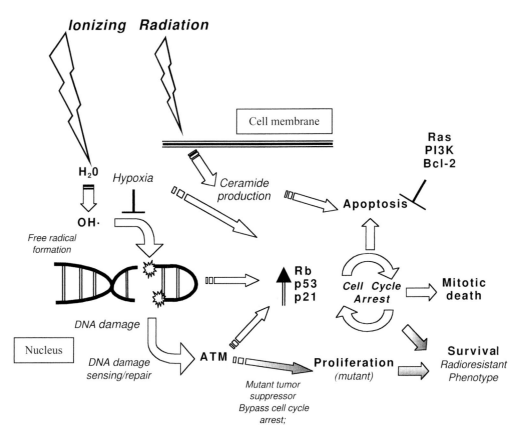

Fig. 1. Simplified overview of cellular effects of ionizing radiation and some mechanisms of radioresistance. Ionizing radiation may induce DNA damage either directly or through generation of free radical sp. Free radicals may cause DNA strand breaks, base damage, or crosslinking. Hypoxia can inhibit the induction of DNA damage by free radicals. Radiation also induces the production of the second messenger ceramide, which may trigger apoptosis. Cellular DNA damage-repair genes, including ATM, are induced following DNA damage—as are cell-cycle control genes such as p21, Rb, and p53. Cell-cycle arrest may follow, during which repair may occur. Mutations in tumor suppressors and cell-cycle control genes may bypass normal cell-cycle arrest and repair following irradiation. Radiosensitive cells will tend to undergo apoptosis, or mitotic death following cell division. Radioresistant cells will continue to proliferate.

various tumor types. In many cases, small increments in total tumor dose results in significant increases in tumor control. Increased dose is also accompanied with increased side-effects to normal tissue. Selective radiosensitization of tumor cells would result in increased tumor control without a corresponding increase in normal tissue effects.

3.2. Hypoxia

At low oxygen tensions (< 2%), radiation sensitivity decreases—an effect attributed to decreased stabilization of free-radical mediated cellular damage *(14)*. Radiosensitivity rises with oxygen tension, an effect referred to as the oxygen enhancement ratio

Table 1
Molecular Lesions in Prostate Cancer

	Normal function	Defect in prostate cancer	XRT response/ clinical predictive value
Tumor Suppressors			
p53	Regulation of cell cycle G1/S checkpoint, apoptosis, response to stress/DNA damage	Mutated in 20–75% of prostate cancers	Mutations associated with radioresistance in some systems May predict for poor clinical response
Rb	Cell-cycle regulation and differentiation	Allelic loss in 27–40% prostate cancers	Mutations associated with radioresistance in some systems
pTEN	Regulation of PI3K cell survival pathway	Decreased expression in 50% of prostate cancers	Overactivity associated with decreased apoptosis in response to radiation
p16 (CDKN2)	Cyclin-dependent kinase inhibitor involved in cell-cycle regulation	Markedly reduced expression in 43% of untreated primary prostate cancers; no alteration in BPH	Loss of expression associated with radioresistance
p21 (waf 1/cip1)	Cyclin-dependent kinase inhibitor	Aberrant overexpression linked to poor prognosis in prostate cancer	Loss of expression/mutant overexpression associated with radioresistance
Oncogenes			
Bcl-2	Inhibition of apoptosis	Uniformly elevated in androgen-independent prostate cancers	Increased expression associated with radioresistance
Ras	GTP-binding proteins involved in growth regulation	Mutated in 2–5% CaP in US men; In Japanese cases CaP ~25% mutated	Associated with poor clinical outcome Associated with radioresistance
Growth factors			
IGFs/IGFBPs	Growth factors/growth factor regulatory proteins	Increased IGF-I levels associated with increased risk of CaP	
TGF-β	Growth factor-growth inhibitory in normal prostate	Tumor progression may involve dysregulation of TGF-B growth inhibition	Associated with increased radioresistance and radiation fibrosis
Detoxification			
ffGSTP1	Detoxification of electrophilic carcinogens	Absent expression secondary to promoter hypermethylation in PIN and 98% of clinical prostate cancers	Inactivation associated with Gleason grade

(OER). Several lines of evidence point to tumor hypoxia as a major clinical determinant of response to radiation therapy. Increased tumor control and survival have been observed when radiation therapy is delivered in conjunction with hyperbaric oxygen for some tumor types *(122)*. Supporting the notion that hypoxia may be relevant to prostate radiotherapy is recent in vivo evidence for the presence of hypoxic regions in prostate tumors *(80)*. Intratumoral pO_2 in patients undergoing either brachytherapy or radical prostatectomy was determined using a microelectrode. A significant association was revealed between the degree of tumor hypoxia and tumor stage. These patients are being evaluated prospectively to determine if tumor hypoxia is a predictor for response to therapy. In tumors of the cervix, decreased oxygenation is a strong independent predictor for decreased radiocurability *(55)*. Surprisingly, in the same group of patients, hypoxia also predicted for poor prognosis, even among untreated patients or those treated with surgery *(54)*. This underscores the potentially broad biological implications of tumor hypoxia and cell redox state, which extend beyond the physicochemical attenuation of radiation response.

Hypoxic cell radiosensitizers are designed to negate the effects of low oxygen tension on radiation sensitivity. Misonidazole is a type of electron-affinic hypoxic cell radiosensitizer. It substitutes for oxygen in cells to "fix" (make permanent) ionizing radiation-induced free-radical damage *(14)*. It is selective for tumor cells simply because of the higher oxygen enhancement ratio in hypoxic cells. In normal cells with their typically higher pO_2, the effect of misonidazole on radiation sensitivity is minimal. Although efficacy in preclinical studies was promising, results in clinical trials in a variety of body sites have not shown clear benefit *(31)*. This is likely to be the result of the relatively low toxicity-limited dose levels attained in clinical trials together with the reoxygenation that occurs between conventionally fractionated radiation. The dose-limiting toxicity of misonidazole is neurological. SR2058, a less toxic alternative to misonidazole in the same class, achieves higher tumor concentrations at an equal injected dose to misonidazole. Despite its improved pharmacology, in an RTOG trial *(70)* for locally advanced prostate cancer, SR2058 showed no effect on biochemical control or survival.

The use of biologically targeted gene therapy approaches may permit improved delivery of hypoxic cell radiosensitizers or hypoxic cell-cytotoxic agents. The identification of a variety of hypoxia-inducible genes *(103)* together with cloning of hypoxia-inducible regulatory regions allows the delivery of hypoxic cell-specific radiosensitizing or cytotoxic drugs in principle.

3.3. Chronic Oxidative Stress

Normal cellular processes, inflammation, and such environmental factors as diet and ionizing radiation may contribute to the formation of reactive oxygen species within cells. In prostate cells, androgen may play a role in increasing cell oxidative stress *(95)*. In most cells, the potentially promutagenic effects of these species are counteracted by free-radical detoxification and DNA repair systems. Substantial evidence supports the idea that elevation of oxidative stress can contribute to tumorigenesis. Increased expression of cyclooxygenase-2 (COX-2), an enzyme involved in arachidonic acid metabolism, results in increased formation of reactive oxygen species. COX-2 overexpression has been observed in human colorectal cancer *(98)*. The ability of specific

COX-2 inhibitors to decrease colorectal polyp formation in both animal models and human studies support the role of chronic oxidative stress in tumorigenesis *(41,85)*.

Mismatch repair genes are involved in the recognition and repair of mismatched nucleotides. Deficiencies in mismatch repair genes such as hMSH2 and hMLH1 result in a mutator phenotype with markedly increased mutation frequencies, both in microsatellite and coding regions. Mutations in these genes are observed in the majority of HNPCC patients, supporting their role in tumorigenesis in vivo. Cells with normal DNA damage sensing and repair mechanisms will typically either undergo repair or apoptosis in response to accumulated mutations. Those with deficiencies in the mismatch repair enzymes, such as hMSH2, show a surprising tolerance to the effects of oxidative stress on the genome. These cells display decreased apoptosis and increased survival following the oxidative stress of low dose rate radiation, thereby permitting cells to survive and accumulate more potentially proneoplastic mutations *(28)*. Conceivably, the tolerance to accumulated mutations and the expected "hypermutability" of these cells may increase the likelihood of the emergence of radioresistant cells. The potential of wild-type hMSH2 and hMLH1 to induce apoptosis when overexpressed in mismatch-repair-deficient or proficient cells suggests that mutations in these genes may also directly diminish the ability of cells to undergo apoptosis in response to oxidative stress *(130)*.

Another important gene involved in protection of the cell from the effects of chronic oxidative stress is GSTP1. The GSTP1 gene product is involved in detoxification of electrophilic carcinogens by conjugation to glutathione, protecting the genome from the potentially mutagenic effects of oxidative stress. The glutathione-S transferase P1 gene is a frequent target for inactivating methylation changes in prostate cancer. The absence of GSTP1-inactivating methylation in normal prostate or BPH, and its presence in PIN and more than 98% of clinical prostate tumors, suggests that it is an early step in prostate tumorigenesis *(71)*. Early studies have revealed that the human prostate cancer cell line LnCaP, which lacks GSTP1 expression secondary to promoter hypermethylation, tolerates the oxidative stress of low dose rate irradiation and accumulates higher levels of the promutagenic oxidized DNA base 8-hydroxyguanine to a greater degree than LnCaP cells engineered to stably express the GSTP1 protein *(27)*. These data suggest an important role for GSTP1 in the modulation of oxidative stress-induced DNA damage. The near uniform inactivation of GSTP1 in PIN and prostate cancers suggests that screening may not be useful in initial therapeutic risk stratification.

3.4. Tumor Suppressors

Tumor suppressor genes, such as p53, retinoblastoma (Rb), p16, and pTEN, show evidence of mutation or aberrant expression in some prostate cancers *(10,58,88, 115,124)*. The tumor suppressor gene p53 encodes a transcription factor involved in regulation of the cell cycle and apoptosis. p53 is thought to play a central role in the response of cells to DNA-damaging agents, such as ionizing radiation *(13)*. Mutations in p53 are widespread in human cancer and are observed in between 20–75% of prostate cancers, more commonly in advanced metastatic tumors *(53)*. Given the prevalence of p53 mutations in tumors, several retrospective studies have been performed to assess the possible clinical relevance to response to radiation therapy.

A recent study *(99)* revealed a striking association between pretreatment expression of p53 and bcl-2 and response to radiotherapy. In a group of predominantly early-stage patients (74% T1C) with average Gleason score of 6.9 and PSA 25.3 ng/mL, the expression of either p53 or bcl-2 was a strong independent predictor for treatment failure—defined as nadir PSA posttreatment >1 ng/mL. 85% of patients with bcl-2-positive pretreatment biopsies failed treatment, while 88% of those with p53 positive pretreatment biopsies failed. The presence of both p53 and bcl-2 expression in a patient was uniformly associated with treatment failure. In another retrospective study, however, pretreatment p53 levels showed no association with cancer-specific survival following radiation therapy *(110)*.

One approach to therapy of p53 mutant radioresistant tumors could be corrective gene therapy to restore wild-type p53. In addition to potentially increasing the radiosensitivity of p53-deficient tumors, overexpressed wild-type p53 is able to inhibit the growth of primary cultures derived from radical prostatectomy specimens—surprisingly, even when p53 status is normal *(3)*. In most tissues, p53 is induced by genotoxic agents, such as ionizing radiation, as part of the cellular DNA-damage response. However, in a majority of normal prostate epithelial cells, p53 induction is not observed in response to ionizing radiation *(42)*, calling into question the importance of p53 to DNA damage repair in the prostate *(29)* and its potential utility as a radiosensitizer. At present, two Phase I clinical trials are underway at UCLA and MD Anderson which utilize intratumoral injections of replication-defective Adp53 for patients with locally-advanced or recurrent prostate cancer, administered without XRT.

Another tumor suppressor, the retinoblastoma gene product (Rb), is involved in regulation of the G1/S cell cycle checkpoint. Allelic loss of Rb is seen in 27–40% of prostate tumors *(89)*. In the prostate cancer cell line DU 145, Rb is functionally absent, and the cells display resistance to radiation or ceramide-induced apoptosis. If Rb expression is restored in these cells, then apoptotic response is restored following radiation and ceramide treatment *(12)*. A recent retrospective study examined levels of Rb, p53, and bcl-2 immunoreactivity prior to radical prostatectomy. Elevated levels of Rb immunoreactivity predicted for improved survival on multivariate analysis *(117)*. Pretreatment p53 and Rb were superior predictors of disease-specific survival when compared to Gleason grade/clinical stage. The effect of Rb mutations on clinical response to radiotherapy has not yet been examined.

Mutations of the tumor suppressor pTEN have been frequently observed in prostate cancer *(88,115,124)*. pTEN is involved in regulation of the PI3K/Akt pathway, a prosurvival cell signalling pathway. The PI3K pathway is a conduit for integration of multiple-signal transduction pathways including *ras* and receptor tyrosine kinases such as EGF-R and the insulin receptor. Increased signaling via PI3K promotes cell survival, decreases apoptosis, and increases radiosensitivity *(65)*. Candidates for effectors downstream in this signaling pathway include GSK-3B/ B–catenin and members of the bcl-2 family. Overactivity of the PI3K pathway, as is seen with inactivating mutations of pTEN, is known to decrease apoptosis in response to cytotoxic agents and radiation. Expression of wild-type pTEN in cells containing mutant pTEN results in increased apoptosis following radiation *(125)*, suggesting the potential use of PI3K inhibitors in biological radiosensitizing strategies.

Analysis of allelic loss on chromosome 11 in prostate cancer led to cloning of the KAI-1 gene *(32)*. Expression of KAI-1 was found to be deficient in prostate cancer metastases, suggesting a possible function as a metastasis suppresser gene. KAI-1 expression can be regulated directly by p53, and recent evidence shows a strong correlation in human prostate tumors of loss of p53 expression and loss of KAI-1 expression *(74)*. The impact of KAI-1 on radiosensitivity has not been reported; screening for KAI-1 could conceivably function as a marker to stratify tumors for risk of dissemination.

3.5. Cell Cycle

Among the regulators of entry into the cell cycle which have shown mutations or aberrant expression in prostate cancer are several cyclin dependent kinase inhibitors. p21WAF1/CIP1 is a cyclin-dependent kinase inhibitor which may be induced in response to cytotoxic stress by both p53-dependent and independent mechanisms. When induced by p53, it may cause cell-cycle arrest at G1 by inhibition of DNA replication. In a murine carcinoma model, the presence of low basal p21 levels was found to correlate with increased radiosensitivity. In these tumors, p21 was induced following irradiation and was followed by induction of bax expression. In tumors with high basal p21 levels, there was no increase from basal p21 levels following irradiation, and no induction of bax expression was observed *(2)*. In a retrospective review of 213 prostate cancer cases, increased levels of p21 were associated with decreased survival *(1)*. In local tumors, p21 expression was an independent predictor of cancer-specific survival together with Gleason grade and T stage.

Another cyclin dependent kinase inhibitor, p16 (CDKN2), shows markedly reduced expression in 43% of untreated primary prostate cancers, but is unaltered in BPH *(15)*. Downregulation by androgen, promoter methylation, or another inactivating mutation may increase progression through the cell cycle *(60,73)*. The loss of p16 expression results in decreased radiosensitivity in several nonprostate cell lines *(37,76,79)*; however, the impact on prostate cancer cell radiosensitivity is unknown.

3.6. Oncogenes and Growth Factors

The oncogene *Bcl*-2 functions in the regulation of apoptosis. Increased levels of Bcl-2 protein result in supresion of apoptosis. Bcl-2 overexpression is noted in the majority of androgen independent prostate cancers *(39)*, suggesting a role in their aggressive phenotype. Overexpression of Bcl-2 in prostate cancer cell lines results in increased resistance to radiation-induced apoptosis, but no change in clonogenic survival in vitro *(66)*. The potential clinical relevance of Bcl-2 overexpression in prostate cancer was evaluated by comparing Bcl-2 and p53 immunopositivity in preirradiation and postirradiation tumor specimens from patients who had failed therapy, to preirradiation specimens from patients who had no evidence of disease failure. Those who failed radiotherapy had 41% Bcl-2 positivity preirradiation compared to 8% in patients with no evidence of postradiation recurrence. These findings support the pursuit of prospective trials to evaluate the predictive value of Bcl-2 expression with respect to response to radiotherapy *(57)*. In another retrospective study, the levels of Bcl-2 and the Bcl-2 homolog bax were examined in pretreatment paraffin sections of radiation responders and nonresponders. While there was no significant difference in stage, Gleason score, or PSA between the two groups, the bcl-2/bax ratio was an independent predictor for response to radiotherapy *(73)*.

Signal transduction through the *ras* signalling pathways contributes to cell survival and may increase tumor radioresistance. Activation of *ras* for signalling requires that it undergo prenylation. Inhibition of prenylation using prenyltransferase inhibitors in cells with oncogenic *H*- or *K-ras* mutations has been demonstrated to increase radiosensitivity as measured with clonogenic survival assays. A recent study showed that the effect of combined radiation treatment with prenyltransferase inhibitors was synergistic in cells with activating *ras* mutations, and additive in those with wild-type *ras. (7)*.

The insulin-like growth factors (IGFs) are potent mitogens for prostate epithelial cells. The ability of IGF-I to activate the androgen receptor, even in the absence of hormone, suggests a potential role in prostate cancer progression *(19,20)*. Decreased IGF-IR mRNA expression has been observed in prostate cancer vs BPH *(116)*. In the TRAMP prostate cancer model, decreased IGF-IR and IGF-2R are seen in androgen-independent and metastatic disease.The role of the IGF-I receptor (IGF-IR) in prostate cancer prognosis or response to radiotherapy is unclear. IGF-IR has been shown to increase radioresistance when overexpressed in fibroblasts. Furthermore, expression of IGF-IR in primary breast tumors predicted for early breast tumor relapse following lumpectomy and radiation *(118)*. These findings warrant further investigation of the effects of IGF-IR expression on response to radiotherapy.

cerbB-2 overexpression is observed in prostate tumors *(45)*. In ovarian cancer cell lines, the use of a single-chain antibody against erbB2 resulted in greater sensitivity to ionizing radiation in vivo, although not in vitro *(109)*. In radioresistant GBM cells, disabling the erbB- receptor signaling results in increased sensitivity to gamma radiation *(86)*. This may be a useful sensitization strategy in the subset of prostate cancers in which erbB-2 is overexpressed. By analogy with the erbB receptor, disabling the EGF-receptor in head and neck cancer cell lines with the monoclonal antibody C225 inhibits proliferation. EGF receptor blockade also induces increased bax and decreased bcl-2 expression, with enhancement of radiosensitivity and increased single dose or fractionated radiation-induced apoptosis. Cells show an accumulation in G1, with a decrease in S-phase fraction by two to threefold *(57)*.

3.7. Gene Therapy Radiosensitizing Strategies

Gene therapy may be used to augment radiation treatment in a variety of ways. Radiation therapy may be spatially targeted with great precision, but gene therapy may be biologically targeted to specific tissue and cell types. The identification of genes uniquely expressed in the prostate, such as probasin, allow for the use of prostate-specific gene therapy strategies. In addition, gene therapy vectors may be designed with a radiation response element incorporated which can limit replication or the expression of a transgene to irradiated tissue—a combination referred to as "radio-genetic therapy" *(48)*.

Recent evidence supports the idea that oncolytic gene therapy using replication-competent vectors may be enhanced by the use of radiation. Greater than expected tumor regression was observed in U-87MG glioma cell xenografts following combined radiation and viral treatment with the herpes simplex virus mutant R3616 (Advani, 1998). In radiated xenografts, viral replication was increased two to fivefold per cell. In unirradiated tumors, virally infected cells were restricted to regions of the xenograft immediately adjacent to the infecting needle track. In radiated tumors, virally infected cells were more widely distributed throughout the xenograft and away from the needle track than unirradiated tumors. Increased doses of virus to unirradiated cells resulted in no increase in viral spread from the vicinity of the needle track, supporting the idea that radiation was facilitating not only viral replication, but viral spread as well.

Gene therapy may also be used to activate a radiosensitizing prodrug such as ganciclovir *(84)*, or 5-fluorocytosine *(51)*. While chemotherapy has thus far been relatively ineffective for prostate cancer, novel combinations of gene therapy and chemotherapy may display synergistic improvements in efficacy. The combination of paclitaxel and gene therapy utilizing an adenovirus expressing p53 under the control of the CMV promoter revealed synergy for the combined modality treatment for a wide variety of tumor cell lines in vitro and in xenografts including the DU-145 prostate cancer cell line *(83)*. Combinations of three modalities have also been demonstrated—radiotherapy, viral-cytopathic (E1B-deleted-Ad), and radiosensitizing double-suicide gene therapy—with marked enhancement in efficacy in vitro with DU-145 cells.

3.8. Biological Therapies: DNA Repair/Apoptosis/Angiogenesis

Another strategy for radiosensitization is enhancement of radiation-induced DNA damage by inhibition of cellular DNA repair. Poly-ADP-ribose-polymerase (PARP) is an enzyme involved in DNA base-excision repair and in the cellular response to DNA damage. PARP regulates chromatin structure through modification of nuclear proteins. Using a PARP-inhibitory compound, a 30–50% increased radiosensitivity is observed in vitro in clonogenic survival assays using rat and human prostate carcinoma cell lines *(100)*.

Another way to enhance the ability of ionizing radiation (IR) to induce apoptosis in prostate cells is through expression of tumor necrosis factor-alpha (TNF-α). Exposure of prostate cancer cells normally resistant to IR-induced apoptosis in vitro to TNF-α and radiation resulted in a substantial increase in apoptotic cell death *(63)*. Were these results in vitro to translate to clinical efficacy, TNF-α could conceivably be delivered intratumorally by either gene therapy or sustained-release form to improve radiation response. Another method to augment IR-induced apoptosis may be through delivery of proapoptotic toxins, such as Pseudomonas exotoxin A, to cells. Pseudomonas exotoxin A modified to display binding specificity to the EGF receptor has been shown to significantly increase radiosensitivity. Treatment with this construct resulted in increased ceramide production and inhibition of protein synthesis *(102)*. Clusterin, also known as SGP-2, is a secreted glycoprotein which inhibits cellular apoptosis. In prostate cancer cells, SGP-2 has been shown to inhibit TNF-induced cytotoxicity *(105)*. Levels of SGP-2 correlate with resistance to apoptotic cell death. Analysis of prostate tumors reveals little or no SGP-2 expression in normal prostate epithelial cells, whereas staining in tumors shows significant correlation with Gleason grade ($p = 0.006$) *(111)*.

Substantial evidence supports the importance of tumor angiogenesis to tumor growth, invasive potential, and metastatic ability. In prostate cancer, the extent of angiogenesis as measured by mean vessel density (MVD) has been shown to be associated with grade *(82)*, tendency for extracapsular extension *(11)*, and incidence of metastases *(123)*. Angiogenesis inhibitors, such as angiostatin or endostatin, administered in animal tumor models have shown marked tumoristatic effects, but are not tumoricidal, and therefore require prolonged administration for efficacy *(8)*. Combined radiation/ antiangiogenesis therapy has been proposed as a means to circumvent the need for prolonged administration of antiangiogenic agents for tumor control. Treatment of four types of tumor cells in vivo—including the PC-3 prostate cancer cell line with a combination of radiation (40 Gy, 5 Gy/d) and systemically administered angiostatin—showed a greater than additive antitumor effect with no increase in normal tissue cytotoxicity *(77)*. A recent study showed that the presence of angiostatin at the time of irradiation was sufficient in itself to cause potentiation of radiation-induced tumor cell kill *(43)*.

3.9. Chemoirradiation

The principal treatment presently used with radiation is androgen suppression. A variety of chemotherapeutic agents with radiosensitizing properties have also been employed together with radiation. For localized disease, chemotherapy has been used in combined modality trials with both external beam radiation and brachytherapy. An RTOG pilot trial evaluated the efficacy of external beam radiation delivered in conjunction with cisplatin, adriamycin, and cytoxan for high-grade localized prostate carcinoma *(90)*. Although no increase in radiation toxicity to the pelvis was observed with this combined modality regimen, the severe myelosuppression associated with the chemotherapy regimen led to discontinuation of the trial. Continuous infusion 5FU has been evaluated in Phase I trial in conjunction with prostate interstitial brachytherapy *(101)*, with no observed increase in acute toxicity. For metastatic disease, chemotherapy has been evaluated in conjunction with radioisotope therapy. Combination therapy of patients with hormone refractory metastatic disease, using Strontium-90 in conjunction with estramustine, has shown promising improvement in time to failure compared to more toxic combination chemotherapy regimens *(22)*.

3.10. New Tools for Systemic Radiation Targeting

No curative treatment presently is available for metastatic prostate cancer. Hormonal therapy, the use of localized radiation or systemic radionuclides, and chemotherapy are all currently used for metastatic disease. While these may provide temporary palliation, patients ultimately fail such therapy because of escape from hormone dependence, or progressive dissemination. Among the traditional barriers to the use of tumor-targeted radioimmunotherapy has been the inability to achieve high and uniform tumor concentrations of radionuclide without normal cell toxicity, and the development of immunity against the antibody conjugate *(107)*. New strategies which may improve the targeting and toxicity profiles of current treatments might exploit prostate specific genes for delivery of radionuclides *(131)*. Conjugation of radioisotopes to prostate specific antibodies has already aided in the determination of localization of recurrent disease and metastatic sites *(33,67)*.

Another potential strategy to improve tumor radionuclide uptake is to exploit the ability of a nonprostate tissue, the thyroid, to concentrate exogenously administered radioactive iodine. Thyroid cells express the sodium-iodide symporter gene, a 634 amino acid protein, which can cause a 20 to 40-fold concentration of administered iodine. Recently, the human NIS gene was cloned and inserted into a vector using a PSA-promoter region to drive expression. This construct was used to successfully induce androgen-dependent iodide uptake in the PSA-expressing prostate cancer cell line LnCaP. These NIS-expressing prostate cancer cells were able to concentrate ^{125}I approx 50-fold *(108)* in the presence of androgen. Given the large number of prostate-unique genes, it should be possible to express the NIS gene specifically in prostate cancer cells without dependence on androgen.

3.11. New Approaches to Limiting Normal Tissue Toxicity

The major long-term adverse effects of radiation for prostate cancer may include decreased potency and damage to the rectum, bladder, and urethra. Prevention of adverse treatment sequelae, and identification of patients at particular risk for late effects, would be a major advancement in therapy. A biological radioprotector in current use is amifostine (WR-2721). Amifostine is itself a prodrug, which is converted by alkaline phosphatase to the active sulfhydryl compound WR-1065. The activated compound may then protect normal cells from radiation injury by scavenging free radicals and depleting oxygen. The selectivity of amifostine for protection of normal cells rather than tumors is hypothesized to result from the decreased vascularity of tumors, decreased activity of alkaline phosphatase in tumor cells, and pH dependence of WR-1065 uptake *(119,121)*. The major dose-limiting toxicities include nausea, emesis, and malaise. In clinical testing, radioprotection of normal tissue has been observed at some sites without evidence of accompanying tumor radioprotection *(78)*.

One way to predict which patients are at particular risk of normal tissue side effects is the detection of lesions in DNA repair pathways. One such group of patients are those with defects in fidelity of DNA repair secondary to mutations in the ATM gene, the gene responsible for the autosomal recessive disease ataxia-telangiectasia. Patients with AT are homozygous for mutations in ATM and show extreme normal tissue radiosensitivity. While AT homozygotes are rare, AT carriers (heterozygotes) comprise 1–2% of the population. Studies to assess the relevance of AT carrier status to radiation sensitivity have been hampered by the difficulty of sequencing the large ATM genome. A recent study evaluated the frequency of mutations in the ATM gene among prostate cancer patients treated with high-dose conformal external beam radiation who subsequently developed proctitis/cystitis. It was found that among the patients with adverse late sequelae *(17)*, mutations in the ATM gene were detected in 17.6%, while among those with no late effects, no mutations were detected *(46)*. These suggestive findings support further studies to identify patients with unfavorable genetic lesions for radiation treatment. Identification of such patients could prospectively allow adjustments to be made in dose, treatment volume, and in therapeutic choice—ie, surgery vs radiation. Lesions in other steps in the DNA repair process could underlie abnormal tissue sensitivity, such as components of DNA dependent protein kinase Ku70 and Ku80, and several recently identified Ku70-binding proteins including XIP-8, testosterone-repressed prostate message-2 (TRPM-2) and clusterin *(126)*.

3.12. Synthesizing the Molecular and the Technical

The identification of individual molecular lesions and the analysis of their role in tumorigenesis, natural history, and radiation response will also guide the development

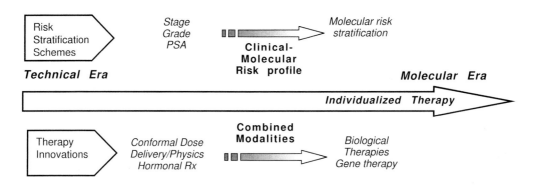

Fig. 2. Transition from the "Technical" to the "Molecular" Era.

and application of new biological therapies for the 21st century. This will be of particular importance for the treatment of metastatic disease, for which current therapies are inadequate. A remarkably diverse range of prostate unique gene expression has been observed, with at least 500 prostate specific expressed sequence tags already identified *(52)*. The process of molecular profiling of individual tumors has the potential to exploit this tumor-specific gene expression to direct tumor-specific delivery of radiopharmaceuticals, biologic therapy, or gene therapy.

The advent of gene chip/proteomics technology is a vital technological development which should facilitate prospective multivariate analysis of genetic/protein alterations and their clinical relevance. As new algorithms for risk stratification emerge during the next few decades, it will be possible to provide the patient with a more accurable risk assessment of extraprostatic disease, radiocurability, and normal tissue radiosensitivity and morbidity. Conceivably, the therapeutic arsenal of the radiation oncologist will come to include a wide range of radiosensitizing and radioprotective biomolecules, vectors, and targeting systems. The prostate cancer patient may be offered combinations of biological/gene therapy with radiation, building upon the efficacy of technical-based treatment innovations developed during the last century.

The combination of clinical and molecular risk stratification should permit "molecular treatment planning." The radiation oncologist of the 21st century should have access to molecular indices of locoregional invasiveness and risk of nodal metastasis to guide the choice of local therapy and radiation treatment port design. Adjuvant systemic treatment may be considered in lesions with high risk of micro-metastatic disease. A major benefit of improved conformal-dose technology developed during the technical era was the capacity for dose escalation. Dose escalation and conformal therapy could be utilized more selectively with individualized prediction of radiocurability. In patients with radiosensitizing gene defects such as mutations in ATM, dose escalation could be avoided. In relatively radioresistant tumors, alternative treatment could be recommended, or conformal high-dose radiation could be combined with a radiosensitizer, gene therapy, or other adjuvant modality for improved local control. The skilled synthesis of current radiotherapy with the new molecular paradigms for therapy and risk stratification (Fig. 2) holds great promise for significant progress in the battle against prostate cancer.

REFERENCES

1. Aaltomaa, S., et al. 1999. Prognostic value and expression of p21(waf1/cip1) protein in prostate cancer. *Prostate* **39:** 8–15.
2. Akimoto, T., et al. 1999. Association of increased radiocurability of murine carcinomas with low constitutive expression of P21WAF1/CIP1 protein. *Int. J. Rad. Oncol. Biol. Phys.* **44:** 413–419.
3. Asgari, K., et al. 1997. Inhibition of the growth of pre-established subcutaneous tumor nodules of human prostate cancer cells by single injection of the recombinant adenovirus p53 expression vector. *Int. J. Cancer* **71:** 377–382.
4. Bagshaw, M. A., H. S. Kaplan, and R. H. Sagerman. 1965. Linear accelerator supervoltage radiotherapy. VII. Carcinoma of the prostate. *Radiology* **85:** 121–129.
5. Barringer, B. S. 1928. Phases of the pathology, diagnosis and treatment of cancer of the prostate. *J. Urol.* 407–411.
6. Batterman, J. J. 1981. The Clinical Application of Fast Neutrons: the Amsterdam Experience. Amsterdam: *Rodipi*.
7. Bernhard, E. J., et al. 1998. Inhibiting Ras prenylation increases the radiosensitivity of human tumor cell lines with activating mutations of ras oncogenes. *Cancer Res.* **58:** 1754–1761.
8. Boehm, T., et al. 1997. Antiangiogenic therapy of experimental cancer does not induce acquired drug resistance. *Nature* **390:** 404–407.
9. Bolla, M., et al. 1997. Improved survival in patients with locally advanced prostate cancer treated with radiotherapy and goserelin. *N. Engl. J. Med.* **337:** 295–300.
10. Bookstein, R., et al. 1993. p53 is mutated in a subset of advanced-stage prostate cancers. *Cancer Res.* **53:** 3369–3373.
11. Bostwick, D. G. and J. W. Aquilina. 1996. Prostatic intraepithelial neoplasia (PIN) and other prostatic lesions as risk factors and surrogate endpoints for cancer chemoprevention trials. *J. Cell Biochem. Suppl.* **25:** 156–164.
12. Bowen, C., S. Spiegel, and E. P. Gelmann. 1998. Radiation-induced apoptosis mediated by retinoblastoma protein. *Cancer Res.* **58:** 3275–3281.
13. Bristow, R. G., S. Benchimol, and R. P. Hill. 1996. The p53 gene as a modifier of intrinsic radiosensitivity: implications for radiotherapy. *Radiother. Oncol.* **40:** 197–223.
14. Chapman, J., et al. 1973. Chemical radioprotection and radiosensitization of mammalian cells growing in vitro. *Radiat. Res.* **56:** 291–306.
15. Chi, S. G., et al. 1997. Frequent alteration of CDKN2 (p16(INK4A)/MTS1) expression in human primary prostate carcinomas. *Clin. Cancer Res.* **3:** 1889–1897.
16. Chuba, P. J., et al. 1996. Hip stiffness following mixed conformal neutron and photon radiotherapy: a dose-volume relationship. *Int. J. Radiat. Oncol. Biol. Phys.* **35:** 693–699.
17. Critz, F. A., et al. 1998. Simultaneous radiotherapy for prostate cancer: 125I prostate implant followed by external beam radiation. *Cancer J. Sci. Am.* **4:** 359–363.
18. Critz, F. A., R. S. Tarlton, and D. A. Holladay. 1995. Prostate specific antigen-monitored combination radiotherapy for patients with prostate cancer. I-125 implant followed by external beam radiation. *Cancer.* **75:** 2383–2391.
19. Culig, Z., et al. 1995. Activation of the androgen receptor by polypeptide growth factors and cellular regulators. *World J. Urol.* **13:** 285–289.
20. Culig, Z., et al. 1995. Androgen receptor activation in prostatic tumor cell lines by insulin-like growth factor-I, keratinocyte growth factor and epidermal growth factor. *Eur. Urol.* **27(Suppl. 2):** 45–47.
21. Curie, M. S. 1904. Recherches sur les substances radioactives, in *These presentee a la Faculte des Sciences de Paris pour obtenir le grade de docteur es sciences physiques,* 2nd ed. Gauthier-Villas, Paris.

22. Dahut, W., et al. 1998. Strontium-89 and estramustine: delaying treatment failure in hormone-refractory prostate cancer. *J. Clin. Oncol.* **17**(Annual Meeting Report).

23. D'Amico, A.V., et al. 1998. Biochemical outcome after radical prostatectomy, external beam radiation therapy, or interstitial radiation therapy for clinically localized prostate cancer. *JAMA* **280**: 969–974.

24. Dattoli, M., et al. 1996. 103Pd brachytherapy and external beam irradiation for clinically localized, high-risk prostatic carcinoma. *Int. J. Radiat. Oncol. Biol. Phys.* **35**: 875–879.

25. Del Regato, J. 1968. Radiotherapy for carcinoma of the prostate. A report from the Committee for the Cooperative Study of Radiotherapy for Carcinoma of the Prostate. Penrose Cancer Hospital: Colorado Springs, CO.

26. Del Regato, J. A. 1967. Radiotherapy in the conservative treatment of operable and locally inoperable carcinoma of the prostate. *Radiology* **88**: 761–766.

27. DeWeese, T., et al. 1998. Inactivation of GSTPI genes provides a survival advantage following oxidative DNA damage in human prostate cancer cells. *Proc. Am. Assoc. Cancer Res.* **39**: 466.

28. DeWeese, T. L., et al. 1998. Mouse embryonic stem cells carrying one or two defective Msh2 alleles respond abnormally to oxidative stress inflicted by low-level radiation. *Proc. Natl. Acad. Sci. USA* **95**: 11,915–11,920.

29. DeWeese, T. L., et al. 1998. Sensitivity of human prostatic carcinoma cell lines to low dose rate radiation exposure. *J. Urol.* **159**: 591–598.

30. Dinges, S., et al. 1998. High-dose rate interstitial with external beam irradiation for localized prostate cancer—results of a prospective trial. *Radiother. Oncol.* **48**: 197–202.

31. Dische, S. 1983. Clinical trials with hypoxic cell sensitizers—the European experience. *Prog. Clin. Biol. Res.* 293–303.

32. Dong, J. T., et al. 1995. KAI1, a metastasis suppressor gene for prostate cancer on human chromosome 11p11.2. *Science* **268**: 884–886.

33. Elgamal, A. A., M. J. Troychak, and G. P. Murphy. 1998. ProstaScint scan may enhance identification of prostate cancer recurrences after prostatectomy, radiation, or hormone therapy: analysis of 136 scans of 100 patients. *Prostate* **37**: 261–269.

34. Engels, H. and A. Wambersie. 1998. Relative biological effectiveness of neutrons for cancer induction and other late effects: a review of radiobiological data. Recent results. *Cancer Res.* **150**: 54–87.

35. Forman, J. D., et al. 1996. Comparison of hyperfractionated conformal photon with conformal mixed neutron/photon irradiation in locally advanced prostate cancer. *Bull. Cancer Radiother.* **83**(Suppl.): 101s–105s.

36. Forman, J. D., et al. 1996. Conformal mixed neutron and photon irradiation in localized and locally advanced prostate cancer: preliminary estimates of the therapeutic ratio. *Int. J. Radiat. Oncol. Biol. Phys.* **35**: 259–266.

37. Fu, X. Y., et al. 1998. Restoration of the p16 gene is related to increased radiosensitivity of p16-deficient lung adenocarcinoma cell lines. *J. Cancer Res. Clin. Oncol.* **124**: 621–666.

38. Fuks, Z., et al. 1991. The effect of local control on metastatic dissemination in carcinoma of the prostate: long-term results in patients treated with 125I implantation. *Int. J. Radiat. Oncol. Biol. Phys.* **21**: 537–547.

39. Furuya, Y., et al. 1995. Androgen ablation-induced programmed death of prostatic glandular cells does not involve recruitment into a defective cell cycle or p53 induction. *Endocrinology* **136**: 1898–1906.

40. George, F. W., et al. 1965. Cobalt-60 telecurietherapy in the definitive treatment of carcinoma of the prostate: a preliminary report. *J. Urol.* **93**: 102–109.

41. Giardiello, F. M., et al. 1993. Treatment of colonic and rectal adenomas with sulindac in familial adenomatous polyposis. *N. Engl. J. Med.* **328**: 1313–1316.

42. Girinsky, T., et al. 1995. Attenuated response of p53 and p21 in primary cultures of human prostatic epithelial cells exposed to DNA-damaging agents. *Cancer Res.* **55**: 3726–3731.

43. Gorski, D. H., et al. 1998. Potentiation of the antitumor effect of ionizing radiation by brief concomitant exposures to angiostatin. *Cancer Res.* **58(24)**: 5686–5689.

44. Green, N., et al. 1984. Improved control of bulky prostate carcinoma with sequential estrogen and radiation therapy. *Int. J. Radiat. Oncol. Biol. Phys.* **10**: 971–976.

45. Gu, K., et al. 1996. Overexpression of her-2/neu in human prostate cancer and benign hyperplasia. *Cancer Lett.* **99**: 185–189.

46. Hall, E. J., et al. 1998. A preliminary report: frequency of A-T heterozygotes among prostate cancer patients with severe late responses to radiation therapy. *Cancer J. Sci. Am.* **4**: 385–389.

47. Hall, E. J. and D. J. Brenner. 1991. The dose-rate effect revisited: radiobiological considerations of importance in radiotherapy. *Int. J. Radiat. Oncol. Biol. Phys.* **21**: 1403–1414.

48. Hallahan, D. E., et al. 1995. Spatial and temporal control of gene therapy using ionizing radiation. *Nat. Med.* **1**: 786–791.

49. Hanks, G. E., et al. 1996. Conformal technique dose escalation for prostate cancer: biochemical evidence of improved cancer control with higher doses in patients with pretreatment prostate-specific antigen > or = 10 NG/ML. *Int. J. Radiat. Oncol. Biol. Phys.* **35**: 861–868.

50. Hanks, G. E., et al. 1999. Survival advantage for prostate cancer patients treated with high-dose three-dimensional conformal radiotherapy. *Cancer J. Sci. Am.* **5**: 152–158.

51. Hanna, N. N., et al. 1997. Virally directed cytosine deaminase/5-fluorocytosine gene therapy enhances radiation response in human cancer xenografts. *Cancer Res.* **57**: 4205–4209.

52. Hawkins, V., et al. 1999. PEDB: the prostate expression database. *Nucleic Acids Res.* **27**: 204–208.

53. Heidenberg, H. B., et al. 1995. Alteration of the tumor suppressor gene p53 in a high fraction of hormone refractory prostate cancer. *J. Urol.* **154**: 414–421.

54. Hockel, M., et al. 1996. Association between tumor hypoxia and malignant progression in advanced cancer of the uterine cervix. *Cancer Res.* **56**: 4509–4515.

55. Hockel, M., et al. 1993. Tumor oxygenation: a new predictive parameter in locally advanced cancer of the uterine cervix. *Gynecol. Oncol.* **51**: 141–149.

56. Holm, H. H., et al. 1983. Transperineal 125 iodine seed implantation in prostatic cancer guided by transrectal ultrasonography. *J. Urol.* **130**: 283–286.

57. Huang, A., et al. 1998. p53 and bcl-2 immunohistochemical alterations in prostate cancer treated with radiation therapy. *Urology* **51**: 346–351.

58. Isaacs, W. B., et al. 1994. Molecular biology of prostate cancer. *Semin. Oncol.* **21**: 514–521.

59. Isaacs, W. B., et al. 1995. Molecular biology of prostate cancer progression. *Cancer Surv.* **23**: 19–32.

60. Jarrard, D. F., et al. 1997. Deletional, mutational, and methylation analyses of CDKN2 (p16/MTS1) in primary and metastatic prostate cancer. *Genes Chromosomes Cancer* **19**: 90–96.

61. Joon, D. L., et al. 1997. Supraadditive apoptotic response of R3327-G rat prostate tumors to androgen ablation and radiation. *Int. J. Radiat. Oncol. Biol. Phys.* **38**: 1071–1077.

62. Kaplan, H. S. and M. A. Bagshaw. 1957. The Stanford medical linear accelerator. III. Application to clinical problems of radiation therapy. *Stanford Med. Bull.* **15**: 141–151.

63. Kimura, K., et al. 1999. Tumor necrosis factor-alpha sensitizes prostate cancer cells to gamma-irradiation-induced apoptosis. *Cancer Res.* **59**: 1606–1614.

64. Konishi, N., et al. 1997. Genetic changes in prostate cancer. *Pathol. Int.* **47(11)**: 735–747.

65. Krasilnikov, M., et al. 1999. Contribution of phosphatidylinositol 3-kinase to radiation resistance in human melanoma cells. *Mol. Carcinog.* **24**: 64–69.

66. Kyprianou, N., et al. 1997. bcl-2 over-expression delays radiation-induced apoptosis without affecting the clonogenic survival of human prostate cancer cells. *Int. J. Cancer* **70:** 341–348.

67. Lamb, H. M. and D. Faulds. 1998. Capromab pendetide. A review of its use as an imaging agent in prostate cancer. *Drugs Aging* **12:** 293–304.

68. Laramore, G. E., et al. 1993. Fast neutron radiotherapy for locally advanced prostate cancer. Final report of Radiation Therapy Oncology Group randomized clinical trial. *Am. J. Clin. Oncol.* **16:** 164–167.

69. Laverdiere, J., et al. 1997. Beneficial effect of combination hormonal therapy administered prior and following external beam radiation therapy in localized prostate cancer. *Int. J. Radiat. Oncol. Biol. Phys.* **37:** 247–252.

70. Lawton, C. A., et al. 1996. Results of a phase II trial of external beam radiation with etanidazole (SR 2508) for the treatment of locally advanced prostate cancer (RTOG Protocol 90-20). *Int. J. Radiat. Oncol. Biol. Phys.* **36:** 673–680.

71. Lee, W. H., et al. 1994. Cytidine methylation of regulatory sequences near the pi-class glutathione S-transferase gene accompanies human prostatic carcinogenesis. *Proc. Natl. Acad. Sci. USA* **91:** 11,733–11,737.

72. Lu, J., C. M. Chuong, and R. B. Widelitz. 1997. Isolation and characterization of chicken beta-catenin. *Gene* **196:** 201–207.

73. Mackey, T. J., et al. 1998. bcl-2/bax ratio as a predictive marker for therapeutic response to radiotherapy in patients with prostate cancer. *Urology* **52:** 1085–1090.

74. Mashimo, T., et al. 1998. The expression of the KAI1 gene, a tumor metastasis suppressor, is directly activated by p53. *Proc. Natl. Acad. Sci. USA* **95:** 11,307–11,311.

75. Mason, K. A. and H. R. Withers. 1977. RBE of neutrons generated by 50 MeV deuterons on beryllium for control of artificial pulmonary metastases of a mouse fibrosarcoma. *Br. J. Radiol.* **50:** 652–657.

76. Matsumura, Y., et al. 1997. Increase in radiation sensitivity of human malignant melanoma cells by expression of wild-type p16 gene. *Cancer Lett.* **115:** 91–96.

77. Mauceri, H. J., et al. 1998. Combined effects of angiostatin and ionizing radiation in antitumour therapy. *Nature* **394:** 287–291.

78. Mehta, M. P. 1998. Protection of normal tissues from the cytotoxic effects of radiation therapy: focus on amifostine. *Semin. Radiat. Oncol.* **8(4 Suppl. 1):** 14–16.

79. Miyakoshi, J., et al. 1997. Increased radiosensitivity of p16 gene-deleted human glioma cells after transfection with wild-type p16 gene. *Jpn. J. Cancer Res.* **88:** 34–38.

80. Movsas, B., et al. 1999. Hypoxic regions exist in human prostate carcinoma. *Urology* **53:** 11–18.

81. Munzenrider, J. E. and N. J. Liebsch. 1999. Proton therapy for tumors of the skull base. *Strahlenther. Onkol.* **175 (Suppl. 2):** 57–63.

82. Mydlo, J. H., et al. 1998. An analysis of microvessel density, androgen receptor, p53 and HER-2/neu expression and Gleason score in prostate cancer. Preliminary results and therapeutic implications. *Eur. Urol.* **34:** 426–432.

83. Nielsen, L. L., et al. 1998. Adenovirus-mediated p53 gene therapy and paclitaxel have synergistic efficacy in models of human head and neck, ovarian, prostate, and breast cancer. *Clin. Cancer Res.* **4:** 835–846.

84. Nishihara, E., et al. 1997. Retrovirus-mediated herpes simplex virus thymidine kinase gene transduction renders human thyroid carcinoma cell lines sensitive to ganciclovir and radiation in vitro and in vivo. *Endocrinology* **138:** 4577–4583.

85. Oshima, M., et al. 1996. Suppression of intestinal polyposis in Apc delta716 knockout mice by inhibition of cyclooxygenase 2 (COX-2). *Cell* **87:** 803–809.

86. O'Rourke, D. M., et al. 1998. Conversion of a radioresistant phenotype to a more sensitive one by disabling erbB receptor signaling in human cancer cells. *Proc. Natl. Acad. Sci. USA* **95:** 10,842–10,847.

87. Partin, A. W., et al. 1997. Combination of prostate-specific antigen, clinical stage, and Gleason score to predict pathological stage of localized prostate cancer. A multi-institutional update (published erratum appears in *JAMA* 1997 Jul 9; **278**: 118). *JAMA* **277**: 1445–1451.

88. Pesche, S., et al. 1998. PTEN/MMAC1/TEP1 involvement in primary prostate cancers. *Oncogene* **16**: 2879–2883.

89. Phillips, S. M., et al. 1994. Loss of the retinoblastoma susceptibility gene (RB1) is a frequent and early event in prostatic tumorigenesis. *Br. J. Cancer* **70**: 1252–1257.

90. Pilepich, M. V., et al. 1986. Adjuvant chemotherapy with adriamycin, cytoxan, and *cis*-platinum in high-grade carcinoma of the prostate treated with definitive radiotherapy (RTOG pilot 81-12). *Am. J. Clin. Oncol.* **9**: 135–138.

91. Pilepich, M. V., et al. 1995. Androgen deprivation with radiation therapy compared with radiation therapy alone for locally advanced prostatic carcinoma: a randomized comparative trial of the Radiation Therapy Oncology Group. *Urology* **45**: 616–623.

92. Pilepich, M., et al. 1998. Phase III Radiation therapy oncology group trial 86-10 of androgen deprivation before and during radiotherapy in locally advanced carcinoma of the prostate. *J. Clin. Oncol.* **17**(Abstract).

93. Radford, I. R. 1986. Evidence for a general relationship between the induced level of DNA double-strand breakage and cell-killing after X-irradiation of mammalian cells. *Int. J. Radiat. Biol. Relat. Stud. Phys. Chem. Med.* **49**: 611–620.

94. Ragde, H., et al. 1998. Ten-year disease free survival after transperineal sonography-guided iodine-125 brachytherapy with or without 45-gray external beam irradiation in the treatment of patients with clinically localized, low to high Gleason grade prostate carcinoma. *Cancer* **83**: 989–1001.

95. Ripple, M. O., et al. 1997. Prooxidant-antioxidant shift induced by androgen treatment of human prostate carcinoma cells. *J. Natl. Cancer Inst.* **89**: 40–48.

96. Roentgen, W. C. 1895. Ueber eine nue Art von Strahlen. *Proceedings of the Wurzburg Phisico-Medical Society*, December 28.

97. Russell, K. J., et al. 1994. Photon versus fast neutron external beam radiotherapy in the treatment of locally advanced prostate cancer: results of a randomized prospective trial. *Int. J. Radiat. Oncol. Biol. Phys.* **28**: 47–54.

98. Sano, H., et al. 1995. Expression of cyclooxygenase-1 and -2 in human colorectal cancer. *Cancer Res.* **55**: 3785–3789.

99. Scherr, D. S., et al. 1999. BCL-2 and p53 expression in clinically localized prostate cancer predicts response to external beam radiotherapy. *J. Urol.* **162**: 12–16 (discussion).

100. Schlicker, A., et al. 1999. 4-Amino-1,8-naphthalimide: a novel inhibitor of poly(ADP-ribose) polymerase and radiation sensitizer. *Int. J. Radiat. Biol.* **75**: 91–100.

101. See, W. A., et al. 1996. Brachytherapy and continuous infusion 5-fluorouracil for treatment of locally advanced, lymph node negative, prostate cancer: a phase I trial. *Cancer* **77**: 924–927.

102. Seetharam, S., et al. 1998. Modulation of apoptotic response of a radiation-resistant human carcinoma by Pseudomonas exotoxin-chimeric protein. *Cancer Res.* **58**: 3215–3220.

103. Semenza, G. L. 1998. Hypoxia-inducible factor 1 and the molecular physiology of oxygen homeostasis. *J. Lab. Clin. Med.* **131**: 207–214.

104. Shipley, W. U., et al. 1995. Advanced prostate cancer: the results of a randomized comparative trial of high dose irradiation boosting with conformal protons compared with conventional dose irradiation using photons alone. *Int. J. Radiat. Oncol. Biol. Phys.* **32**: 3–12.

105. Sintich, S. M., et al. 1999. Cytotoxic sensitivity to tumor necrosis factor-alpha in PC3 and LNCaP prostatic cancer cells is regulated by extracellular levels of SGP-2 (clusterin). *Prostate* **39**: 87–93.

106. Slater, J. D., et al. 1999. Conformal proton therapy for early-stage prostate cancer. *Urology* **53:** 978–984 (discussion).

107. Slovin, S. F., et al. 1998. Interferon-gamma and monoclonal antibody 131I-labeled CC49: outcomes in patients with androgen-independent prostate cancer. *Clin. Cancer Res.* **4:** 643–651.

108. Spitzweg, C., et al. 1999. Prostate-specific antigen (PSA) promoter-driven androgen-inducible expression of sodium iodide symporter in prostate cancer cell lines. *Cancer Res.* **59:** 2136–2141.

109. Stackhouse, M. A., et al. 1998. Radiosensitization mediated by a transfected anti-erbB-2 single-chain antibody in vitro and in vivo. *Int. J. Radiat. Oncol. Biol. Phys.* **42:** 817–822.

110. Stattin, P., et al. 1996. Pretreatment p53 immunoreactivity does not infer radioresistance in prostate cancer patients. *Int. J. Radiat. Oncol. Biol. Phys.* **35:** 885–889.

111. Steinberg, J., et al. 1997. Intracellular levels of SGP-2 (Clusterin) correlate with tumor grade in prostate cancer. *Clin. Cancer Res.* **3:** 1707–1711.

112. Sternick, E. S., ed. 1997. *The Theory and Practice of Intensity Modulated Radiation Therapy.* Advanced Medical Publishing: Madison, WI.

113. Stromberg, J. S., et al. 1997. Conformal high dose rate iridium-192 boost brachytherapy in locally advanced prostate cancer: superior prostate-specific antigen response compared with external beam treatment. *Cancer J. Sci. Am.* **3:** 346–352.

114. Suit, H. D. 1992. Local control and patient survival. *Int. J. Radiat. Oncol. Biol. Phys.* **23:** 653–660.

115. Suzuki, H., et al. 1998. Interfocal heterogeneity of PTEN/MMAC1 gene alterations in multiple metastatic prostate cancer tissues. *Cancer Res.* **58:** 204–209.

116. Tennant, M. K., et al. 1996. Protein and messenger ribonucleic acid (mRNA) for the type 1 insulin-like growth factor (IGF) receptor is decreased and IGF-II mRNA is increased in human prostate carcinoma compared to benign prostate epithelium. *J. Clin. Endocrinol. Metab.* **81:** 3774–3782.

117. Theodorescu, D., et al. 1997. p53, bcl-2 and retinoblastoma proteins as long-term prognostic markers in localized carcinoma of the prostate. *J. Urol.* **158:** 131–137.

118. Turner, B. C., et al. 1997. Insulin-like growth factor-I receptor overexpression mediates cellular radioresistance and local breast cancer recurrence after lumpectomy and radiation. *Cancer Res.* **57:** 3079–3083.

119. van der Vijgh, W. J. and G. J. Peters. 1994. Protection of normal tissues from the cytotoxic effects of chemotherapy and radiation by amifostine (Ethyol): preclinical aspects. *Semin. Oncol.* **21(5 Suppl. 11):** 2–7.

120. Verhey, L. J. 1999. Comparison of three-dimensional conformal radiation therapy and intensity-modulated radiation therapy systems. *Semin. Radiat. Oncol.* **9:** 78–98.

121. Wasserman, T. H. 1994. Radiotherapeutic studies with amifostine (Ethyol). *Semin. Oncol.* **21(5 Suppl. 11):** 21–25.

122. Watson, E. R., et al. 1978. Hyperbaric oxygen and radiotherapy: a Medical Research Council trial in carcinoma of the cervix. *Br. J. Radiol.* **51:** 879–887.

123. Weidner, N., et al. 1993. Tumor angiogenesis correlates with metastasis in invasive prostate carcinoma. *Am. J. Pathol.* **143:** 401–409.

124. Whang, Y. E., et al. 1998. Inactivation of the tumor suppressor PTEN/MMAC1 in advanced human prostate cancer through loss of expression. *Proc. Natl. Acad. Sci. USA* **95:** 5246–5250.

125. Wick, W., et al. 1999. PTEN gene transfer in human malignant glioma: sensitization to irradiation and CD95L-induced apoptosis. *Oncogene* **18:** 3936–3943.

126. Yang, C. R., et al. 1999. Isolation of Ku70-binding proteins (KUBs). *Nucleic Acids Res.* **27:** 2165–2174.

127. Young, H. H. and W. A. Frontz. 1917. Some new methods in the treatment of carcinoma of the lower genito-urinary tract with radium. *J. Urol.* **1:** 505–541.
128. Zelefsky, M. J., et al. 1999. Long term tolerance of high dose three-dimensional conformal radiotherapy in patients with localized prostate carcinoma. *Cancer* **85:** 2460–2468.
129. Zelefsky, M. J. and W. F. Whitmore, Jr. 1997. Long-term results of retropubic permanent 125-iodine implantation of the prostate for clinically localized prostatic cancer. *J. Urol.* **158:** 23–29; discussion 29,30.
130. Zhang, H., et al. 1999. Apoptosis induced by overexpression of hMSH2 or hMLH1. *Cancer Res.* **59:** 3021–3027.
131. Zhang, S., et al. 1998. Expression of potential target antigens for immunotherapy on primary and metastatic prostate cancers. *Clin. Cancer Res.* **4:** 295–302.
132. Zietman, A. L., et al. 1997. The effect of androgen deprivation and radiation therapy on an androgen-sensitive murine tumor: an in vitro and in vivo study. *Cancer J. Sci. Am.* **3:** 31–36.

Table 2
Combination Chemotherapy Trials in Hormone Refractory
Prostate Cancer: Pre-PSA Era

Regimen	# Patients	Response %	Reference(s)
Cyclophosphamide/Cisplatin/Doxorubicin	40	5–33	*58,59*
Cyclophosphamide/Cisplatin/Prednisone	22	0	*60*
Cyclophosphamide/MTX/5-FU	15	7	*61*
Cyclophosphamide/Doxorubicin/BCl	27	26	*62*
Cyclophosphamide/Doxorubicin	93	0–32	*63–67*
Cyclophosphamide/5-FU	13	8	*64*
Estramustine/Prednimustine	54	2	*35*
Estramustine/Cisplatin	42	0	*10*
Estramustine/Vincristine	4	0	*18*
Doxorubicin/Methotrexate/5-FU	160	0–48	*68–71*
Chlorambucil/Prednisone	11	0	*72*
Carboplatin/Epirubicin/Etoposide	12	25	*73*
Cisplatin/Mitoxantrone	44	12	*74*

standard measurable disease criteria as well as an evaluation of prostatic-acid phosphotase, recalcification of osteolytic lesions, and resolution of osteoblastic sites of disease. However, this created further problems. Osseous metastases can be difficult to quantitate, and bone scans as a measure of disease response are not reliable. Because of this, patients were determined to have responded if they were "clinically stable." Response came to mean one of several different things; either a reduction in objective tumor size, an improvement in well being, or a decrease in a surrogate marker. Many clinical investigators remained skeptical of the ability to reproducibly assess response to chemotherapy in this group of patients.

3. THE PRESENT: CHEMOTHERAPY IN THE ERA OF PSA

The arrival of PSA ushered in a new era in the treatment of prostate cancer. The assay was simple to perform, reproducible, and readily available. A number of early trials included PSA decline as a marker of response along with more traditional measurements. Research into the treatment of hormone refractory prostate cancer accelerated. Also, a broader patient population was now included in the trials. Patients were no longer required to have measurable soft-tissue disease; patients with only bone disease could be included and assessed by PSA response. A number of trials using PSA decline as a marker of tumor response have demonstrated increased response rates. Response rates for each of these "first-generation" regimens is about 50%. The pessimism associated with chemotherapy for hormone refractory prostate cancer has diminished. In fact, in its guidelines for the management of prostate cancer, the National Comprehensive Cancer Network (NCCN) suggests a trial of chemotherapy as a treatment option for advanced disease. The five regimens suggested by the NCCN represent the "state of the art" at the end of the 20th century in the chemotherapy of hormone refractory disease (Table 3).

Table 3
Present Chemotherapy for Hormone Refractory Prostate Cancer

Regimen	Schedule	PSA response	Soft-tissue response	Reference
Ketoconazole	1200 mg/d	55%	58%	*85*
Doxorubicin	20 mg/m^2 iv over 24 q wk			
Vinblastine	4 mg/m^2 weekly × 6	54–61%	14–40%	*81,88,89*
Estramustine	600 mg/m^2 × 42 d			
Etoposide	50 mg/m^2/d × 21 d	39–58%	45–53%	*91–93*
Estramustine	10 mg/kg/d × 21 d			
Mitoxantrone	12 mg/m^2 iv q 21 d	33%	NA	*79*
Prednisone	10 mg daily			
Paclitaxel	120 mg/m^2 iv over 96 h q 3 wk	53%	44%	*102*
Estramustine	600 mg/m^2/d continuously			

3.1. PSA as a Marker of Response

PSA, a 34-kDa protein produced almost exclusively by the prostate and prostate cancer cells, has been demonstrated to be a sensitive and specific marker of response following surgery and radiation therapy for localized prostate cancer *(74,117)*. More recently, it has been used as an indicator of disease and response to therapy in patients with metastatic disease. PSA has been used since 1992 as an indicator of response in a number of trials of cytotoxic agents in hormone refractory prostate cancer.

Several trials have shown a direct relationship between decline in PSA and shrinkage of bidimensional measurable tumor. A trial of weekly epirubicin in 39 HRPC patients with bidimensional measurable disease demonstrated a positive trend between declining PSA and reduction in measurable tumor *(12)*. Declines in PSA have also been correlated with improved quality of life in HRPC patients *(108)*.

PSA response has also been investigated as a prognostic tool. Kelly and colleagues analyzed PSA response in 110 patients treated in seven sequential HRPC protocols at Memorial Sloan Kettering *(47)*. Utilizing a landmark analysis, they found a longer median survival rate for patients who experienced at least a 50% decline in PSA at 60 d from the start of treatment. A multivariate analysis of prognostic factors found a greater than 50% decline in PSA along with the natural log of the LDH to be the two most significant variables in predicting survival. In a trial of estramustine phosphate and vinblastine, patients who experienced a PSA decline of greater than 50% on three successive measurements were found to have significantly prolonged overall and progression-free survival *(34)*. A landmark analysis of 114 patients enrolled in two trials of estramustine and etoposide demonstrated that a PSA decline of greater than 50% from baseline at 8 wk into therapy was associated with improved survival *(100)*. Median survival for patients with and without a greater than 50% decline in PSA was 91 wk and 38 wk, respectively. A PSA decline of 50% or more has also been associated with prolonged survival in patients treated with megesterol acetate and suramin *(17,27)*.

A reduction of pretreatment PSA by 50% at 8 wk of therapy is a useful predictor for survival and disease response for most cytotoxic agents. The use of PSA with differentiating agents, antigrowth-factor agents, gene therapy, and immunotherapy has not yet been determined. In addition, no absolute value of pretreatment PSA has yet been correlated with disease response or survival.

3.2. Current Chemotherapy Regimens

3.2.1. Ketoconazole and Doxorubicin

The combination of doxorubicin and ketoconazole has been evaluated in a Phase II trial *(97)*. Thirty-nine patients who had progressed following initial hormone therapy were treated with weekly infusions of doxorubicin (20 mg/m^2 over 24 h) and daily ketoconazole (1200 mg daily). Patients received hydrocortisone only at the time of developing clinical adrenal insufficiency; 63% required this intervention at some time during the therapy. A PSA decline of greater than 50% from baseline was seen in 21 of 38 (55%) assessable patients. Seven of the twelve patients (58%) with bidimensional measurable disease demonstrated a partial response.

Therapy was complicated by the development of significant acral erythema and stomatitis in 29% of patients. This symptom did not require cessation of therapy, and resolved with the discontinuation of doxorubicin. Upon resolution, the doxorubicin was restarted and the reaction did not recur. Also, two patients with a history of coronary artery disease experienced sudden death while on therapy. One other patient experienced congestive heart failure. Seventeen patients (45%) required hospitalization for complications.

3.2.2. Vinblastine and Estramustine

Vinblastine has yielded minimal response as a single agent in HRPC *(19)*. However, the combination of vinblastine and estramustine has demonstrated synergistic cytotoxicity in preclinical models of prostate cancer *(5)*. Based on this interaction, the combination (vinblastine 4 mg/m^2 weekly accompanied by estramustine phosphate 600 mg/m^2 or 10 mg/kg daily for 6 wk followed by a 2-wk rest period) has been tested in clinical trials of patients with hormone refractory prostate cancer *(3,34,95)*. Response rates of 14–40% were demonstrated for patients with bidimensional measurable disease. PSA declines of greater than 50% were found in 54–61% of patients. The therapy was well tolerated. One trial demonstrated that patients who experienced a greater than 50% decline in PSA on three separate occasions had significantly prolonged overall and progression-free survival *(34)*.

3.2.3. Etoposide and Estramustine

Both estramustine and etoposide exert an effect through the nuclear matrix, and the interaction of these two agents has been studied *(78)*. In vitro, a combination of the two drugs has been demonstrated to have enhanced cytotoxicity and to impair DNA synthesis at the level of the nuclear matrix. In vivo, a combination of the two drugs was more effective at suppressing tumor growth than either agent alone.

The synergistic interaction between these two agents formed the basis for a Phase II trial *(81)*. Both agents were given orally (estramustine 15/mg/kg/d in four divided doses and etoposide 50 mg/m^2/d in two divided doses) for 3 wk with a 1-wk rest period. Of the eighteen patients with bidimensional measurable disease, 50% had objective responses: three complete and six partial. A PSA decline of greater than 50% from baseline was demonstrated in 55% of patients. Estramustine caused significant nausea in 29% of patients, and two patients withdrew secondary to this toxicity. A second trial examined the combination but used a lower dose of estramustine (10 mg/kg/d) *(80)*. This trial enrolled 62 patients and demonstrated a PSA decline of greater than 50% from baseline in 39% of patients and objective partial responses in 8 of 15 (53%) patients with measurable disease. Toxicity was similar, although the regimen was more tolerable for patients with less nausea. Median survival was 14 mo. A third trial using an even lower dose of estramustine (140 mg three times a day) with etoposide (50 mg/m^2/d) in 56 patients demonstrated similar results *(22)*. Forty-five percent of 33 patients with bidimensional measurable disease achieved an objective response: five complete and ten partial responses. A PSA decline of greater than 50% from baseline was seen in 58% of patients. Median survival was 13 mo.

The combined results of the three trials demonstrate soft-tissue responses in 45–53% of patients, PSA declines of greater than 50% in 39–58%, and median survival of 52–56 wk.

Currently, it is our practice to treat patients with 280 mg estramustine three times a day and etoposide 50 mg twice a day. Patients are instructed to take the estramustine with food while avoiding calcium-rich products (milk, yogurt, ice cream, calcium-containing antacids) which can interfere with absorption *(32)*. This regimen produces mild nausea, but is generally well tolerated.

3.2.4. Mitoxantrone and Prednisone

Mitoxantrone is a semisynthetic anthracenedione with some structural similarity to doxorubicin. Early studies of single-agent mitoxantrone demonstrated modest activity with good toleration of the drug *(44,76)*. These observations led to a trial of mitoxantrone in HRPC using palliative endpoints as response criteria. Moore and colleagues conducted a Phase II study of 27 patients using mitoxantrone (12 mg/m^2 iv every 21 d) and prednisone (10 mg/d continuously) *(63)*. The primary endpoints were quality of life, pain indices, and analgesic usage. A complete response was the resolution of all disease-related symptoms. A palliative partial response was defined to be a 50% reduction in analgesic usage with no increase in pain, or a decrease by two points in a six-point pain scale with no increase in analgesic usage. Progression was defined as either an increase in analgesic use, an increase by one in the six-point pain scale, or new bone pain requiring palliative radiotherapy. Patients who did not meet either of these criteria were labeled as having stable disease. Using these palliative response criteria, 36% of patients experienced a complete response, 44% experienced a partial response, and 20% had stable disease. Overall, there was a modest reduction in analgesic usage. Quality-of-life analyses revealed decreases in pain throughout treatment; social functioning also improved. However, there was no improvement in overall quality of life. Serious toxicity was limited to hematologic; however, no patients required hospitalization.

A larger randomized trial using similar palliative endpoints and definitions of response compared the combination of mitoxantrone (12 mg/m^2 every 21 d) and prednisone (10 mg/d continuously) to prednisone alone *(108)*. In this trial of 161 men with hormone refractory prostate cancer, the primary endpoint was achieved in 29% of the mitoxantrone/prednisone patients and 12% of the prednisone-alone patients. The median duration of response for the mitoxantrone/prednisone arm (43 wk) was significantly longer than the prednisone-alone arm (18 wk). Patients who demonstrated a response had significant improvement in quality-of-life scales measuring overall well-being.

3.2.5. Paclitaxel and Estramustine

Paclitaxel and estramustine, two drugs with demonstrated antimicrotubule activity, possess different mechanisms of action. Estramustine has been demonstrated to promote inappropriate microtubule disassembly, with accompanying cytotoxicity *(16)*. Conversely, paclitaxel inhibits normal microtubule disassembly and thereby induces cytotoxicity *(88)*.

A Phase II trial of paclitaxel alone in 24 patients with hormone refractory prostate cancer demonstrated only one objective response *(87)*. However, the combination of paclitaxel and estramustine phosphate has demonstrated synergistic cytotoxicity in both animal and human prostate cancer cell lines *(79,105)*. Hudes and colleagues utilized this synergism to conduct a trial of estramustine phosphate (600 mg/m^2/d, continuously) and paclitaxel (120 mg/m^2 by 96 h continuous infusion every 21 d) in 34 hormone refractory prostate cancer patients *(35)*. The preclinical activity of the combination was verified in this patient population. Four of nine patients (44%) with measurable disease demonstrated an objective response (two-thirds with liver metastasis and two-sixths with lymph node disease). A PSA decline of greater than 50% from baseline was achieved in 17 of 32 (53%) evaluable patients. Median response duration was 37 wk, with a median survival time of 69 wk. Notably, all patients continued to have testicular androgen suppression during the trial.

4. THE NEXT STEP: NEW APPROACHES

4.1. New Chemotherapy Regimens

The five regimens of the NCCN guidelines represent a significant step forward in the treatment of hormone refractory prostate cancer. In general, the response rates are 50% for PSA and 40–50% for soft tissue disease. Several new combinations have demonstrated higher response rates and will most likely be the foundation for future investigation (Table 4).

4.1.1. Paclitaxel, Estramustine, and Etoposide

In addition to its effect at the nuclear matrix, estramustine has an effect against microtubules. The drug has been shown to promote microtubule disassembly through interaction with microtubule-associated proteins and tubulin *(16,106)*. Paclitaxel achieves its antineoplastic effect through interaction with microtubules. The microtubules formed in the presence of paclitaxel are extraordinarily stable and dysfunctional *(88)*. Preclinical studies of the combination of estramustine and paclitaxel have shown a synergistic inhibition on prostate cancer cell growth *(79,105)*. These preclinical studies demonstrate that estramustine potentiates the effect of agents which act independently at the nuclear matrix (i.e., etoposide) and with microtubules (i.e., paclitaxel). Preclinical cytotoxicity assays, both in vitro and in vivo, demonstrate an increased effect for the three-drug combination compared to any two-drug combination *(79)*.

Table 4
Emerging Chemotherapy for Hormone Refractory Prostate Cancer

Regimen	Schedule	PSA response %	Soft-tissue response %	Reference
Paclitaxel	135 mg/m^2 on d 2	65	45	*104*
Estramustine	50 mg/m^2/d × 14 d			
Etoposide	10 mg/kg/d × 14 d			
Ketoconazole	1200 mg/d on wk 1,3,5	67	75	*105*
Doxorubicin	20 mg/m^2 iv over 24 h/wk on wk 1,3,5			
Vinblastine	5 mg/m^2 weekly on wk 2,4,6			
Estramustine	520 mg/d on wk 2,4,6			
Docetaxel	60–70 mg/m^2 on d 2	58–63	28–56	*108,109*
Estramustine	10 mg/kg/day on d 1–5			

The three-drug combination was evaluated in a Phase II trial of 40 patients with hormone refractory prostate cancer *(101)*. The regimen consisted of estramustine 10 mg/kg/d and etoposide 50 mg/m^2/d for the first 14 d of a 21-d cycle along with paclitaxel 135 mg/m^2 on d 2. Ten of 22 patients (45%) with bidimensional measurable disease experienced a soft-tissue response; nine of these were partial and one was complete. Twenty-six patients (65%) had a PSA decline of greater than 50% from baseline, with 16 patients showing a decrease of greater than 75%. The median duration of response was 3.2 mo, with a maximum of 8.7 mo. The regimen was tolerated with neutropenia as the most common event. Three patients developed deep venous thrombosis. Quality-of-life analysis found no decline in overall measures during therapy.

4.1.2. Alternating Weekly Chemohormonal Therapy

Another novel approach to chemotherapy involves the use of concurrent chemo-hormonal therapy. Patients with disease progression on one regimen often respond to another regimen. This observation was the foundation for an approach involving alternating weekly regimens *(30)*. The two components used both had hormonal agents as part of the treatment to ensure continued hormonal suppression. The approach involved alternating cycles of doxorubicin (20 mg/m^2 over 24 h) and ketoconazole (1200 mg daily) on wk 1, 3, and 5. During wk 2, 4, and 6 patients received vinblastine (5 mg/m^2) and estramustine (140 mg by mouth 3 times/d). A PSA decline of greater than 50% was seen in 67% of patients. Sixteen patients had measurable soft-tissue disease; 75% of these demonstrated a response (11 partial and 1 complete). The median duration of response was 8 mo. The therapy was well tolerated; peripheral edema was the most common side effect.

4.1.3. Docetaxel and Estramustine

Docetaxel, a semisynthetic taxane, has been evaluated in preclinical models of prostate cancer. Prostate cancer cell lines are highly sensitive to docetaxel—the IC$_{50}$ for LNCaP and PC-3 cells is approx 2 nM *(43)*. In vivo, the combination of docetaxel and estramustine was more effective at suppressing tumor growth than docetaxel alone in the Dunning rat prostate adenocarcinoma model *(43)*. Also, microtubule stabilization is more efficient with docetaxel relative to paclitaxel *(21)*.

A Phase I trial investigated the maximum tolerated dose (MTD) for the combination of docetaxel and estramustine *(77)*. In this trial, estramustine was administered over the first five days rather than continuously. Docetaxel was administered on day 2 and the dosage was increased from 40 mg/m^2 up to 80mg/m^2. Patients were divided into two categories based upon prior therapy (either minimal or extensive). The MTD for the minimally pretreated group was 70 mg/m^2, and for the extensively pretreated group it was 60 mg/m^2. Overall, 63% of patients experienced a decline in PSA of greater than 50%. The response was most dramatic in the patients with minimal prior treatment. In this group, 70% of patients had declines of greater than 50% in PSA, with five patients having normalization of their PSA levels. Analgesia use was discontinued in 50% of patients who required pain relief prior to treatment. Soft-tissue responses were seen in 28% (5/18) of patients with bidimensional measurable disease.

A CALGB trial treated hormone refractory prostate cancer patients with estramustine 10 mg/kg/d for 5 d, docetaxel 70 mg/m^2 on day 2 and low-dose daily hydrocortisone over a 21-d cycle *(90)*. Preliminary results demonstrate a PSA response rate of 58% (11/19 patients) and a soft-tissue response rate of 56% (5/9 patients). Notably, a majority of the PSA responses (7/11) were greater than 75%.

Another study evaluating the combination used a standard dose of docetaxel (70 mg/m^2) but substituted the 5-d estramustine treatment course with a 1-d dose (280 mg every 6 h for 5 doses) *(98)*. The response rates in this trial were 31% (4/13) for PSA decline and 29% (2/7) for soft-tissue response. Although patient selection makes comparison of Phase II trials difficult, the decreased response rate seen in this trial suggests that a longer rather than shorter course of estramustine is preferable.

Further studies of the combination of docetaxel and estramustine are ongoing, and hopefully will confirm the activity of this regimen as well as the proper dose and duration of therapy for both drugs.

4.2. Systemic Treatment for Early-Stage Disease

Another novel approach that will be more fully investigated in the coming years entails administering systemic therapy in the earlier stages of disease. This approach has been studied with the use of androgen suppression prior to prostatectomy or following radiation therapy in patients with early-stage disease. Neoadjuvant hormonal therapy has failed to demonstrate prolonged disease-free survival in patients treated with prostatectomy *(114)*. However, adjuvant androgen suppression has been associated with both prolonged disease-free progression and overall survival in patients with locally-advanced prostate cancer treated with radiation therapy *(11)*. Investigators are now beginning to evaluate the addition of chemotherapy to traditional treatments for early-stage prostate cancer.

4.2.1. Neoadjuvant Chemotherapy and Radiation Therapy

The development of regimens with increased activity has allowed the role of neoadjuvant chemotherapy prior to definitive radiation therapy for locally advanced prostate cancer to be investigated. Estramustine has been demonstrated to enhance the cytotoxicity of radiation for prostate cancer cell lines, human xenograft tumors growing in nude mice, and in the Dunning rat prostate adenocarcinoma model *(29,89,113)*. Also, chronic estramustine therapy is effective in suppressing testosterone to castration levels in a majority of patients *(9,45)*. Both of these attributes make estramustine an attractive agent in combination with radiation therapy.

Weekly estramustine and vinblastine have been tested as concurrent treatments with radiation therapy for locally advanced prostate cancer *(48)*. This regimen produced a biochemical control rate of 48% at 5 yr, and was well tolerated with no significant increase in toxicity.

The neoadjuvant administration of estramustine (10 mg/kg/d) and etoposide (500 mg/ms2) followed by concurrent single-agent estramustine (10 mg/kg/d) during definitive radiotherapy has been studied in 13 patients with locally-advanced prostate cancer *(7)*. PSA values fell from a median of 35 ng/mL to a value of 2.6 ng/mL following the induction of chemotherapy. The chemotherapy was well tolerated; the development of a deep venous thrombosis in one patient was the major toxicity. One patient experienced a local relapse. Four patients had a prostate biopsy 18 mo after completion of treatment, and one showed evidence of residual disease. All other patients remain in biochemical control. Although this approach appears to be well tolerated, the efficacy of the regimen needs to be established. This information will be available as this study matures and other trials are initiated.

4.2.2. Neoadjuvant Chemotherapy and Prostatectomy

The feasibility of neoadjuvant chemotherapy is beginning to be investigated. Researchers at M.D. Anderson treated 33 patients with locally advanced prostate cancer with neoadjuvant chemotherapy (alternating doxorubicin/ketoconazole and vinblastine/estramustine) for two cycles prior to prostatectomy *(82)*. Following chemotherapy, pelvic lymph node dissection was uncomplicated, but the prostatic dissection off the rectal wall was more difficult secondary to chemotherapy-induced changes. There was no increase in postoperative complications. All of the patients achieved an undetectable PSA nadir, and 26 patients remain recurrence-free. This study has demonstrated the feasibility of neoadjuvant chemotherapy. However, the impact of relapse-free survival will need to be determined to ensure that the more difficult prostate resection has not affected relapse rates.

4.3. Cytoreduction Followed by Chronic Maintenance Therapy

Another novel theoretical approach involves the combination of chemotherapy and a novel agent to suppress the regrowth of the residual malignant cells. The chemotherapy regimens developed are effective at reducing the tumor burden in patients with hormone refractory disease. However, the disease is not eradicated. The eventual regrowth of chemotherapy-resistant disease is the natural history of the disease. This approach would involve the administration of chemotherapy to reduce the tumor to a minimal size. Once the tumor has been cytoreduced, a single agent or a combination of agents could be administered to control the tumor's growth. The ideal agent in this setting would limit tumor growth while exhibiting minimal toxicity. No agent currently fits into this category. However, antiangiogenesis, signal transduction inhibitors, and matrix metalloprotease inhibitors all offer the potential of finding a role in this setting. This approach currently exists in theory alone, but future research will certainly utilize the paradigm in hopes of obtaining long-term control of tumor growth for patients with hormone refractory prostate cancer.

5. CONCLUSION

An enormous effort has been invested in understanding the role of chemotherapy in patients with hormone refractory prostate cancer. The advent of PSA as a marker of disease has brought about an acceleration in this research during the last decade. Chemotherapy regimens are currently available which can reduce the burden of disease. Response rates are improving, and patients are demonstrating clinical improvement. Phase III studies will investigate whether the use of chemotherapy in this setting offers an improvement in survival. Encouraged by the improvements in patients with advanced disease, researchers are now investigating the use of chemotherapy in early-stage prostate cancer. Also, the combination of chemotherapy with novel tumor growth-suppressing agents offers a new paradigm for the management of hormone refractory prostate cancer in the 21st century.

REFERENCES

1. Ansfield, F. J., J. Schroeder, and A. R. Curreri. 1962. Five years clinical experience with 5-fluorouracil. *JAMA* **181:** 295–299.
2. Atkins, J. N., H. B. Muss, D. Case, et al. 1991. High-dose 24-hour infusion of 5-fluorouracil in metastatic prostate cancer. A phase II trial of the Piedmont Oncology Association. *Am. J. Clin. Oncol.* **14:** 526–529.
3. Attivissimo, L. A., J. V. Fetten, and W. Kreis. 1996. Symptomatic improvement associated with combined estramustine and vinblastine chemotherapy for metastatic prostate cancer. *Am. J. Clin. Oncol.* **19:** 581–583.
4. Babaian, R. J. and S. D. Hsu. 1984. Chemotherapy of hormone refractory carcinoma of prostate with 5-fluorouracil, adriamycin, and mitomycin C. *Urology* **23:** 272–275.
5. Batra, S., R. Karlsson, and L. Witt. 1996. Potentiation by estramustine of the cytotoxic effect of vinblastine and doxorubicin in prostatic tumor cells. *Int. J. Cancer* **68:** 644–649.
6. Beckley, S., L. Z. Wajsman, N. H. Slack, and G. P. Murphy. 1981. Chemotherapy in metastatic, hormone refractory prostatic cancer using chlorambucil in combination with prednisolone versus conjugate, prednimustine (Leo 1031). *Urology* **17:** 446–448.
7. Ben-Josef, E., S. Han, W. Mertens, et al. 1999. Neoadjuvant estramustine/etoposide followed by concurrent estramustine and definitive radiotherapy for locally advanced prostate cancer. *Proc. Annu. Meet. Am. Soc. Clin. Oncol.* **18:** A1238.
8. Berry, J. and R. N. MacDonald. 1982. Cisplatin, cyclophosphamide and prednisone therapy for stage D prostatic cancer. *Cancer Treat. Rep.* **66:** 1403–1404.
9. Bishop, M. C., C. Selby, and M. Taylor. 1985. Plasma hormone levels in patients with prostatic carcinoma treated with diethylstilbestrol and estramustine. *Br. J. Urol.* **57:** 542–547.
10. Blumenstein, B., E. D. Crawford, J. H. Saiers, R. L. Stephens, S. E. Rivkin, and C. A. Coltman Jr. 1993. Doxorubicin, mitomycin C and 5-fluorouracil in the treatment of hormone refractory adenocarcinoma of the prostate: a Southwest Oncology Group study. *J. Urol.* **150:** 411–413.
11. Bolla, M., D. Gonzalez, P. Warde, et al. 1997. Improved survival in patients with locally advanced prostate cancer treated with radiotherapy and goserelin. *N. Engl. J. Med.* **337:** 295–300.
12. Brausi, M., W. G. Jones, S. D. Fossa, et al. 1995. High dose epirubicin is effective in measurable metastatic prostate cancer: a phase II study of the EORTC Genitourinary Group (see comments). *Eur. J. Cancer* **31A:** 1622–1626.
13. Bui, N. B., J. Chauvergne, R. Brunet, P. Richaud, C. Lagarde, and M. Le Guillou. 1986. Metastatic cancer of the prostate: phase II study of spirogeranium (NSC 192965). *Bull. Cancer (Paris)* **73:** 65–67.

14. Canobbio, L., D. Guarneri, L. Miglietta, A. Decensi, F. Oneto, and F. Boccardo. 1993. Carboplatin in advanced hormone refractory prostatic cancer patients. *Eur. J. Cancer* **29A:** 2094–2096.

15. Catane, R., J. H. Kaufman, S. Madajewicz, A. Mittelman, and G. P. Murphy. 1978. Prednimustine therapy for advanced prostatic cancer. *Br. J. Urol.* **50:** 29–32.

16. Dahllof, B., A. Billstrom, F. Cabal, and B. Hartley-Asp. 1993. Estramustine depolymerizes microtubules by binding to tubulin. *Cancer Res.* **53:** 4573–4581.

17. Dawson, N. A., S. Halabi, V. Hars, E. J. Small, and N. J. Vogelzang. 1999. Prostate specific antigen decline as a predictor of survival: Cancer and Leukemia Group B 9181. *Proc. Annu. Meet. Am. Soc. Clin. Oncol.* **18:** A1209.

18. deKernion, J.B. and A. Lindner. 1984. Chemotherapy of hormonally unresponsive prostatic carcinoma. *Urol. Clin. N. Am.* **11:** 319–326.

19. Dexeus, F., C. J. Logothetis, M. L. Samuels, E. Hossan, and A. C. Von Eschenbach. 1985. Continuous infusion of vinblastine for advanced hormone refractory prostate cancer. *Cancer Treat. Rep.* **69:** 885–886.

20. Dexeus, F. H., C. Logothetis, M. L. Samuels, et al. 1986. Phase II study of spirogeranium in metastatic prostate cancer. *Cancer Treat. Rep.* **70:** 1129–1130.

21. Diaz, J. F. and J. M. Andreu. 1993. Assembly of purified GDP-tubulin into microtubules induced by taxol and taxotere: reversibility, ligand stoichiometry and competition. *Biochemistry* **32:** 2747–2755.

22. Dimopoulos, M. A., C. Panopoulos, C. Bamia, et al. 1997. Oral estramustine and oral etoposide for hormone refractory prostate cancer. *Urology* **50:** 754–758.

23. Drelichman, A., R. Brownlee, and M. Al-Sarraf. 1981. Phase II study of hexamethylmelamine for disseminated prostatic carcinoma. *Cancer Clin. Trials* **4:** 309–312.

24. Drelichman, A., D. A. Decker, M. Al-Saraff, and C. B. Dhabuwala. 1982. M-AMSA in disseminated prostatic carcinoma: a phase II study. *Cancer Treat. Rep.* **66:** 1993–1994.

25. Drelichman, A., J. Oldford, and M. Al-Sarraf. 1985. Evaluation of cyclophosphamide, adriamycin and *cis*-platinum (CAP) in patients with disseminated prostatic carcinoma. A phase II study. *Am. J. Clin. Oncol.* **8:** 255–259.

26. Eisenberger, M. A. 1988. Chemotherapy for prostate cancer. *NCI Monographs* **7:** 151–163.

27. Eisenberger, M., M. Meyer, P. Lenehan, et al. 1999. Suramin induced decrease in PSA is associated with prolonged objective progression-free and overall survival in hormone refractory prostate cancer. *Proc. Annu. Meet. Am. Soc. Clin. Oncol.* **18:** A1208.

28. Eisenberger, M. A., R. Simon, and P. J. O'Dwyer. 1985. A re-evaluation of non-hormonal cytotoxic chemotherapy in the treatment of prostatic carcinoma. *J. Clin. Oncol.* **3:** 827–841.

29. Eklov, S., J. E. Westlin, G. Rikner, and S. Nilsson. 1994. Estramustine potentiates the radiation effect in human prostate tumor transplant in nude mice. *Prostate* **24:** 39–45.

30. Ellerhorst, J. A., S. Tu, R. J. Amato, et al. 1997. Phase II trail of alternating weekly chemohormonal therapy for patients with androgen-independent prostate cancer. *Clin. Cancer Res.* **3:** 2371–2376.

31. Fuse, H., Y. Muraishi, Y. Fujishiro, and T. Katayama. 1996. Etoposide, epirubicin and carboplatin in hormone refractory prostate cancer. *Int. Urol. Nephrol.* **28:** 79–85.

32. Gunnarsson, P. O., T. Davidsson, S. B. Andersson, C. Backman, and S. A. Johansson. 1990. Impairment of estramustine phosphate absorption by concurrent intake of milk and food. *Eur. J. Clin. Pharmacol.* **38:** 189–193.

33. Hansen, R., T. Moynihan, P. Beatty, et al 1991. Continuous systemic 5-fluorouracil infusion in refractory prostatic cancer. *Urology* **37:** 358–361.

34. Hudes, G. R., R. Greenberg, R. L. Krigel, et al. 1992. Phase II study of estramustine and vinblastine, two microtubule inhibitors, in hormone refractory prostate cancer. *J. Clin. Oncol.* **10:** 1754–1761.

35. Hudes, G. R., F. Nathan, C. Khater, et al. 1997. Phase II trial of 96-hour paclitaxel plus oral estramustine phosphate in metastatic hormone refractory prostate cancer. *J. Clin. Oncol.* **15**: 3156–3163.

36. Huggins, C. and C. Hodges. 1941. Studies on prostatic cancer. I: The effect of castration, of estrogen and of androgen injection on serum phosphatases in metastatic carcinoma of the prostate. *Cancer Res.* **1**: 293–297.

37. Huggins, C., W. W. Scott, and C. V. Hodges. 1941. Studies on prostatic cancer III. The effects of fever, of deoxycorticosterone and of estrogen on clinical patients with metastatic carcinoma of the prostate. *J. Urol.* **46**: 997–1001.

38. Huggins, C., R. E. Stevens, and C. Hodges. 1941. Studies on prostatic cancer. II: The effects of castration on advanced carcinoma of the prostate gland. *Arch. Surg.* **43**: 209–223.

39. Hussain, M. H., K. J. Pienta, B. G. Redman, G. D. Cummings, and L. E. Flaherty. 1994. Oral etoposide in the treatment of hormone refractory prostate cancer. *Cancer* **74**: 100–103.

40. Ihde, D. C., P. A. Bunn, M. H. Cohen, et al. 1980. Effective treatment of hormonally-unresponsive metastatic carcinoma of the prostate with adriamycin and cyclophosphamide. Methods of documenting tumor response and progression. *Cancer* **45**: 1300–1310.

41. Izbicki, R. M., M. H. Amer, and M. Al-Sarraf. 1979. Combination of adriamycin and cyclophosphamide in the treatment of metastatic prostatic carcinoma. *Cancer Treat. Rep.* **63**: 999–1001.

42. Jones, W. G., S. D. Fossa, L. Denis, et al. 1983. An EORTC phase II study of vindesine in advanced prostate cancer. *Eur. J. Cancer Clin. Oncol.* **19**: 583–588.

43. Kamradt, J. M., M. A. Walsh, S. K. Brumfield, J. F. Williams, and K. J. Pienta. 1999. Docetaxel and estramustine: activity in preclinical models of prostate cancer. *Proc. Annu. Meet. Am. Assoc. Cancer Res.* **40**: A1553.

44. Kantoff, P. W., C. Block, L. Letvak, and M. George. 1993. 14-day continuous infusion of mitoxantrone in hormone refractory metastatic adenocarcinoma of the prostate. *Am. J. Clin. Oncol.* **16**: 489–491.

45. Karr, J. P., Z. Wajsman, R. Y. Kirdani, G. P. Murphy, and A. A. Sandberg. 1980. Effects of diethylstilbestrol and estramustine phosphate on serum sex hormone binding globulin and testosterone levels in prostate cancer patients. *J. Urol.* **124**: 232–236.

46. Kasimis, B. S., E. M. Moran, J. B. Miller, et al. 1983. Treatment of hormone-resistant metastatic carcinoma of the prostate with 5-FU, doxorubicin and mitomycin (FAM): a preliminary report. *Cancer Treat. Rep.* **67**: 937–939.

47. Kelly, W. K., H. I. Scher, M. Mazumdar, V. Vlamis, M. Schwartz, and S. D. Fossa. 1993. Prostate-specific antigen as a measure of disease outcome in metastatic hormone-refractory prostate cancer. *J. Clin. Oncol.* **11**: 607–615.

48. Khil, M. S., J. H. Kim, L. J. Bricker, and J. C. Cerny. 1997. Tumor control of locally advanced prostate cancer following combined estramustine, vinblastine and radiation therapy. *Cancer J. Sci. Am.* **3**: 289–296.

49. Kuss, R., S. Khoury, F. Richard, et al. 1980. Estramustine phosphate in the treatment of advanced prostatic cancer. *Br. J. Urol.* **52**: 29–33.

50. Kuzel, T. M., M. S. Tallman, D. Shevrin, et al. 1993. A phase II study of continuous infusion 5-fluorouracil in advanced hormone refractory prostate cancer. An Illinois Cancer Center Study. *Cancer* **72**: 1965–1968.

51. Lerner, H. J. and T. R. Malloy. 1977. Hydroxyurea in stage D carcinoma of prostate. *Urology* **10**: 35–38.

52. Lloyd, R. E., S. E. Jones, S. E. Salmon, et al. 1976. Combination chemotherapy with adriamycin (NSC-123127) and cyclophosphamide (NSC-26271) for solid tumors: a phase II trial. *Cancer Treat. Rep.* **60**: 77–83.

53. Loening, S. A., S. Beckley, M. F. Brady, et al. 1983. Comparison of estramustine phosphate, methotrexate and *cis*-platinum in patients with advanced, hormone refractory prostate cancer. *J. Urol.* **129:** 1001–1006.

54. Loening, S. A., W. W. Scott, J. deKernion, et al. 1981. A comparison of hydroxyurea, methyl-chloroethyl-cyclohexy-nitrosourea and cyclophosphamide in patients with advanced carcinoma of the prostate. *J. Urol.* **125:** 812–816.

55. Logothetis, C. J., M. L. Samuels, A. C. Von Eschenbach, et al. 1983. Doxorubicin, mitomycin-C and 5-fluorouracil (DMF) in the treatment of metastatic hormonal refractory adenocarcinoma of the prostate, with a note on the staging of metastatic prostate cancer. *J. Clin. Oncol.* **1:** 368–379.

56. Madsen, E. L., L. Bastholt, K. Bertelsen, C. Rose, and E. S. Nielsen. 1992. Weekly oral idarubicin in advanced prostatic cancer. A phase II study. *Acta Oncol.* **31:** 337–340.

57. Mahjoubi, M., M. Azab, M. Ghosn, C. Theodore, and J. P. Droz. 1990. Phase II trial of ifosfamide in the treatment of metastatic hormone refractory patients with prostatic cancer. *Cancer. Invest.* **8:** 477–481.

58. Merrin, C.E. 1979. Treatment of genitourinary tumors with *cis*-diammineplatinum (II): Experience in 250 patients. *Cancer Treat. Rep.* **63:** 1579–1589.

59. Merrin, C. E. and S. Beckley. 1979. The treatment of estrogen-resistant stage D carcinoma of the prostate with *cis*-diamminedichloroplatinum. *Urology* **13:** 267–272.

60. Merrin, C., W. Etra, Z. Wajsman, et al. 1976. Chemotherapy of advanced carcinoma of the prostate with 5-fluorouracil, cyclophosphamide and adriamycin. *J. Urol.* **115:** 86–88.

61. Mittleman, A., S. K. Shukla, and G. P. Murphy. 1976. Extended therapy of stage D carcinoma of the prostate with oral estramustine phosphate. *J. Urol.* **115:** 409–412.

62. Moore, G. E., I. D. J. Bross, and R. Ausman. 1968. Effects of 5-fluorouracil (NSC-19893) in 389 patients with cancer. Eastern Clinical Drug Evaluation Program. *Cancer Chemother. Rep.* **52:** 641–653.

63. Moore, M. J., D. Osoba, K. Murphy, et al. 1994. Use of palliative end points to evaluate the effects of mitoxantrone and low-dose prednisone in patients with hormonally resistant prostate cancer. *J. Clin. Oncol.* **12:** 689–694.

64. Moore, M. R., S. D. Graham, R. Birch, and L. Irwin. 1987. Phase II evaluation of mitoguazone in metastatic hormone-resistant prostate cancer: a Southeastern Cancer Study Group trial. *Cancer Treat. Rep.* **71:** 89–90.

65. Moore, M. R., M. B. Troner, and P. DeSimone. 1986. Phase II evaluation of weekly cisplatin in metastatic hormone-resistant prostate cancer. A Southeastern Cancer Study Group trial. *Cancer Treat. Rep.* **70:** 541–542.

66. Murphy, G. P., R. P. Gibbons, D. E. Johnson, et al. 1977. A comparison of estramustine phosphate and streptozotocin in patients with advanced prostatic carcinoma who have had extensive radiation. *J. Urol.* **118:** 288–291.

67. Murphy, G. P., R. P. Gibbons, D. E. Johnson, et al. 1979. The use of estramustine and prednimustine versus prednimustine alone in advanced metastatic prostatic cancer patients who have received prior irradiation. *J. Urol.* **121:** 763–765.

68. Murphy, G. P., R. L. Priore, and P. T. Scardino. 1988. Hormone refractory metastatic prostatic cancer treated with methotrexate, cyclophosphamide plus adriamycin, *cis*-platinum plus 5-fluorouracil plus cyclophosphamide. National Prostatic Cancer Project randomized trial. *Urology* **32:** 33–40.

69. Murphy, G. P. and N. H. Slack. 1980. Response criteria for the prostate of the USA National Prostatic Cancer Project. *Prostate* **1:** 375–382.

70. Muss, H. B., V. Howard, F. Richards, et al. 1981. Cyclophosphamide versus cyclophosphamide, methotrexate and 5-fluorouracil in advanced prostatic cancer: a randomized trial. *Cancer* **47:** 1949–1953.

71. Natale, R. B., A. Yagoda, and R. C. Watson. 1982. Phase II trial of AMSA in prostatic cancer. *Cancer Treat. Rep.* **66:** 208–209.

72. O'Bryan, R. M., L. H. Baker, and J. F. Gottlieb. 1977. Dose response evaluation of Adriamycin in human neoplasia. *Cancer* **39:** 1940.

73. O'Bryan, R. M., J. K. Luce, and R. W. Talley. 1973. Phase II evaluation of Adriamycin in human neoplasia. *Cancer* **32:** 1–8.

74. Oesterling, J. E., D. W. Chan, and J. Epstein. 1988. Prostate specific antigen in preoperative and postoperative evaluation of localized prostatic cancer treated with radical prostatectomy. *J. Urol.* **139:** 766–772.

75. Osborne, C. K., B. A. Blumenstein, E. D. Crawford, G. R. Weiss, R. M. Bukowski, and N. R. Larrimer. 1992. Phase II study of platinum and mitoxantrone in metastatic prostate cancer: a Southwest Oncology Group Study. *Eur. J. Cancer* **28:** 477–478.

76. Osborne, C. K., A. Drelichman, D. D. Von Hoff, and E. D. Crawford. 1983. Mitoxantrone: modest activity in a phase II trial in advanced prostate cancer. *Cancer Treat. Rep.* **67:** 1133–1135.

77. Petrylak, D. P., R. B. MacArthur, J. O'Connor, et al. 1999. Phase I trial of docetaxel with estramustine in androgen-independent prostate cancer. *J. Clin. Oncol.* **17:** 958–967.

78. Pienta, K. J. and J. E. Lehr. 1993. Inhibition of prostate cancer growth by estramustine and etoposide: evidence for interaction at the nuclear matrix. *J. Urol.* **149:** 1622–1625.

79. Pienta, K. J., H. Naik, and J. E. Lehr. 1996. Effect of estramustine, etoposide and taxol on prostate cancer cell growth in vitro and in vivo. *Urology* **48:** 164–170.

80. Pienta, K. J., B. G. Redman, R. Bandekar, et al. 1997. A phase II trial of oral estramustine and oral etoposide in hormone refractory prostate cancer. *Urology* **50:** 401–407.

81. Pienta, K. J., B. Redman, M. Hussain, et al. 1994. Phase II evaluation of oral estramustine and oral etoposide in hormone refractory adenocarcinoma of the prostate. *J. Clin. Oncol.* **12:** 2005–2012.

82. Pisters, L., C. A. Pettaway, P. Troncoso, L. D. Finn, J. W. Slaton, and C. J. Logothetis. 1999. Preoperative chemotherapy and hormonal therapy followed by radical prostatectomy for locally advanced prostate cancer. *Proc. Annu. Meet. Am. Soc. Clin. Oncol.* **18:** A1212.

83. Presant, C.A., A. Van Amburg, C. Klahr, and G. E. Metter. 1980. Chemotherapy of advanced prostatic cancer with adriamycin, BCNU and cyclophosphamide. *Cancer* **46:** 2389–2392.

84. Qazi, R. and J. Khandekar. 1983. Phase II study of cisplatin for metastatic prostatic carcinoma. An Eastern Cooperative Oncology Group study. *Am. J. Clin. Oncol.* **6:** 203–205.

85. Rangel, C., H. Matzkin, and M. S. Soloway. 1992. Experience with weekly doxorubicin (adriamycin) in hormone refractory stage D2 prostate cancer. *Urology* **39:** 577–582.

86. Rossof, A. H., R. W. Talley, and R. Stephens. 1979. Phase II evaluation of *cis*-dichlorodiammineplatinum(II) in advanced malignancies of the genitourinary and gynecologic organs: a Southwest Oncology Group study. *Cancer Treat. Rep.* **63:** 1557–1564.

87. Roth, B. J., B. Y. Yeap, G. Wilding, B. Kasimis, D. McLeod, and P. J. Loehrer. 1993. Taxol in advanced, hormone refractory carcinoma of the prostate. A phase II trial of the Eastern Cooperative Oncology Group. *Cancer* **72:** 2457–2460.

88. Rowinsky, E. K. and R. C. Donehower. 1995. Paclitaxel (Taxol). *New Engl. J. Med.* **332:** 1004–1014.

89. Ryu, S., M. Gabel, M. S. Khil, Y. J. Lee, S. H. Kim, and J. H. Kim. 1994. Estramustine: a novel radiation enhancer in human carcinoma cells. *Int. J. Radiat. Oncol. Biol. Phys.* **30:** 99–104.

90. Savarese, D. M., M. Taplin, B. Marchesni, et al. 1999. A phase II study of docetaxel, estramustine and low dose hydrocortisone in hormone refractory prostate cancer: CALGB 9780. *Proc. Annu. Meet. Am. Soc. Clin. Oncol.* **18:** A1234.

91. Scher, H. I., C. Sternberg, W. D. Heston, et al. 1986. Etoposide in prostatic cancer: experimental studies and phase II trial in patients with bidimensionally measurable disease. *Cancer Chemother. Pharmacol.* **18:** 24–26.

92. Scher, H. I., A. Yagoda, T. Ahmed, and R. C. Watson. 1985. Methylglyoxal-bis (guanylhydrazone) in hormone-resistant adenocarcinoma of the prostate. *J. Clin. Oncol.* **3:** 224–228.

93. Schmidt, J. D., W. W. Scott, R. P. Gibbons, et al. 1979. Comparison of procarbazine, imadzole-carboxamide and cyclophosphamide in relapsing patients with advanced carcinoma of the prostate. *J. Urol.* **121:** 185–189.

94. Scott, W. W., R. P. Gibbons, D. E. Johnson, et al. 1976. The continued evaluation of the effects of chemotherapy in patients with advanced carcinoma of the prostate. *J. Urol.* **116:** 211–213.

95. Seidman, A. D., H. I. Scher, D. Petrylak, D. D. Dershaw, and T. Curley. 1992. Estramustine and vinblastine: use of prostate specific antigen as a clinical trial end point for hormone refractory prostatic cancer. *J. Urol.* **147:** 931–934.

96. Seifter, E., P. Bunn, M. Cohen, et al. 1984. A trial of combination chemotherapy followed by hormonal therapy for previously untreated metastatic carcinoma of the prostate. *J. Clin. Oncol.* **4:** 1365–1373.

97. Sella, A., R. Kilbourn, R. Amato, et al. 1994. Phase II study of ketoconazole combined with weekly doxorubicin in patients with androgen-independent prostate cancer. *J. Clin. Oncol.* **12:** 683–688.

98. Sinibaldi, V. J., M. A. Carducci, S. Moore-Cooper, et al. 1999. A phase II study evaluating a one day course of estramustine phosphate and docetaxel in patients with hormone refractory prostate cancer. *Proc. Annu. Meet. Am. Soc. Clin. Oncol.* **18:** A1239.

99. Slack, N.H. and G. P. Murphy. 1983. A decade of experience with chemotherapy for prostate cancer. *Urology* **22:** 1–7.

100. Smith, D. C., R. L. Dunn, M. S. Strawderman, and K. J. Pienta. 1998. Change in serum prostate specific antigen as a marker of response to cytotoxic therapy for hormone-refractory prostate cancer. *J. Clin. Oncol.* **16:** 1835–1843.

101. Smith, D. C., P. Esper, M. Strawderman, B. Redman, and K. J. Pienta. 1999. Phase II trial of oral estramustine, oral etoposide and intravenous paclitaxel in hormone refractory prostate cancer. *J. Clin. Oncol.* **17:** 1664–1671.

102. Soloway, M. S., S. Beckley, M. F. Brady, et al. 1983. A comparison of estramustine phosphate versus *cis*-platinum alone versus estramustine phosphate plus *cis*-platinum in patients with advanced hormone refractory prostate cancer who had extensive irradiation to the pelvis or lumbosacral area. *J. Urol.* **129:** 56–61.

103. Soloway, M. S., J. B. deKernion, R. P. Gibbons, et al. 1981. Comparison of estramustine phosphate and vincristine alone or in combination for patients with advanced, hormone refractory, previously irradiated carcinoma of the prostate. *J. Urol.* **125:** 664–667.

104. Soloway, M. S., R. M. Shippel, and M. Ikard. 1979. Cyclophosphamide, doxorubicin hydrochloride and 5-fluorouracil in advanced carcinoma of the prostate. *J. Urol.* **122:** 637–639.

105. Speicher, L. A., L. Barone, and K. D. Tew. 1992. Combined antimicrotubule activity of estramustine and taxol in human prostatic carcinoma cell lines. *Cancer Res.* **52:** 4433–4440.

106. Stearns, M. E., and K. D. Tew. 1988. Estramustine binds MAP-2 to inhibit microtubule assembly in vitro. *J. Cell Sci.* **89:** 331–341.

107. Stephens, R. L., C. Vaughn, M. Lane, et al. 1984. Adriamycin and cyclophosphamide versus hydroxyurea in advanced prostatic cancer. A randomized Southwest Oncology Group study. *Cancer* **53:** 406–410.

108. Tannock, I. F., D. Osoba, M. R. Stockler, et al. 1996. Chemotherapy with mitoxantrone plus prednisone or prednisone alone for symptomatic hormone-resistant prostate cancer: a Canadian randomized trial with palliative end points. *J. Clin. Oncol.* **14:** 1756–1764.

109. Torti, F., D. Aston, and B. L. Lum. 1983. Weekly doxorubicin in endocrine refractory carcinoma of the prostate. *J. Clin. Oncol.* **1:** 477–482.
110. Trump, D. L., J. C. Marsh, L. K. Kvols, et al. 1990. A phase II trial of carboplatin (NSC 241240) in advanced prostate cancer, refractory to hormonal therapy. An Eastern Cooperative Oncology Group pilot study. *Invest. New Drugs* **(8 Suppl. 1):** S91–S94.
111. Veronesi, A., V. Dal Bo, G. Lo Re, et al. 1989. Mitomycin C treatment of advanced, hormone-resistant prostatic carcinoma: a phase II study. *Cancer Chemother. Pharmacol.* **23:** 115–116.
112. Walther, P. J., S. D. Williams, M. Troner, F. A. Greco, R. Birch, and L. H. Einhorn. 1986. Phase II study of etoposide for carcinoma of the prostate. *Cancer Treat. Rep.* **70:** 771–772.
113. Widmark, A., J. E. Damber, A. Bergh, and R. Henriksson. 1994. Estramustine potentiates the effects of irradiation on the Dunning (R3327) rat prostatic adenocarcinoma. *Prostate* **24:** 79–83.
114. Wieder, J. A. and M. S. Soloway. 1998. Incidene, etiology, location, prevention and treatment of positive surgical margins after radical prostatectomy for prostate cancer. *J. Urol.* **160:** 299–315.
115. Yagoda, A. and D. Petrylak. 1993. Cytotoxic chemotherapy for advanced hormone-refractory prostate cancer. *Cancer* **71:** 1098–1109.
116. Yagoda, A. R., R. C. Watson, and R. B. Natalie. 1979. A critical analysis of response criteria in patients with prostatic cancer treated with *cis*-diamminechloride platinumII. *Cancer* **44:** 1553–1562.
117. Zagars, G. K. and A. C. Von Eschenbach. 1993. Prostate specific antigen. An important marker for prostate cancer treated by external beam radiation therapy. *Cancer* **72:** 538–548.

25

The Role of Small Bioactive Peptides and Cell Surface Peptidases in Androgen Independent Prostate Cancer

Joel B. Nelson, MD

1. INTRODUCTION

At current rates of diagnosis, a man in the United States has a one-in-five chance that invasive prostate cancer will develop in his lifetime *(69)*. This rate is nearly twice that of lung cancer and three times that of colorectal cancer. Death from prostate cancer is the second leading cause of death from cancer in men in the United States. Almost every man with advanced prostate cancer will undergo androgen ablation therapy and in time, most will progress. The central characteristic of fatal prostate cancer is androgen independence. These facts were established in 1941, when therapeutic castration was first described *(53,54)*, and, unfortunately, still hold true as the 1990s drew to a close. Historically, there has been an inverse relationship between efforts to maximize the efficacy of hormonal therapy for prostate cancer and the outcomes of those efforts: thousands of patients studied and billions of dollars spent repeatedly show hormonal therapy to have dramatic—yet ultimately ineffective—therapeutic effects *(67)*. Although a number of growth and survival factors have been implicated in the androgen independent phenotype of prostate cancer, there has been no translation of these findings to effective therapy *(87)*.

In some androgen independent prostate cancers, neuroendocrine gene products are expressed, usually as scattered cells or nests of cells throughout the tumor *(33)*. Neuroendocrine cells are characterized by secretory granules rich in neuropeptides, such as chromogranin A. These cells are normally dispersed in the prostate, and may function as paracrine mediators of secretory epithelial function, much like a "soluble nervous system." It is the continued expression or reexpression of this phenotype in prostate cancer that has led to investigation of these neuroendocrine gene products as mediators of androgen independent disease *(1,5,26,34,36,51,104)*. This chapter is not confined to the classic neuroendocrine phenotype (which, in its small cell or carcinoid manifestations represents a fraction of prostate cancers)—it examines a recent series of related observations about the role of the small bioactive peptides bombesin, endothelin-1 (ET-1), and neurotensin in prostate cancer. These peptides—which have compelling biological

From: *Prostate Cancer: Biology, Genetics, and the New Therapeutics*
Edited by: L. W. K. Chung, W. B. Isaacs, and J. W. Simons © Humana Press Inc., Totowa, NJ

effects in prostate cancer—act through specific, high-affinity heptahelical, G-protein-coupled receptors *(12,25,28,61,80,105)*. The enzyme responsible for the degradation of these peptides, endopeptidase 24.11, is decreased in androgen independent prostate cancer *(90)*: this loss of local peptide regulation may enhance cancer progression. Caveolin, the protein component of the plasma membrane structure caveolae, are associated with G-protein coupled receptors *(74)*. Caveolin expression is increased in androgen-independent prostate cancer, and in certain models is inversely related to androgen sensitivity *(82,119)*. Collectively, these observations may provide a broader understanding of androgen independent prostate cancer. Excitement for targeting these pathways in therapy has been fueled by early clinical trial results: the use of an endothelin-receptor antagonist has resulted in both objective and subjective responses.

2. BOMBESIN/GASTRIN RELEASING PEPTIDE

Bombesin is a bioactive 14 amino acid peptide originally isolated from the skin of the European frog *Bombina bombina (4,39)*. Gastrin Releasing Peptide (GRP), the 27 amino acid mammalian counterpart *(75)*, has been found to produce many of the same biological properties, including induction of small cell lung *(18,27,114)*, breast *(83)* and colon cancer *(81)* proliferation. Bombesin/GRP peptides mediate a wide spectrum of activities by binding to specific, heptahelical G-protein coupled receptors, and inducing signal transduction via rapid mobilization of intracellular calcium *(17,46,49, 71,101,113)*. Three bombesin-like receptors have been identified and cloned.

In human prostate cancer, the addition of bombesin to culture media stimulated growth in a dose-dependent fashion (0.1 nm to 10 nm): this effect was specifically inhibited by an antibody against GRP *(16)*. High affinity (K_d 10^{-11} M) receptors for bombesin/GRP have been identified on prostate cancer cell lines *(9,96)*; by Northern blot analysis, only the GRP receptor mRNA is expressed *(7)*. By *in situ* hybridization, GRP receptor mRNA was expressed in both normal luminal and basal cells and in prostate cancers. Levels of GRP mRNA expression were variable in the cancers (ranging from intense to no staining), while normal tissues has consistently low levels of staining *(11)*. The bombesin/GRP peptides are capable of triggering rapid calcium mobilization in prostate cancer cell lines *(111)*: in PC-3 (an androgen independent line), an acute, reversible desensitization to additional stimulation was observed *(48)*. Bombesin increased invasion of PC-3 and LNCaP (androgen sensitive prostate cancer cell lines) into reconstituted basement membrane (Matrigel) *(50)*; in PC-3, the effects of bombesin are mediated in part by tyrosine phosphylation of a focal adhesion kinase (pp125[FAK]) *(8,9)*. Indeed, bombesin has been shown to increase expression of the proteolytic enzyme urokinase plasminogen activator, and to stimulate production of matrix metalloproteases (MMP-9) *(40)*. These activities are important in the degradation of the extracellular matrix observed in the metastatic pathway (Fig. 1).

A number of bombesin/GRP antagonists have been shown to inhibit tumor growth in rat and human prostate cancer xenograft models *(59,76,92,93)*. The combination of luteinizing hormone releasing hormone (LHRH) agonists and antagonists enhanced the effects of the bombesin antagonists. Cytotoxic bombesin analogs acting as doxorubicin carriers have also been developed: one of these agents, an analog of doxorubicin (2-pyrrolino-DOX), potently inhibited the growth of PC-3 cells (IC_{50} 3.6×10^{-10} M)

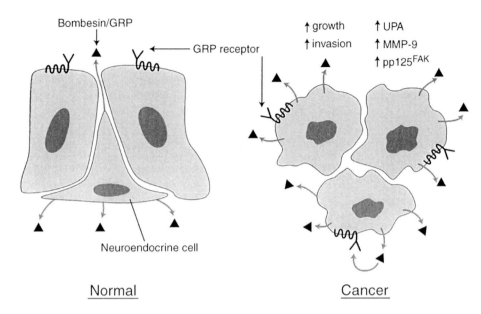

Fig. 1. Bombesin/Gastrin Releasing Peptide expression in the normal prostate and in prostate cancer. Reprinted with permission from ref. *89*, p. 89 by courtesy of Marcel Dekker, Inc.

(79). These data support the translation of bombesin/GRP antagonists alone, or as carriers for other classic cytotoxic agents, into clinical trials.

3. ENDOTHELIN-1

Endothelin-1, first isolated from porcine endothelial cells (hence the name), is the most potent endogenous vasoconstrictor known. Unlike its nearest competitor, angiotensin II (endothelin-1 is about ten times more potent on a molar basis), endothelin-1 has prolonged effects *(118)*. The endothelin family contains several 21 amino acid members, all characterized by two defining disulphide bridges *(56)*: ET-1, ET-2, and ET-3 and the Sarafotoxins (isolated from the venom of the Israeli burrowing asp, *Atractaspis engaddensis*) *(64,65,107)*. These ligands bind to the endothelin receptors ET_A and ET_B, with varying affinity *(55)*. The endothelins are identical in all mammals and most higher vertebrates; the endothelin receptors are also very similar.

Endothelin-1 is produced by many different cell types *(97)*, including prostatic epithelium *(70)*: almost all the secretory columnar epithelium produces ET-1. It should be noted that the pattern of ET-1 expression is unique among the other bioactive peptides discussed in this chapter, which have scattered, scant, or undetectable expression in the normal prostate. Indeed, the concentration of immunoreactive ET-1 are highest in seminal fluid—about 500 times greater than the concentration in circulation *(70)*. Endothelin-1 expression has been demonstrated in prostatic tissues in vivo *(70)* and by prostate cells in culture *(110)*. The endothelin receptor expression is greatest in prostatic stroma, at a density 35-fold greater than $\alpha 1$-adrenergic binding sites *(62)*, although ET_A and ET_B binding sites are present on prostatic epithelial cells *(45,63,66,72,112)*.

Every prostate cancer cell line tested produces ET-1 mRNA and protein *(84)*. A majority of men (*n* = 79) with androgen refractory prostate cancer had abnormally elevated plasma ET-1 concentration *(84)*. All primary prostate cancer and 14 of 16 prostate cancer metastases were uniformly positive for ET-1 expression by immunohisto-chemistry *(85)*.

Exogenous ET-1 was a mitogen for prostate cancer cell lines in vitro *(52,84,85)*. The direct growth-promoting effects are modest, but ET-1 also synergized the proliferative effects of other peptide growth factors in certain prostate cancer cell lines *(13,85)*. Ligands for G-protein coupled receptors, like ET-1, can transactivate other more classic, mitogenic pathways: ET-1 induces rapid tyrosine phosphorylation of epidermal growth-factor receptor in Rat-1 cells, in the absence of epidermal growth factor itself *(30)*. The effects of ET-1 on prostate cancer cells appear to be mediated through the ETA receptor subtype exclusively: the addition of an ET_A receptor antagonist blocked the growth-promoting effects of ET-1 *(85)*. Endothelin-1 also elevates intracellular calcium in several prostate cancer cell lines *(111)*.

Benign prostatic epithelium predominantly express the ET_B receptor subtype *(63)*. In prostate cancer cells, however, the ET_B receptor is not expressed; in both primary and metastatic prostate tumors, expression of the ET_B receptor is reduced *(85)*. Since ET_B is the receptor responsible for clearance *(43)* and regulation of ET-1 *(120)*, loss of ET_B may contribute to increased local and systemic ET-1 concentration. The ET_B receptor gene *(EDRNB)* contains a CpG in the promoter region *(10)*; inactivation of gene transcription by hypermethylation of CpG islands has been demonstrated for a number of genes associated with carcinogenesis *(6,14,58,73)*. Indeed, in 70% of the prostate cancers studied, the CpG island of the *EDNRB* gene is methylated *(86)*. Normal tissues show no methylation. The prostate cancer cell line LNCaP also has a frame-shift mutation in exon 4 of the *EDNRB* gene, but to date, no other *EDNRB* mutations have been found in other prostate cancers (Nelson, J. B., unpublished data). Based on these data, therefore, blocking ET-1 action in prostate cancer should be done through the ET_A receptor, since the ET_B receptor is frequently silenced.

Other malignancies express endothelin-1, including breast, pancreas, and colon. Along with prostate cancer, these tumors are characterized by an acinar and ductal architecture often associated with a local desmoplastic reaction *(37,68,98,106,116,117)*. The common osteoblastic response of bone to metastatic prostate cancer is considered to be secondary to tumor-derived factors acting in a paracrine fashion. Endothelin-1 is a mitogen for osteoblasts *(103,108,109)*, and has been shown to inhibit osteoclast function *(2)*, which further enhances the formation of an osteosclerotic lesion over an osteolytic one. In a matrix-induced bone forming system *(94,95)*, ET-1 increased alkaline phosphatase activity (used as an index of new formation) *(84)*. Using another osteoblastic model system, stable transfection of an ET-1 overexpression vector increased the area of new bone formation, and chronic administration of an ETA receptor antagonist decreased new bone formation *(88)*. Collectively, these data support a potential role for ET-1 in the osteoblastic response of bone to metastatic prostate cancer.

The pain associated with metastatic prostate cancer is often severe and debilitating; much of the focus of care in advanced disease is directed at relieving pain. Endothelin-1—like the homologous snake venom—induces pain *(29)*. In several animal models of pain, ET-1 was noxious *(31,35)*, and endothelin receptor antagonists had analgesic qualities. Using a selective ET_A receptor antagonist, given either intraperitoneal or

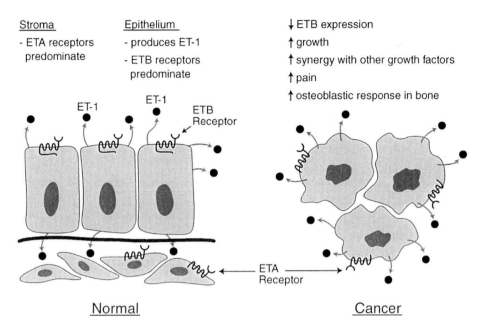

Fig. 2. Endothelin-1 and endothelin receptor expression in the normal prostate and prostate cancer. Reprinted with permission from ref. *89*, p. 90 by courtesy of Marcel Dekker, Inc.

orally, the abdominal constrictor response (a well-characterized pain response) of mice to ET-1 was completely inhibited (Nelson, J. B., unpublished data). Based on these findings (Fig. 2), clinical trials using endothelin receptor antagonists to relieve pain were initiated.

ABT-627, the racemic version of a highly potent and selective ET_A receptor antagonist (A-127722, ET_A *Ki* 0.069 nm, ET_B *Ki* 139 nm) *(89)*, was studied in two Phase I clinical trials at the Johns Hopkins Oncology Center and in the Netherlands. This orally bioavailable compound has a prolonged ET_A inhibition profile which allows once-a-day dosing *(89)*. These 28-d, open label dose escalation studies examined the toxicity, tolerability, and pharmacokinetics of ABT-627 in men with progressive hormone refractory prostate cancer. Most patients were heavily pretreated. Secondary endpoints were pain relief and PSA response. Patients with other ET-1-producing adenocarcinomas were also enrolled. If patients had subjective or objective responses, they were eligible for an extension study.

In the Phase I studies, ABT-627 was very well tolerated; mild to moderate headache was the most common side effect. In 70% (7/10) of patients with pain requiring narcotics, ABT-627 reduced pain (as measured by the visual analog scale), and in several patients narcotic use declined. In 68% (15/22) of men, PSA dropped, ranging from <5–90%. Of the patients eligible for the extension study, 66% (28/42) enrolled; of this group, 57% (16/28) had objective disease progression. It should be noted these data are from a short-term open label study, and the results should be viewed cautiously. Nevertheless, these compelling findings support further examination of endothelin blockade in men with prostate cancer.

Two randomized double blind placebo controlled Phase II studies using ABT-627 are underway. One is designed to study pain relief, the other to study time to progression. Preliminary results from these trials were gathered in the fall of 1999.

4. NEUROTENSIN

Like BN/GRP and ET-1, neurotensin (NT) is a small peptide with 13 amino acids *(19)*. Neurotensin is part of a family of peptides characterized by a high degree of homology at the carboxyl-terminus *(21,77)*, with activities as both neurotransmitters and gastrointestinal regulatory peptides *(15,20,42)*. Neurotensin is trophic for rat intestine *(115)* and pancreas *(41)* in vivo, and acts as a mitogen for small cell lung cancer cells *(32)* and pancreatic cancer cells *(57)* in vitro.

The expression of neurotensin by prostate cancer was first described in a patient who suffered from watery diarrhea *(60)*. Neurotensin concentration were elevated in the serum and tumors (primary prostate carcinoma and liver metastases) of this patient. Unlike ET-1—which is uniformly expressed by benign prostatic epithelium— neurotensin is usually not expressed by the normal prostate *(47)*. The androgen sensitive prostate cancer cell line LNCaP has been found to produce and secrete neurotensin following androgen withdrawal *(100)*. The same cell line expressed the neurotensin receptor (both with and without androgen), but only the androgen deprived cells had a growth response to exogenous neurotensin. In the androgen independent prostate cancer cell line PC-3, neurotensin was not found in conditioned media or cell lysates, and neurotensin mRNA was absent by RT-PCR *(99)*. The PC-3 cell line expresses neurotensin receptors of both high and low affinity (K_d 40 pm and 300 pm, respectively) *(99)*. Exogenous neurotensin stimulated growth in a bell-shaped dose response (fold increase ~ 1.8, maximum effect 0.1 nm); the neurotensin receptor antagonist SR48692 completely blocked the mitogenic effect *(99)* (Fig. 3).

Interestingly, neurotensin was stable in the androgen independent PC-3 cultures *(99)* and in androgen depleted LNCaP cultures *(100)*, but was completely degraded in LNCaP cultures containing androgen *(78)*. These data suggest an androgen induction of metalloprotease activity which is lost with androgen withdrawal or independence. Neurotensin is a substrate for several proteases found in abundance in the prostate gland, including neutral endopeptidase 24.11 (NEP), metalloendopeptidase 3.4.24.15, and angiotensin-converting enzyme (ACE) 3.4.15.1. High levels of NEP were detected in LNCaP cells, but not in the androgen-independent PC-3 or DU-145 cell lines *(78)*. Neurotensin degradation was rapid by LNCaP: this effect was blocked by phosphoramidon, an inhibitor of NEP *(78)*. Therefore, the loss of normal metabolism of a mitogenic factor in the androgen depleted or androgen independent phenotype provides another mechanism of prostate cancer progression.

5. NEUTRAL ENDOPEPTIDASE 24.11

Neutral endopeptidase 24.11 is a zinc dependent cell surface enzyme *(3,44,102)* expressed by benign prostatic epithelial cells *(38)* that cleaves and inactivates bioactive peptides, including bombesin, endothelin-1, and neurotensin (Fig. 4). Total NEP enzyme activity from normal prostate homogenates was more than twice that of ACE *(38)*. Loss of NEP activity could result in increased concentration of these bioactive and mitogenic peptides (Fig. 4), as demonstrated by the inverse relationship between

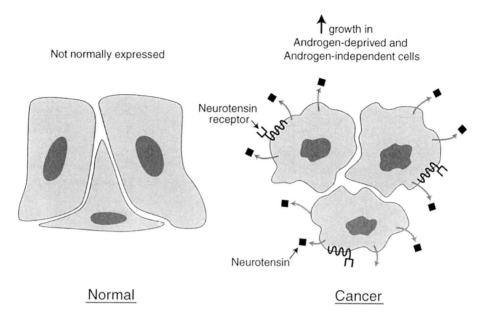

Fig. 3. Neurotensin and neurotensin receptor expression in prostate cancer. Reprinted with permission from ref. *89*, p. 91 by courtesy of Marcel Dekker, Inc.

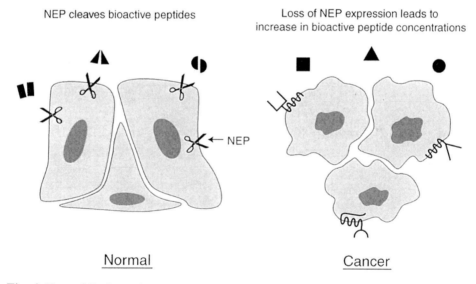

Fig. 4. Neutral Endopeptidase 24.11 (NEP) expression in the normal prostate and reduced expression in prostate cancer. Reprinted with permission from ref. *89*, p. 92 by courtesy of Marcel Dekker, Inc.

neurotensin concentration and NEP activity. Whether NEP inactivation contributed to androgen independent prostate carcinogenesis and progression is an intriguing possibility.

Support for a role of NEP loss in androgen independent progression was recently presented in a series of straightforward observations *(90)*. First, NEP expression and activity were found only in the androgen sensitive prostate cancer cell line LNCaP, but not in three androgen independent prostate cancer cell lines (confirming the work of others). Second, reintroduction of NEP (either by stable NEP transfection or addition of exogenous NEP) inhibited androgen independent prostate cancer cell growth. Third, inhibition of NEP activity by phosphoramidon increased anchorage independent growth in LNCaP. Fourth, androgen withdrawal resulted in decreased NEP expression and activity. Finally, prostate cancer biopsies obtained from men who were hormonally naive ($n = 6$) had greater NEP expression then men who were hormone refractory ($n = 9$). In some cases, the NEP gene appears to be hypermethylated in the promoter region (Nanus, D. M., personal communication). Together, these data support the hypothesis of an association of androgen independent prostate cancer and loss of NEP, and they also suggest a central role of NEP in limiting the effects of alternative growth promoting peptides in prostate cancer progression. Loss of NEP may also contribute to the increased plasma ET-1 concentration in men with androgen independent prostate cancer. Restoration of NEP activity—with the benefit of metabolizing several pathogenic peptides—is an attractive therapeutic target in prostate cancer.

6. CAVEOLIN

All the bioactive active peptides discussed here act through heptahelical, G-protein coupled receptors. Enhancement of these receptor signaling pathways or their components may be important in androgen independent disease. Caveolin is the major structural protein of caveolae *(74)*. Structurally and functionally, caveolae are like a cellular satellite dish: the curved invaginations of the plasma membrane are associated with a host of signal transduction pathways, including G-protein coupled receptors *(74)*. For example, the ET_A receptor is localized within caveolae *(23)*; ET-1 binding induces rapid endocytosis of ET_A and ET-1 *(24)*. Caveolae are abundant in endothelium, adipocytes, smooth muscle, and fibroblasts *(74)*.

Recently, an association between prostate cancer progression and caveolin was identified. Mouse caveolin was increased in metastases-derived prostate cancer cell lines compared to genetically matched primary prostate cancer cell lines *(119)*. In human tissues, caveolin expression was rare in benign prostatic epithelium, but increased in prostatic carcinoma metastatic to lymph nodes *(119)*.

In a model of prostate cancer in which androgen independent pathways allow survival, an inverse relationship between androgen sensitivity and the elements of androgen resistance is expected. This type of relationship was recently demonstrated between androgen sensitivity and caveolin expression in a metastatic mouse prostate cancer model. A reduction in caveolin expression increased the sensitivity of cell lines or tumors to androgen withdrawal *(82)*. Androgen independent mouse prostate cancer cells had increased caveolin expression, and overexpression of caveolin reduced the sensitivity of cells to androgen withdrawal *(82)*. Yet caveolin expression is decreased in the androgen depleted phenotype of two human prostate cancer cell lines (LNCaP, LAPC-4), and reintroduction of exogenous dihydrotestosterone increased caveolin expression *(91)*. Nevertheless, alterations in caveolin expression and function provide another possible pathway for the study of androgen independent prostate cancer progression (Fig. 5).

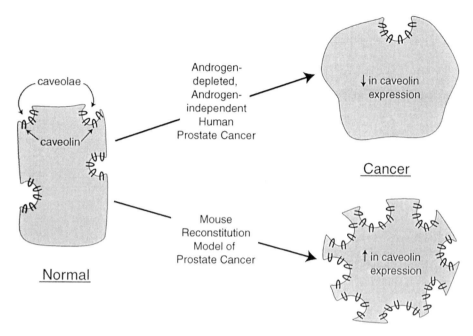

Fig. 5. Caveolin expression in androgen-depleted human prostate cancer is reduced compared to normal prostatic epithelium, whereas caveolin expression increases in the androgen independent mouse reconstitution model of prostate cancer. Reprinted with permission from ref. *89*, p. 93 by courtesy of Marcel Dekker, Inc.

7. CONCLUSION

The propensity of prostate cancer to survive despite androgen withdrawal continues to plague efforts to cure the disease. Recent advances have identified the roles of bioactive peptides, their receptors, and cell surface peptidases in this lethal phenotype of prostate cancer, and therapeutic interventions based on this new understanding are now being developed.

ACKNOWLEDGMENT

This article has been previously published in *Cancer Investigation*, and is reprinted with permission by courtesy of Marcel Dekker, Inc.

REFERENCES

1. Abrahamsson, P. 1996. Neuroendocrine differentiation and hormone refractory prostate cancer. *Prostate* (**Suppl.**)6: 3–8.
2. Alam A. S. M. T., A. Gallagher, V. Shankar, et al. 1992. Endothelin inhibits osteoclastic bone resorption by a direct effect on cell motility: implications for the vascular control of bone resorption. *Endocrinology* 130: 3617–3624.
3. Almenoff, J. and M. Orlowski. 1983. Membrane-bound kidney neutral metalloendopeptidase: interaction with synthetic substrates, natural peptides, and inhibitors. *Biochemistry* 22: 590–598.

4. Anastasi, A., V. Erspamer, and M. Bucci. 1971. Isolation and structure of bombesin and alytesin, two analogous active peptides from the skin of European amphibians *Bombyna* and *Alytes. Experimentia* **27:** 166–167.

5. Angelsen, A., U. Syversen, M. Stridsberg, et al. 1997. Use of neuroendocrine serum markers in the follow-up of patients with cancer of the prostate. *Prostate* **31:** 110–117.

6. Antequera, F., B. Boyes, and A. P. Bird. 1990. High levels of *de novo* methylation and altered chromatin structure at CpG islands in cell lines. *Cell* **62:** 503–514.

7. Aprikian, A. G., K. Han, S. Chevalier, et al. 1996. Bombesin specfically induces intracellular calcium mobilization via gastrin-releasing peptide receptors in human prostate cancer cells. *J. Mol. Endocrinol.* **16:** 297–306.

8. Aprikian, A. G., L. Tremblay, K. Han, et al. 1997. Bombesin stimulates the motility of human prostate carcinoma cells through tyrosine phosphorylation of focal adhesion kinase and of integrin-associated proteins. *Int. J. Cancer* **72:** 498–504.

9. Aprikain, A. G., K. Han, L. Guy, et al. 1998. Neuroendocrine differentiation and the bombesin/gastrin-releasing peptide family of neuropeptides in the progression of human prostate cancer. *Prostate* **(Suppl.)8:** 52–61.

10. Aria, H., K. Nakao, K. Takaya, et al. 1993. The human endothelin-B receptor gene: structural organization and chromosomal assignment. *J. Biol. Chem.* **268:** 3463–3470.

11. Bartholdi, M. F., J. M. Wu, H. Pu, et al. 1998. *In situ* hybridization for gastrin-releasing peptide receptor (GRP receptor) expression in prostatic carcinoma. *Int. J. Cancer* **79:** 82–90.

12. Battey, J. F., J. M. Way, M. J. Corjay, et al. 1991. Molecular cloning of the bombesin/gastrin-releasing peptide receptor from Swiss 3T3 cells. *Proc. Natl. Acad. Sci. USA* **88:** 395–399.

13. Battistini, B., P. Chailler, P. D'Orleans-Juste, et al. 1993. Growth regulatory properties of endothelins. *Peptides* **14:** 385–399.

14. Baylin, S. B., M. Makos, J. J. Wu, et al. 1991. Abnormal pattern of DNA methylation in human neoplasia: potential consequences for tumor progression. *Cancer Cells* **3:** 383–390.

15. Blackburn, A. M., D. R. Fletcher, and S. R. Bloom. 1980. Effect of neurotensin on gastric function in man. *Lancet* **1:** 987–989.

16. Bologna, M., C. Festuccia, P. Muzi, et al. 1989. Bombesin stimulates growth of human prostatic cancer cells *in vitro. Cancer* **63:** 1714–1720.

17. Bunn, P. A., D. G. Dienhart, D. Chan, et al. 1990. Neuropeptide stimulation of calcium flux in human lung cancer cells: delineation of alternative pathways. *Proc. Natl. Acad. Sci. USA* **87:** 2162–2166.

18. Carney, D. N., F. Cutitta, T. W. Moody, et al. 1987. Selective stimulation of small cell lung cancer clonal growth by bombesin and gastrin-realeasing peptide. *Cancer Res.* **47:** 821–825.

19. Carraway, R. and S. E. Leeman. 1973. The isolation of a new hypotensive peptide, neurotensin, from bovine hypothalamus. *J. Biol. Chem.* **248:** 6854–6861.

20. Carraway, R., and S. E. Leeman. 1976. Characterization of radioimmunoassayable neurotensin in the rat: its differential distribution in the central nervous system, small intestine and stomach. *J. Biol. Chem.* **251:** 7045–7052.

21. Carraway, R. E., S. P. Mitra, and D. E. Cochrane. 1987. Structure of a biologically active neurotensin-related peptide obtained from pepsin treated albumins. *J. Biol. Chem.* **262:** 5968–5973.

22. Casey, M. L., W. Byrd, and P. C. MacDonald. 1992. Massive amounts of immunoreactive endothelin in human seminal fluid. *J. Clin. Endocrinol. Metabol.* **74:** 223–225.

23. Chun, M., U. K. Liyanage, M. P. Lisanti, et al. 1994. Signal transduction of a G protein-coupled receptor in caveolae: colocalization of endothelin and its receptor with caveolin. *Proc. Natl. Acad. Sci. USA* **91:** 11,728–11,732.

24. Chun, M., H. Y. Lin, Y. I. Henis, et al. 1995. Endothelin-induced endocytosis of cell surface ET_A receptors: endothelin remains intact and bound to the ET_A receptor. *J. Biol. Chem.* **270:** 10,855–10,560.

25. Corjay, M. H., D. J. Dobrzanski, J. M. Way, et al. 1991. Two distinct bombesin receptor subtypes are expressed and functional in human lung carcinoma cells. *J. Biol. Chem.* **266:** 18,771–18,779.

26. Cussenot, O., J. M. Villette, A. Valeri, et al. 1996. Plasma neuroendocrine markers in patients with benign prostatic hyperplasia and prostatic carcinoma. *J. Urol.* **155:** 1340–1343.

27. Cutitta, F., D. N. Carney, J. Mulshine, et al. 1985. Bombesin-like peptides can function as autocrine growth factors in human small cell lung cancer. *Nature* **316:** 823–826.

28. Cyr, C., K. Huebner, T. Druck, et al. 1991. Cloning and chromosomal localization of a human endothelin ET_A receptor. *Biochem. Biophys. Res. Commun.* **181:** 184–190.

29. Dahlof, B., D. Gustafsson, T. Hedner, et al. 1990. Regional haemodynamic effects of endothelin-1 in rat and man: unexpected adverse reactions. *J. Hypertens.* **8:** 811–817.

30. Daub, H., F. U. Weiss, C. Wallasch, et al. 1996. Role of transactivation of the EGF receptor in signalling by G-protein-coupled receptors. *Nature* **379:** 557–560.

31. Davar, G., G. Hans, M. U. Fareed, et al. 1998. Behavioral signs of acute pain produced by application of endothelin-1 to rat sciatic nerve. *Neuroreport* **13:** 2279–2283.

32. Davis, T. P., H. S. Burgess, S. Crowell, et al. 1989. β-endorphin and neurotensin stimulate *in vitro* clonal growth of human SCLC cells. *Eur. J. Pharmacol.* **161:** 283–285.

33. Deftos, L., S. Nakada, D. Burton, et al. 1996. Immunoassay and immunohistology studies of chromogranin A as a neuroendocrine marker in patients with carcinoma of the prostate. *Urology* **48:** 58–62.

34. Deftos, L. J. and P. Abrahamsson. 1998. Granins and prostate cancer. *Urology* **51:** 141–145.

35. De-Melo, J. D., C. R. Tonussi, P. D'Orleans-Juste, et al. 1998. Articular nociception induced by endothelin-1, carrageenan and LPS in naive and previously inflamed knee-joints in the rat: inhibition by endothelin receptor antagonists. *Pain* **77:** 261–269.

36. di Sant'Agnese, P. A. 1998. Neuroendocrine differentiation in prostatic carcinoma: an update. *Prostate* **8S:** 74–79.

37. Economos, K., P. C. Macdonald, and M. L. Casey. 1992. Endothelin-1 gene expression and biosynthesis in human endometrial HEC-1A cancer cells. *Cancer Res.* **52:** 554–557.

38. Erdös, E. G., W. W. Schulz, J. T. Gafford, et al. 1985. Neutral metalloendopeptidase in human male genital tract: comparison to angiotensin I-converting enzyme. *Lab. Invest.* **52:** 437–447.

39. Erspamer, V., G. F. Erspamer, M. Inselvini, et al. 1972. Occurrence of bombesin and alytesin in extracts of the skin of three European discoglossid frogs and pharmacological actions of bombesin on extravascular smooth muscle. *Br. J. Pharmacol.* **45:** 333–3348.

40. Festuccia, C., F. Guerra, S. D'Ascenzo, et al. 1998. *In vitro* regulation of pericellular proteolysis in prostatic tumor cells treated with bombesin. *Int. J. Cancer* **75:** 418–431.

41. Feurle, G. E., B. Muller, and E. Rix. 1987. Neurotensin induces hyperplasia of the pancreas and growth of the gastric antrum in rats. *Gut* (**Suppl.**)**28:** 19–23.

42. Fletcher, D. R., A. M. Blackburn, T. E. Adrian, et al. 1981. Effect of neurotensin on pancreatic function in man. *Life Sci.* **29:** 2157–2161.

43. Fukahiro, T., T. Fujikawa, S. Ozaki, et al. 1994. Clearance of circulating endothelin-1 by ET_B receptors in rats. *Biochem. Biophys. Res. Commun.* **199:** 1461–1465.

44. Gafford, J. T., R. A. Skidgel, E. G. Erdös, et al. 1983. Human kidney "enkephalinase," a neutral metaloendopeptidase that cleaves active peptides. *Biochemistry* **22:** 3265–3275.

45. Galetti, T. P., G. P. Rossi, A. Belloni, et al. 1996. Localization of endothelin receptors A and B in normal human prostate and BPH. *J. Urol.* **155:** 463A.

46. Ghatei, M. A., R. T. Jung, J. C. Stevenson, et al. 1982. Bombesin action on gut hormones and calcium in man. *J. Clin. Endocrinol. Metab.* **54:** 980–985.

47. Gu, J., M. Polak, L. Probert, et al. 1983. Peptidergic innervation of the human male genital tract. *J. Urol.* **130:** 386–391.

48. Han, K., J. Viallet, S. Chevalier, et al. 1997. Characterization of intracellular calcium mobilization by bombesin-related neuropeptides in PC-3 human prostate cancer cells. *Prostate* **31:** 53–60.

49. Heikkila, R., J. B. Trepel, F. Cuttitta, et al. 1987. Bombesin-related peptides induce calcium mobilization in a subset of human small cell lung cancer cell lines. *J. Biol. Chem.* **262:** 16,456–16,460.

50. Hoosein, N. M., C. J. Logothetis, and L. W. K. Chung. 1993. Differential effects of peptide hormones bombesin, vasoactive intestinal polypeptide and somatostatin analog RC-160 on the invasive capacity of human prostatic carcinoma cells. *J. Urol.* **149:** 1209.

51. Hoosein, N., M. Abdul, R. McCabe, et al. 1995. Clinical significance of elevation of neuroendocrine factors and interleukin-6 in metastatic prostate cancer. *Urol. Oncol.* **1:** 246–254.

52. Hsu, J.-Y. and M. Pfahl. 1998. ET-1 expression and growth inhibition of prostate cancer cells: a retoid target with novel specificity. *Cancer Res.* **58:** 4817–4822.

53. Huggins, C. and C. V. Hodges. 1941. Studies on prostatic cancer: I. The effects of castration, of estrogen and androgen injection on serum phosphatases in metastatic carcinoma of the prostate. *Cancer Res.* **1:** 293–303.

54. Huggins, C., R. E. Stevens, and C. V. Hodges. 1941. Studies on prostatic cancer: II. The effects of castration on advanced carcinoma of the prostate gland. *Arch. Surg.* **43:** 209–223.

55. Huggins, S. P., J. T. Pelton, and R. C. Miller. 1993. The structure and specificity of endothelin receptors: their importance in physiology and medicine. *Pharmacol. Ther.* **59:** 55–123.

56. Inoue, A., M. Yanagisawa, S. Kimura, et al. 1989. The human endothelin family: three structurally and pharmacologically distinct isopeptides predicted by three separate genes. *Proc. Natl. Acad. Sci. USA* **86:** 2863–2867.

57. Ishizuka, J., C. M. Townsend, J. C. Thompson, et al. 1993. Neurotensin regulates growth of human pancreatic cancer. *Ann. Surg.* **217:** 439–446.

58. Jones, P. A. 1996. DNA methylation errors and cancer. *Cancer Res.* **56:** 2463–2467.

59. Jungwirth, A., J. Pinski, G. Galvan, et al. 1997. Inhibition of growth of androgen-independent DU-145 prostate cancer *in vivo* by luteinizing hormone releasing hormone antagonist cetrolix and bombesin antagonists RC-3940-II and RC-3950-II. *Eur. J. Cancer* **33:** 1141–1148.

60. Kapuscinski, M., A. Shulkes, D. Read, et al. 1990. Expression of neurotensin in endocrine tumors. *J. Clin. Endocrinol. Metab.* **70:** 100–106.

61. Kitabgi, P., F.Checler, J. Maxella, et al. 1985. Pharmacology and biochemistry of neurotensin receptors. *Rev. Clin. Basic Pharm.* **5:** 397–486.

62. Kobayashi, S., R. Tang, B. Wang, et al. 1994. Binding and functional properties of endothelin receptor subtypes in the human prostate. *Mol. Pharmacol.* **45:** 306–311.

63. Kobayashi, S, R. Tang, B. Wang, et al. 1994. Localization of endothelin receptors in the human prostate. *J. Urol.* **151:** 763–766.

64. Kochva, E., C. C. Viljoen, and D. P. Botes. 1982. A new type of toxin in the venom of snakes of the genus *Atractaspis* (Atractaspidinae). *Toxicon* **20:** 581–592.

65. Kochva, E., A. Bdolah, and Z. Wollberg. 1993. Sarafotoxins and endothelins: evolution, structure and function. *Toxicon* **31:** 541–568.

66. Kondo, S., T. Morita, and Y. Tashima. 1994. Endothelin receptor density in human hypertrophic and non-hypertrophic prostate tissue. *Tohoku J. Exp. Med.* **172:** 381–384.

67. Kozlowski, J. M., and J. T. Grayhack. 1991. Carcinoma of the prostate, in *Adult and Pediatric Urology* (Gillenwater, J. Y., J. T. Grayhack, S. S. Howards, and J. W. Duckett, eds.), Mosby-Year Book, St. Louis, MO, pp. 1277–1393.

68. Kusuhara, M., K. Yamaguchi, K. Nagasaki, et al. 1990. Production of endothelin in human cancer cell lines. *Cancer Res.* **50:** 3257–3261.

69. Landis, S. H., T. Murray, S. Bolden, et al. 1998. Cancer Statistics, 1998. *CA Cancer J. Clin.* **48:** 6–29.

70. Langenstroer, P., R. Tang, E. Shapiro, et al. 1993. Endothelin-1 in the human prostate: tissue levels, source of production and isometric tension studies. *J. Urol.* **149:** 495–499.

71. Lebacg-Verheyden, A. M., J. Trepel, E. A. Sausville, et al. 1990. Peptide growth factors and their receptors. *Handbook Exp. Pharmacol.* **95:** 71–124.

72. Le Brun, G., F. Moldovan, P. Aubin, et al. 1996. Identification of endothelin receptors in normal and hyperplastic human prostate tissues. *Prostate* **28:** 379–384.

73. Lee, W.-H., R. A. Morton, J. I. Epstein, et al. 1994. Cytidine methylation of regulatory sequences near the π-class glutathione S-transferase gene accompanies human prostatic carcinogenesis. *Proc. Natl. Acad. Sci. USA* **91:** 11,733–11,737.

74. Lisanti, M. P., P. E. Schere, J. Vidugiriene, et al. 1994. Characterization of caveolin-rich membrane domains isolated from an endothelial-rich source: implications for human disease. *J. Cell Biol.* **126:** 111–126.

75. McDonald, T. J., H. Jornvall, G. Hilsson, et al. 1979. Characterization of a gastrin releasing peptide from porcine non-antral gastric tissue. *Biochem. Biophys. Res. Commun.* **90:** 227–233.

76. Milovanovic, S. R., S. Radulovic, K. Groot, et al. 1992. Inhibition of growth of PC-82 human prostate cancer line xenografts in nude mice by bombesin antagonist RC-3095 or combination of agonist [D-Trp^6]-luteinizing hormone-releasing hormone and somatostatin analog RC-160. *Prostate* **20:** 269–280.

77. Mogard, M. H., R. Kobayashi, C. F. Chen, et al. 1986. The amino acid sequence of kinetensin, a novel peptide isolated from pepsin-treated human placenta: homology with human serum albumin, neurotensin and angiotensin. *Biochem. Biophys. Res. Commun.* **136:** 983–988.

78. Moody, T. W., C. A. Mayr, T. J. Gillespie, et al. 1998. Neurotensin is metabolized by endogenous proteases in prostate cancer cell lines. *Peptides* **19:** 253–258.

79. Nagy, A., P. Armatis, R.-Z. Cai, et al. 1997. Dosing, synthesis, and *in vitro* evaluation of cytotoxic analogs of bombesin-like peptides containing doxorubicin or its intensely potent derivative, 2-pyrrolinodoxorubicin. *Proc. Natl. Acad. Sci. USA* **94:** 652–656.

80. Nakamuta, M., R. Takayanagi., Y. Sakai, et al. 1991. Cloning and sequence analysis of a cDNA encoding human non-selective type of endothelin receptor. *Biochem. Biophys. Res. Commun.* **177:** 34–39.

81. Narayan, S., E. R. Spindel, N. H. Rubin, et al. 1992. A potent bombesin receptor antagonist inhibits bombesin-stimulated growth of mouse colon cancer cells *in vitro*: absence of autocrine effects. *Cell Growth Differ.* **3:** 111–118.

82. Nasu, Y., T. L. Timme, G. Yang, et al. 1998. Suppression of caveolin expression induces androgen sensitivity in metastatic androgen insensitive mouse prostate cancer cells. *Nat. Med.* **4:** 1062–1064.

83. Nelson, J., M. Donnelly, B. Walker, et al. 1991. Bombesin stimulates proliferation of human breast cancer cells in culture. *Br. J. Cancer* **63:** 933–936.

84. Nelson, J. B., S. P. Hedican, D. J. George, et al. 1995. Identification of endothelin-1 in the pathophysiology of metastatic adenocarcinoma of the prostate. *Nat. Med.* **1:** 944–949.

85. Nelson, J. B., K. Chan-Tack, S. P. Hedican, et al. 1996. Endothelin-1 production and decreased endothelin B receptor expression in advanced prostate cancer. *Cancer Res.* **56:** 663–668.

86. Nelson, J. B., W.-H. Lee, S. H. Nguyen, et al. 1997. Methylation of the 5′ CpG island of the endothelin B receptor gene is common in human prostate cancer. *Cancer Res.* **57:** 35–37.

87. Nelson, J. B. 1998. Alternatives to death: understanding androgen independent prostate cancer. *Nat. Med.* **4:** 1011–1012.

88. Nelson, J. B., S. H. Nguyen, J. R. Wu-Wong, et al. 1999. New bone formation in an osteoblastic tumor model is increased by endothelin-1 overexpression and decreased by endothelin A receptor blockade. *Urology* **53:** 1063–1069.

89. Nelson, J. B. and M. A. Carducci. 2000. Small bioactive peptides and cell surface peptidases in androgen-independent prostate cancer. *Cancer Investigation.* **18:** 87–96.

90. Papandreou, C. N., B. Usmani, Y. Geng, et al. 1998. Neutral endopeptidase 24.11 loss in metastatic human prostate cancer contributes to androgen-independent progression. *Nat. Med.* **4:** 50–57.

91. Pflug, B. R., R. Reiter, and J. B. Nelson. 1999. Caveolin expression is decreased following androgen deprivation in human prostate cancer cell lines. *Prostate* **40:** 269–273.

92. Pinski, J., G. Halmos, K. Szepeshazi, et al. 1993. Antagonists of bombesin/gastrin-releasing peptide as adjuncts to agonists of luteinizing hormone-releasing hormone in the treatment of experimental prostate cancer. *Cancer* **72:** 3263–3270.

93. Pinski, J., H. Reile, G. Halmos, et al. 1994. Inhibitory effects of somatostatin analogue RC-160 and bombesin/gastrin-releasing peptide antagonist RC-3095 on the growth of the androgen-independent Dunning R-3327-AT-1 rat prostate cancer. *Cancer Res.* **54:** 169–174.

94. Reddi, A. H., and C. Huggins. 1972. Biochemical sequences in the transformation of normal fibroblasts in adolescent rats. *Proc. Natl. Acad. Sci. USA* **69:** 1601–1605.

95. Reddi, A. H. and N. E. Sullivan. 1980. Matrix-induced endochondral bone differentiation influence of hypophysectomy, growth hormone, and thyroid-stimulating hormone. *Endocrinology* **107:** 1291–1299.

96. Reile, H., P. E. Armatis, and A. V. Schally. 1994. Characterization of high-affinity receptors for bombesin/gastrin releasing peptide on the human prostate cancer cell lines PC-3 and DU-145: internalization of receptor bound ^{125}I-(Tyr^4) bombesin by tumor cells. *Prostate* **25:** 29–38.

97. Rubanyi, G. M., and M. A. Polokoff. 1994. Endothelins: molecular biology, biochemistry, pharmacology, physiology, and pathophysiology. *Pharmacol. Rev.* **46:** 325–415.

98. Schrey, M. P., K. V. Patel, and N. Tezapsidis. 1992. Bombesin and glucocorticoids stimulate human breast cancer cells to produce endothelin, a paracrine mitogen for breast stromal cells. *Cancer Res.* **52:** 1786–1790.

99. Seethalakshmi, L., S. P. Mitra, P. R. Dobner, et al. 1997. Neurotensin receptor expression in prostate cancer cell line and growth effect of NT at physiological concentrations. *Prostate* **31:** 183–192.

100. Sehgal, I., S. Powers, B. Huntley, et al. 1994. Neurotensin is an autocrine trophic growth factor stimulated by androgen withdrawal in human prostate cancer. *Proc. Natl. Acad. Sci. USA* **91:** 4673–4677.

101. Severi, C., R. T. Jensen, V. Erspamer, et al. 1991. Different receptors mediate the action of bombesin-related peptides on gastric smooth muscle cells. *Am. J. Physiol.* **260:** G683–G690.

102. Shipp, M. A., J. Vijayaraghavan, E. V. Schmidt, et al. 1989. Common acute lymphoblastic leukemia antigen (Calla) is active neutral endopeptidase 24.11 ("enkephalinase"): direct evidence by cDNA transfection analysis. *Proc. Natl. Acad. Sci. USA* **86:** 297–301.

103. Shioide, M. and M. Noda. 1993. Endothelin modulates osteopontin and osteocalcin messenger ribonucleic acid expression in rat osteoblastic osteosarcoma cells. *J. Cell Biochem.* **53:** 176–180.

104. Sim, S., A. Glassman, J. Ro, et al. 1996. Serum calcitonin in small cell carcinoma of the prostate. *Ann. Clin. Lab. Sci.* **26:** 487–495.

105. Spindel, E. R., E. Giladi, P. Brehm, et al. 1990. Cloning and functional characterization of a complementary DNA encoding the murine fibroblast bombesin/gastrin-releasing peptide receptor. *Mol. Endocrinol.* **4:** 1956–1963.

106. Suzuki, N., H. Matsumoto, C. Kitada, et al. 1989. Production of endothelin-1 and big-endothelin-1 by tumor cells with epithelial-like morphology. *J. Biochem.* **106:** 736–741.

107. Takasaki, C., M. Yanagisawa, S. Kimura, et al. 1988. Similarity of endothelin to snake venom toxin. *Nature* **335:** 303.

108. Takuwa, Y., Y. Ohue, N. Takuwa, et al. 1989. Endothelin-1 activates phospholipase C and mobilizes Ca^{2+} from extra- and intracellular pools in osteoblastic cells. *Am. J. Physiol.* **257:** E797–803.

109. Takuwa, Y., T. Masaki, and K. Yamashita. 1990. The effects of the endothelin family peptides on cultured osteoblastic cells from rat calvariae. *Biochem. Biophys. Res. Conmmun.* **170:** 998–1005.

110. Walden, P. D., M. Ittmann, M. E. Monaco, et al. 1998. Endothelin-1 production and agonist activites in cultured prostate-derived cells: implications for regulation of endothelin bioactivity and bioavailability in prostatic hyperplasia. *Prostate* **34:** 241.

111. Wasilenko, W. J., J. Cooper, A. J. Palad, et al. 1997. Calcium signaling in prostate cancer cells: evidence for multiple receptors and enhanced sensitivity to bombesin/GRP. *Prostate* **30:** 167–173.

112. Webb, M. L., C.-C. Chao, M. Rizzo, et al. 1995. Cloning and expression of an endothelin receptor subtype B from human prostate that mediates contraction. *Mol. Pharmacol.* **47:** 730–737.

113. Weber, H. C., L. L. Hampton, R. T. Jensin, et al. 1998. Structure and chromosomal localization of the mouse bombesin receptor subtype 3 gene. *Gene* **211:** 125–131.

114. Weber, S., J. E. Zuckerman, D. G. Bostwich, et al. 1985. Gastrin releasing peptide is a selective mitogen for small cell lung carcinoma *in vitro*. *J. Clin. Invest.* **75:** 306–309.

115. Wood, J. G., H. D. Hoang, L. J. Bussjaeger, et al. 1988. Neurotensin stimulates growth of small intestine in rats. *Am. J. Physiol.* **255:** 813–817.

116. Yamashita, J., M. Ogawa, H. Egami, et al. 1992. Abundant expression of immunoreactive endothelin-1 in mammary phyllodes tumor: possible role of endothelin 1 in the growth of stromal cells in phyllodes tumor. *Cancer Res.* **52:** 4046–4049.

117. Yamashita, J., M. Ogawa, K. Nomura, et al. 1993. Interleukin 6 stimulates the production of immunoreactive endothelin 1 in human breast cancer cells. *Cancer Res.* **53:** 464–467.

118. Yanagisawa, M., H. Kurihara, S. Kimura, et al. 1988. A novel potent vasoconstrictor peptide produced by vascular endothelial cells. *Nature* **332:** 411–415.

119. Yang, G., L. D. Truong, T. L. Timme, et al. 1998. Elevated expression of caveolin is associated with prostate and breast cancer. *Clin. Cancer Res.* **8:** 1873–1880.

120. Yohn, J. J., C. Smith, T. Stevens, et al. 1994. Autoregulation of endothelin-1 secretion by cultured human keratinocytes via the endothelin B receptor. *Biochim. Biophys. Acta* **1224:** 454–458.

26

Development of Dendritic Cell-Based Prostate Cancer Vaccine

Benjamin A. Tjoa, PhD and Gerald P. Murphy, MD, DSc

1. INTRODUCTION

Current prostate cancer treatments include surgery, radiotherapy, chemotherapy, and hormone therapy. Efforts in early detection of prostate cancer—which include serum prostate specific antigen (PSA) screening and digital rectal examination—have allowed for diagnoses of the disease at its earliest stages. Treatment strategies such as radical prostatectomy and local radiotherapy are largely successful for patients with clinically localized prostate cancer *(14,32,64)*. Brachytherapy is an example of a novel method to introduce radioisotopes to localized cancer tissues *(40)*. This method implants radioactive seeds directly into tumor sites, minimizing exposure to surrounding tissues. A 10-yr follow-up study involving brachytherapy treatment of 152 consecutive patients with clinically organ confined prostate carcinoma reported a disease-free rate of 64% *(41)*. However, up to one-third of patients initially diagnosed with clinically localized disease and treated with conventional treatments may eventually develop metastases *(20)*.

At this time, available treatments for metastatic prostate cancer have failed to demonstrate significant curative potential *(20,39)*. Androgen reduction therapy is commonly used to control metastatic growth. This strategy can be achieved by surgical removal of the testes (bilateral orchiectomy) or by administration of antiandrogens and/or luteinizing hormone releasing hormone (LHRH) agonists *(19,51)*. While hormone sensitive tumor cells are effectively controlled, hormone refractory clones often emerge after the course of hormonal therapy. At this point, radiation therapy has a palliative role, and chemotherapy has been relatively ineffective in the treatment of patients with hormone refractory prostate cancer *(19,20)*. Thus, there is a need for ongoing research into the development of new therapeutic approaches to prostate cancer.

The immune system is capable of recognizing and rejecting autologous tumor cells. This is suggested by cases of spontaneous remission of various cancers *(25)*, and the presence of infiltrating leukocytes—a majority of which consist of T cells *(33,42,47)*. Furthermore, there is a direct correlation between immunosuppresion and increased incidence of certain malignancies—e.g., Epstein-Barr virus (EBV)-associated lymphomas, Kaposi's sarcoma, and cervical cancer *(5)*. However, the very existence of cancer and its inevitable progression without treatment demonstrate the inefficiency of this natural defense against tumors, and the ability of neoplastic cells to evade immune-

From: *Prostate Cancer: Biology, Genetics, and the New Therapeutics*
Edited by: L. W. K. Chung, W. B. Isaacs, and J. W. Simons © Humana Press Inc., Totowa, NJ

surveillance. Thus, the major objective of immunotherapeutic approaches is to augment the effectiveness and efficiency of the immune response against malignant tissues.

2. CANCER IMMUNOTHERAPY

Immunotherapeutic approaches to cancer treatment can generally be categorized into passive and active immunotherapy. The former involves administration of activated immune system effector component into cancer patients—e.g., cancer specific antibodies, lymphokine-activated killer (LAK) cells, and tumor infiltrating lymphocytes (TIL) *(30,53)*. This approach is often combined with administration of cytokines that augment immune function—e.g., interleukin-2 (IL-2) and interferon-γ *(46,62)*.

2.1. Active Immunotherapy: Cancer Vaccine

The second approach, active immunotherapy, involves vaccination of patients with agents that elicit activation of tumor specific T cells, the major cellular immune-effector component. Early efforts in cancer vaccine studies involved the use of irradiated tumor specimens or tumor cells derived from the patient (autologous), or from other individuals (allogeneic) to inoculate cancer patients with the hope of generating a therapeutic immune response *(52)*. Discoveries and characterizations of cancer antigens have provided well-defined targets for T-cell attack *(63)*.

Ideal targets of cancer specific immunotherapy are antigens expressed by neoplastic cells (cancer specific antigens), but not by normal cells. These are often identified as products of mutated oncogenes or tumor suppressor genes (e.g., mutated *ras* or p53 peptides) *(63)*. However, most of the human cancer antigens characterized today are also expressed at a lower level by normal cells (cancer-associated antigens). These antigens can further be classified into tissue specific antigens and shared/common antigens expressed by various cancer types. One may argue that immune tolerance for these "self" antigens acquired during development could reduce the effectiveness of cancer-associated antigens as cancer vaccine candidates *(21)*.

Few prostate cancer associated antigens that could potentially be used as targets for specific immunotherapy have been identified. The short list includes tissue specific antigens such as PSA, prostatic acid phosphatase (PAP), and prostate specific membrane antigen (PSMA) *(8,18,65)*. MUC-1 is an example of a shared/common cancer-associated antigen. It is a glycoprotein secreted by glandular organs such as breast, ovary, colon, and prostate. In malignant cells, an underglycosylated form of mucin is overexpressed over the entire surface of the cell. Clinical trials involving the administration of mucin-1 (MUC-1) peptide vaccine were conducted at the Memorial Sloan-Kettering Cancer Center in New York *(55)*. Twenty patients with increasing PSA values observed after primary therapies participated in this study. All patients generated IgM and IgG response after three immunizations. High titers for MUC-1 peptides were maintained for more than 46 wk, and the rate of PSA increase may have diminished in some patients *(55)*.

Advances in molecular biology have made it possible to isolate and characterize the genes that code for antigens which may be responsible for the spontaneous regression of cancer. These antigens are termed cancer rejection antigens. For example, melanoma specific TIL clones have been used to screen complementary DNA (cDNA) libraries from the original tumor in an attempt to identify specific antigens responsible for tumor rejection *(45)*. These rejection antigens are potentially more effective targets for immunotherapeutic modalities.

The main objective of cancer vaccine administration is to elicit activation of cancer specific T cells, which can attack cancer cells in vivo. T cells recognize their target cells through a heterodimeric membrane-bound protein known as the T-cell receptor (TCR). TCR recognizes short peptide antigens bound to human histocompatibility leukocyte antigen (HLA) molecules expressed by target cells *(28,67)*. Thus, it is important to identify the peptide/HLA complexes that form the T-cell epitopes. With the recent availability of known peptide motifs of HLA binding, it has been possible to predict the composition of short peptides with high affinities for certain HLA molecules from the amino acid sequence of tumor antigens *(6)*. Clinical trials with synthetic HLA-specific peptides have been conducted with some success for several cancers *(1,4,48)*.

3. ADJUVANTS: THE SECOND COMPONENT OF A CANCER VACCINE

The term "adjuvant" is derived from the Latin word *adjuvare*, which means "to help." Any material that helps augment the immune response to antigens is referred to as an adjuvant. Adjuvants have been used with conventional vaccines to elicit strong and long-lasting immune response *(12)*. Various adjuvants used in cancer vaccine studies include: bacterial products (e.g., Bacillus Calmette Guerin *[BCG]*, cholera and diphtheria toxins, and Detox [monophosphoryl lipid A cell wall skeleton from *Mycobacterium phlei*, squalane oil, and Tween80]), carrier proteins (e.g., keyhole limpet hemocyanin [KLH]), liposomes, saponin-derived products (e.g., QS21, and immunostimulating complexes [ISCOMS]), and various cytokines (e.g., IL-2, IL-4, interferon-α [IFN-α], IFN-β, IFN-γ, and granulocyte macrophage colony stimulating factor [GM-CSF]) *(9,13,15,43)*.

One of the more recent advances in cancer vaccine studies has been the use of autologous antigen-presenting cells (APCs) as an adjuvant to present tumor antigens to patients' T cells *(23,31)*. APCs are members of the hematopoetic cell family that have unique capabilities to present antigens to T cells. The rationale for using cells that are specialized for antigen presentation is that these cells should provide all factors necessary for initiation of the immune response, including those that are not yet defined *(23,31)*. Dendritic cells (DCs)—a type of APC known for efficient antigen presentation—have recently been utilized as vehicles to deliver antigens in several cancer vaccine studies, including melanoma and follicular B-lymphoma *(17,38)*. Our group at Northwest Hospital in Seattle, WA recently completed Phase I and II prostate cancer clinical trials involving the administration of DCs and HLA-A2-specific peptides derived from prostate specific membrane antigen (PSMA) *(34,35,37,60,61)*. These studies will be discussed further in subsequent sections.

4. DENDRITIC CELL-BASED PROSTATE CANCER VACCINE

Two main components of this cancer vaccine are **antigens** as specific targets, and **autologous dendritic cells** as adjuvant that help deliver and present these antigens for attack by components of the immune system. Phase I and II clinical trials conducted at the Northwest Hospital in Seattle, WA utilized two HLA-A2-specific peptides from PSMA. PSMA is a 750 amino acid membrane-bound protein expressed by prostate epithelial cells *(18)*. One of the monoclonal antibodies (MAbs) specific for PSMA (7E11-C5.3) is used in a prostate cancer imaging method (ProstaScint®, Cytogen Corp., Princeton, NJ) *(16)*. Elevated expression of PSMA was detected in hormone refractory prostatic carcinoma *(22)*. In addition, levels of PSMA are elevated in the serum of hormone refractory advanced prostate cancer patients *(36)*.

The second vaccine component, dendritic cells (DCs) originate in the bone marrow. During an early stage of their maturation process, DCs migrate to nonlymphoid tissues such as the epidermal layer of the skin, the respiratory and gastrointestinal systems, and the interstitial regions of several solid organs *(2,26)*. At this stage, DCs possess unique capabilities for antigen uptake and processing *(2)*. Antigen capture is facilitated by a high level of micropinocytosis as well as mannose receptor mediated uptake of macromolecules *(50)*.

DCs are an important accessory cell for the stimulation of both T-cell subsets (cytotoxic T lymphocytes and helper T cells) *(10)*. In vivo studies indicate that DCs furnish all the needed signals to stimulate naïve T cells. These signals include presentation of antigenic peptides by the major histocompatibility complex proteins (MHC) for recognition by the T-cell receptor molecules, as well as the binding of costimulatory molecules on the DCs to their receptors on the T-cell surface *(66)*. Potent T-cell reactivity can be provoked using very low DC:T-cell ratios (1:50–1:200) *(66)*.

The study of DC-based immunotherapeutics has received a big boost from the improvement of isolation and culture methods. DCs lack most of the markers typical of other leukocyte populations (e.g., CD3, CD14, CD15, CD16, and CD19, which are markers for T cells, macrophage/monocytes, granulocytes, natural killer, and B cells, respectively) *(56)*. Thus, DCs can be isolated directly from blood by negative selection, using a cocktail of the lineage specific MAbs *(57)*. Alternatively, DCs may be cultured from CD34+ hematopoietic progenitor cells from human umbilical cords and bone marrow, or CD14+ monocytes isolated from peripheral blood *(3,44,49,59)*. Various cytokines have been utilized for propagation, including granulocyte macrophage colony stimulating factor (GM-CSF), interleukin-4 (IL-4), and tumor necrosis factor alpha (TNF-α) *(3,44,49,59)*. In addition, in vivo administration of Fms-like tyrosine kinase ligand (Flt-3 ligand), a potent enhancer of hematopoietic differentiation from several lineage precursors, has been shown to significantly increase the number of DCs in mice *(27)*.

Various experiments involving in vivo administration of DCs pulsed with tumor-associated antigens for rejection of tumors have been conducted in mice. One of the initial studies using a mouse sarcoma model demonstrated a 50% survival rate in mice given splenic DCs, compared with 0% survival in animals that did not receive DCs. However, mice receiving DCs pulsed with tumor antigens did not have improved survival. The authors postulated that pulsing before injection blocks the DCs with nonspecific antigens, whereas more specific antigens were acquired in vivo *(24)*. Other reports, however, showed successful prevention of tumor growth in vivo by administration of DCs pulsed with various antigens, including autologous tumor fragments, idiotype IgM in a B-cell tumor system, and OVA peptides against an OVA-transduced tumor cell line *(7,11,29)*.

Clinical trials involving DC-based cancer vaccines with several types of cancers, including follicular-B lymphoma and melanoma, have recently been reported *(17,38)*. Our group has completed prostate cancer clinical trials with cultured autologous DCs pulsed with HLA-A2 PSMA-specific peptides.

5. PHASE I CLINICAL TRIAL: ASSESSMENT OF SAFE ADMINISTRATION OF AUTOLOGOUS DCs AND PSMA PEPTIDES

The Phase I study examined the administration of HLA-A2-specific PSMA peptides (PSM-P1 and PSM-P2), autologous DCs, and PSM-P1 and -P2 pulsed autologous DCs to 51 patients with advanced hormone refractory prostate cancer *(37)*. The majority of these patients (39/51) were in stage D2 ($T_4N_{1-3}M_{1a-c}$), according to AJCC cancer-staging system. Many of them were anemic, and had undergone various treatments which resulted in an impaired immune competency.

All participants received four infusion cycles of the test substances over 6-wk intervals. At the completion of four cycles of infusions, the maximum tolerated dose was not achieved. Significant acute and chronic toxicity were not observed in all doses of test substances, except for mild to moderate cases of hypotension without pulse change during the time of infusion *(37)*.

Patients were monitored for cellular immune modulation to the appropriate PSMA peptides (PSM-P1 or -P2). An increased cellular response was observed within the HLA-A2-positive subjects who were infused with DCs pulsed with PSM-P1 or -P2 *(37)*. Patient clinical response was analyzed based on National Prostate Cancer Project (NPCP) criteria and a minimum of 50% reduction of serum PSA levels. Seven partial responders were observed *(37,60)*. Average PSA levels showed an significant increase in the nonresponder group, while a decrease was observed in the seven partial responders *(60)*.

6. PHASE II CLINICAL TRIAL: ASSESSMENT OF EFFICACY OF ADMINISTRATION OF AUTOLOGOUS DCs PULSED WITH PSMA PEPTIDES

Our Phase II trial began in January 1997 and initially enrolled 107 subjects. Participants in this study included 66 patients with hormone refractory metastatic prostate cancer (group A). One-half of group A participants (33/66) were participants in the previous Phase I study who had requested to be enrolled in the Phase II trial (group A-I). The other half of the participants were new subjects with no previous immunotherapy study (group A-II). Group B included 41 patients with evidence of local recurrence after failure of a primary treatment (e.g., slowly rising PSA, positive prostate biopsy, or detection of pelvic lymph node on a ProstaScint® scan). Study participants received a total of six infusions of autologous DCs pulsed with PSM-P1 and -P2 at 6-wk intervals. With each infusion, one-half of study subjects received a 7-d course of sc injection of GM-CSF as systemic adjuvant.

Thirty-three patients with metastatic prostate cancer who participated in the Phase I study (group A-I) were the first group to complete the Phase II study. Based on the NPCP criteria and 50% reduction in PSA, nine of the 33 subjects (27.3%) were identified as partial responders *(61)*. Eleven patients (33.3%) exhibited no significant change during the Phase II trial. Thirteen patients exhibited disease progression. Seven patients died during the study. Among the nine partial responders, four were also

Table 1
Summary of Phase II Trial Clinical Evaluation[a]

	Group A-II Subjects admitted with hormone refractory metastatic prostate cancer	Group B Subjects admitted with suspected local recurrence of prostate cancer
Number of evaluable subjects	25	37
Number of deceased subjects	9	0
Percent deceased	36%	0%
Number of responders	8	11
Percent responders	32%	30%
Number of no change	1	8
Percent no change	4%	22%
Number of progression	16	18
Percent progression	64%	49%

[a]This table was reproduced with permission from Murphy, G. P., et al., *Prostate.* **38:** 73–78, 1999 *(34)*, and Murphy, G. P., et al., *Prostate* **39:** 54–59, 1999 *(36)*.

responders in the Phase I study. A majority of the partial responders exhibited improvements in general immune response as assessed using delayed-type hypersensitivity (DTH) skin test to recall antigens. This Phase I/II study encompassed an average total period of 613 d. Twelve of nineteen subjects (63%) with stage D_2 hormone refractory prostate cancer metastases survived a period of over 600 d (median survival period was 608 d) *(61)*.

Group A-II and B subjects completed all scheduled infusions as of September 1998. These groups were evaluated for response to treatment using the NPCP criteria, 50% reduction in PSA, and significant improvement in a repeat ProstaScint® scan. Addition of the ProstaScint® scan comparisons as a response criteria allowed for evaluation of patient nodal disease status.

Within group A-II, 32% of the study population showed diseased regression. These included two patients (8%) who were complete responders (CR) and six patients (24%) who were partial responders (PR). One patient exhibited no significant change (NC), while 16 patients (64%) showed disease progression (P) *(34)*. Ten group B participants (27%) were partial responders (PR) and one subject (3%) was a complete responder (CR). Eight patients (22%) showed no significant change (NC), and 18 patients (49%) showed disease progression *(35)*. The summary of clinical evaluations for groups A-II and B is shown in Table I. Within these two study groups, 31% (19/62) of total evaluable participants was identified as partial or complete responders. No significant difference in clinical response was observed in patients who received the sc GM-CSF injection with their DC/peptide infusion compared to those who only received DC/peptide infusions *(54)*.

In order to evaluate whether the responses were durable or not, study participants were given periodic follow-up evaluations following the conclusion of the study *(54)*. Since the majority of response was identified with repeat ProstaScint® or bone scans, the response duration was calculated starting from the end of the clinical trial until a disease progression was diagnosed. The average duration of response was 149 d for group A-II, and 187 d for group B. A majority of the responders (11/19, or 58%) were still responsive at the end of the most recent follow-up period *(58)*. This study suggests that the majority of the responses identified in the various groups appear to be durable.

7. CONCLUSION AND FUTURE DIRECTIONS

This chapter examines progress in the development of a DC-based vaccine for cancer of the prostate gland. Vaccine therapy may provide an alternative therapy for patients with hormone refractory metastatic prostate cancer. The administration of dendritic cells pulsed with PSMA peptides has induced cellular immune responses against the tumor with virtually no adverse effects.

Future studies in this field should include the use of other available prostate antigens, including the full-length PSMA protein, discovery of novel prostate cancer specific antigens as new targets, and optimization of vaccine delivery, as well as studies involving therapies which combine conventional procedures and immunotherapy. In the future, these modalities may provide an additional therapy for advanced prostate cancer.

ACKNOWLEDGMENTS

The authors thank the staff of Northwest Hospital Day Surgery/Short Stay Unit, especially Nancy Martin, Sharon Vitolo, Frances Seemann, and Lanelle Bentz. We wish to pay tribute to Dr. Donald S. Coffey, who is completing 40 successful years at the Brady Urological Institute and the Johns Hopkins Medical Institutions. This work was supported in part by the CaP CURE foundation, the Rontell foundation, the Phi Beta Psi Sorority, and the John Jolly and Stanley McNaughton families of Seattle, Washington.

REFERENCES

1. Alexander, M., M. L. Salgaller, E. Celis, A. Sette, W. A. Barnes, S. A. Rosenberg, et al. 1996. Generation of tumor-specific cytolytic T lymphocytes from peripheral blood of cervical cancer patients by in vitro stimulation with a synthetic human papillomavirus type 16 E7 epitope. *Am. J. Obstet. Gynecol.* **175:** 1586–1593.
2. Austyn, J. 1996. New insights into the mobilization and phagocytic activity of dendritic cells. *J. Exp. Med.* **180:** 1287–1292.
3. Berhard, H., M. L. Disis, S. Heimfeld, S. Hand, J. R. Gralow, and M. A. Cheever. 1995. Generation of immunostimulatory dendritic cells from human CD34+ hematopoietic progenitor cells of the bone marrow and peripheral blood. *Cancer Res.* **55:** 1099–1104.
4. Cormier, J. N., M. L. Salgaller, T. Prevette, K. C. Barracchini, L. Rivoltini, N. P. Restifo, et al. 1997. Enhancement of cellular immunity in melanoma patients immunized with a peptide from MART-1/Melan A. *Cancer J. Sci. Am.* **3:** 37–44.

5. DeVita, Jr., V. 1997. Principles of chemotherapy, in *Cancer Principles & Practice of Oncology* (DeVita, Jr., S. Hellman, and S. Rosenberg, eds.), Lippincott, Philadelphia, PA, p. 276.

6. Engelhard, V. H. 1994. Structure of peptides associated with class I and class II MHC molecules. *Annu. Rev. Immunol.* **12:** 181–207.

7. Flamand, V., T. Sornasse, K. Thielemans, C. Demanet, M. Bakkus, H. Bazin, et al. 1994. Murine dendritic cells pulsed in vitro with tumor antigen induce tumor resistance in vivo. *Eur. J. Immunol.* **24:** 605–610.

8. Foti, A. G., J. F. Cooper, H. Herschman, and R. R. Malvaez. 1977. Detection of prostatic cancer by solid-phase radioimmunoassay of serum prostatic acid phosphatase. *N. Engl. J. Med.* **297:** 1357–1361.

9. Fung, P. Y. S., M. Madej, R. R. Koganty, and B. M. Longenecker. 1992. Active specific-immunotherapy of a murine mammary adenocarcinoma using a specific tumor-associated glycoconjugate. *Cancer Res.* **50:** 4308–4311.

10. Grabbe, S., S. Beissert, T. Schwarz, and R. D. Granstein. 1995. Dendritic cells as initiators of tumor immune responses: a possible strategy for tumor immunotherapy? *Immunol. Today* **16:** 117–121.

11. Grabbe, S., S. Bruvers, R. L. Gallo, T. L. Knisely, R. Nazareno, and R. D. Grandstein. 1991. Tumor antigen presentation by murine epidermal cells. *J. Immunol.* **146:** 3656–3661.

12. Gupta, R. K. and G. R. Siber. 1995. Adjuvants for human vaccines—current status, problems, and future prospects. *Vaccine* **13:** 1263–1276.

13. Gupta, R. K., C. L. Varanelli, P. Griffin, D. F. Wallach, and G. R. Siber. 1996. Adjuvant properties of non-phospholipid liposomes (Novasomes) in experimental animals for human vaccine antigens (published erratum appears in *Vaccine* 1996 Jun;**14[8]:**1). *Vaccine* **14:** 219–225.

14. Hanks, G., J. Krall, A. Hanlon, S. Asbell, M. Pilepich, and J. Owen. 1994. Patterns of care and RTOG studies in prostate cancer: long-term survival, hazard rate observations, and possibilities of cure. *Int. J. Radiat. Oncol. Biol. Phys.* **28:** 39–45.

15. Helling, F., S. Zhang, A. Shang, S. Adluri, M. Calves, R. Koganty, et al. 1995. GM2-KLH conjugate vaccine: increased immunogenicity in melanoma patients after administration with immunological adjuvant QS-21. *Cancer Res.* **55:** 2783–2788.

16. Horoszewicz, J. S., E. Kawinski, and G. P. Murphy. 1987. Monoclonal antibodies to a new antigenic marker in epithelial prostate cells and serum of prostatic cancer patients. *Anticancer Res.* **7:** 927–936.

17. Hsu, F. J., C. Benike, F. Fagnoni, T. M. Liles, D. Czerwinski, B. Taidi, et al. 1996. Vaccination of patients with B-cell lymphoma using autologous antigen-pulsed dendritic cells. *Nat. Med.* **2:** 52–28.

18. Israeli, R. S., C. T. Powell, J. G. Corr, W. R. Fair, and W. Heston. 1993. Molecular cloning of a complementary DNA encoding a prostate-specific membrane antigen. *Cancer Res.* **54:** 1807–1811.

19. Iverson, P. 1998. Orchidectomy and oestrogen therapy revisited. *Eur. Urol.* **34(Suppl.):** 7–11.

20. Jones, G., C. Mettlin, G. Murphy, P. Guinan, H. Herr, D. Hussey, et al. 1995. Patterns of care for carcinoma of the prostate gland; results of a national survey of 1984 and 1990. *J. Am. Coll. Surg.* 545–554.

21. Kappler, J., N. Roehm, and P. T. Marrack. 1987. Cell tolerance by clonal elimination in the thymus. *Cell* **49:** 273–280.

22. Kawakami, M. and J. Nakayama. 1997. Enhanced expression of prostate-specific membrane antigen gene in prostate cancer as revealed by in situ hybridization. *Cancer Res.* **15:** 2321–2324.

23. Knight, S. C. and A. J. Stagg. 1993. Antigen-presenting cell types. *Curr. Opin. Immunol.* **5:** 374–382.

24. Knight, S. C., R. Hunt, C. Dore, and P. B. Medawar. 1985. Influence of dendritic cells on tumor growth. *Proc. Natl. Acad. Sci. USA* **82:** 4495–4497.

25. Krikorian, J., C. Portlock, D. Cooney, and S. Rosenberg. 1980. Spontaneous regression of non-Hodgkin's lymphoma. A report of nine cases. *Cancer* **46:** 2093–2099.

26. Lindhout, E., C. G. Figdor, and G. J. Adema. 1998. Dendritic cells: migratory cells that are attractive. *Cell Adhes. Commun.* **6:** 117–123.

27. Maraskovsky, E., McKenna, H., and Brasel, K. 1995. In vivo administration of Flt3 ligand but not G-CSF nor GM-CSF results in the generation of large numbers of dendritic cells in mice. *Blood* **86:** 423a (Abstract 1680).

28. Marrack, P. and J. Kappler. 1987. The T cell receptor. *Science* **238:** 1073–1079.

29. Mayordomo, J. I., T. Zorina, W. J. Storkus, L. Zitvogel, C. Celluzzi, L. D. Falo, et al. 1995. Bone marrow-derived dendritic cells pulsed with synthetic tumour peptides elicit protective and therapeutic antitumour immunity. *Nat. Med.* **1:** 1297–1302.

30. Melder, R. J., T. L. Whiteside, N. L. Vujanovic, J. C. Hiserodt, and R. B. Herberman. 1988. A new approach to generating antitumor effectors for adoptive immunotherapy using human adherent lymphokine-activated killer cells. *Cancer Res.* **48:** 3461–3469.

31. Mellman, I., S. J. Turley, and R. M. Steinman. 1998. Antigen processing for amateurs and professionals. *Trends Cell Biol.* **8:** 231–237.

32. Middleton, R., J. Smith, R. Melzer, and P. Hamilton. 1986. Patient survival and local recurrence rate following radical prostatectomy for prostatic carcinoma. *J. Urol.* **136:** 422–424.

33. Mitropoulos, D., S. Kooi, J. Rodriguez-Villanueva, and C. D. Platsoucas. 1994. Characterization of fresh (uncultured) tumour-infiltrating lymphocytes (TIL) and TIL-derived T cell lines from patients with renal cell carcinoma. *Clin. Exp. Immunol.* **97:** 321–327.

34. Murphy, G. P., B. A. Tjoa, S. J. Simmons, J. Jarisch, V. A. Bowes, H. Ragde, et al. 1999. Infusion of dendritic cells pulsed with HLA-A2-specific prostate-specific membrane antigen peptides: a phase II prostate cancer vaccine trial involving patients with hormone-refractory prostate cancer. *Prostate* **38:** 73–78.

35. Murphy, G. P., B. A. Tjoa, S. J. Simmons, H. Ragde, M. Rogers, A. Elgamal, et al. 1999. Phase II prostate cancer vaccine trial: report of a study involving 37 patients with disease recurrence following primary treatment [In Process Citation]. *Prostate* **39:** 54–59.

36. Murphy, G., H. Ragde, G. Kenny, R. Barren III, S. Erickson, B. Tjoa, et al. 1995. Comparison of prostate specific membrane antigen, and prostate specific antigen levels in prostatic cancer patients. *Anticancer Res.* **15:** 1473–1480.

37. Murphy, G., B. Tjoa, H. Ragde, G. Kenny, and A. Boynton. 1996. Phase I clinical trial: T cell therapy for prostate cancer using autologous dendritic cells pulsed with HLA-A0201-specific peptides from prostate-specific membrane antigen. *Prostate* **29:** 371–380.

38. Nestle, F. O., S. Alijagic, M. Gilliet, Y. Sun, S. Grabbe, R. Dummer, et al. 1998. Vaccination of melanoma patients with peptide- or tumor lysate-pulsed dendritic cells. *Nat. Med.* **4:** 328–332.

39. Oh, W. K. and P. W. Kantoff. 1998. Management of hormone refractory prostate cancer: current standards and future prospects. *J. Urol.* **160:** 1220–1229.

40. Ragde, H. 1997. Brachytherapy (seed implantation) for clinically localized prostate cancer. *J. Surg. Oncol.* **64:** 79–81.

41. Ragde, H., A. Elgamal, P. Snow, J. Brandt, A. Bartolucci, B. Nadir, et al. Ten-year disease free survival after transperineal sonography-guided iodine-125 brachytherapy with or without 45-gray external beam irradiation in the treatment of patients with clinically localized, low to high Gleason grade prostate carcinoma. *Cancer* **83:** 989–1001.

42. Ralfkiaer, E., K. Hou-Jensen, K. Gatter, D. Drzewiecki, and D. Mason. 1987. Immuno-histological analysis of the lymphoid infiltrate in cutaneous malignant melanomas. *Virchows Arch.* **410:** 355–361.

43. Ravindranath, M. H., D. L. Morton, and R. F. Irie. 1989. An epitope common to ganglio-sides O-acetyl-GD3 and GD3 recognized by antibodies in melanoma patients after active specific immunotherapy. *Cancer Res.* **49:** 3891–3897.

44. Romani, N., D. Reider, M. Heuer, S. Ebner, and E. Kempgen. 1996. Generation of mature dendritic cells from human blood. An improved method with special regard to clinical applicability. *J. Immunol. Methods* **196:** 137–151.

45. Rosenberg, S. A. 1996. Development of cancer immunotherapies based on identification of the genes encoding cancer regression antigens. *J. Natl. Cancer Inst.* **88:** 1635–1644.

46. Rosenberg, S. A., B. S. Packard, P. M. Aebersold, D. Solomon, S. L. Topalian, S. T. Toy, et al. 1988. Use of tumor-infiltrating lymphocytes and interleukin-2 in the immunotherapy of patients with metastatic melanoma. A preliminary report. *N. Engl. J. Med.* **319:** 1676–1680.

47. Ruiter, D. J., A. K. Bhan, T. J. Harrist, A. J. Sober, and M. Mhim-Jr. 1982. Major histo-compatibility antigens and mononuclear inflammatory infiltrate in benign nevomelanocytic proliferation and malignant melanoma. *J. Immunol.* **129:** 2808–2815.

48. Salgaller, M. L., F. M. Marincola, J. N. Cormier, and S. A. Rosenberg. 1996. Immunization against epitopes in the human melanoma antigen gp100 following patient immunization with synthetic peptides. *Cancer Res.* **56:** 4749–4757.

49. Sallusto, F. and A. Lanzavecchia. 1994. Efficient presentation of soluble antigen by cul-tured human dendritic cells is maintained by granulocyte/macrophage colony-stimulating factor plus interleukin 4 and downregulated by tumor necrosis factor alpha. *J. Exp. Med.* **179:** 1109–1118.

50. Sallusto, F., M. Cella, C. Danieli, and A. Lanzavecchia. 1995. Dendritic cells use macropinocytosis and the mannose receptor to concentrate macromolecules in the major histocompatibility complex class II compartment: downregulation by cytokines and bacte-rial products [see comments]. *J. Exp. Med.* **182:** 389–400.

51. Scher, H. I., G. Steineck, and W. K. Kelly. 1995. Hormone-refractory (D3) prostate cancer: refining the concept. *Urology* **46:** 142–148.

52. Sedlacek, H. 1994. Vaccination for treatment of tumors: a critical comment. *Critical Rev. Oncog.* **5:** 555–587.

53. Siegall, C. B. 1994. Targeted toxins as anticancer agents. *Cancer* **74:** 1006–1012.

54. Simmons, S. J., B. A. Tjoa, M. Rogers, A. Elgamal, G. M. Kenny, H. Ragde, et al. 1999. GM-CSF as a systemic adjuvant in a phase II prostate cancer vaccine trial. *Prostate* **39:** 291–297.

55. Slovin, S. F., W. K. Kelly, and H. I. Scher. 1998. Immunological approaches for the treat-ment of prostate cancer. *Sem. Urol. Oncol.* **16:** 53–59.

56. Steinman, R. M. 1991. The dendritic cell system and its role in immunogenicity. *Annu. Rev. Immunol.* **9:** 271–296.

57. Thomas, R., L. S. Davis, and P. E. Lipsky. 1993. Isolation and characterization of human peripheral blood dendritic cells. *J. Immunol.* **150:** 821–829.

58. Tjoa, B. A., S. J. Simmons, A. Elgamal, M. Rogers, H. Ragde, G. M. Kenny, et al. 1999. Follow-up evaluation of a phase II prostate cancer vaccine trial. *Prostate* **40:** 125–129.

59. Tjoa, B., S. Erickson, R. Barren III, H. Ragde, G. Kenny, A. Boynton, et al. 1995. In vitro propagated dendritic cells from prostate cancer patients as a component of prostate cancer immunotherapy. *Prostate* **27:** 63–69.

60. Tjoa, B., S. Erickson, V. Bowes, H. Ragde, G. Kenny, O. Cobb, et al. 1997. Follow-up evaluation of prostate cancer patients with autologous dendritic cells pulsed with PSMA peptides. *Prostate* **32:** 272–278.

61. Tjoa, B., S. Simmons, V. Bowes, H. Ragde, M. Rogers, A. Elgamal, et al. 1998. Evaluation of phase I/II clinical trials in prostate cancer with dendritic cells and PSMA peptides. *Prostate* **36:** 39–44.
62. Topalian, S., D. Solomon, F. P. Avis, A. E. Chang, D. L. Freerksen, W. M. Linehan, et al. 1988. Immunotherapy of patients with advanced cancer using tumor-infiltrating lymphocytes and recombinant interleukin-2: A pilot study. *J. Clin. Oncol.* **6:** 839–853.
63. Urban, J. L. and H. Schreiber. 1992. Tumor antigens. *Ann. Rev. Immunol.* **10:** 617–644.
64. Walsh, P. C., A. W. Partin, and J. I. Epstein. 1994. Cancer control and quality of life following anatomic radical retropubic prostatectomy. Results at 10 years. *J. Urol.* **152:** 1831–1836.
65. Wang, M., L. Valenzuela, G. Murphy, and T. Chu. 1979. Purification of a human prostate-specific antigen. *Investig. Urol.* **17:** 159–163.
66. Young, J. W. and R. M. Steinman. 1990. Dendritic cells stimulate primary human cytolytic lymphocyte response in the absence of CD4+ helper T cells. *J. Exp. Med.* **171:** 1315–1332.
67. Zinkernagel, R. M. and P. C. Doherty. 1974. Restriction of in vitro T cell-mediated cytotoxicity in lymphocytic choriomeningitis within a syngeneic or semiallogeneic system. *Nature* **248:** 701,702.

27

Antiprogression Agents for Prostate Cancer

Hadley M. Wood and Michael A. Carducci, MD

1. ANTIPROGRESSION AGENTS FOR PROSTATE CANCER

Pharmacological treatments that inhibit tumor progression or induce malignant reversion are broadly defined as antiprogression agents, also known as differentiation therapies. Differentiation therapy has proven most successful for the treatment of acute promyelocytic leukemia, and is now being extensively investigated for treatment of colon, breast, and prostate cancer (PCA). Other classes of treatments used to slow the progression of PCA reduce the ability of cells to enter or leave the vasculature (antimetastatics) or limit the ability of the tumor to signal growth of new vasculature (anti-angiogenics). These and other classes of drugs are discussed elsewhere in this book. This chapter discusses the use of differentiation therapies for the treatment of PCA.

Treatment strategies that prolong survival in androgen independent prostate cancer (AIPCA) are rare. For many men, the toxicities caused by chemotherapy only add to the distress of having cancer, especially when the survival benefit is unclear. With a reduced toxicity profile and a growing potential for slowing the progression of advanced disease, differentiation therapies offer an alternative to chemotherapy.

Whether differentiation of a cancer cell represents the malignant transformation in reverse is unknown. Research suggests that these agents may induce terminal differentiation (arrest in G_0), may induce differentiation to a mature cell with cellular functions and a growth pattern similar to nonmalignant cells, or may trigger an apoptotic cascade, making the drugs cytostatic as well as cytotoxic. In advanced prostate cancer, measuring the differentiating vs apoptotic effects of these agents is difficult, as metastatic disease is characterized by broad cellular population heterogeneity. Differentiation agents may not induce terminal differentiation, yet as maturational agents, they may still benefit patients if the agent can decrease the proliferative rate, the agent can attenuate the ability to invade or metastasize, the agent can convert a heterogeneous population to a more homogeneous population, and/or the agent can enhance the therapeutic index of other forms of antitumor therapy.

The use of differentiating agents for advanced stages of cancer has been troubled by discrepancy between in vitro concentration needed for activity and those achieved in vivo. Agents such as hexamethylene bisacetamide (HMBA) or dimethylsulfoxide (DMSO) have significant toxicities below a bioactive concentration, which has prevented further development (2). Butyrate has not been clinically useful because its

From: *Prostate Cancer: Biology, Genetics, and the New Therapeutics*
Edited by: L. W. K. Chung, W. B. Isaacs, and J. W. Simons © Humana Press Inc., Totowa, NJ

metabolism is too rapid and an appropriate formulation is not yet available. All-trans-retinoic acid (ATRA) has proven successful in remission induction of acute promyelocytic leukemia, particularly when it is followed with systemic chemotherapy. However, as discussed here, attempts to use ATRA for the treatment of AIPCA has been largely unsuccessful thus far.

The antiprogression agents discussed throughout this chapter have been divided into families of agents based on their mechanisms of action. These include: metabolites of vitamin A and its analogs, short-chain fatty acids (phenylacetate and phenylbutarate), peroxisome proliferator activated receptor (PPAR) agonists, vitamin D and its analogs, polyamine inhibitors, and hybrid polar compounds.

2. METABOLITES OF VITAMIN A AND ANALOGS

It has long been known that vitamin A, its synthetic analogs, and metabolites (retinoids) are critical effectors of nuclear receptors that control cell growth, differentiation, and apoptosis. In 1983, while investigating the ability of retinoic acid (RA) to induce alkaline phosphatase activity in cells derived from rat prostatic adenocarcinoma, Reese et al. noted that the RA-treated cells occupied more space on the culture dish surface, indicating that the treatment induced morphological changes in the culture cells *(77)*. In 1993, Peehl et al. harvested normal, BPH, and malignant prostates from human subjects and grew the samples in a serum-free medium. They then demonstrated that clonal growth of prostate epithelial cells was inhibited when treated with (RA) >3 nm (through a 10-d incubation period). At this concentration, morphological changes were also noted. These changes included the production of widely spaced cells that lacked intracellular bodies. These data provided a strong indication that the retinoids play a role in prostate cell differentiation and apoptosis, and set off a flurry of further investigation *(73)*.

The nuclear receptors that interact with retinoids fall into two classes: the retinoid X receptors (RXRs) and the retinoic acid receptors (RARs). Each of these classes has three known subtypes (α,β,γ) and numerous isoforms. The RXRs are the most versatile of the known nuclear receptors, acting as one of a dimer pair in conjunction with a number of other receptor types. These include: other RXRs, RARs, vitamin D receptors (VDR), thyroid hormone receptors (TR), and peroxisome proliferator-activated receptors (PPARs). RARs are only known to dimerize with RXRs. As shown in Fig. 1, activation of these different nuclear receptor dimers have been shown to exhibit a distinct yet redundant influence on cellular activity. The RXR-RAR, RXR-PPAR, and the RXR-VDR receptors are known to induce differentiation when activated. Many vitamin A metabolites bind nonspecifically to both the RAR and RXR receptors, stimulating a combination of responses from the cell that may conflict with the desired outcome—for example, apoptosis as well as proliferation *(16)*. All-trans-retinoic acid showed early promise in some in vitro studies of PCA cell lines, but other in vitro studies produced evidence that some strains of LNCaP (hormone dependent cell line) experienced proliferation rather than the intended antiproliferative effects *(24)*. In Phase II clinical trials, ATRA was found to demonstrate minimal effectiveness in reducing pain and PSA levels in hormone refractory PCA because of a failure of drug delivery associated with enhanced clearance of the drug after a few days of treatment *(15,100)*.

Current research in retinoid use entails identification and testing of subclass-specific synthetic analogs that act on only the desired nuclear receptor to limit toxicity and unwanted effects that may be caused by the drug cross-reacting with another similar nuclear receptor. Dietary fenretinide (4HPR) (a synthetic retinoid) is effective in reducing both the incidence and mass of *ras+myc*-induced tumors in a mouse prostate reconsititution system *(92)*. A Phase II clinical trial in which patients with negative prestudy biopsies were treated with fenretinide for twelve 28-d cycles was terminated early when over one-third (*n* = 8/22) of the patients were discovered to have positive prostate biopsies. However, the authors noted that the study subjects had a mean initial PSA = 8.6 ng/mL (range 4.3–20.9 ng/mL), which put these individuals in the highest risk group for developing clinical disease. They suggested that the number of positive biopsies may have been the result of poor sensitivity of the initial screening test, and noted that the sample size was not large enough to provide sufficient statistical power to draw reasonable conclusions *(74)*. A more recent Phase II chemoprevention study measured the effect of treatment with and without 4HPR on patients for 3 wk prior to radical prostatectomy. This study reported no statistically significant differences in the biomarkers measured on the treatment group as compared to the control group *(101)*. Although clinical trials with 4HPR have failed to demonstrate an antiproliferative effect thus far, investigation into the use of this drug for treatment of both early and advanced disease continues.

Other synthetic retinoids have been tested only in vitro and show some potential. A synthetic retinoid, CD-271, that selectively activates the RARγ subtype nuclear receptor has shown increased antiproliferative effects on the DU-145 as compared to ATRA *(53)*. Another synthetic retinoid, CD-437, caused 100% and 60% inhibition of growth in vitro in LNCaP and PC-3 cells respectively, suggesting that this drug may be applicable to both hormone refractory and hormone dependent prostate carcinomas *(46)*. Neither of these synthetic analogs has yet been tested in vivo.

Other clinical applications of retinoids for the treatment of advanced PCA have combined retinoid treatment with other differentiation and/or chemotherapeutic drugs. The use of alpha-interferon (IFN) and 13-*cis*-retinoic acid (13*cis* RA) has been applied with some success on other solid tumors, including renal cell *(64)*, cervical *(48)*, and skin *(49)*. DiPaola et al. explored the use of combination therapy of 13*cis*RA and IFN in AIPCA patients. Twenty-six percent of the patients had a partial decrease in PSA (50% decrease, maintained for at least 1 mo, and these patients had significant increases in TGF-β1 at 1 mo of therapy *(19)*. Currently, the same group is conducting a Phase I/II study treating AIPCA patients with IFN and 13*cis*RA followed by paclitaxel. Preliminary data demonstrate that this combination treatment is well tolerated, and suggest than an antiproliferative effect may be achieved *(20)*. Treatment protocols that combine multiple differentiation therapies are under investigation.

The mechanism through which retinoids act is an active area of investigation. As discussed here, retinoid receptors belong to a superfamily of nuclear receptors that act as transcription factors when induced by ligand. They bind to regulatory sequences of DNA known as hormone responsive elements (HREs), which modulate gene transcription. Several genes have been proposed as targets of retinoid HREs, and it is likely that these and others yet undiscovered may all contribute to the changes that occur at the cellular level in response to treatment with retinoids. The p21$^{\text{waf1/cip1/sid1}}$ (p21) gene and the endothelin-1 (ET-1) gene are two examples of genes that are affected by retinoid HREs. Treatment with both vitamin D and RA induces p21, which is believed to be responsible for cellular arrest in G_1 by inhibiting entry into the S phase. Liu et al. showed that this gene is an RAR-responsive target gene that acts in response to RAR-RXR heterodimer activation. They identified a RA-responsive element in the promotor region of p21 *(50)*. Hsu et al. have suggested that retinoids suppress endothelin-1 (ET-1) expression through specific binding sites in the promotor region of that gene, and attributed the differential effects of various retinoids to differential binding of these promotor sites *(37)*. Nelson et al. have demonstrated that ET-1 is PCA mitogen, and that the most common endothelin receptor—ETB—is not expressed in PCA cell lines *(66)*. They found increased cytidine methylation of portions of the ETB gene (CpG island sequences) in 5 of 5 PCA cell lines, in 15 of 21 primary PCA tissues, and in 8 of 14 prostate metastases. Postulating that ETB may inhibit production of ET-1 and mediate ET-1 clearance, they suggested that this mechanism may account for increased ET-1 in PCA *(67)*.

Notably, one drug—Liarozole (R75251)—inhibits the cytochrome p450-system that metabolizes RA, thereby increasing tissue concentration of RA. This drug—known as a retinoic acid metabolism-blocking agent (RAMBA)—was the first in its class to be extensively tested for clinical use. Liarozole was administered to 55 AIPCA patients. In over one-half of the patients, pain was reported to improve and PSA declined in 41% of the subjects, respectively *(18)*. Similar results were obtained in a larger study (*n* = 100) published a year later *(17)*. However, the significant side effects and only moderate efficacy demonstrated by this drug have shifted the focus of investigation and development of RAMBA drugs to more potent, less toxic successors. A second-generation RAMBA—R116010—has demonstrated greater potency and fewer side effects than Liarozole in rat models and is currently in early clinical trials. Early data suggest that this drug has fewer negative side effects when compared with Liarozole, but further trials are needed to assess potency *(8)*.

3. SHORT-CHAIN FATTY ACIDS

This class of differentiating agents includes the bioactively stable analogs of sodium butyrate (NaBu), phenylbutyrate (PB), and phenylacetate (PA). Both of these drugs have been used for some time in treatment of patients with disorders of urea metabolism. Shortly after publishing their findings on the effects of RA on prostatic cell-culture growth, Reese et al. explored the effect of butyrate and short-chain fatty acids on similar cell cultures. Butyrate proved to be more potent than RA at inducing alkaline phosphatase activity and suppressed cell growth at concentration above 5 mm. They also noted important morphological changes that occurred within the butyrate-treated cultures. The cells, which normally grow in a disorganized fashion, associated into parallel tracts, suggesting that morphological changes were induced *(78)*.

Active investigation into effects of PA on PCA cell lines began in the early 1990s, when Samid et al. found that PA-treated PC3, DU145, and LNCaP cell lines lost their ability to invade a reconstituted basement membrane and showed diminished ability to form tumors when transplanted into athymic mice *(83)*. This finding triggered investigation into the in vivo effects of these short-chain fatty acids. A Phase I study published a year later measured the safety of treatment with a bolus followed by a 14-d infusion of PA. The study reported dose-limiting toxicity and minimal effectiveness in relieving bone pain and reducing PSA values *(97)*.

Because of the apparent limitations of PA in vivo, the focus of investigation turned to PB. PB was found to be 1.5–2.5 times more active at inhibiting growth and inducing apoptosis than PA at clinically achievable doses, and exposure of cancer cell lines to PB caused 50-60% of the cells to undergo apoptosis *(10,76)*. PB induces G_1/G_0 arrest in treated PCA cells within 24 h of exposure. The p21 protein is induced two to threefold over control, as determined by immunoblotting, and topoisomerase IIα is downregulated over a 48-h period. PB-treated PCA cells also demonstrate increased and multiple acetylated forms of histone H4 using histone separation by triton-acetic acid-urea electropheresis. Prolonged PB exposure (7 d) inhibits telomerase activity in the LNCaP cell line *(98)*. These molecular effects of PB on gene expression are probably affected through alterations in chromatin condensation, favoring genes promoting the differentiated phenotype. Variations were demonstrated in the cellular response to PB in athymic mice treated with the LNCaP and LuCaP 23 cell lines. Terminal differentiation was induced in a time and dose-dependent manner, and apoptosis was induced at concentration at and above 2.5 mm *(58)*.

Two Phase I clinical trials of PB have been completed based on this preclinical data. In the first study, PB was administered by infusion for 120 h on an every 3-wk schedule, and the second trial used oral PB given three times daily. In both studies, peak concentrations of PB were above 1.5–2.5 mm. On the continuous infusion schedule, the PB concentration remained above 0.5 mm, a therapeutic threshold defined by preclinical studies for the duration of the infusion when administered at 410 mg/kg/d. On the oral schedule, PB concentration remained above the 0.5 mm level for 4 h after each oral dosing. 5/19 (iv schedule) and 4/11 (oral schedule) patients with heavily pretreated hormone refractory PCA had stable disease for greater than 6 mo in these Phase I studies. *(9)* PSA levels typically rose during the 5-d infusion schedule and dropped to baseline when patients were off the agent. This effect on PSA had been noted in preclinical models and was expected. These single-agent Phase I studies are encouraging, but suggest that combination strategies may increase the disease stabilization fraction.

Some investigators have tested the affects of combining PA or PB with more traditional therapies. Phenylbutyrate was found to have additive cytotoxic effects on human neuroblastoma cell lines when used in combination with vincristine, although not with doxorubicin, etoposide, or cisplatin *(75)*. In vitro studies demonstrated that pretreatment with either PA or PB before radiation therapy significantly increased radiosensitivity and induced G_1 phase arrest. The increased radiosensitivity was accompanied by increased activity of antioxidant enzymes and a decline in intracellular glutathione levels *(62)*. Unpublished in vivo data comparing the antiproliferative effects of combining 13cisRA and PB and planned clinical trials for this combination treatment are discussed in a later section of this chapter.

Several mechanisms of action for the short-chain fatty acids have been postulated. A growing body of evidence suggests that these mechanisms are most likely not mutually exclusive. Two accepted mechanisms of action for these compounds are histone hyperacetylation and activation of the PPAR nuclear receptor.

3.1. Hyperacetylation of Histones

Phenylbutyrate has been proven to maintain histones in a hyperacetylated state, presumably as a result of histone deacetylase inhibition. Enhanced acetylation of the H4 histone has been associated with increased binding of transcription factors *(102)*, DNA fragmentation *(44)*, and increased production of proteins such as caspase-3, which trigger the apoptotic cascade *(57)*. Other studies have provided data to suggest that increased acetylation of histones upregulates gamma globulin production, which may enhance the immune response *(40,56)*. Using a hyperacetylating agent similar to PB, trichostatin A, Van Lint et al. reported that expression of approx 2% of the genes they investigated were affected by histone deacetylase inhibitors *(102)*. Sowa et al. found a close correlation between the amount of histone hyperacetylation that occurs (in response to Trichostatin A) and the expression of the p21 gene promotor, independent of the p53 gene *(95)*. Using the breast cancer cell line, MCF-7, Gorospe et al. found that enhanced expression of p21 by PA leads to dephosphorylation of the retinoblastoma (Rb) protein—which is associated with tumor suppression *(29)*. Another recent study reported the expression of carboxypeptidase A3 (CPA3) in response to treatment of PC3 cell lines with NaBu. Although the role of this protein has not yet been established, expression of CPA3 is one step in the p21 induction pathway that is induced by hyperacetylation *(38)*. PB and PA, as well as other aromatic fatty acids, have also been implicated as PPAR agonists.

4. PEROXISOME PROLIFERATOR ACTIVATED RECEPTOR AGONISTS

PPARs are nuclear receptors that form heterodimers with RXRs to function as transcription factors. PPARs are largely responsible for regulating transcription of proteins that control lipid metabolism, transport, and storage. Three subclasses of receptors have been identified. Affectors of the PPARγ receptor have proven to be most promising for inducing differentiation. The ability to induce terminal differentiation in human liposarcoma cells through activation of the PPARγ-RXRα was demonstrated by Tontonoz in 1997. Using thiazolidinedione antidiabetic drugs as activators of the PPARγ subunit and LG268—a ligand specific for RXRα—an additive effect on differentiation of liposarcoma cell lines was demonstrated *(99)*. Further research has investigated the use of PPAR agonists to induce differentiation in several types of cancer cell lines, including breast *(23,65)*, colorectal *(41,82)*, liver *(5)*, prostate *(43,76)* and monocytic leukemia *(108)*.

Research suggests that the human PPAR nuclear receptor is activated by PB and PA, in addition to other aromatic short-chain fatty acids *(76)*. PPARs are known to upregulate expression of enzymes responsible for β-oxidation of fatty acids, a process that involves sequential transfer of acetyl-CoA groups. These enzymes have not been shown to be linked to the histone acetylation that is also known to occur in response to treatment with short-chain fatty acids.

Kubota et al. reported that PC-3 cells expressed high levels of the PPARγ receptor, while normal prostate cells did not. In response to treatment with troglitazone and other thiazolidinedione derivatives, the investigators showed potent antiproliferative effects in PC-3 cell cultures. Interestingly, although morphological changes were readily apparent in these cells using light and electron microscopy, the markers of differentiation and cell-cycle response that they measure showed no significant changes *(43)*. A Phase II clinical trial that treated both androgen dependent and hormone refractory PCA men with troglitazone reported some limited success on a small sample size (*n* = 13 evaluable for response) *(94)*. Larger controlled clinical trials of these PPARγ-activating drugs are needed to adequately determine whether they are of clinical use in carcinomas expressing the PPARγ receptor.

5. VITAMIN D AND ANALOGS

In 1990, Schwartz et al. noted that the major known risk factors for clinical PCA—i.e., old age, African-American race, and residence in northern latitudes—are all associated with low serum levels of vitamin D *(85)*. They hypothesized that vitamin D maintains the differentiated phenotype of prostate cells, and that insufficient levels of vitamin D allowed progression of subclinical cancers to clinical disease. Two years later, Hanchette and Schwartz released epidemiological evidence that further supported their theory: they reported finding a close inverse correlation ($p < 0.0001$) between latitudinal geographic distribution of 3073 counties in the United States and PCA mortality *(32)*. Schwartz's hypothesis relating levels of vitamin D and risk for PCA was validated in 1993 by Corder et al. Using data from 181 men diagnosed with PCA from whom serum samples had been collected and analyzed for $1,25(OH)_2D3$ and $25(OH)D3$ (a metabolic precursor), and comparing these data to age and race-matched controls, they found a significant ($p = 0.002$) relationship between serum $1,25(OH)_2D3$ concentration and incidence of PCA. Serum concentration of $1,25(OH)_2D3$ appeared to be a good predictor of risk for palpable and anaplastic tumors in men over the age of 57. However, serum concentration of $25(OH)D3$ did not show a strong relationship to PCA risk *(13)*. More recent studies have reported a strong relationship between intake of calcium and risk for PCA, and have attributed this effect to calcium lowering circulating $1,25(OH)_2D3$ *(11,28)*. In an attempt to understand the basis of vitamin D's action on PCA cells and develop clinical applications for treatments using vitamin D, researchers began to investigate the molecular effects of vitamin D on PCA cell lines.

Miller et al. identified receptors for vitamin D in the androgen dependent cell line, LNCaP. They also showed that physiologic concentration of $1,25(OH)_2D3$, the biologically active form of vitamin D, were mitogenic, whereas in concentration at or above 10^{-8} M, cellular differentiation is promoted *(61)*. Skowronski et al. substantiated these findings in 1993, when they reported all three of the commonly investigated PCA cell lines—LNCaP, PC-3, and DU145—expressed receptors for $1,25(OH)_2D3$. Interestingly, physiological levels inhibited proliferation of only the LNCaP and the PC-3 cell lines, not DU-145, and treatment with $1,25(OH)_2D3$ caused dose-dependent secretion of PSA in the LNCaP cell line *(90)*. The antiproliferative effects of $1,25(OH)_2D3$ were demonstrated on primary cultures harvested from normal, BHP, and malignant prostate samples by Peehl et al. They noted that epithelial cell as well as fibroblast growth was inhibited by treatment with $1,25(OH)_2D3$ although epithelial cells showed a greater response than fibroblasts *(72)*.

Because of the undesirable hypercalcemia induced by treatment with $1,25(OH)_2D3$, research on the use of vitamin D in treating PCA began to compare the less calcemic analogs and combination therapies to $1,25(OH)_2D3$. Schwartz et al. tested three such analogs (1,25-Dihydroxy-16-ene-cholecalciferal [Ro24-2637], 1,25-Dihydroxy-16,23E-diene-cholecalciferol [Ro24-2201], 25-Hydroxy-16,23E-diene-cholecalciferol [Ro24-2287]) on PCA cell lines, and compared their effects to those obtained using $1,25(OH)_2D3$. They found significant inhibition of proliferation using all three of the analogs. Unlike Miller et al., who reported differentiation occurring at high concentrations of $1,25(OH)_2D3$, the Schwartz study noted antiproliferative effects at all concentrations tested. Although Schwartz et al. used an experimental method that was different from the method used by Skowronski in 1993, they also noted that the PC-3 and LNCaP cell lines responded to physiological levels of the analogs, whereas DU-145 did not *(86)*. In a later study, Schwartz et al. surprisingly found that DU-145, the most highly invasive of the three cell lines, was the only cell line in which invasiveness was significantly affected by treatment with $1,25(OH)_2D3$ and 1,25-Dihydroxy-16-ene-23-yne-cholecalciferol (16-23-D) *(87)*. These findings suggest that although DU-145 may not show antiproliferative effects at physiological concentration, the cell line does demonstrate antimetastatic effects in vitro when treated with vitamin D or 16-23-D. A study conducted by Skowronski et al. in 1995 compared the effect of vitamin D analogs in ligand binding tests. They demonstrated the following order of potency: EB-1089>$1,25(OH)_2D3$>MC-903>1,24,25-(OH)3D3>22-oxacalcitriol>Ro24-2637>25-OH-D3. Their tests showed that although binding to the VDR is necessary for action of these analogs, additional factors significantly contribute to the magnitude of biological response. This was especially apparent in the testing of the synthetic analogs, where binding affinity did not directly correlate with biological potency *(91)*. Hedlund et al. reported that the vitamin D analogs, Ro 23-7553, Ro 24-5531, and Ro 25-6760, induced secretion of PSAP and PSA in vitro, further suggesting that the antiproliferative effects were attributable to induction of differentiation vs apoptosis *(34)*.

Animal studies have further substantiated the role that vitamin D and its analogs play in PCA proliferation. Using the noncalcemic analog, 16-23-D3, Schwartz et al. treated athymic mice inoculated with the PC-3 cell line and compared them with controls. The experimental cohort demonstrated no evidence of toxicity and a modest decrease in mean tumor volume when compared with the controls *(84)*. Lucia et al. measured the incidence of invasive tumors of the seminal vesicle and anterior prostate in tumor-promoted Lobund-Wistar rats given diets supplemented with RO24-5531, tamoxifen, and Fenretinide. They reported reduced invasive tumor incidence with all three agents *(54)*. Getzenberg et al. demonstrated the antimetastatic effects of both $1,25(OH)_2D3$ and a less hypercalcemic analog, Ro25-6760, on MLL and AT2 rats *(27)*. Others have investigated the use of EB1089 on MLL rats, and found reduced tumor size and reduced incidence of lung metastases, but both increased serum calcium (EB1089 less so than $1,25(OH)_2D3$) *(6,51)*.

Like the other differentiating agents already discussed, there has been some attempt to combine vitamin D analogs with chemotoxic compounds for treatment of advanced PCA. Pretreatment of mice with squamous cell carcinomas with Ro23-7553 before treatment with cisplatin demonstrated enhanced cytotoxic effects, even at a low dose of cisplatin, as compared to treatment with cisplatin alone. This combination also demonstrated increased tumor regrowth delay *(47)*.

Clinical trials have demonstrated that $1,25(OH)_2D3$ every other day at doses of 10 µg results in dose-limiting hypercalcemia ($n = 3/3$), but doses less than 10 µg showed little toxicity *(93)*. Still, the search continues for a vitamin D analog that provides greater antiproliferative (and antimetastatic) effects without inducing hypercalcemia. Schwartz reported α-hydroxylase activity in the two hormone refractory PCA cell lines (PC-3, DU-145), suggesting that administration of 25-OHD3, a $1,25(OH)_2D3$ precursor, may limit the invasiveness of advanced PCA *(88)*. 1α-OHD2, a less calcemic similar prodrug, has been tested in Phase I clinical trials on more than 17 patients with AIPCA. The drug has been well tolerated, although hypercalcemia varying from mild to severe was induced in three patients. Mild hyperphosphatemia and mild to moderate anemia, leukopenia, and thrombocytopenia were also noted in some of the study patients. No significant hepatotoxicity was seen. Phase II results of 1α-OHD2 clinical studies at the University of Wisconsin are anticipated shortly.

The mechanism of action exerted by vitamin D on PCA cells is still under investigation. As noted here, the VDR associates with RXR to act as a heterodimeric nuclear receptor. Investigators have demonstrated that different PCA cell lines exhibit different antiproliferative effects, and although the concentration of VDR receptors expressed by the particular cell line suggests that they play a role in determining the efficacy of $1,25(OH)_2D3$ in inducing differentiation, other factors also play a role in determining this. PC-3 and DU-145, which contain low levels of VDR, demonstrate the least amount of inhibition. LNCaP, with higher VDR content, exhibited higher growth inhibition in response to treatment with $1,25(OH)_2D3$ *(33,110)*. In a later study, treatment of LNCaP cell line with $1,25(OH)_2D3$ demonstrated the accumulation of cells in G_1/G_0, accompanied by decreased phosphorylation of the retinoblastoma (Rb) protien, decreased cyclin-dependent kinase (CDK) inhibitor p21, and decreased CDK2. The investigators attributed the reduced p21 protein to translational or posttranslational modifications that occurred as a result of treatment, because the reduced levels of CDK inhibitor demonstrated were not accompanied by reduced p21 mRNA *(109)*. Bookstein et al. noted very low levels of Rb expression in the DU-145 cell line, suggesting that treatment with $1,25(OH)_2D3$ may not be effective, whereas PC-3 and LNCaP both express Rb *(7)*. The relationship between treatment of LNCaP cell lines with $1,25(OH)_2D3$ and expression of PSA is consistent with induction of differentiation (G_1/G_0 stasis) *(61,90)*.

Interesting investigations into the interaction between steroids and $1,25(OH)_2D3$ on PCA cell lines have provided further insight into the potential mechanism of action of vitamin D. Zhao et al. reported identification of a link between dihydrotestosterone (DHT) and the antiproliferative effects of $1,25(OH)_2D3$ by demonstrating that the androgen receptor (AR) is upregulated in response to treatment with $1,25(OH)_2D3$ in androgen-dependent cell lines *(106)*. Hsieh et al. reported increased concentration of AR in the nucleus following treatment with $1,25(OH)_2D3$, and suggested that vitamin D may promote translocation of AR from the cytosol to the nucleus *(36)*. Addition of dexamethasone to $1,25(OH)_2D3$ treatments reduced cell survival in vitro and reduced tumor size in vivo for squamous cell carcinoma. Also, reduced calcemic effects were noted with the use of dexamethasone. The investigators attributed the apparent increased antitumor effects to upregulation of the VDR receptor *(105)*. These studies suggest a potentially significant interaction between steroid receptors and VDRs, although the exact mechanism of these interactions has not yet been described. Further work must be done to determine how each of the known PCA cell lines respond to treatment with 1,25(OH)$_2$D3 at the molecular level and—more importantly—how clinicians can diagnostically determine whether a PCA patient will be responsive to such treatment.

Work both in the laboratory and in the clinic on vitamin D and its analogs continues today, especially with regard to the use of this class of drugs in combination with other treatments. Like the other differentiating agents already discussed, successful monotherapy with any of these treatments seems unlikely. In the final section of this chapter, we examine the future of differentiating agents—using these agents in combination to maximize therapeutic benefit.

6. POLYAMINE INHIBITORS

Because polyamines are ubiquitous and essential for cell survival, investigators have attempted to limit or inhibit polyamine synthesis to reduce cycling of highly proliferative cancer cells. Difluoromethylornithine (DFMO) is an irreversible inhibitor of the initial enzymatic step (ornithine decarboxylase, ODC) in polyamine synthesis. DFMO has shown the greatest success in prevention of epithelial cancers, including colon, skin, breast, and urinary bladder. Most human and rodent cell cultures respond to treatment with DFMO with reduced levels of putrescine and spermidine and unaffected levels of spermine. This was demonstrated by Meyskens et al. in clinical trial that measured the chemoprevention effects of low levels of DFMO on patients who had undergone surgical removal of one or more adenomatous colon polyps *(59)*. However, in PCA cell lines, spermine is the major polyamine.

Because spermine and spermidine concentration are higher in the prostate than in most other tissues in the body, the potential for DFMO and other inhibitors of polyamine synthesis to be effective antiproliferative agents for PCA is enticing. The ability of DMFO to inhibit ODC activity and tumor growth in the prostate was demonstrated both in vitro and in vivo in 1982 *(35)*. Additionally, epidemiological and laboratory studies have suggested that there is a correlation between consumption of green tea (which contains ODC-reducing compounds) and reduced incidence of various cancers, including PCA *(1,71)*. Using a polyphenolic mixture extracted from green tea, Gupta et al. demonstrated reduced ODC activity in the LNCaP cell line and in a rat model. Because polyphenols extracted from green tea have demonstrated selective growth inhibition of cancer cell lines, Gupta et al. postulated that treatment with these compounds may only reduce ODC activity in PCA cells and spare normal cells *(31)*.

A significant limiting side effect noted with the use of DMFO is ototoxicity. Additional side effects include diarrhea, abdominal pain, and nausea, as well as moderate anemia, leukopenia, and thrombocytopenia. Although clinical trials have demonstrated only gastrointestinal symptoms at levels of DMFO as high as 3.75 g/m^2 every 6 h *(30)*, research into the use of DMFO today is largely in the chemoprevention arena. Because this potential for low levels of DMFO over the long term for chemoprevention remains, an effort has been made to identify "safe" levels of DMFO. In a multicenter study, Loprinzi et al. reported no significant toxicity in treatment of 35 patients for 1 yr or more with does of DFMO ranging from 0.125–1.0 g per d *(52)*. A review of the current status of the development of this drug as a chemopreventive agent is provided by Meyskens and Gerner *(60)*.

Because of the limitations of DFMO, recent investigation in this area has turned toward the development of less toxic, more potent polyamine inhibitors. Eiseman et al. investigated the effect of 1,12-diaziridinyl-4,9-diazadodecance (BIS), a spermine analog, on PC-3 and DU-145 cell lines. They demonstrated an apparent dose-dependent apoptic effect and increased radiosensitivity of BIS-treated cell cultures. Using immunodeficient mice, they examined the in vivo effects of the drug and found BIS-mediated tumor regression via induction of apoptosis *(21)*. Another novel drug, methylacetylenic putrescine (MAP), was administered to mice xenografted with various cancer cell lines, including human thyroid carcinoma (BHT-101), mouse lymphoma (P388), human breast carcinoma (MCF-7 and MDA-MB-231). Although some arrest in G_1 reported at low doses, nonapoptotic programmed cell death was noted at high doses. The investigators also reported that treatment of breast cancer cell lines with MAP induced complete inhibition of ODC and demonstrated 10 times greater potency than DMFO *(70)*.

As spermidine and spermine are associated with proliferation and differentiation in prostate cells, some investigators have suggested the use of these compounds as markers of PCA progression. Cipolla et al. demonstrated a correlation between erythrocytic polyamine concentration and BPH and PCA proliferation and metastases. They suggest using erythrocytic polyamines as markers for measuring progression of PCA *(12)*. Recommending that measurement of ODC in prostatic serum may be an effective method of early detection and monitoring the efficacy of treatments, Mohan et al. demonstrated increased levels of ODC in prostatic fluid of PCA patients as compared to those with benign tissue *(63)*. The potential to use radiolabeled polyamines in radiographic (PET) imaging of prostate carcinomas has been demonstrated, and represents another means by which polyamines can be used in characterizing and following PCA progression *(39)*.

Interestingly, there is a relationship between androgen receptor and ODC activity. Crozat et al. demonstrated increased expression of the ODC mRNA and enzyme in androgen-stimulated prostate, kidney, and seminal vesicle cells. This effect was attributed to a somewhat weak androgen responsive element (ARE) in the ODC promotor *(14)*. If and how this interaction between AR and ODC impacts the clinical use of androgen dependent vs androgen independent PCA has yet to be discovered.

7. HYBRID POLAR COMPOUNDS

The ability of hybrid polar compounds to induce differentiation has been recognized for a long time. Over 20 years ago, it was reported that treating cultured murine erythroleukemia cells (MELCs) with hexamethylene bisacetamide (HMBA) caused a transient rise and fall in intracellular diacylglycerol, followed by increased protein kinase C (PKC) activity. A prolonged G_1 phase, which was followed by terminal differentiation, was noted in about 15% of the cells after the first cell division, and in nearly all of the cells after 5 or 6 more cell cycles *(25)*. Most of the research on this class of agents has since focused on HMBA and how it effects growth of MELC cell lines. Differentiation effects were associated with accumulation of histone H10, modulation of the

activity of cyclins and cyclin dependent kinases, and hypophosphorylation of Rb
(42,69,80). Although the in vitro evidence supporting the ability of HMBA to
induce differentiation was strong, clinical trials demonstrated its severe limitations. A
Phase II clinical trial published in 1992 reported some limited success in using continuous infusions of HMBA to induce complete or partial remission in about one-third of
the subjects (9/28 patients), but significant thrombocytopenia and the drug's short half-
life hindered its practicality for widespread use *(2)*.

A resurgence in research interest in this class of drugs has occurred, as second-
generation hybrid polar compounds have been shown to be several thousand times
more potent than HMBA. These drugs include suberolanilide hydroxamic acid (SAHA)
and *m*-carboxycinamic acid *bis*-hydroxamide (CBHA), among others. There are apparent differences between the ways that CBHA and SAHA act to induce differentiation
as compared to HMBA. Richon et al. reported that HMBA-induced differentiation
depends on downregulation of the *c-myb* gene, a regulator of the G_1 checkpoint. SAHA
and CBHA induce differentiation without downregulation of *c-myb* protein. Whereas
HMBA is effective at the mmol range, SAHA and CBHA are effective in the μmol
range *(81)*.

Recent evidence into the mechanisms of action of CBHA and HMBA suggests that
they may be more like the short-chain fatty acids than their predecessor, HMBA. These
drugs are known inhibitors of histone deacetylases, and SAHA has been demonstrated
to induce hyperacetylation of H4 (like PB), whereas HMBA does not. Furthermore,
MELCs resistant to SAHA are also resistant to Trichostatin A, a hyperacetylating agent.
Of the 150 differentiation inducers tested, only those with one or more hydroxamic
acid moieties inhibited histone deacetylase activity and caused accumulation of
hyperacetylated H4 in culture *(79)*. There is also recent evidence that SAHA directly
affects ribosomal proteins, although how this relationship impacts translation of specific differentiation-inducing proteins and whether there is a relationship between this
effect and the histone hyperacetylating effects have not yet been elucidated *(104)*.

The similarities between the second-generation hybrid polar compounds and the
short-chain fatty acids make these drugs a curiosity for treatment of advanced PCA.
However, little research has been conducted on the effects of these drugs on any solid
tumor cell lines, much less PCA specifically. As the pharmacokinetics and safety of
SAHA and CBHA are further investigated, the likelihood of these agents being used in
treating advanced prostate cancer will be assessed.

8. OTHER ANTIPROGRESSION AGENTS

Several other agents—most of them extracted from products with which an epidemiological connection to reduced cancer risk has been established—are also under
investigation. Extracts of milk thistle known as flavenoids have demonstrated some
encouraging results. Flavenoids are believed to increase intracellular glucuronidation
of testosterone, thereby inhibiting testosterone stimulated release of PSA by LNCaP
cell cultures *(96)*. These agents also have been shown to induce G_1 arrest in both hormone-dependent (LNCaP) and hormone refractory (DU-145) cell lines by decreasing
levels of cyclin D, CDK4, and CDK6, and increasing levels of p21, p27, and bound
CDK2. The growth inhibition effects demonstrated were dose and time-dependent and
were shown to be the result of differentiation rather than apoptosis. *(111,112)*.

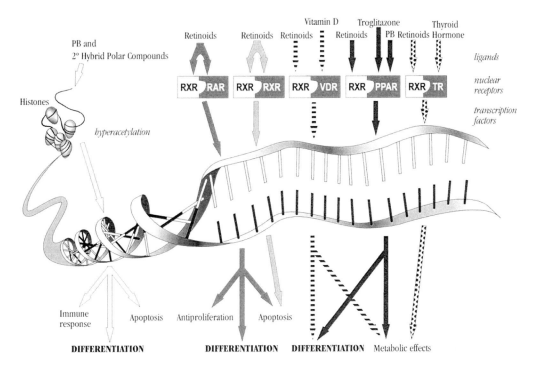

Fig. 1. Antiproliferation drug pathways. Vitamin A derivatives (retinoids), vitamin D and analogs (vitamin D), thiazolidinedione derivatives (troglitazone), and phenylbutarate (PB) all activate heterodimeric nuclear receptors that modulate gene expression to induce differentiation. Other cellular responses (apoptosis, antiproliferation, etc.) are also induced, as indicated. Histone hyperacetylation is induced by PB and second-generation hybrid polar compounds and results in altered gene expression and protein expression favoring differentiation by undetermined pathways.

An isoflavone extracted from soybeans called genestein has also been shown to inhibit growth and induce apoptosis in LNCaP cell lines *(68)*. Other studies have shown that genestein also inhibits BPH histoculture growth with doses ranging from 1.25–10 µg *(26)*.

In 1992, the ability of cAMP to induce expression of active TGF-β2 by PC-3 cells was demonstrated *(3)*. Further investigation revealed that both cAMP analogs and phosphodiesterase inhibitors induced terminal differentiation in the LNCaP and PC-3 cell lines *(4)*. The ability of pituitary adenylyl cyclase activating polypeptide (PACAP), and other agents that elevate cAMP, to inhibit PCA tumor growth in mice has recently been demonstrated *(45)*.

9. COMBINING DIFFERENTIATION TREATMENTS

As the investigation of differentiation therapies expands, it has become clear that multiple agents can induce differentiation through alternative pathways. The connection between these pathways is still largely speculative. It has been demonstrated that these agents alternatively bind to their respective subunits of heterodimeric nuclear receptors (represented in Fig. 1). This appears to be one level at which some of these antiproliferation agents may synergistically act to upregulate transcription of the proteins necessary for differentiation. We have discussed how some of the agents known to induce differentiation demonstrate differential hyperacetylation of histones, which may provide another level of additive antiproliferation effects when two are used in combination. As our understanding of how each of these agents specifically influences the cascade of events that leads to differentiation unfolds, the relationship among antiproliferation agents may become clearer. Despite the lack of concrete evidence linking mechanisms of action for multiple antiproliferation agents, it is becoming increasingly evident that combinations of differentiation agents can indeed provide a synergistic effect.

Most combination therapies studied have included one retinoid and another differentiation agent. For example, Elstner et al. investigated the growth inhibition effects of vitamin D analogs (CB1093, KH1060, KH1266, and CB1267) used in combination with 9cisRA on the LNCaP cell line. They reported that the combination of CB1267 and 9cisRA was the most effective at limiting colony growth in vitro *(22)*. A synergistic effect on growth inhibition of LNCaP cell line was also demonstrated using 1,25(OH)$_2$D3 in combination with 9*cis*RA *(107)*. As discussed here, the drug Liarozole mimics the effects of RA by reducing the rate of metabolism of endogenous retinoids. Because Liarozole acts by modulating p450 enzymes, Ly et al. postulated that it would also inhibit metabolism of 24-hydroxylase, an enzyme that is highly expressed in DU-145 cell lines. They demonstrated that a combination of Liarozole and 1,25(OH)$_2$ D3 provided a synergistic antiproliferative effect on the DU-145 cell line, increasing the half-life of 1,25(OH)$_2$D3 and amplifying expression of the VDR. This combination has not yet been evaluated in clinical trials *(55)*.

In 1995, Sidell et al. examined the effect of treatment with PA and RA independently and then in combination on human neuroblastoma cell lines. They found that these drugs interact synergistically both in terms of the number of cells responding and in the differentiating effect induced *(89)*. Our own unpublished data provide encouraging evidence that a combination of PB and 13*cis*RA provide a synergistic antitumor effect. Using nude mice with LNCaP, PC-3 and Dunning G-cell tumor xenografts, the PB/13cisRA combination therapy either significantly slows (PC-3) or entirely stops (LNCaP and G-cell) tumor growth as compared to either of the agents used singly. Using a matrigel assay, the combination also demonstrates antiangiogenic effects. Clinical trials using this combination of agents are being developed and implemented.

10. CONCLUSION

This chapter provides only a brief overview of the current state of investigation and development of differentiation therapies. The process of defining the utility of a specific anticancer agents—first in vitro, then in animal models, and finally in clinical trials—can be long and often disappointing. Yet recent work in the field of antiproliferation agents has been encouraging. With the use of PSA screening and greater societal attention to PCA, most PCA patients live long asymptomatic lives between when their disease is first diagnosed and when it becomes debilitating. Differentiation therapies, particularly in combination with each other, are demonstrating encouraging antitumor effects and a decrease in side effects in advanced PCA. Certainly, the earlier these agents are administered to PCA patients, the greater potential there is for diminishing the rate of cell proliferation and metastases. The hope of many in this area of research is to develop drugs that will provide an effective, low-toxicity first-line treatment for patients with newly-diagnosed PCA.

REFERENCES

1. Ahmad, N., D. K. Feyes, A. L. Nieminen, R. Agarwal, and H. Mukhtar. 1997. Green tea constituent epigallocatechin-3-gallate and induction of apoptosis and cell cycle arrest in human carcinoma cells. *J. Natl. Cancer Inst.* **89:** 1881–1886.
2. Andreeff, M., R. Stone, J. Michaeli, C. W. Young, W. P. Tong, H. Sogoloff, et al. 1992. Hexamethylene bisacetamide in myelodysplastic syndrome and acute myelogenous leukemia: a phase II clinical trial with a differentiation-inducing agent. *Blood* **80:** 2604–2609.
3. Bang, Y. J., S. J. Kim, D. Danielpour, M. A. O'Reilly, K. Y. Kim, C. E. Meyers, et al. 1992.Cyclic AMP induces transforming growth factor beta 2 gene expression and growth arrest in the human androgen-independent prostate carcinoma cell line PC-3. *Proc. Natl. Acad. Sci. USA* **89:** 3556–3560.
4. Bang, Y. J., F. Pirnia, W. G. Fang, W. K. Kang, O. Sartor, L. Whitesell, et al. 1994. Terminal neuroendocrine differentiation of human prostate carcinoma cells in response to increased intracellular cyclic AMP. *Proc. Natl. Acad. Sci. USA* **91:** 5330–5334.
5. Bayly, A. C., N. J. French, C. Dive, and R. A. Roberts. 1993. Non-genotoxic hepatocarcinogenesis in vitro: the FaO hepatoma line responds to peroxisome proliferators and retains the ability to undergo apoptosis. *J. Cell Sci.* **104:** 307–315.
6. Blutt, S. E., T. J. McDonnell, and N. L. Weigel. 1997. Effects of 1,25-dihydroxyvitamin D3 on cell cycle distribution and apoptosis of LNCaP cells. *In Proc. Ann. Meet. Am. Assoc. Cancer Res.*
7. Bookstein, R., J. Y. Shew, P. L. Chen, P. Scully, and W. H. Lee. 1990. Suppression of tumorigenicity of human prostate carcinoma cells by replacing a mutated RB gene. *Science* **247:** 712–715.
8. Bowden, C. J., P. De Porre, W. Wouters, and K. Snoeck. 1998. Second generation RAMBA (Retinoic Acid Metabolism Blocking Agent), in *Workshop on Clinical Application of Differentiation Therapy.* Houston, Texas.
9. Carducci, M., M. K. Bowlling, M. Eisenberger, V. Sinibaldi, T. Chen, D. Noe, et al. 1997. Phenylbutyrate (PB) for refractory solid tumors" Phase I clinical and pharmacologic evaluation of intravenous and oral PB. *Anticancer Research* **17:** 3972.
10. Carducci, M. A., J. B. Nelson, K. M. Chan-Tack, S. R. Ayyagari, W. H. Sweatt, P. A. Campbell, et al. 1996. Phenylbutyrate induces apoptosis in human prostate cancer and is more potent than phenylacetate. *Clin. Cancer Res.* **2:** 379–387.
11. Chan, J. M., E. Giovannucci, S. O. Andersson, J. Yuen, H. O. Adami, and A. Wolk. 1998. Dairy products, calcium, phosphorus, vitamin D, and risk of prostate cancer. *Cancer Causes Control* **9:** 559–566.
12. Cipolla, B., F. Guille, B. Quemener, J. M. Leveque, J. P. Moulinoux, and B. Lobel. 1992. The diagnostic value of erythrocyte polyamines (EPA) in prostatic adenocarcinoma (PA): apropos of 100 patients." *Prog. Urol.* **2:** 50–57.
13. Corder, E. H., H. A. Guess, B. S. Hulka, G. D. Friedman, M. Sadler, R. T. Vollmer, et al. 1993. Vitamin D and prostate cancer: a prediagnostic study with stored sera. *Cancer Epidemiol. Biomark. Prev.* **2:** 467–472.
14. Crozat, A., J. J. Palvimo, M. Julkunen, and O. A. Janne. 1992. Comparison of androgen regulation of ornithine decarboxylase gene expression in rodent kidney and accessory sex organs. *Endocrinology* **130:** 1131–1144.
15. Culine, S., A. Kramar, J. P. Droz, and C. Theodore. 1999. Phase II study of all-trans retinoic acid administered intermittently for hormone refractory prostate cancer. *J. Urol.* **161:** 173–175.

16. Davies, P. J. A. and S. M. Lippman. 1996. Biologic basis of retinoid pharmacology: implications for cancer prevention and therapy. *Adv. Oncol.* **12:** 2–10.

17. Denis, L., F. Debruyne, P. De Porre, and J. Bruynseels. 1998. Early clinical experience with liarozole (Liazal) in patients with progressive prostate cancer. *Eur. J. Cancer* **34:** 469–475.

18. Dijkman, G. A., P. Fernandez del Moral, J. Bruynseels, P. de Porre, L. Denis, and F. M. Debruyne. 1997. Liarozole (R75251) in hormone-resistant prostate cancer patients. *Prostate* **33:** 26–31.

19. DiPaola, R. S., R. E. Wiess, K. B. Cummings, F. M. Kong, R. L. Jirtle, M. Anscher, et al. 1997. Effect of 13-cis-retinoic acid and alpha-interferon on transforming growth factor beta 1 in patients with rising prostate-specific. *Clin. Cancer Res.* **3:** 1999–2004.

20. DiPaola, S., R. Mohmed, D. Toppmeyer, E. Rubin, P. Medina, S. Goodin, et al. 1999. bcl-2 modulation with 13-cis retinoic acid, alpha interferon and paclitaxel in vitro and in patients with prostate cancer and advanced malignancy. *In Proc. Am. Soc. Clin. Oncol.* 323a.

21. Eiseman, J. L., F. A. Rogers, Y. Guo, J. Kauffman, D. L. Sentz, M. F. Klinger, et al. 1998. Tumor-targeted apoptosis by a novel spermine analogue, 1,12-diazridinyl-4,9-diazadodecane, results in therapeutic eficacy and enhanced radiosensitivity of human prostate cancer. *Cancer Res.* **58:** 4864–4870.

22. Elstner, E., M. J. Campbell, R. Bunker, P. Shintaku, L. Binderup, D. Heber, et al. 1999. Novel 20-epi-viatmin D3 analog combined with 9-cis-retinoic acid markedly inhibits colony growth of prostate cancer cells. *Prostate* **40:** 141–149.

23. Elstner, E., C. Muller, K. Koshizuka, E. A. Williamson, D. Park, H. Asou, et al. 1998. Ligands for peroxisome proliferator-activated recetprogamma and retinoic acid receptor inhibit growth and induce apoptosis of human breast cancer cells in vitro and in BNX mice. *Proc. Natl. Acad. Sci. USA* **95:** 8806–8811.

24. Esquenet, M. , J. V. Swinnen, W. Heyns, and G. Verhoeven. 1997. LNCaP prostatic adenocarcinoma cells derived from low and high passage numbers display divergent responses not only to androgens but also to retinoids. *Steroid Biochem. Molec. Biol.* **62:** 391–399.

25. Fibach, E., R. C. Reuban, R. A. Rifkind, and P. A. Marks. 1977. Effect of hexamethylene bisacetamide on the commitment to differentiation of murine erythroleukemia cells. *Cancer Res.* **37:** 440–444.

26. Geller, J., L. Sionit, C. Partido, L. Li, X. Tan, T. Youngkin, et al. 1998. Genistein inhibits the growth of human-patient BPH prostate cancer in histoculture. *Prostate* **34:** 75–79.

27. Getzenberg, R. H., B. W. Light, P. E. Lapco, B. R. Konety, A. K. Nangia, J. S. Acierno, et al. 1997. Vitamin D inhibition of prostate adenocarcinoma growth and metastasis in the Dunning rat prostate model system. *Urology* **50:** 999–1006.

28. Giovannucci, E. 1998. Dietary influences of 1,25 (OH)2 vitamin D in relation to prostate cancer: a hypothesis. *Cancer Causes Control* **9:** 567–582.

29. Gorospe, M., S. Shack, K. Z. Guyton, D. Samid, and N. J. Holbrook. 1996. Up-regulation and functional role of p21Waf1/Cip1 during growth arrest of human breast carcinoma MCF-7 cells by phenylacetate. *Cell Growth Differ.* **7:** 1609–1615.

30. Griffin, C. A., M. Slavik, S. C. Chien, J. Hermann, G. Thompson, O. Blanc, et al. 1987. Phase I trial and pharmacokinetic study of intravenous oral alpha-diflouromethylornithine. *Invest. New Drugs* **5:** 177–186.

31. Gupta, S., N. Ahmad, R. R. Mohan, M. M. Husain, and H. Mukhtar. 1999. Prostate cancer chemoprevention by green tea: in vitro and in vivo inhibition of testosterone-mediated induction of ornithine decarboxylase. *Cancer Res.* **59:** 2115–2120.

32. Hanchette, C. L. and G. G. Schwartz. 1992. Geographic patterns of prostate cancer mortality. Evidence for a protective effect of ultraviolet radiation. *Cancer* **70:** 2861–2869.

33. Hedlund, T. E., K. A. Moffatt, and G. J. Miller. 1996. Vitamin D receptor expression is required for growth modulation by 1 alpha, 25-dihydroxyvitamin D3 in the human prostatic carcinoma cell line ALVA-31. *J. Steroid Biochem. Mol. Biol.* **58:** 277–288.

34. Hedlund, T. E., K. A. Moffatt, M. R. Uskokovic, and G. J. Miller. 1997. Three synthetic vitamin D analogues induce prostate-specific acid phosphatase and prostate-specific antigen while inhibiting the growth of human prostate cancer cells in a vitamin D receptor-dependent fashion. *Clin. Cancer Res.* **3:** 1331–1338.

35. Heston, W. D., D. Kadmon, D. W. Lazan, and W. R. Fair. 1982. Copenhagen rat prostatic tumor ornithine decarboxylase activity (ODC) and the effect of the ODC inhibitor alpha-difluoromethulornithine. *Prostate* **3:** 383–389.

36. Hseih, T. and J. M. Wu. 1997. Induction of apoptosis and altered nuclear/cytoplasmic distribution of the androgen receptor and prostate-specific antigen by 1alpha, 25-dihydroxyvitamin D3 in androgen-responsive LNCaP cells. *Biochem. Biophys. Res. Commun.* **23:** 539–544.

37. Hsu, J. Y. and M. Pfahl. 1997. ET-1 expression and growth inhibition of prostate cells: a retinoid target with novel specificity. *Cancer Res.* **58:** 4817–4822.

38. Huang, H., C. P. Reed, J. S. Zhang, V. Shridhar, L. Wang, and D. I. Smith. 1999. Carboxypeptidase A3 (CPA3): a novel gene highly induced by histone deacetylase inhibitors during differentiation of prostate epithelial cancer cells. *Cancer Res.* **59:** 2981–2988.

39. Hwang, D. R., C. J. Mathias, M. J. Welch, A. H. McGuire, and D. Kadmon. 1990. Imaging prostate derived tumors with PET and N-(3-(18F) fluoropropyl) putrescine. *Int. J. Radiat. Appl. Instrum.* **17:** 525–532.

40. Kawamoto, T., E. Gohda, H. Iji, M. Fujiwara, and I. Yamamoto. 1998. SKW 6.4 cell differentiation induced by interleukin 6 is stimulated by butyrate. *Immunopharmacology* **40:** 119–130.

41. Kitamura, S., Y. Miyazaki, Y. Shinomura, S. Kondo, S. Kanayama, and Y. Matsuzawa. 1999. Peroxisome proliferator-activated receptor gamma induces growth arrest and differentiation markers of human colon cancer cells. *Jpn. J. Cancer Res.* **90:** 75–80.

42. Kiyokawa, H., L. Ngo, T. Kurosaki, R. A. Rifkind, and P. A. Marks. 1992. Changes in p34cdc2 kinase activity and cyclin A during induced differentiation of murine erythroleukemia cells. *Cell Growth Differ.* **3:** 377–383.

43. Kubota, T., K. Koshizuka, E. A. Williamson, H. Asou, J. W. Said, S. Holden, et al. 1998. Ligand for peroxisome proliferator-activated receptor gamma (troglitazone) has potent antitumor effect against human prostate cancer both in vitro and in vivo. *Cancer Res.* **58:** 3344–3352.

44. Lee, E., T. Furukubo, T. Miyabe, A. Yamauchi, and K. Kariya. 1996. Involvement of histone hyperacetylation in triggering DNA fragmentation of rat thymocytes undergoing apoptosis. *FEBS Lett.* **395:** 183–187.

45. Leyton, J., T. Coelho, D. H. Coy, S. Jakowlew, M. J. Birrer, and T. W. Moody. 1998. PACAP(6-38) inhibits the growth of prostate cancer cells. *Cancer Lett.* **125:** 131–139.

46. Liang, J. Y., J. A. Fontana, J. N. Rao, J. V. Ordonez, M. I. Dawson, B. Shroot, et al. 1999. Synthetic retinoid CD437 induces S-phase arrest and apoptosis in human prostate cancer cells LNCaP and PC-3. *Prostate* **38:** 228–236.

47. Light, B. W., W. D. Yu, M. C. McElwain, D. M. Russell, D. L. Trump, and C. S. Johnson. 1997. Potentiation of cisplatin antitumor activity using a vitamin D analogue in a murine squamous cell carcinoma model system. *Cancer Res.* **57:** 3759–3764.

48. Lippman, S. M., J. J. Kavanagh, M. Paredes-Espinoza, F. Delgadillo-Madrueno, P. Paredes-Casillas, W. K. Hong, et al. 1992. 13-cis-retinoic acid plus interferon alpha-2a: highly active systemic therapy for squamous cell carcinoma of the cervix. *J. Natl. Cancer Inst.* **84:** 241–245.

49. Lippman, S. M., D. R. Parkinson, L. M. Itri, R. S. Weber, S. P. Schantz, D. M. Ota, et al. 1992. 13-cis-retinoic acid and interferon alpha-2a: effective combination therapy for advanced squamous cell carcinoma of the skin. *J. Natl. Cancer Inst.* **84:** 235–241.

50. Liu, M., A. Iavarone, and L. P. Freedman. 1996. Transcriptional activation of the human p21 (WAF1/CIP1) gene by retinoic acid receptor. Correlation with retinoid induction of U937 cell differentiation. *J. Biol. Chem.* **27:** 31,723–31,728.

51. Lokeshwar, B. L., G. G. Schwartz, M. G. Selzer, K. L. Burnstein, S. H. Zhuang, N. L. Block, et al. 1997. Inhibition of prostate cancer metastasis in vivo: a comparison of 1,23-dihydroxyvitamin D (calcitriol) and EB1089. *Cancer Epidemiol. Biomark. Prev.* **8:** 241–248.

52. Loprinzi, C. L., E. M. Messing, J. R. O'Fallon, M. A. Poon, R. R. Love, S. K. Quella, et al. 1996. Toxicity evaluation of difluoromethylornithine: doses for chemoprevention trials. *Cancer Epidemiol. Biomark. Prev.* **5:** 371–374.

53. Lu, X. P., A. Fanjul, N. Picard, B. Shroot, and M. Pfahl. 1999. A selective retinoid with high activity against an androgen-resistant prostate cancer cell type. *Int. J. Cancer* **80:** 272–278.

54. Lucia, M. S., M. A. Anzano, M. V. Slayter, M. R. Anver, D. M. Green, M. V. Shrader, et al. 1995. Chemopreventive activity of tamoxifen, N-(4-hydroxyphenyl) retinamide, and the vitamin D analogue Ro24-5531 for androgen-promoted carcinomas of the rat seminal vesicle and prostate. *Cancer Res.* **55:** 5621–5627.

55. Ly, L. H., X. Y. Zhao, L. Holloway, and D. Feldman. 1999. Liarozole acts synergistically with 1alpha,25-dihydroxyvitamin D3 to inhibit growth of DU 145 human prostate cancer cells by blocking 24-hydroxylase activity. *Endocrinology* **140:** 2071–2076.

56. McCaffrey, P. G., D. A. Newsome, E. Fibach, M. Yoshida, and M. S. Su. 1997. Induction of gamma-globin by histone deacetylase inhibitors. *Blood* **90:** 2075–2083.

57. Medina, V., B. Edmonds, G. P. Young, R. James, S. Appleton, and P. D. Zalewski. 1997. Induction of caspase-3 protease activity and apoptosis by butyrate and trichostatin A (inhibitors of histone deacetylase): dependence on protein synthesis and synergy with a mitochondrial/cytochrome c-dependent pathway. *Cancer Res.* **57:** 3697–3707.

58. Melchior, S. W., L. Brown, J. Quinn, R. A. Santussi, P. H. Lange, and R. L. Vessella. 1997. Effects of phenylbutyrate on cell cycle and apoptosis in human prostate cancer cells. *In Proc. Annu. Meet. Am. Assoc. Cancer Res.*

59. Meyskens, F. L., S. S. Emerson, D. Pelot, H. Meshkinpour, L. R. Shassetz, J. Einspahr, et al. 1994. Dose de-escalation chemoprevention trial of alpha-difluoromethylornithine in patient with colon polyps. *J. Natl. Cancer Inst.* **86:** 1122–1130.

60. Meyskens, F. L. and E. W. Gerner. 1999. Development of difluoromethylornithine (DFMO) as a chemoprevention agent. *Clin. Cancer Res.* **5:** 945–951.

61. Miller, G. J., G. E. Stapleton, J. A. Ferrar, M. S. Luica, S. Pfister, T. E. Hedlund, et al. 1992. The human prostatic carcinoma cell line LNCaP expresses biologically active, specific receptors for 1 alpha, 25-dihydroxyvitamin D3. *Cancer Res.* **52:** 515–520.

62. Miller, A. C., T. Whittaker, A. Thibault, and D. Samid. 1997. Modulation of radiation response of human tumour cells by the differentiation inducers, phenylacetate and phenylbutarate. *Int. J. Radiat. Biol.* **72:** 211–218.

63. Mohan, R. R., A. Challa, S. Gupta, D. G. Bostwick, N. Ahmad, R. Agarwal, et al. 1999. Overexpression of ornithine decarboxylase in prostate cancer and prostatic fluid in humans. *Clin. Cancer Res.* **5:** 143–147.

64. Motzer, R. J., L. Schwartz, T. M Law, B. A. Murphy, A. D. Hoffman, A. P. Albino, et al. 1995. Interferon alfa-2a and 13-cis-retionid acid in renal cell carcinoma: antitumor activity in a phase II trial and interactions in vitro. *J. Clin. Oncol.* **13:** 1950–1957.

65. Mueller, E., P. Sarraf, P. Tontonoz, R. M. Evans, K. J. Martin, M. Zhang, et al. 1998. Terminal differentiation of human breast cancer through PPAR gamma. *Mol. Cell* **1:** 465–470.

66. Nelson, J. B., K. Chan-Tack, S. P. Hedican, S. R. Magnuson, T. J. Opgenorth, G. S. Bova, et al. 1996. Endothelin-1 production and decreased endothelin B receptor expression in advanced prostate cancer. *Cancer Res.* **56:** 663–668.

67. Nelson, J. B., W. H. Lee, S. H. Nguyen, D. F. Jarrard, J. D. Brooks, S. R. Magnuson, et al. 1997. Methylation of the 5′ CpG island of the endothelin B receptor gene is common in human prostate cancer. *Cancer Res.* **51:** 35–37.

68. Onozawa, M., K. Fukuda, M. Ohtani, H. Akaza, T. Sugimura, and K. Wakabayashi. 1998. Effects of soybean isoflavones on cell growth and apoptosis of the human prostatic cancer cell line LNCaP. *Jpn. J. Clin. Onc.* **28:** 360–363.

69. Osborne, H. B. and A. Chabanas. 1984. Kinetics of histone H10 accumulation and commitment to differentiation in murine erythroleukemia cells. *Exp. Cell Res.* **152:** 449–458.

70. Palyi, I., T. Kremmer, A. Kalnay, G. Turi, R. Mihalik, K. Bencsik, et al. 1999. Effects of methylacetylenic putrescine, an ornithine decarboxylase inhibitor and potential novel anticancer agent, on human and mouse cancer cell lines. *Anticancer Drugs* **10:** 103–111.

71. Paschka, A. G., R. Butler, and C. Y. Young. 1998. Induction of apoptosis in prostate cancer cell lines by the green tea component, (1)-epigallocatechin-3-gallate. *Cancer Lett.* **130:** 1–7.

72. Peehl, D. M., R. J. Skowronski, G. K. Leung, S. T. Wong, T.v A. Stamey, and D. Feldman. 1994. Antiproliferative effects of 1,25-dihydroxyvitamin D3 on primary cultures of human prostatic cells. *Cancer Res.* **54:** 805–810.

73. Peehl, D. M., S. T. Wong, and T. A. Stamey. 1993. Vitamin A regulates proliferation and differentiation of human prostatic epithelial cells. *Prostate* **23:** 69–78.

74. Peinta, K. J., P. S. Esper, F. Zwas, R. Krzewminski, and L. E. Flaherty. 1997. Phase II chemoprevention trial of oral fenretinide in patients at risk for adenocarcinoma of the prostate. *Am. J. Clin. Oncol.* **20:** 36–39.

75. Pelidis, M. A, M. A. Carducci, and J. W. Simons. 1998. Cytotoxic effects of sodium phenylbutyrate on human neuroblastoma cell lines. *Int. J. Oncol.* **12:** 889–893.

76. Pineau, T., W. R. Hudgins, L. Liu, L. C. Chen, T. Sher, F. J. Gonzalex, et al. 1996. Activation of a human peroxisome proliferator-activated receptor by the antitumor agent phenylacetate and its analogs. *Biochem. Pharmacol.* **52:** 659–667.

77. Reese, D. H., B. Gordon, H. G. Gratzner, A. J. Claflin, T. I. Malinin, N. L. Block, et al. 1983. Effect of retinoic acid on the growth and morphology of a prostatic adenocarcinoma cell line cloned for the retinoid inducibility of alkaline phosphatase. *Cancer Res.* **43:** 5443–5450.

78. Reese, D. H., H. G. Gratzner, N. L. Block, and V. A. Politano. 1985. Control of growth, morphology, and alkaline phosphatase activity by butyrate and related short-chain fatty acids in the retinoid-responsive 9-1C rat prostatic adenocarcinoma cell. *Cancer Res.* **45:** 2308–2313.

79. Richon, V. M., S. Emiliani, E. Verdin, Y. Webb, R. Breslow, R. A. Rifkind, et al. 1998. A class of hybrid polar inducers of transformed cell differentiation inhibits histone deacetylases. *Proc. Natl. Acad. Sci. USA* **95:** 3003–3007.

80. Richon, V. M., R. A. Rifkind, and P. A. Marks. 1992. Expression and phosphorylation of the retinoblastoma protein during induced differentiation of murine erythroleukemia cells. *Cell Growth Differ.* **3:** 413–420.

81. Richon, V. M., Y. Webb, R. Merger, T. Sheppard, B. Jursic, L. Ngo, et al. 1996. Second generation hybrid polar compounds are potent inducers of transformed cell differentiation. *Proc. Natl. Acad. Sci. USA* **93:** 5705–5708.

82. Saez, E., P. Tontonoz, M. C. Nelson, J. G. Alvarex, U. T. Ming, S. M. Baird, et al. 1998. Activators of the nuclear receptor PPARgamma enhance colon polyp formation. *Nat. Med.* **4:** 1058–1061.

83. Samid, D., S. Shack, and C. E. Myers. 1993. Selective growth arrest and phenotypic reversion of prostate cancer cells in vitro by nontoxic pharmacological concentrations of phenylacetate. *J. Clin. Investig.* **91:** 2288–2295.

84. Schwartz, G. G., C. C. Hill, T. A. Oeler, M. J. Becich, and R. R. Mahnson. 1995. 1,25-Dihydroxy-16-ene-23-yne-vitamin D3 and prostate cancer cell proliferation in vivo. *Urology* **46:** 365–369.

85. Schwartz, G. G. and B. S. Hulka. 1990. Is vitamin D deficiency a risk factor for prostate cancer? *Anticancer Res.* **10:** 1307–1311.

86. Schwartz, G. G., T. A. Oeler, M. R. Uskokovic, and R. R. Bahnson. 1994. Human prostate cancer cells: inhibition of proliferation by vitamin D analogues. *Anticancer Res.* **14:** 1077–1081.

87. Schwartz, G. G., M. H. Wang, M. Zang, R. K. Singh, and G. P. Siegal. 1997. 1 alpha, 25-dihydroxyvitamin D (calcitriol) inhibits the invasiveness of human prostate cancer cells. *Cancer Epidemiol. Biomark. Prev.* **6:** 727–732.

88. Schwartz, G. G., L. W. Whitlatch, T. C. Chen, B. L. Lokeshwar, and M. F. Holick. 1998. Human prostate cancer cells synthesize 1,25-dihydroxyvitamin D3 from 25-dihydroxyvitamin D3. *Cancer Epidemiol. Biomark. Prev.* **7:** 391–395.

89. Sidell, N., R. Wada, G. Han, B. Chang, S. Shack, T. Moore, et al. 1995. Phenylacetate synergizes with retinoic acid in inducing the differentiation of human neuroblastoma cells. *Int. J. Cancer* **60:** 507–514.

90. Skowronski, R. J., D. M. Peehl, and D. Feldman. 1993. Vitamin D and prostate cancer: 1,25 dihydroxyvitamin D3 receptors and actions in human prostate cancer cell lines. *Endocrinology* **132:** 1952–1960.

91. Skowronski, R. J., D. M. Peehl, and D. Feldman. 1995. Actions of vitamin D3, analogs on human prostate cancer cell lines: comparison with 1,25-dihydroxyvitamin D3. *Endocrinology* **136:** 20–26.

92. Slawin, K., D. Kadmon, S. H. Park, P. T. Scardino, M. Anzano, M. B. Sporn, et al. 1993. Dietary fenreinide, a synthetic retiniod, decreases the tumor incidence and the tumor mass of ras+ myc-induced carcinomas in the mouse prostate reconstitution model system. *Cancer Res.* **53:** 4461–4465.

93. Smith, D. C., C. S. Johnson, C. C. Freeman, J. Muindi, J. W. Wilson, and D. L. Trump. 1999. A phase I trial of calcitriol (1,25-dihydroxycholecalciferol) in patients with advanced malignancy. *Clin. Cancer Res.* **5(6):** 1339–1345.

94. Smith, M., E. Mueller, G. Demtri, D. Kaufman, W. Oh, J. Jacobsen, et al. 1999. Preliminary results: Phase II trial of troglitazone for androgen dependent (AD) and androgen independent (AI) prostate cancer. *Proc. Am. Soc. Clin. Oncol.* **18:** 328a.

95. Sowa, P. T. Orita, S. Minamikawa, K. Nakano, T. Mizuno, H. Nomura, et al. 1997. Histone deacetylase inhibitor activates the WAF1/Cip1 gene promotor through Sp1 sites. *Biochem. Biophys. Res. Commun.* **241:** 142–150.

96. Sun, X. Y. and J. M. Phang. 1997. Biochanin A, a dietary flavenoid, reduces PSA levels in LNCaP prostate cancer cells by modulating testosterone metabolism. *In Proc. Annu. Meet. Am. Assoc. Cancer Res.* **38.**

97. Thibault, A., M. R. Cooper, W. D. Figg, D. J. Venzon, A. O. Sartor, A. C. Tompkins, et al. 1994. A phase I and pharmacokinetic study of intravenous phenylacetate in patients with cancer. *Cancer Res.* **54:** 1690–1694.

98. Tong, K. P., G. David-Beabes, A. Meeker, J. Bucci, T. DeWeese, and M. Carducci. 1997. Phenylbutyrate (PB) has plieotropic effects on gene transcription and inhibits telomerase activity in human prostate cancer. *Anticancer Res.* **17:** 3953.

99. Tontonoz, P., S. Singer, B. M. Forman, P. Sarraf, J. A. Fletcher, C. D. Fletcher, et al. 1997. Terminal differentiation of human liposarcoma cells induced by ligands for peroxisome proliferator-activated receptor gamma and the retinoid X receptor. *Proc. Natl. Acad. Sci. USA* **94:** 237–241.

100. Trump, D. L., D. C. Smith, D. Stiff, A. Adedoyin, R. Day, R. R. Bahnson, et al. 1997. A phase II trial of all-trans-retioic acid in hormone-refractory prostate cancer: a clinical trial with detailed pharmacokinetic analysis. *Cancer Chemother. Pharmacol.* **39:** 349–356.

101. Urban, D., R. Myers, U. Manne, H. Weiss, J. Mohler, D. Perkins, et al. 1999. Evaluation of biomarker modulation by fenretinide in prostate cancer patients. *Eur. Urol.* **35:** 429–238.

102. Van Lint, C., S. Emiliani, and E. Verdin. 1996. The expression of a small fraction of cellular genes is changed in response to histone hyperacetylation. *Gene Expr.* **5:** 245–253.

103. Vettese-Dadey, M., P. A. Grant, T. R. Hebbes, C. Crane-Robinson, C. D. Allis, and J. L. Workman. 1996. Acetylation of histone H4 plays a primary role in enhancing transcription factor binding to nucleosomal DNA in vitro. *EMBO J.* **15:** 2508–2518.

104. Webb, Y., X. Zhou, L. Ngo, V. Cornish, J. Stahl, H. Erdjument-Bromage, et al. 1999. Photoaffinity labeling and mass spectrometry identify ribosomal protein S3 as a potential target for hybrid polar cytodifferentiation agents. *J. Biol. Chem.* **274:** 14,280–14,287.

105. Yu, W. D., M. C. McElwain, R. A. Modzelewski, D. M. Russell, D. C. Smith, D. L. Trump, et al. 1998. Enhancement of 1,25-dihydroxyvitamin D3-mediated antitumor activity with dexamethasone. *J. Natl. Cancer Inst.* **90:** 134–141.

106. Zhao, X. Y., L. H. Ly, D. M. Peehl, and D. Feldman. 1997. 1 alpha,25-dihydroxyvitamin D3 actions in LNCaP human prostate cancer cells are androgen-dependent. *Endocrinology* **138:** 3290–3298.

107. Zhao, X. Y., L. H. Ly, D. M. Peehl, and D. Feldman. 1999. Induction of androgen receptor 1alpha,25-dihydroxyvitamin D3 and 9-cis retinoic acid in LNCaP human prostate cancer. *Endocrinology* **140:** 1205–1212.

108. Zhu, L., B. Gong, C. L. Bisgaier, M. Aviram, and R. S. Newton. 1998. Induction of PPARgamma1 expression in human THP-1 monocytic leukemia cells by 9-cis-retinoic acid is associated with cellular growth suppression. *Biochem. Biophys. Res. Commun.* **251:** 842–848.

109. Zhuang, S. H. and K. L. Burnstein. 1998. Antiproliferative effect of 1alpha, 25-dihydroxyvitamin d3 in human prostate cancer cell line LNCaP involves reduction of cyclin-dependent kinase 2 activity and persistent G1 accumulation. *Endocrinology* **138:** 1197–1207.

110. Zhuang, S. H., G. G. Schwartz, D. Cameron, and K. L. Burnstein. 1997. Vitamin D receptor content and transcriptional activity do not fully predict antiproliferative effects of vitamin D in human prostate cancer cell lines. *Mol. Cell Endocrinol.* **126:** 83–90.

111. Zi, X., A. W. Grasso, H. J. Kung, and R. Agarwal. 1998. A flavenoid antioxidant, silymarin, inhibits activation or erbB1 signaling and induces cyclin-dependent kinase inhibitors, G1 arrest, and anticarcinogenic effects in human prostate carcinoma DU-145 cells. *Cancer Res.* **58:** 1920–1929.

112. Zi, X. and R. Agarwal. 1999. Silibinin decreases prostate-specific antigen with cell growth inhibition via G1 arrest, leading to differentiation of prostate carcinoma cells: implications for prostate cancer intervention. *Proc. Natl. Acad. Sci. USA* **96:** 7490–7495.

28

Human Gene Therapy for Urological Oncology

Fernando Ferrer, MD, Jonathan W. Simons, MD, and Ronald Rodriguez, MD

You have to see what you are not looking for to be truly creative.

> **Donald S. Coffey, PhD,** *Orient Restaurant, Towson, Maryland, January 23, 1996*

A young mind can solve insolvable problems—at any age.

> **Andrew S. Grove, PhD,** *AACR Special Conference on Prostate Cancer, Palm Springs, California, 2 December, 1998*

1. INTRODUCTION

Gene therapy is the pharmacologic use of the digital code in recombinant genetic materials (DNA or RNA) to reverse, ameliorate, or cure human disease. In this context, gene therapy can be applied to organs or cells in vivo, or to tissue removed ex vivo and subsequently administered to the patient after the cells have been genetically modified. Early gene therapeutics were based on the ex vivo paradigm. This was caused by low efficiencies of gene transfer which required selection of transfected clones with a coselectable marker gene, and regulatory concerns about monitoring effects of gene transfer on cells prior to infusion into patients. Donated bone-marrow hematopoietic cells were engineered to produce adenosine deaminase (ADA), in order to correct ADA gene deficiency and reverse a severe underlying immune deficiency syndrome (SCIDS) *(17)*. With continued advances in gene vectors and delivery systems, it is likely that in vivo approaches will become more clinically practicable. Dividing current gene therapeutic strategies into ex vivo and in vitro facilitates discussion on their current state of research and development in urological oncology.

2. EX VIVO

2.1. Tumor Cell Vaccines

Many initial urologic applications of gene therapy have been primarily based on tumor vaccination strategies and ex vivo gene transfer (*7,28,37*; Fig. 1). Anticancer

From: *Prostate Cancer: Biology, Genetics, and the New Therapeutics*
Edited by: L. W. K. Chung, W. B. Isaacs, and J. W. Simons © Humana Press Inc., Totowa, NJ

**Primary Culture (Autologous) or Permanently
Established, Antigenically Similar Cell Line (Allogeniec)**

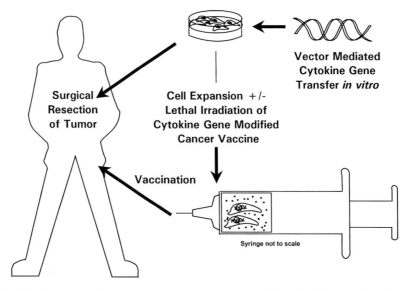

Fig. 1. Ex vivo gene therapy: cancer cells are transduced with a particular cytokine, UV-irradiated, and then sc injected as a vaccination. The paracrine secretion of cytokines activate antigen presenting cells (e.g., dendritic cells or macrophages) against native tumor antigens, which then process and present these antigens to the patient's T cells—stimulating a tumor specific immunity against the cancer cells at distant sites.

vaccines rely on presenting tissue or cancer specific antigens to elicit a systemic immune response. The therapeutic assumption is that even poorly immunogenic tumors express antigens which can be recognized when a patient has metastatic cancer if new immune responses are primed against these antigens. A major research goal has been to stimulate tumor associated antigen recognition using cytokine gene transfer into whole tumor cell vaccines. Advances in molecular immunology have allowed the use of immune system-activating genes as drugs in gene therapy strategies *(7,28,37)*. Cytokines are the critical activation peptides of immune responses to infection and cancer. One approach entails harvesting tumor cells from the patient, and genetically modifying the tumor cells and lethally irradiating them so that they may be administered as a vaccine. Once reintroduced into a host, these irradiated cells have no potential for tumorogenesis, as they are committed to cell death. However, by producing immunomodulatory cytokines in the context of tumor cell death, they augment the helper T-cell response. This results can drive enhanced tumor cell recognition and cell killing by the immune system at metastatic sites in experimental models. This approach has been used in various urologic malignancies with modest, but encouraging initial results.

Several preliminary studies have centered around enhanced expression of interleukin-2 (IL-2) and the T cell costimulatory factor HLA-B7. IL-2 is a potent promotor of antigen specific T-lymphocyte differentiation and proliferation that is normally produced by helper T cells. Initial work using systemic infusion of IL-2 into patients with renal-cell carcinoma suggested a potential therapeutic benefit through enhanced tumor surveillance *(7,28)*. Subsequently, the concept of gene manipulation of native host cells to overexpress critical immunostimulatory polypeptides (cytokines) has evolved *(7,11,28,37)*.

The HLA-B7 family of T-cell costimulatory factors is a new and exciting discovery in tumor immunology. HLA-B7 molecules are found on the surface of antigen-presenting cells and interact with their cognate receptors, CD-28 or CTLA4, on the surface of T cells, to either up or downregulate T-cell proliferation. HLA-B7 ligand binding is essential to T lymphocyte stimulation, and failure of HLA-B7 binding to the CD-28 receptor can result in a diminished immunologic response (anergy) *(3,11,21)*.

Conversely, HLA-B7 binding to the CTLA4 receptor results in inhibition of the T-cell response. In a series of provocative experiments, Kwon and colleagues capitalized on this dual regulation of T-cell stimulation by augmenting their tumor vaccination strategy with anti-CTLA4 antibodies in a transgenic mouse model of metastatic prostate cancer *(3)*. In these experiments, mice receiving ip injections of anti-CTLA4 antibodies had substantial delays in tumor growth compared to controls. In one animal, actual tumor rejection occurred. In the same report, these authors showed that genetically altering pTC1 (TRAMP-derived prostate cancer cells) to overexpress HLA-B7 resulted in tumor rejection in a murine model. Together, these findings highlight the important role of the HLA-B7 costimulatory pathway in tumor immunology, and indicate future directions for tumor vaccination strategies. When combined with GM-CSF gene transduced vaccines, the anti-CTLA4 antibody treatment appeared to have the greatest antineoplastic activity, suggesting that both priming antigen specific T-cell responses and sustaining them therapeutically to attack tumors are possible with experimental gene transfer (Allison, personal communication, 1999).

Treatment of superficial TCC of the bladder with Bacille Calmette-Guerin (BCG)— an enhancer of antitumor immune response—has also demonstrated results. As such, TCC appears to be an ideally suited target for anticancer vaccine strategies. Using liposomal transfection of IL-2 or HLA-B7 gene complexes, Larchian and colleagues transfected ex vivo modified TCC cells into mice bearing orthotopic tumors *(22)*. Mice treated with IL-2 alone had a twofold increased survival time compared to control mice. More impressively, 75% of mice receiving combined therapy with IL-2 or HLA-B7 had durable complete remissions. Clinical trials using ex vivo therapy in humans for TCC may be expected in the future, but have not been presented for NIH regulatory review.

Ex vivo cytokine gene transduced tumor cell vaccines were initially explored in animal models for prostate cancer, as extensively reviewed recently *(28)*. Utilizing the Dunning rat R3327 Mat-Ly-Lu model, transfection using a retroviral vector of IL-2 was performed. These cells were then lethally irradiated and introduced into syngeneic rats as vaccines. Mat-Ly-Lu was an interesting model, as it is poorly immunogenic, and unlike some murine tumor cell lines vaccinations with irradiated untransduced Mat-Ly-Lu cells, it could not confer either protective immunity or impact on pre-established experimental metastases *(32,42)*. Yet, animals treated with GM-CSF gene-transduced tumor vaccines had T-cell mediated regression of their primary lesions and immunologic protection from subsequent tumor outgrowth challenges. A similar strategy was also utilized in the rat model, using murine granulocyte macrophage colony stimulating factor (GM-CSF) and retroviral gene transfer.

GM-CSF has emerged as a cytokine with significant potency in the induction of an antitumor immune response. Interest in its use stems from an understanding of how powerful this immunostimulatory molecule can be in stimulating antigen presentation of tumor-associated peptides. Much of this recognition is the result of research on gene transfer as a form of molecule pharmacology, rather than a pre-existing model of immune response pathways *(7,28,37)*. GM-CSF is the most potent stimulator of dendritic cell (DC) maturation from hematopoietic progenitors yet identified *(42)*. Dendritic cells are a unique type of antigen-presenting cell which are specialized for both CD-4 (MHC Class II) and CD-8 (MHC Class I) peptide presentation to prime robust T-cell responses to infections. Activated DCs can present tumor vaccine-associated antigens they have processed to both CD4 (helper) and CD8 (cytolytic) T-cells in the draining lymph node of the vaccination sites (Fig. 1.), activating a systemic tumoricidal immune response. The name DC is derived from the fact that they appear as dendrites with multiple pseudopods when examined microscopically. Irradiated GM-CSF transduced tumor cell vaccines activate quiescent DCs and macrophages at the vaccine site, which then capture prostate tumor cell vaccine antigens, process them, and present antigen peptides on their surfaces. Compared head-to-head with over 15 other cytokines, GM-CSF is the most potent cDNA identified in conferring systemic antineoplastic immune responses to poorly immunogenic tumors. DCs are the most potent antigen presenting cell (APC) in the immune system and—thanks in large measure to cytokine gene therapy research—are the central cell type which most tumor immunotherapy approaches are attempting to optimally activate using gene-transfer biotechnologies *(7,28,37)*.

Initial studies utilizing GM-CSF in animal models that showed tumoricidal activity against preestablished tumor burdens led to the first human gene therapy trial for prostate cancer using the high efficiency, replication defective retroviral vector MFG *(28)*. In this phase I trial, eight patients were vaccinated with autologous, GM-CSF-secreting, irradiated prostate cancer cells. Tumor vaccines were prepared from ex vivo transduction of surgically harvested cells derived at radical prostatectomy and expanded for 4–7 wk in primary culture. The treatment concept tested for the first time in humans with prostate cancer was that paracrine expression of GM-CSF by gene transduced, autologous prostate cancer vaccines could elicit systemic immune responses against autologous tumor cells *(38)*. Patients with metastatic prostate cancer discovered at anatomic prostatectomy were treated. Vaccine site biopsies demonstrated infiltrates of DC and macrophages, confirming in the patients that cells critical in tumor-antigen presentation were recruited to vaccination sites following treatment. No PSA responses were noted, and vaccine cell yields were limiting and did not allow effects of repeated vaccinations to be tested. Yet, new T-cell responses were noted to challenge with irradiated, untransfected, autologous prostate tumor cells at delayed hypersensitivity sites. The posttreatment histology in patients was strikingly consistent with the mixed Th-1 and Th-2 subendothelial, eosinophilic vasculitis responses consistently generated in preclinical models *(16)*. Moreover, new oligoclonal, high titer antibodies from B-cell responses to prostate cancer and normal prostate epithelial-associated antigens were noted after vaccination in these patients, suggesting for the first time that not only T-cell tolerance, but B-cell tolerance to prostate cancer associated antigens may be broken by GM-CSF gene-transduced prostate cancer vaccines that load antigens on dendritic cells in vivo. Side effects in this group were limited to pruritis, erythema, and swelling of the vaccination site for 3–4 d. The entire treatment was safe in outpatients. These data suggested for the first time in humans that both systemic T-cell and B-cell immune responses can be generated by GM-CSF-transduced PCA vaccines which activate dendritic cell tumor associated antigen presentation, and provided in a single, small clinical trial a rationale for expanded clinical development of this therapeutic strategy for adjuvant therapy following surgery or radiation therapy.

While a variety of cytokine-based gene approaches are being explored (i.e., TNF-α, interferon (IFN), IL-4, HLA-B7), experience with ex vivo vaccine therapy for renal-cell carcinoma have similarly centered around immune induction by IL-2 or GM-CSF. Initial studies performed in mice supported the ability of IL-2 to inhibit growth of renal cell carcinoma in this model. As such, current clinical trials utilizing ex vivo approaches with IL-2 have been proposed.

The group at Hopkins has also completed a clinical trial testing safety, involving 16 patients treated with ex vivo autologous GM-CSF gene therapy *(36)*. In this phase I clinical trial, patients were randomized to receive escalating vaccine cell doses of lethally irradiated, autologous RCC cells expanded in short-term culture and transduced with human GM-CSF or control nontransduced cells. No significant vaccine-related toxicities were observed in these patients. Intradermal injection site biopsy confirmed distinctive macrophage, dendritic-cell (DC), eosinophil, neutrophil, and T-cell infiltrates *(36)*. One patient was noted to have a clinical partial response for 7 mo, but recurred in sites of pulmonary metastases which did not fully regress with three vaccinations. Unfortunately, there were no additional vaccine cells left for subsequent booster injections. Indeed, it was not ex vivo gene transfer, but tumor vaccine cell yield which limited the ability of the study to test the molecular effects of a long schedule of booster injections in patients. Modeled on the Hopkins experience showing both safety and clinical activity in the institution's first human gene therapy clinical trial, larger doses of GM-CSF gene transduced, autologous RCC vaccines are being tested in patients with stage IV RCC in the first human gene therapy trial in Japan (K. Tani, P.I.).

Like laboratory research, translational research in human gene therapy clinical pharmacology advances from research on hypotheses which were tested and found to be incorrect as well as correct. While valuable lessons have been learned from these initial experiences with ex vivo gene therapy using tumor cell vaccines, significant limitations exist. First, ex vivo autologous vaccine strategies require obtaining a host tumor sample, which usually necessitates a surgical procedure or either the primary of metastatic tumor. Expansion of the host tumor cell line to the minimally required dose level is expensive and often unreliable for ultimate yield with current bioprocessing technology. It is still the rare exception rather than the rule that primary prostate cancers can be turned into immortal, stable tumor cell lines. These factors limit the practicality of this technique for executing large phase III trials, which would be required to reduce ex vivo gene transduced tumor vaccines to clinical practice in urological oncology.

In an attempt to overcome these limitations, newer approaches for ex vivo vaccine therapy utilizing allogeneic tumor cells are being developed *(37)*. These new approaches involve the use of irradiated, immortalized, allogeneic tumor cell lines which have been genetically engineered to overexpress specific important tumor antigens. The next step is to express by gene transfer critical levels of the immunostimulatory cytokine of choice, and then develop these into a vaccine with an infinite supply. The choice is critical; allogeneic tumor vaccine cell lines selected must share as many candidate antigens as the metastatic tumors encountered in the clinic. This strategy eliminates the need to harvest cells from individual patients, and thereby simplifies production in the biotechnology sector *(28)*. It also allows an early clinical developmental exploration of dose, schedule, and duration of total treatment that has not been possible with autologous, irradiated, cytokine gene transduced vaccines *(16,36)*. Early evidence suggests that longer schedules of booster vaccinations with GM-CSF gene transduced allogeneic prostate cancer vaccines in humans continue to generate clinically measurable antineoplastic immune responses (Simons and Nelson, unpublished observations).

Attempts with gene transfer research to improve on the antineoplastic immune responses activated by GM-CSF gene transduced vaccines have not been restricted to the tumor vaccine cell. New ex vivo strategies are utilizing DC as target cells for gene manipulation. It has become possible to study the therapeutic effects of transfecting defined antigen cDNAs into DCs using improved vector systems for ex vivo gene transfer. The definition of DC biology for therapeutic manipulation has been critical to this approach. Dendritic cells develop from precursor cells derived from the bone marrow. Once in the blood, three types of DC precursors can be found—$CD14^+$ monocytes, $CD11c^+$ and $CD11^-$ cells *(27)*. These precursor cells are immunologically quiescent, and must be activated before they can participate in the immunologic cascade. DC are involved in both the innate (nonlymphocyte) and adaptive (lymphocyte-mediated) immune responses. The innate immune system specializes in recognition of nonprocessed antigens, whereas the adaptive system relies on antigen recognition and processing. In adoptive immunity—a subtype of adaptive system—immunity to disease is conferred to previously nonimmune individuals by transfer of cells that have been activated against certain peptide antigens. DC-based anticancer strategies revolve primarily around adoptive strategies at this time *(37)*.

Three types of dendritic cells (APC) are currently defined: Langerhans' cells of the skin, interstitial cells, and cells of lymphoid origin. Dendritic cells in peripheral tissues are constantly sampling antigens; however, they have little capacity to elicit a T-cell response. After antigen internalization by the DC and peptide breakdown, the cell begins the process of maturation, whereby the antigenic peptide fragments are processed and presented on its cell surface MHC molecules to circulating T cells. DC maturation in vivo involves the influence of various cytokines, and occurs within the lymphatic system. Once in the lymphatic system, DC come into contact with and activate T cells, and then generate a potent immunologic response to antigens which have become "dangerous" to the host *(40)*.

To date, the role of DC therapy has been explored in bladder, renal, and prostate carcinomas in urological oncology research *(41)*. In transitional cell carcinoma of the bladder, DC have been identified in tumor areas. An association between diminished *DC* activation and higher grade tumors has also been noted *(41)*. The urological research group at the University of Innsbruck, Austria have pioneered novel clinical approaches to ex vivo gene therapy for RCC, and have done much to advance DC-based therapy in general by conducting translational clinical research trials with molecular endpoints as well as clinical ones. They have recently reported on their initial data utilizing "pulsed" DC therapy in a group of patients with metastatic renal cell carcinoma in which treatment was well tolerated, and both molecular and clinical responses were observed *(15)*. In their study, peripheral mononuclear cells were harvested from patients and cultured in GM-CSF and IL-4 to prime them for antigen uptake and presentation. Interleukin-4 is a multifunctional cytokine that plays a critical role in the regulation of immune responses, and is critical for DC activation in biological activities including regulation of antibody production and inflammation and other immune cascade functions. After this, cells were pulsed with autologous tumor lysate and Keyhole-Limpet Hemocyanin (KLH) was added as a tracking antigen. These cells were then activated with a combination of TNF-α and PGE2 to produce a subpopulation of mature DC which was reinfused into patients. Patients were treated after nephrectomy with three infusions at monthly intervals. Using this approach, the authors reported no serious side effects, presented case histories of patients with KLH antigen T-cell responses proving activation of the entire axis, and also reported a clinical patient response with a substantial reduction of tumor burden *(14,15,40)*.

Salgallar and colleagues have reported their experience using pulsed DC therapy in patients with advanced prostate cancer. Using this approach, a pulsed exposure of dendritic cells to certain fragments of the prostate-specific membrane antigen (PSMA) is performed, and DCs are collected from leukopheresis. Such "pulsed-dendritic cells" are then redelivered to the patient. A phase I study of 51 patients with prostate cancer (including control groups) revealed that the therapy was well tolerated, and transient hypotension was the only major side effect *(31)*. This study was limited by its nature as a phase I study and its nonhomogeneous study population with regard to tumor stage. In addition, some patients had undergone a variety of previous therapies—including second line hormonal therapy—and had varying baseline immunologic status. Nonetheless, 7 of 51 patients had partial responses, as defined by a decrease in PSA of greater than 50% following infusions of peptide-loaded DCs. Using acid phosphatase as the model antigen, Small and Valone (UCSF and Dendreon, respectively) have tested acid phosphatase pulsed DCs that have been infused in patients with hormone refractory prostate cancer. Notably, a dose response is suggested between T-cell CTL responses to the acid phosphatase antigen and DC dose infused. (Small, personal communication). Given the safety of this approach, a pivotal trial to test improvement in survival for hormone refractory (D3) patients is being planned *(39)*.

Currently, all DC strategies require ex vivo cell peptide loading, activation, and subsequent maturation and infusion. This requires autologous DC precursor harvests by leukopheresis. At this time, DC activation/maturation is usually induced using TNF α and PGE2. Exposure to these cytokines causes activated DC cells to downregulate their endocytotic activities and express markers of maturation such as CD83 antigen. The DC also undergo exposure to desired antigens, thus enhancing immune response against specific cells (i.e., PSMA). Once reinfused into patients, these cells convey an immune enhancing activity.

While clearly promising as an avenue for translational research, currently available gene therapy strategies applied to immunotherapy all suffer from some inherent limitations. The most significant limitation appears to be the definition of the critical tumor-associated antigens for each urological cancer approached. The new genomics tools may assist within clinical trials to identify antigens involved in clinical response. Moreover, it seems imperative to apply additional pharmacologic concepts to sustain antineoplastic immune responses once they are generated. For example, it is in the nature of all immune responses—both B-cell and T-cell mediated—to be counterregulated as soon as the threat of infection is addressed. As a chronic presentation of tumor associated antigens, metastatic cancers may require maintenance of immune responses for years. This could be particularly true for activated DCs, either by use of GM-CSF gene-transduced vaccines or use of gene-loaded DCs with defined tumor associated antigens. New molecular concepts and both molecular and clinical evidence in translational clinical trials of broken immunologic tolerance to a specific case of cancer is not the same as consistent remissions from cancer, but it points the way towards ultimately achieving this end.

3. IN VIVO GENE THERAPY

Effective in vivo gene therapy relies on the successful transfer of genetic information to living cells *in situ* to achieve a therapeutic benefit. This is accomplished by delivering the DNA or RNA in a vehicle that allows efficient gene transfer. Such vehicles include liposomes, viruses, DNA, and ternary complexes of DNA and viruses. Table 1 lists the more commonly applied vehicles for gene transfer, and their advantages and disadvantages. In general, the choice of vehicle depends largely on the goal of the therapy and the size of the gene to be delivered. Transient expression may be preferable for certain cancer applications, but is suboptimal for correcting enzymatic deficiencies. Liposomes and naked DNA approaches can facilitate larger segments of DNA, but are less efficient in gene transfer than viral methods. Even within viral vectors, there are significant differences in the method and temporal expression of gene transfer. Retroviruses integrate into the host genome and thus have longer term expression; however, such integration raises the possibility of incidental activation of neighboring proto-oncogenes or disruption of tumor suppressor genes—either of which in theory could result in the formation of de novo tumors. However, this theoretical risk has not yet been encountered as toxicity in any clinical trial, to our knowledge. Adenoviral based vectors bypass this concern by maintaining their DNA completely in an episomal form (i.e., no integration), but as a result the gene expression is transient in nature. Moreover, most viruses are highly immunogenic, thus limiting the efficiency of repeated gene transfer and expression.

4. PHARMACOLOGY OF IN VIVO CANCER GENE THERAPY

The current principles and practice of in vivo human gene therapy for urological oncology are best comprehensively assessed using classical pharmacology concepts. For any given dose of an agent, there is a certain potential efficacy and toxicity, as with any novel antineoplastic agent described in this book. Slight increases in the dose may cause significant increases in toxicity, with only minor increases in efficacy. It is this

Table 1
NIHRAC/FDA Reviewed and Initiated Human Gene Therapy Trials in Prostate Cancer[a]

Vector	Gene	PI	Strategy	App.date
Retrovirus	GM-CSF	Simons	Exvivo; vaccine	8/3/94
Retrovirus	IL-2 + g-IFN	Gansbacher	Ex vivo; vaccine	5/14/95
Retrovirus	(-) myc	Steiner	In vivo; intraprost.	9/30/95
Vaccinia	PSA	Chen	In vivo; vaccine	9/22/95
Adenovirus	RSV-TK	Scardino	In vivo; intraprost.	1/29/96
Vaccinia	PSA	Kufe	In vivo; vaccine	9/18/96
Vaccinia	PSA	Sanda	In vivo; vaccine	5/13/97
Retrovirus	GM-CSF	Simons	Ex vivo; vaccine	9/9/97
Adenovirus	wt p53	Belldegrun	In vivo; vaccine	9/17/97
Adenovirus	wt p53	Logothetis	In vivo; intraprost.	11/6/97
Adenovirus	PSA-E1A (oncolytic)	Simons	In vivo; intraprost.	6/19/98
Adenovirus	Osteocalcin-TK	Gardiner	In vivo; *intratumor/bone*	7/99

[a]Source: http://www.nih.gov/od/orda/protocol.htm. Prostate Cancer Human Gene Therapy Clinical Trials Initiated. Both ex vivo and in vivo trials are shown. Data obtained from the National Institutes of Health Office of Recombinant DNA Activities. For updates *see* http://www.nih.gov/od/oba.

ratio of efficacy to toxicity that determines the therapeutic index. Efficacy in gene therapy refers specifically to achieving the desired effect, and is directly related to the efficiency of gene transfer, the potency of the gene in achieving its intended goal, and the ability of the agent to overcome host and tumor specific defense mechanisms. Toxicity, or untoward biological effects, are for the most part a consequence of nonspecific interactions. For example, viremia (manifested by fever, malaise, and myalgia), host immune activation (e.g., prostatitis after intratumoral injection of a gene therapeutic for prostate cancer), viral infection of unintended cells, nonspecific activation of gene expression, hepatotoxicity, and hematotoxicity were all described in 1999 in meetings. Peer review and long-term clinical follow-up will be needed. Possible genetic rearrangements between the vector and the host may result in undetermined consequences—although no evidence for this exists, and this possibility has been very closely monitored by the FDA in multiple clinical trials of retroviral and adenoviral mediated gene transfer. Optimization of the therapeutic index can be achieved by shifting the toxicity curve far to the right (increasing dose to kill/dose to cure), thus allowing higher doses and presumably better efficacy without untoward side effects. Alternatively, increasing the per-vector molecular potency carrying therapeutic genes and improving biodistribution of delivery can shift the dose response curve to the left, allowing a lesser dose to accomplish more for a particular patient.

The single most difficult problem currently facing the human gene therapist in urological oncology remains the overall poor efficiency of gene transfer *in situ*. This is particularly true in the experimental therapeutics of systemically delivering antineoplastic vectors to distant metastases. Methods are being developed to overcome this problem, including development of less immunogenic viral vectors, development of liposomes which can evade the first-pass response from the reticular endothelial system (stealth liposomes), and the development of highly cell specific vectors which require less dose at the metastatic site to achieve cytoreduction. For example, current adenovirus vectors bind to cells by virtue of a receptor present in nearly all eukaryotic cells—referred to as the Coxsackie and Adenovirus Receptor (CAR) (2). Once the virus has initiated binding, internalization is facilitated by the interaction of the viral penton base protein with cell surface alpha-v-integrins *(24)*. However, if the virus could be altered so that it binds to a particular cell-surface protein found only in prostate tumors, then the toxicity curve would be shifted to the right, and much higher doses of virus could be administered to saturate the prostate cell surface receptors. Such tumor markers are being actively studied for targeting experimental therapeutics. Other methods of minimizing toxicity include the use of tissue specific promoters *(9)*. In the case of prostate cancer, several promoters exist, including the prostate specific antigen promoter and its enhancer *(33)*, the prostate specific membrane antigen promoter *(26)*, the rat probasin promoter *(10)*, and the human glandular kallikrein (hK2) *(34)* promoter, among others.

5. HUMAN EXPERIENCE IN UROLOGICAL ONCOLOGY USING HUMAN GENE THERAPY

For ethical reasons, early recombinant DNA investigation in oncology has been restricted until very recently to patients with advanced, metastatic, often end-stage cancers to establish safety. This has been the case in genitourinary cancer as well. It was the original concept of the NIH Recombinant DNA Advisory Committee that this was ethically sound, as the risks of recombinant DNA clinical research could not be projected. Not surprisingly given its incidence and the enormous impact of the private philanthropic sector (i.e., the CaPCure Foundation), most human gene transfer clinical trials have been in prostate cancer. Both ex vivo and in vivo prostate cancer clinical trials (most, through 1999, are phase I trials) are summarized in Table 1. It is anticipated that clinical trial reports from some of these trials, when the safety and efficacy data has matured—will greatly shape the clinical gene therapy research of the first decade of the 21st century.

Most in vivo preclinical studies have been directed at eliminating cancer cells either by correcting an underlying defect which may have led to oncogenesis (e.g., p53, C-CAM1 or RB expression) or by direct cytotoxicity of a suicide-type gene. In the case of overexpression of p53 wild-type protein in p53 mutant tumors, cell death via apoptosis can be observed. Emphasis has been placed on well-characterized suicide genes, which have included herpes simplex virus thymidine kinase *(12)*, cytosine deaminase *(1)*, and the purine nucleoside phosphorylase *(23)*. These activate prodrugs which are given systemically into direct inhibitors of DNA synthesis. Differential killing of tumor vs normal cells is achieved by increased DNA replication in the tumor cells. High levels of activated cytotoxic molecules are achieved in a transfected area of tumor. Other antineoplastic cDNAs are available as candidate cytoreductive genes for cancer gene therapy in genitourinary oncology. Naturally occurring inhibitors of protein synthesis—such as diphtheria toxin, ricin, or the Pseudomonas exotoxin-A—

also represent alternative cytotoxins with the additional advantage of cell cycle independence *(30)*.

A newer form of cancer gene therapy has emerged using oncolytic viruses, which are selectively replication-competent viruses that lyse cancer cells by virtue of their replication cycles *(18)*. Several different applications of vector systems and genetic engineering of the viruses have been employed. These oncolytic vectors can be activated by several different pathways which distinguish the tumor from the normal cell. For example, the presence of a mutant p53 gene *(13)* can be used to drive cytotoxic Adenovirus type 5 replication. This is achieved by engineering a deletion in a critical sequence of the E1B gene of the Ad5 genome. (Onyx 015, Onyx) This generates a replication-attenuated virus which preferentially replicates in p53 mutant prostate cancer cells in vitro, as well as other tumor cells. Alternatively, Ad5 can be made tissue type, transcriptionally target-specific for replication. A clear example is the use of PSA enhancer and promoter *(29)* sequences to drive viral replication restricted to intracelluar, prostate-unique transcription factors. CN 706 and CN786, (Calydon), CN706 (PSE-E1a), and CN787 (PSE-E1a/probasin-E1b) have striking antineoplastic activities in vitro and in vitro, and are selective for PSA expressing human prostate cancer lines *(29,45)*. Oncolytic vectors have been expanded to genetic engineering of attenuated herpes virus vectors, which have a differential ability to replicate in tumor vs normal tissue on the basis of ribonucleotide reductase levels by deletions in the ICP 34.5 gene and insertional mutagenesis of the ICP6 gene (G207, Neurovir). This replication-attenuated HSV vector is remarkably cytotoxic against LnCAP, and PSA-expressing cell lines in vitro and in vitro. The advantage of oncolytic vectors such as ON015, CN706, CN787, and G207 is that lower doses can be delivered in situ, with propagation of the virus resulting in a higher total dose at the site of interest. It may also be possible to achieve a therapeutic benefit with only a single dose schedule. Preclinical models of this strategy have been very promising *(29)*. Early clinical trial results are expected to mature for CN706 in 2000 based on phase I evaluation in patients with radiation recurrent prostate cancer when the virus is given as brachytherapy using stereotactic, transperineal, ultrasound directed injections. A similar clinical development pathway is anticipated for G207 (R. Martuza, personal communication). One unifying concept—as originally described by the Hopkins group (Simons et al.) for replication restricted adenoviral vectors and the Georgetown group (Martuza et al.) for replication restricted herpes simplex virus vectors is that oncolytic vectors kill hormone refractory human prostate cancer clones independent of cell cycle. Thus, the dose from a single treatment is amplified with waves of oncolytic vector replication in vivo, and the host immune responses to this can only be truly measured in early clinical trials which are ongoing. Interestingly, oncolytic vectors can be modeled for treatment as a form of ultrasound directed brachytherapy in radiation and hormone refractory recurrent local prostate cancer.

Attacking the critically supporting stroma with cytoreductive gene therapy approaches has also developed into a research avenue for early human investigation. Chung and colleagues at the University of Virginia have developed a C-42-2 PSA-expressing LnCAP bone metastasis model, and tested osteocalcin driven TK Ad5 vectors to kill the osteoblastics responses that support the prostate tumor as well as the tumor itself.

Early clinical evaluation has centered on direct injection of the OC-TK virus into bone metastases *(6,20,35)*.

6. AVENUES FOR CURRENT AND FUTURE RESEARCH

Toxicology considerations have driven current urological clinical trials to include only patients with advanced cancers whose tumor burdens may be beyond the reach of any known type of treatment. However, gene therapy has been rapidly developing as a treatment modality for earlier stage cancers as well as benign disease. In many cases, it will require testing earlier in the disease course to truly assess effectiveness. The safety of GM-CSF gene transduced tumor vaccines allows consideration of larger, adjuvant therapy trials in outpatients following urologic surgery. In addition, recent applications of human gene therapy in clinical trials including cystic fibrosis *(44)*, muscular dystrophy *(25)*, peripheral vascular disease, and coronary artery disease suggest that safety allows further scientific and clinical development for benign diseases in urology *(4)*. Indeed, benign disease may ultimately prove to be one of the most common models for gene therapeutics in the long term. For example, it is possible that the same gene therapy vectors developed for prostate cancer may also prove useful for the treatment of benign prostatic hypertrophy (BPH). Gene therapy delivery of nitric-oxide synthase (NOS) intracorporally may provide an alternative treatment for erectile dysfunction for those patients who are not candidates for Viagra. Preclinical models of NOS delivery by adenovirus are already in development *(5,8)*. Methods of promoting nerve regeneration by gene therapy directed secretion of nerve growth factors may prove to be a useful adjunct in radical prostatectomy or radical cystectomy. Women with urinary incontinence and intrinsic sphincteric deficiency may be candidates for gene therapy utilizing nerve and skeletal muscle growth factors locally. Finally, severe recurrent stone disease may be amenable to treatment by gene therapeutic approaches. For example, defective transport mechanisms, which are responsible for the lack of reabsorption of the dibasic amino acids (including cystine), may be reconstituted to a degree sufficient to prevent further stone formation. Alternatively, increased secretion of inhibitors of stone formation may be easily achieved in the renal tubules, thus reducing the likelihood of a variety of urinary stones.

Currently, most research must be focused primarily on improved vector development for applications in urological disease. In particular, improved gene transfer *in situ* is necessary if we ever expect to achieve strong responses in nononcologic applications. Methods of augmenting current vector efficacy can also be achieved by combination strategies. Thus, efforts are being directed at radiosensitization, chemosensitization, and various combination strategies which may help optimize gene therapy efficacy. For example, certain differentiation therapies may help sensitize tumors to activate prostate specific promoters, thus increasing the pool of cells susceptible to promoter specific treatments. This may be a particularly important issue in those patients who have developed non-PSA secreting tumors or who have androgen insensitive prostate cancer. Finally—since the immune system plays a role both in the modulation of gene transfer and expression—it may be necessary in the future to pharmacologically "manage" the immune response to allow optimal gene transfer and gene expression during the time it is desired.

An entire academic research culture exploring gene therapy as a branch of experimental therapeutics and a biotechnology industry of gene therapeutic applications has emerged the decade following the first administration of a gene transduced human cell to a human with disease. The pace has been staggering. Some "hot" ideas in the mid1990s have failed as clinical leads by 2000, and the first FDA-approved human gene therapy is an unachieved milestone for the field. Translational clinical trials, testing concepts in the relevant species—*Homo sapiens* with cancer—have begun to inform both basic and clinical research fundamentally, bridging the two. Cancer genomics promises to disclose entire new classes of targets for the cancer gene therapist. Thus, we have only begun to explore the possibilities using our knowledge of genetics to treat disease with genes. To quote the scholar Donald S. Coffey, to whom this book is dedicated: "If the past helps predict the future, we are most likely to *underestimate* the pace and impact of our progress in the future."

7. ACKNOWLEDGEMENTS

The authors wish to thank the patients, their families, and the staff and faculty of the Johns Hopkins Prostate Cancer Human Gene Therapy Laboratory and Translational Research Program for their contributions to this manuscript. Particular appreciation is expressed for the research support of the NIH Special Program of Research Excellence in Prostate Cancer, (Donald S. Coffey, P.I.) Sanskar Longrifle Gift for Prostate Cancer Gene Therapy Research, CaPCure Foundation Clinical Trials Consortuim, and Little Round Top Graphics.

REFERENCES

1. Austin, E. A. and B. E. Huber. 1993. A first step in the development of gene therapy for colorectal carcinoma: cloning, sequencing, and expression of *Escherichia coli* cytosine deaminase. *Mol. Pharmacol.* **43:** 380–387.
2. Bergelson, J. M., J. Cunningham, G. Droguett, et al. 1997. Isolation of a common receptor for Coxsackie B viruses and adenoviruses 2 and 5. *Science* **275:** 1320–1323.
3. Chambers, C. A., M. Kuhns, and J. Allison. 1999. Cytotoxic T lymphocyte antigen-4 (CTLA-4) regulates primary and secondary peptide-specific CD4(+) T cell responses. *Proc. Natl. Acad. Sci. USA* **96:** 8603–8608.
4. Chao, J. and L. Chao. 1997. Experimental kallikrein gene therapy in hypertension, cardiovascular and renal diseases. *Pharmacol. Res.* **35:** 517–522.
5. Christ, G. J. and A. Melman. 1998. The application of gene therapy to the treatment of erectile dysfunction. *Int. J. Impot. Res.* **10:** 111–112.
6. Chung, L. W., C. Kao, R. Sikes, and H. Zhau. 1997. Human prostate cancer progression models and therapeutic intervention. *Hinyokika Kiyo* **43:** 815–820.
7. Dranoff, G. 1998. Cancer gene therapy: connecting basic research with clinical inquiry. *J. Clin. Oncol.* **16:** 2548–2556.
8. Garban, H., D. Marquez, T. Magee, et al. 1997. Cloning of rat and human inducible penile nitric oxide synthase. Application for gene therapy of erectile dysfunction. *Biol. Reprod.* **56:** 954–963.
9. Gotoh, A., S. Ko, T. Shirakawa, et al. 1998. Development of prostate-specific antigen promoter-based gene therapy for androgen-independent human prostate cancer. *J. Urol.* **160:** 220–229.

10. Greenberg, N. M., F. DeMayo, P. Sheppard, et al. 1994. The rat probasin gene promoter directs hormonally and developmentally regulated expression of a heterologous gene specifically to the prostate in transgenic mice. *Mol. Endocrinol.* **8:** 230–239.

11. Greenfield, E. A., K. Nguyen, and V. Kuchroo. 1998. CD28/B7 costimulation: a review. *Crit. Rev. Immunol.* **18:** 389–418.

12. Hall, S. J., M. Sanford, G. Atkinson, and S. Chen. 1998. Induction of potent antitumor natural killer cell activity by herpes simplex virus-thymidine kinase and ganciclovir therapy in an orthotopic mouse model of prostate cancer. *Cancer Res.* **58:** 3221–3225.

13. Heise, C., A. Sampson-Johannes, A. Williams, et al. 1997. ONYX-015, an E1B gene-attenuated adenovirus, causes tumor-specific cytolysis and antitumoral efficacy that can be augmented by standard chemotherapeutic agents (see comments). *Nat. Med.* **3:** 639–645.

14. Holtl, L., C. Rieser, C. Papesh, R. Ramoner, G. Bartsch, and M. Thurnher. 1998. CD83+ blood dendritic cells as a vaccine for immunotherapy of metastatic renal-cell cancer. *Lancet* **352:** 1358.

15. Holtl, L., C. Rieser, C. Papesh, R. Ramoner, M. Herold, H. Klocker, C. Radmayr, A. Stenzl, G. Bartsch, and M. Thurnher. (1999). Cellular and humoral immune responses in patients with metastatic renal cell carcinoma after vaccination with antigen pulsed dendritic cells. *J. Urol.* **161:** 777–782.

16. Hung, K., R. Hayashi, A. Lafond-Walker, C. Lowenstein, D. Pardoll, and H. Levitsky. 1998. The central role of CD4(+) T cells in the antitumor immune response. *J. Exp. Med.* **188:** 2357–2368.

17. Kantoff, P. W., D. Kohn, H. Mitsuya, et al. 1996. Correction of adenosine deaminase deficiency in cultured human T and B cells by retrovirus-mediated gene transfer. *Proc. Natl. Acad. Sci. USA* **83:** 6563–6567.

18. Kirn, D. H. and F. McCormick. 1996. Replicating viruses as selective cancer therapeutics. *Mol. Med. Today* **2:** 519–527.

19. Kirn, D., T. Hermiston, and F. McCormick. 1998. ONYX-015: clinical data are encouraging (letter). *Nat. Med.* **4:** 1341–1342.

20. Koeneman, K. S., F. Yeung, and L. Chung. 1999. Osteomimetic properties of prostate cancer cells: a hypothesis supporting the predilection of prostate cancer metastasis and growth in the bone environment. *Prostate* **39:** 246–261.

21. Kwon, E. D., A. Hurwitz, B. Foster, et al. 1997. Manipulation of T cell costimulatory and inhibitory signals for immunotherapy of prostate cancer. *Proc. Natl. Acad. Sci. USA* **94:** 8099–9103.

22. Larchian, W. A., K. Roberson, C. Robertson, E. Gilboa, W. Heston, and W. Fair. 1997. Liposomal mediated gene transfer in bladder cancer cells. *J. Urol.* **157:** 1196A.

23. Martiniello-Wilks, R., J. Garcia-Aragon, M. Daja, et al. 1998. In vivo gene therapy for prostate cancer: preclinical evaluation of two different enzyme-directed prodrug therapy systems delivered by identical adenovirus vectors. *Hum. Gene Ther.* **9:** 1617–1626.

24. Mathias, P., T. Wickham, M. Moore, and G. Nemerow. 1994. Multiple adenovirus serotypes use alpha v integrins for infection. *J. Virol.* **68:** 6811–6814.

25. Moisset, P. A., D. Skuk, I. Asselin, et al. 1998. Successful transplantation of genetically corrected DMD myoblasts following ex vivo transduction with the dystrophin minigene. *Biochem. Biophys. Res. Commun.* **247:** 94–99.

26. O'Keefe, D. S., S. Su, D. Bacich, et al. 1998. Mapping, genomic organization and promoter analysis of the human prostate-specific membrane antigen gene (In Process Citation). *Biochim. Biophys. Acta* **1443:** 113–127 (MEDLINE record in process).

27. Palucka, K. and J. Banchereau. 1999. Linking innate and adaptive immunity. *Nat. Med.* **5:** 868–870.

28. Pardoll, D. M. 1998. Cancer vaccines. *Nat. Med.* **(5 Suppl. 4):** 525–531.

29. Rodriguez, R., E. Schuur, H. Lim, et al. 1997. Prostate attenuated replication competent adenovirus (ARCA) CN706: a selective cytotoxic for prostate-specific antigen-positive prostate cancer cells. *Cancer Res.* **57:** 2559–2563.

30. Rodriguez, R., H. Lim, L. Bartkowski, et al. 1998. Identification of diphtheria toxin via screening as a potent cell cycle and p53-independent cytotoxin for human prostate cancer therapeutics. *Prostate* **34:** 259–269.

31. Salgaller, M. L., B. Tjoa, P. Lodge, et al. 1998. Dendritic cell-based immunotherapy of prostate cancer. *Crit. Rev. Immunol.* **18:** 109–119.

32. Sanda, M. G., S. Ayyagari, E. Jaffee, J. Epstein, S. Clift, L. Cohen, et al. 1994. Demonstration of a rational strategy for human prostate cancer gene therapy. *J. Urol.* **151:** 622–628.

33. Schuur, E. R., G. Henderson, L. Kmetec, et al. 1996. Prostate-specific antigen expression is regulated by an upstream enhancer. *J. Biol. Chem.* **271:** 7043–7051.

34. Shan, J. D., K. Porvari, M. Ruokonen, et al. 1997. Steroid-involved transcriptional regulation of human genes encoding prostatic acid phosphatase, prostate-specific antigen, and prostate-specific glandular kallikrein. *Endocrinology* **138:** 3764–3770.

35. Shirakawa, T., S. Ko, T. Gardner, J. Cheon, T. Miyamoto, A. Gotoh, L. Chung, and C. Kao. 1998. In vivo suppression of osteosarcoma pulmonary metastasis with intravenous osteocalcin promoter-based toxic gene therapy. *Cancer Gene Ther.* **5:** 274–280.

36. Simons, J. W., E. Jaffee, C. Weber, H. Levitsky, W. Nelson, M. Carducci, et al. 1997. Bioactivity of autologous irradiated renal cell carcinoma vaccines generated by ex vivo granulocyte-macrophage colony-stimulating factor gene transfer. *Cancer Res.* **57:** 1537–1546.

37. Simons, J. W. and B. Mikhak. 1998. Ex-vivo gene therapy using cytokine-transduced tumor vaccines: molecular and clinical pharmacology. *Semin. Oncol.* **25:** 661–676.

38. Simons, J. W., B. Mikhak, J. Chang, A. DeMarzo, M. Carducci, M. Lim, et al. 1999. Induction of immunity to prostate cancer antigens: results of a clinical trial of vaccination with irradiated autologous prostate tumor cells engineered to secrete granulocyte-macrophage colony-stimulating factor using ex vivo gene transfer. *Cancer Res.* **59:** 5160–5168.

39. Small, E. J., D. Reese, and N. Vogelzang. 1999. Hormone-refractory prostate cancer: an evolving standard of care. *Semin. Oncol.* **(5 Suppl. 17) 266:** 1–7.

40. Thurnher, M., C. Reiser, L. Holtl, et al. 1998. Dendritic cell based immunotherapy of renal cell carcinoma. *Urol. Int.* **61:** 67–71.

41. Troy, A. J., P. Davidson, C. Atkinson, et al. 1999. CD1A dendritic cells predominate in transitional cell carcinoma of bladder and kidney but are minimally activated. *J. Urol.* **161:** 1962–1967.

42. Vieweg, J., F. Rosenthal, R. Bannerji, W. Heston, W. Fair, B. Gansbacher, and E. Gilboa. 1994. Immunotherapy of prostate cancer in the Dunning rat model: use of cytokine gene modified tumor vaccines. *Cancer Res.* **54:** 1760–1765.

43. Walker, J. R., K. McGeagh, P. Sundaresan, T. Jorgensen, S. Rabkin, and R. Martuza. 1999. Local and systemic therapy of human prostate adenocarcinoma with the conditionally replicating herpes simplex virus vector G207. *Hum. Gene Ther.* **10:** 2237–2243.

44. Whitsett, J. A., C. Dey, B. Stripp, et al. 1992. Human cystic fibrosis transmembrane conductance regulator directed to respiratory epithelial cells of transgenic mice. *Nat. Genet.* **2:** 13–20.

45. Yu, D. C., Y. Chen, M. Seng, J. Dilley, and D. Henderson. 1999. The addition of adenovirus type 5 region E3 enables calydon virus 787 to eliminate distant prostate tumor xenografts. *Cancer Res.* **59:** 4200–4203.

29

Chemoprevention Trials for Prostate Cancer

Peter Greenwald, MD, DrPH, and Ronald Lieberman, MD

1. INTRODUCTION

Prostate cancer is the fourth most frequent cancer among men worldwide *(40)*. Given the magnitude of the prostate cancer burden, considerable efforts have been made by the scientific research community to improve our understanding of the factors that contribute to prostate cancer risk and to develop approaches to modify those factors. Age, race, family history, and the presence of certain genetic polymorphisms, all are risk factors for prostate cancer that clearly cannot be modified *(13)*. Prostate cancer incidence increases dramatically with age *(46)*; in the United States, African-American men are at greater risk than whites *(46)*. Heritable effects may account for as much as one-third of prostate cancer risk *(1)*; and genetic polymorphisms in the vitamin D receptor *(24,25,52)*, the androgen receptor *(24)*, N-acetyltransferase (NAT1) *(16)*, and certain glutathione S-transferases (GSTs) *(45)* likely contribute to variations in prostate cancer risk among individuals. Hormones—both sex hormones and insulin-like growth factors (particularly IGF-I)—may also influence the risk of prostate cancer. Evidence indicates that cumulative exposure of the prostate to androgens—including testosterone and dihydrotestosterone (DHT)—contributes to prostate cancer development *(9,57)*.

Although these factors are important in determining an individual's risk for developing prostate cancer, they do not tell the whole story. Geographical and temporal patterns of incidence and mortality for this disease clearly support a strong environmental component in prostate cancer etiology. Japanese and Chinese men who immigrate to the United States have lower incidence and mortality rates for prostate cancer than US whites, but higher rates than men in their homelands *(21,39,49,59)*, supporting a link between cancer development and environmental factors. For example, the following age-adjusted incidence rates were reported for 1980: Japanese men in Japan (6.3/100,000), Japanese men in Hawaii (31.2/100,000), and white men in Hawaii (58.3/100,000) *(39)*. Furthermore, temporal trends indicate that the incidence of prostate cancer is still increasing worldwide; yet mortality rates—which increased in birth cohorts until about 1900—show little change in subsequent birth cohorts *(7,39)*.

The likelihood that environmental factors play a role in prostate cancer development leads to the supposition that the effects of such factors can be modified by appropriate preventive strategies to reduce risk. Because diet is a lifestyle choice that can be

From: *Prostate Cancer: Biology, Genetics, and the New Therapeutics*
Edited by: L. W. K. Chung, W. B. Isaacs, and J. W. Simons © Humana Press Inc., Totowa, NJ

readily modified, the possible etiologic role of diet in prostate cancer risk has received considerable attention. Available evidence makes a credible case for a diet-prostate cancer relationship, and provides important leads for the identification of substances that show promise for protection against cancer. In brief, dietary fat, meat, dairy products, and calcium appear to increase the risk of prostate cancer, whereas vitamin D, phytoestrogens, selenium, vitamin E, fructose, and tomato-based foods (rich in lycopene) may protect against the disease. A comprehensive review of dietary fat and prostate cancer by Kolonel and colleagues *(30)* concluded that evidence exists for a dietary fat-prostate cancer association, but data are inconclusive and nonspecific regarding types of fat. Because fat is just one component of complex foods such as meat and dairy products, the independent contributions to risk of other dietary components and their interactions with fat can complicate data interpretation. One recent study in a low-risk population in China reported an increased risk of prostate cancer for saturated fat ($OR = 2.9$) and unsaturated fat ($OR = 3.3$) for the highest quartile of intake *(32)*. Giovanucci reviewed the association of dairy products with increased prostate cancer risk—as well as the evidence linking a high circulating level of 1,25-dihydroxyvitamin D (1,25-D) with reduced risk—and formulated the hypothesis that these relationships may be linked *(18)*. Specifically, high levels of calcium and phosphorus from dairy products and sulfur-containing amino acids from animal protein (which lower blood pH) lower the circulating 1,25-D level. Also, high fructose consumption may affect calcium and phosphate balance, resulting in stimulated 1,25-D production *(18,20)*. An evaluation of the epidemiologic literature on tomatoes, tomato products, and lycopene found consistent evidence of an inverse relationship with prostate cancer risk *(19)*, and a recent study of plasma from men enrolled in the Physician's Health Study found that plasma lycopene (highest quintile) was related to lower risk for aggressive prostate cancers ($OR = 0.56$) and for all prostate cancers ($OR = 0.75$) *(17)*. Although the benefits of tomatoes are often attributed to lycopene, other compounds in tomatoes may also contribute to a cancer-protective effect. Consumption of soy milk—rich in phytoestrogens such as genistein and daidzein—more than once a day was associated with a 70% reduction in prostate cancer risk in a prospective study of Seventh-Day Adventist men *(26)*. One case-controlled study of phytoestrogen intake and prostate cancer risk showed protective effects for genistein ($OR = 0.71$), daidzein ($OR = 0.57$), and coumestrol ($OR = 0.48$) *(51)*. A recent study of selenium levels in toenails—also among men enrolled in the Physician's Health Study—reported a reduced risk of advanced prostate cancer ($OR = 0.35$) at the highest quintile *(58)*. Clinical trial secondary endpoint results, discussed here, showed a clear reduction in prostate cancer incidence by supplementation with selenium *(10)* and α-tocopherol (vitamin E) *(23)*.

Prevention strategies in cancer research can be carried out through both public health and medical interventions. Until fairly recently, effective agents for cancer prevention were not available. Consequently, many in the scientific community regarded prevention strategies as being valuable and appropriate only in the area of public health, and not in clinical investigations in a medical setting. Now that significant advances have been made in identifying, developing, and testing defined natural substances and synthetic agents that have potential either to prevent cancer initiation or to inhibit or reverse the progression of premalignant lesions to invasive cancer, a pharmacologic

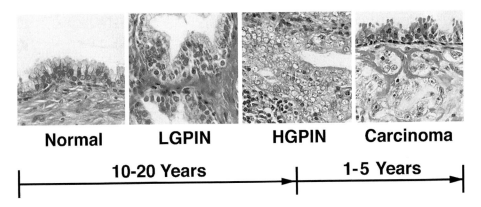

Fig. 1. The stages and timeline of human prostate carcinogenesis are shown. The natural history reflects a pathobiological continuum, beginning with normal-appearing glandular epithelium that evolves over time into dysplasia/prostatic intraepithelial neoplasia (PIN) and finally progresses to invasive adenocarcinoma.

approach for cancer prevention in the medical arena has become realistic. Although this innovative approach, named chemoprevention, is still in the early stages of development, various cancer sites—including prostate, breast, colon, lung, bladder, cervix, oral cavity, esophagus, skin, and liver—have been targeted in preclinical and clinical chemoprevention research, with promising results. Our knowledge of prostate cancer risk factors and precursor lesions makes this disease a prime target for chemoprevention trials. NCI-sponsored Phase I, II, and III chemoprevention trials for prostate cancer are underway.

2. RATIONALE AND GENERAL PRINCIPLES

The rationale for chemoprevention as an interventional strategy relates to the natural history of prostate carcinogenesis. The developmental cascade of initiation, promotion, and progression of sporadic prostate cancer is characterized by a long latency phase that lasts 30–40 yr, and corresponds to a biologic continuum of progressive genetic (e.g., loss of heterozygosity on chromosomes 8 and 10), epigenetic (e.g., hypermethylation of GST-P1, loss of p27), and biochemical changes (elevated prostatic-specific antigen [PSA] and IGF-1) and finally phenotypic abnormalities, culminating in precancerous lesions and invasive cancer (Fig. 1).

Clinical, epidemiologic, and histopathologic (autopsy) studies demonstrate that precursor lesions and/or disease-specific markers, for example, high-grade prostatic intraepithelial neoplasia (HGPIN), develop at least a decade before the onset of invasive adenocarcinoma, primarily in the posterolateral aspects of the peripheral zones *(48)*. New evidence for the existence of earlier lesions that precede HGPIN includes atypical adenomatous hyperplasia in the transitional zones and proliferative inflammatory atrophy in the peripheral zones associated with HGPIN.

This natural history of prostate cancer—combined with PSA screening and serial monitoring—provides multiple opportunities for local and systemic interventions that represent preventive interventional niches for agent approval by regulatory agencies (e.g., the Food and Drug Administration) and study populations for definitive chemo-prevention trials.

The public health aspects of prostate cancer (approx 200,000 new cases and 40,000 deaths annually) and the recent trends of reduced prostate specific mortality associated with active PSA screening serve to underscore the value of developing effective preventive interventions that can be applied earlier in the evolution of prostate cancer *(47)*.

One systematic approach is exemplified by the Chemoprevention Research Program of the Division of Cancer Prevention (DCP) at the National Cancer Institute (NCI). This integrated program involves four research areas: rational agent development; intermediate endpoint biomarkers and validated surrogate endpoints; well-defined target cohorts (i.e., high-risk populations with genetic and/or acquired risk); and clinical trial designs guided by the primary hypothesis and the clinical phase of development *(28)*.

Levels of evidence for chemoprevention trials involve sequential evaluation of a promising agent in a prescribed scientific/regulatory schema that begins with testing in preclinical models and then proceeds through traditional clinical trial phases—Phase I (safety and pharmacokinetics), Phase II (clinical/biologic activity), Phase III (efficacy and safety), and Phase IV (pharmacoepidemiology of adverse drug effects).

2.1. Rational Agent Development and Preclinical Models

One of the levels of evidence for selecting agents to be evaluated in patients for primary or secondary prostate cancer prevention is predicated on data derived from preclinical models. The lead may come from epidemiologic studies (e.g., soy isoflavones, lycopene), previous clinical experience in adjuvant and advanced settings (antiandrogens, antiestrogens), secondary endpoint analyses from recent randomized Phase III prevention trials (e.g., vitamin E and selenium), or—increasingly—new molecular pharmacologic, high-throughput, chemical-biologic screens (*ras* farnesylation inhibitors, tyrosine kinase inhibitors). Regardless of the setting, promising agents are tested for antitumor activity (efficacy) in vitro in prostate cell lines and in vivo in rodent models of prostate cancer.

A summary of recent in vitro studies using human prostatic epithelial cell lines from investigator-initiated and contract research supported by the DCP is shown in Table 1. A summary of recent in vivo studies using rodent models of prostate cancer supported by the DCP is shown in Table 2.

2.2. Promising Chemopreventive Agents in Clinical Trials

There are more than a dozen classes of novel agents in clinical trials (shown in Table 3) that hold promise as modulators of promotion and progression and, thus, for preventing the development of early invasive prostate cancer and/or clinically aggressive cancer *(34,29)*. Several agents are being evaluated in Phase III treatment trials, for example, bicalutamide, luteinizing hormone-releasing hormone agents, selective estrogen-receptor modulator-3, 545416, vitamin D analogs, 9-cis-retinoic acid, tarqretin, and glitazones. Some of these agents are being evaluated in nonprostate epithelial targets. Such agents include cyclooxygenase-2 (COX-2) inhibitors, which are being evaluated in precancerous lesions of the colon, bladder, esophagus, and skin; difluoromethylornithine (DFMO), which is being evaluated in precancerous lesions of the colon, bladder, breast,

Table 1
In Vitro Screening of Chemoprevention Agents in Human Cells[a][b]

HPV-18 Immortalized High-Grade Prostatic Epithelial Neoplasia (HGPIN) Cells		
Agent	Effect	Dose
Oltipraz	Blockage of EGF, bEGF, and IGF-1 stimulated growth	10 µL
Genistein	Blockage of EGF, bEGF, and IGF-1 stimulated growth	40 µL
13-*cis*-Retinoic acid	Blockage of EGF, bEGF, and IGF-1 stimulated growth	1 µ*M*
Oltipraz	Blocked growth by >85% after 72 h	10 µL (IC50 = 1–5 µ*M*)
Genistein	Blocked growth by >85% after 72 h	40 µM (IC50 = 20 µ*M*)
ATRA	Blocked growth by >85% after 72 h	1 µ*M* (IC50 = 0.1 µ*M*)
13-*cis*-Retinoic acid	Blocked growth by >85% after 72 h	1 µ*M* (IC50 = 0.1 µ*M*)
Oltipraz	Apoptosis	(LD50 = 20 µ*M*)
Genistein	Apoptosis	(LD50 = 1 µ*M*)
13-*cis*-Retinoic acid	Apoptosis	(LD50 = 3 µ*M*)
4-HPR	Apoptosis	(LD50 = 1 µ*M*)

[a]Conducted under contracts NCI-CN-55137 and NCI-CN-75122.
[b]Key: ATRA = all-trans-retinoic acid; EGF = epidermal growth factor; IGF = insulin-like growth factor; 4-HPR = *N*-(4-hydroxyphenyl) retinamide.

and cervix; and *N*-(4-hydroxyphenyl)retinamide (4-HPR), which is being evaluated in the bladder, breast, skin, and cervix.

2.3. Endpoints and Biomarkers in Chemoprevention Trials

Endpoints used in chemoprevention trials are guided by the level of scientific regulatory evidence required in the clinical phase of development. Clinical evaluation is divided into three sequential phases. In Phase I, standard endpoints are safety (maximum tolerated dose), pharmacologic (pharmacokinetics, including bioavailability, biodistribution to the target organ, clearance, and limited pharmacodynamics related to the mechanism of action [e.g., inhibition of prostaglandins]), and modulation of selected intermediate endpoint biomarkers (proliferation, apoptosis, change in PSA). In Phase II (hypothesis-generating), standard endpoints are demonstration of dose-dependent modulation of intermediate endpoint biomarkers (IIA) and modulation/correlation of biomarkers with histologic regression (IIB). In Phase III (hypothesis testing), standard endpoints are substantiation of clinical benefit through either reduction in cancer incidence and/or modulation of a surrogate endpoint (SE) and validation of this SE. Furthermore, quality-of-life parameters—both global and disease-specific instruments—are becoming important endpoints and outcome measures in chemoprevention trials.

Table 2
Agents Evaluated for Efficacy in the Prevention of Prostate Cancer in the WU[a] Rat[b]

Agent	Dose Levels (mg/kg diet)	Activity	Reference
9-*cis*-Retinoic acid	100	Active	McCormick et al.,
	50	Active	1999 *(37)*
9-*cis*-Retinoic acid (delayed administration)	100	In progress	—
Dehydroepiandrosterone	2,000	Active	McCormick et al.,
	1,000	Active	1995 *(35)*
Dehydroepiandrosterone (delayed administration)	2,000	Active	Rao et al., 1997 *(44)*
Liarozole fumarate	160	Marginal	Rao et al., 1996
	120	Marginal	*(43)*
N-(4-hydroxyphenyl)retinamide	391	Inactive	McCormick et al., 1998 *(36)*
L-Selenomethionine	3.0	Inactive	McCormick et al.,
	1.5	Inactive	1999 *(37)*
DL-α-Tocopherol acetate	4,000	Inactive	McCormick et al.,
	2,000	Inactive	1999 *(37)*
α-Difluoromethylornithine	2,000	Inactive	Rao et al., 1996
	1,000	Inactive	*(43)*
Oltipraz	250	Inactive	Rao et al., 1996
	125	Inactive	*(43)*

[a]Key: WU = Wistar-Unilever.
[b]Reprinted with permission from *Eur. Urol.* 1999. **35:** 464–467 (Karger).

Currently, several classes of intermediate endpoint biomarkers, listed in Table 4, are being evaluated as candidate SEs and prognostic factors *(29,33)*. These include: histologic markers, such as HGPIN, and histomorphometric parameters identified by computer-assisted image analysis (CAIA), such as nuclear chromatin texture features; tissue/cellular features, such as proliferation index, apoptotic index, and angiogenesis; molecular/genetic features, such as expression of oncogene/tumor suppressor genes and receptors (p53, bcl-2, c-erb-b2); *(4)* biochemical alterations in secreted proteins, (serum PSA free/total, IGF-1, IGF-binding protein [BP]-3); and markers of oxidative stress (oxidation products of DNA, lipids, and protein) that can be detected in various body fluids, including serum, peripheral blood leukocytes, and urine, and in the breath.

2.4. Validation of Surrogate Endpoints and Accelerated Agent Approval

The rationale for using SEs, expressed whenever possible as continuous variables, in contrast to clinical discrete endpoints such as cancer incidence or time to events (i.e., disease-free survival and mortality), relates to efficiency and economics. SE can reduce sample size and shorten study duration, and may improve the precision of estimates of the treatment effect. Validation of an SE can be achieved in the context of a Phase III randomized, controlled trial in which the primary clinical endpoint is closely correlated with the candidate SE and the relationship to pathogenesis is understood.

Table 3
Natural and Synthetic Agents for Prostate Cancer Chemoprevention[a]

Agent	Class/mechanism	Clinical phase of development
Finasteride	Antiandrogen ($\downarrow$ DHT)	III
Analogs	Steroid 5-α-reductase inhibitor (type 1 and 2)	I, II
Flutamide	Antiandrogen	II
Bicalutamide	Androgen receptor blockade	III*
LHRH agents	Medical castration	II, III*
Tamoxifen	Selective estrogen receptor modulators	II, III
Toremifene	Estrogen receptor isotypes	II, III*
SERM-3	(α, β)	I, II, III*
Selenium	Antioxidant	II, III
— L-selenomethionine	Glutathione peroxidase	
— Selenized yeast	(proapoptosis)	
Vitamin E (D-α-tocopherol)	Antioxidant (lipid peroxidation)	I, II, III
Lycopene (carotenoid)	Antioxidant	I, II
Genistein	Soy isoflavones	I, II
Daidzein	(tyrosine kinase inhibitors)	I, II
SU-101/5416	Tyrosine kinase inhibitors (antiangiogenesis-PDGF, VEGF)	I, II,III*
Tea extracts	Green tea polyphenols	I, II
Epigallocatechin gallate	(antiinitiation/promotion)	
Dithiolethiones	Phase 2 enzyme inducers	I, II
Sulforaphane	(modulators of GSH and GSTs)	
N-acetyl-l-cysteine		
Difluoromethylornithine	Antiproliferation (ornithine decarboxylase inhibitor)	I, II, III
Vitamin D/analogs	Differentiation inducer	I, II, III*
(1-α-hydroxyvitamin D$_2$	(vitamin D receptor [RXR])	
9-*cis*-Retinoic acid	Retinoid RAR/RXR ligand	I, II, III*
Targretin	Selective RXR ligand	I, II, III*
Sulindac sulfone	NSAID metabolite	I, II, III
Celecoxib	COX-2 inhibitor	II, III
R-Flurbiprofen	NSAID isomer (proapoptosis)	I, II
SCH66336	*Ras* inhibitors	I, II
FTI-276	(farnesyl transferase)	
L-744832		
Perillyl alcohol/analogs	Monoterpenes (proapoptosis)	I, II
Rezulin (glitazones)	Thiazolidinedione analogs (PPAR γ)	II, III*
4-HPR	Insulin dependent growth factor-1	I, II, III
Tamoxifen	modulation	
Vitamin D analogs		

[a]Key: COX-2 = cyclooxygenase-2; DHT = dihydrotestosterone; GSH = glutathione; GST = glutathione-*S*-transferase; 4-HPR = *N*-(4-hydroxy-phenyl)retinamide; LHRH = luteinizing hormone-releasing hormone; NSAID = nonsteroidal antiinflammatory drug; PDGF = platelet-derived growth factor; PPAR = peroxisome proliferation activation receptor; RAR = retinoic acid receptor; RXR = retinoic acid X receptor; SERM = selective estrogen receptor modulator; VEGF = vascular endothelial growth factor.
*Refers to Phase III treatment trials.

Table 4
Intermediate Endpoint Biomarkers for Prostate Cancer[a]

Class	Biomarker
Histologic	Field changes (malignancy-associated changes; CAIA)
	Precursor dysplastic lesions (AAH, PIA)
	Intraepithelial neoplasia (HGPIN)
Cellular	Proliferation (Ki-67, PCNA, BrdU)
	Apoptosis (apoptotic bodies, bcl-2/bax, PARP-3)
	Differentiation (cytokeratins, PSA)
	Angiogenesis (VEGF, BFGF/receptors, CD31/34, PSMA)
	Telomerase
Molecular/	Gene mutations and loci (P53, 8P, HPC-1, HPC-X)
Genetic	Gene alterations (hypo-hypermethylation of GSTs)
	Chemical DNA adducts
	Differential gene expression (cDNA microarrays)
	Modified protein expression (proteomics)
Biochemical/	Blood or tissue levels of antigens (PSA, HK-2)
Regulatory	Markers of oxidative stress (DNA, lipids, proteins)
Factors	Growth factors/receptors (IGF-1/IGFBP-3, TGFs, EGFR, c-erb-2)
	Enzyme activity/products (ODC/polyamines, COX-2/prostaglandins)
	Nuclear receptors (AR, ER, RAR/RXR, PPAR)
Noninvasive	TRUS (PSA density)
Radioimaging	MRI/MRS (metabolic profiles of choline/citrate ratios)

[a]Key: AAH = atypical adenomatous hyperplasia; AR = androgen receptor; BFGF = basic fibroblast growth factor; BrdU = 5′-bromodeoxyuridine; CAIA = computer-assisted image analysis; COX-2 = cyclooxygenase-2; EGFR = epidermal growth factor receptor; ER = estrogen receptor; GST = glutathione-*S*-transferase; HGPIN = high-grade prostatic intraepithelial neoplasis; HK-2 = human kallikrein; HPC = human prostate cancer; IGF = insulin dependent growth factor; IGFBP = insulin dependent growth factor binding protein; MRI/MRS = magnetic resonance imaging/magnetic resonance spectroscopy; ODC = ornithine decarboxylase; PARP-3 = Poly-ADP-Ribose-Polymerase; PCNA = proliferating-cell nuclear antigen; PIA = prostatic inflammatory atrophy; PPAR = peroxisome proliferation activation receptor; PSA = prostate specific antigen; PSMA = prostate specific membrane antigen; RAR = retinoic acid receptor; RXR = retinoic acid X receptor; TGF = transforming growth factor; TRUS = transrectal ultrasound; VEGF = vascular endothelial growth factor.

Once validated, an SE can accelerate new agent registration, because it can serve as the primary endpoint in Phase IIB/Phase III trials as noted in the Code of Federal Regulations 314.510. It is anticipated that incorporation of an SE will facilitate efficient, small (n = 50–200) proof-of-principle trials and, after the development of validated SEs, intermediate-sized (n = 200–1000) definitive chemoprevention trials. At present, incidence reduction Phase III trials are required. Criteria for statistical validation of an SE have been proposed by Prentice *(42)*. The original concept of the SE having to explain the entire treatment effect has evolved toward the use of statistical modeling to estimate the fraction (e.g., 75%) of the observed treatment effect explained by the changes in the SE.

Although HGPIN and serum PSA (PSA velocity) are two potential SEs for prostate chemoprevention trials, neither has been definitively validated. In the case of HGPIN,

Table 5
Study Populations for Primary and Secondary Prostate Cancer Prevention Trials

1. General population: >55 yr, prostate specific antigen (PSA) <3 ng/mL, negative DRE[a]
2. Familial/hereditary (≥ two first-degree relatives)
3. Borderline PSA
4. Persistently elevated PSA and negative biopsy
5. High-grade prostatic intraepithelial neoplasia (two negative serial biopsies within 6 mo)
6. Early prostate cancer (low tumor vol; Gleason score <7; PSA <15)
7. Organ-confined (T1c/T2) high-risk (Gleason score >7; PSA >15)
8. Postradical prostatectomy and rising PSA

[a]Key: DRE = digital rectal examination.

there are technical problems related to sampling of the prostate gland. Repeat sextant biopsies in subjects with known high-risk disease markers such as HGPIN frequently fail to show HGPIN, although they commonly show prostate cancer (35–50% probability of cancer in many series).

In the case of PSA, a clear unequivocal correlation with clinical course—such as reduction in cancer incidence or time to either progression or survival—has been difficult to demonstrate. Although a recently reported clinical trial of the novel nonsteroidal antiinflammatory drug (NSAID) sulindac sulfone showed significant changes in PSA velocity in high-risk subjects with rising PSA after prostate cancer surgery *(41)*, correlation with clinical benefit—such as either time to progression or a delay in medical management—has not yet been observed. Nevertheless, the cohort of subjects with persistently elevated PSA and a negative biopsy could provide a clinical model to correlate changes in PSA velocity and clinical outcomes (incidence of prostate cancer).

2.5. Clinical Cohorts and Target Populations for Chemoprevention Trials

A general schema for target study populations for primary (general population) and secondary (HGPIN) chemoprevention efficacy trials for prostate cancer is shown in Table 5. As previously noted, target populations for chemoprevention trials arise from the biologic continuum underlying prostate carcinogenesis. A series of clinical trial designs incorporating these high-risk cohorts provides a number of excellent opportunities to conduct efficient chemoprevention trials.

2.6. Representative Clinical Models (Cohorts) and Trial Designs

The probability of cancer risk of the target study population is a key parameter that influences the chemopreventive clinical trial design in terms of the choice of the interventional agent (width of the acceptable therapeutic index), control regimen (placebo vs active control), sample size/statistical power, and the primary endpoint (*see* Table 6).

The population-based, primary Prostate Cancer Prevention Trial (PCPT), which compares finasteride to placebo, requires a very large cohort (about 18,000 men greater than age 55 with a PSA < 3 ng/mL and a negative digital rectal examination [DRE]) and an end-of-intervention biopsy to detect the clinical endpoint of a 25% reduction in period prevalence of biopsy-proven prostate cancer in 7 yr with approx 90% power. This relates to the underlying risk probability of prostate cancer in this population,

Table 6
Representative Cohorts and Trial Design for SE and Cancer Incidence Endpoint Chemoprevention in Prostate[a]

Cohort	Study size	Statistical power (α)	Treatment effect	Primary endpoint
Risk based on age >55 yr (PSA <3 ng/mL, negative DRE)	18,000	90% (0.05)	25% Decrease in cancer incidence	Prostate cancer incidence at 7 yr of treatment
Family history of >2, first-degree relatives (PSA <4 ng/mL)	1250	80% (0.05)	33% Decrease in cancer incidence; 33% Decrease in proportion with elevated PSA velocity	5-yr cumulative risk of prostate cancer
PSA >4 ng/mL (no cancer detected on biopsy)	700	80% (0.05)	50% Decrease in cancer incidence; 50% Decrease in PSA trajectory	Prostate cancer incidence at 4–5 yr of treatment
HGPIN (with no cancer detected on two sextant biopsies)	200–450	93% (0.05)	33/40% Decrease in cancer incidence	Prostate cancer incidence at 1–3 yr of treatment
Watchful waiting (Gleason <7, PSA >4)	220	80% (0.05)	50% Decrease in PSA velocity	PSA and time to progression (4–5 yr)
Postradical prostatectomy, rising PSA	130	80% (0.05)	50% Decrease in PSA trajectory	PSA level after 1 yr of treatment and time to progression

[a]All studies randomized, controlled, and blinded.

which is estimated to be about 1% per yr based on data from the Surveillance, Epidemiology, and End Results (SEER) Program *(15)*.

Randomized, controlled trials of an interventional agent, such as the antiandrogen flutamide or selenium in high-risk cohorts with HGPIN, will require only 200–450 subjects to detect the primary endpoint of a 33–40% reduction in period prevalence of biopsy-proven prostate cancer in 1–3 yr with 90% power. The marked reduction in sample size required to detect a clinically significant change in prostate cancer incidence in cohorts with HGPIN relates to the high probability of HGPIN progressing to cancer (e.g., 50% in 2 yr) and its association with a subsequent diagnosis of invasive prostate cancer within the next 1–3 yr *(6)*.

Subjects with persistently elevated PSA and a negative biopsy represent a cohort with intermediate cancer risk. For this cohort, several studies have shown that the probability of a subsequent diagnosis of prostate cancer is in the range of 20–25% over the next 3–5 yr *(27)*. A trial design in this intermediate risk group involving 700–1000 subjects appears sufficient to detect a 45–50% reduction in the period prevalence of biopsy-proven prostate cancer and a 50% reduction in PSA velocity in 4–5 yr with 80–85% power. This latter design offers the opportunity to validate PSA velocity as an SE for cancer incidence reduction in this setting with the caveat that the interventional agent does not have an intrinsic effect on PSA secretion and/or serum PSA levels.

2.7. Rational Combinations and Factorial Designs

The principle of combination therapy is guided by improving the therapeutic index (increasing efficacy and decreasing toxicity) by using lower doses of each agent with different or complementary mechanisms of action and by avoiding overlapping toxicities. Rational combinations include the micronutrients vitamin E and selenium—which will be combined in a 2×2 factorial design (e.g., SELECT—Selenium and Vitamin E Clinical Trial). Factorial designs are especially well-suited to evaluate antioxidant combinations, because the agents can be given together without significant dose modification, and the design allows for study of more than one agent concurrently. In cases where two agents are expected to show at least additive effects, there is a significant gain in power because the effective sample size is doubled for the combination analysis compared with each alone *(8)*.

Clearly, it would be informative to evaluate several doses of each micronutrient (vitamin E and/or selenium and/or lycopene in a randomized, placebo-controlled Phase II trial to define an optimal dosing regimen, explore potential drug-drug interactions (pharmacokinetic and pharmacodynamic), and assess changes in markers of oxidative stress in serum and in the prostate. Other rational combinations include combining an antiandrogen with an antiestrogen, antiproliferative, or proapoptotic agent.

3. ONGOING PHASE I, II, AND III CHEMOPREVENTION TRIALS IN PROSTATE COHORTS

Table 7 lists Phase I, II, and III clinical trials in high-risk prostate cohorts with chemopreventive agents currently sponsored by the DCP. These trials are evaluating more than 12 agents. Phase II proof-of-principle studies predominate. These studies seek to validate that the experimental agent modulates the putative molecular target; for example, selective COX-2 inhibitors modulate COX-2 dependent prostaglandins.

Table 7
NCI Division of Cancer Prevention Sponsored or Funded Prostate Cancer Chemoprevention Trials[a]

Agent	Cohort (treatment period)	Sample size	Endpoints
		Phase I Trials	
Lycopene	Pilot: tomato paste/oil in normal subjects; no control (single dose)	25	Carotenoid pharmacokinetics, safety
Lycopene	Multidose: African-American males with elevated PSA and negative biopsy; placebo control (12 wk)	18	Pharmacokinetics, safety, drug-effect measurements (markers of oxidative stress)
Soy Isoflavones	Single dose: normal subjects; no control	30	Pharmacokinetics, safety, MTD
Soy Isoflavones	Multidose: normal subjects, stage C or D prostate cancer patients; placebo control (3 mo)	30	Multidose pharmacokinetics, safety, PSA
		Phase II Trials	
DFMO	Scheduled for prostatectomy (stage A or B prostatic carcinoma or bladder cancer without prostatic carcinoma and scheduled for cystprostatectomy); observation control (14 d)	25	Drug effect measurements—ODC activity (skin and prostate), polyamine levels (prostate); histopathology (TRUS-guided biopsies)
DFMO± Flutamide (2 × 2 design)	Scheduled for prostate cancer surgery or brachytherapy; observation control (4–8 wk)	30	Histopathology, polyamine levels, nuclear polymorphism, ploidy proliferation biomarkers (PCNA, Ki-67)
Flutamide	Patients with high-grade PIN; placebo control (12 mo)	212	Cancer incidence, PIN grade, nuclear polymorphism, nucleolar size, ploidy; other endpoints—PCNA, angiogenesis, apoptosis, LOH chromosome 8, growth factor, PSA
Flutamide + Leuprolide	Scheduled for radical prostatectomy; observation control (12 wk)	126	PIN grade and incidence, nuclear polymorphism, nucleolar size, ploidy; proliferation biomarkers—S-phase fraction, bcl-2 angiogenesis, apoptosis
Flutamide ± Finasteride, Toremifene	Scheduled for radical prostatectomy; observation control (4–8 wk)	80	PIN grade and incidence, nuclear polymorphism, nuclear size, ploidy; proliferation biomarkers-S-phase fraction, angiogenesis, apoptosis
4-HPR	Scheduled for prostate cancer surgery; placebo control (4–8 wk)	36	Histopathology–PIN grade, nuclear polymorphism, nucleolar polymorphism, ploidy; proliferation biomarkers—PCNA, Ki-67; differentiation biomarkers—Lewis$^\gamma$ antigen; genetic/ regulatory biomarkers—p53, EGFR, TGFα

Agent/Trial	Population; design	N	Endpoints
Selenized Yeast	Watchful waiting (early prostate cancer); placebo control (45 mo)	220	PSA velocity, time to progression
Soy Isoflavones	Scheduled for prostate cancer surgery; placebo control (3–6 wk)	72	Tissue isoflavone levels; intermediate biomarkers—CX43, Rb, p53, p21, bcl-2, bax, cyclin D1, CDK5, CDK6, EGFR, MIB-1, E-cadherin
Vitamin D Analog ($1\alpha D_2$)	Scheduled for prostate cancer surgery; placebo control (4–6 wk)	60	Proliferation (MIB-1), apoptosis (TUNEL), PSA, microvessel density, nuclear morphometry, VEGF, BFGF, TGFβ, PSA, PSMA
COX-2 Inhibitor	Scheduled for prostate cancer surgery; placebo control (6–8 wk)	60	PGE-2 modulation, histology, oxidized DNA bases, apoptosis, proliferation, p21, p27
Soy Protein	Men with rising PSA after prostate cancer surgery; milk protein control (8 mo)	130	PSA velocity, time to PSA failure
Soy Protein	Prostate cancer patients at high risk for biochemical failure postsurgery; milk protein control (2 yr)	220	PSA velocity, circulating prostate-cancer cells (PSM-RT/PCR)

Phase III Trials

Agent/Trial	Population; design	N	Endpoints
Selenized Yeast	Nonmelanoma skin cancer patients, low selenium areas in US; placebo control (4.5 yr)	1312	PSA levels, biopsy-proven prostate cancer, long-term follow-up
l-Selenomethionine	High-grade PIN; placebo control (3 yr)	450	Cancer incidence; intermediate biomarkers—nuclear morphometry, Ki-67, apoptosis
PCPT-1 Finasteride vs Placebo	Normal males, age >55, PSA <3 ng/ml (7 years)	18,500	PCA incidence; Multiple secondary and tertiary endpoints
PCP-2 SELECT Selenium ± Vitamin E ± vs Placebo	Normal males, age >50 (AAM), age >55 (CM), PSA <4 ng/ml 2 × 2 factorial design (7 years)	34,000	PCA incidence; Multiple secondary and tertiary endpoints

[a]Key: AAM = African-American male; BFGF = basic fibroblast growth factor; CM = Caucasian male; DFMO = difluoromethylornithine; EGRF = epidermal growth-factor receptor; LOH = locus of heterozygosity; MTD = minimum tolerated dose; ODC = ornithine decarboxylase; PCA = prostate cancer; PCNA = proliferating-cell nuclear antigen; PGE = prostaglandin E; PIN = prostatic intraepithelial neoplasia; PSA = prostate-specific antigen; PSMA = prostate-specific membrane antigen; TGF = transforming growth factor; TRUS = transrectal ultrasound; VEGF =vascular endothelial growth factor.

Some agents, such as selenium and flutamide, are being evaluated in both Phase II and Phase III trials. Several pilot Phase II trials in high-risk prostate cohorts with chemoprevention agents have been published. These include studies with DFMO *(38)*, 4-HPR *(54)*, finasteride *(11)*, and lycopene (Kucuk, personal communication). The finasteride and lycopene trials were not sponsored by the NCI. It is anticipated that as Phase I/II proof-of-principle studies on advanced prostate cancer are completed for the new generation of noncytotoxic agents, there will be a strong rationale to move these agents into earlier cohorts for chemoprevention-oriented trials. Examples of new noncytotoxic agents include novel NSAIDs (COX-2 inhibitors, sulindac sulfone), *ras* inhibitors, tyrosine kinase inhibitors, isoflavones, and vitamin D analogs.

4. PUBLISHED CLINICAL TRIAL RESULTS

In Phase III trials, the study populations generally are healthy and without symptoms. Large numbers of subjects are required to detect a difference in incidence, because the effect size of prevention is small, and subjects must be followed for many years, because measured outcomes generally include cancer-specific survival, all-cause survival, and quality-of-life. Consequently, Phase III chemoprevention trials require significant economic and human resources *(53,55)*.

Recent findings in two large-scale chemoprevention trials in which prostate cancer was a secondary endpoint—a trial of selenium supplementation for nonmelanoma skin cancer and the Alpha-Tocopherol, Beta-Carotene Cancer Prevention Study (ATBC Study)—suggest that dietary supplements of selenium and vitamin E (α-tocopherol) may prevent prostate cancer *(10,23)*. In men with a history of nonmelanoma skin cancer, selenium supplementation was associated with a marked reduction in the incidence of total prostate cancer ($RR = 0.37$), local disease ($RR = 0.42$), and advanced disease ($RR = 0.27$) after 4.4 yr of supplementation and 6.2 yr of follow-up *(10)*. The protective effect was stronger in patients under 65 yr ($RR = 0.09$) than in patients over 65 yr ($RR = 0.49$). Analysis of follow-up data from the ATBC Study found a 36% decrease in prostate cancer incidence and a 41% decrease in mortality from prostate cancer among men receiving vitamin E *(23)*. Only a 16% decrease in incidence was observed for men receiving a combination of vitamin E and β-carotene; incidence in the β-carotene alone group increased by 20%. However, β-carotene decreased the risk of prostate cancer by 32% among nondrinkers, whereas the risk among drinkers increased 25%, 42%, and 40% by tertiles. It is unclear how alcohol might influence a protective effect of β-carotene. In the ATBC Study, a protective effect of vitamin E was evident in clinical prostate cancer, but not in latent cancer—suggesting a role for vitamin E in the transformation of latent cancer *(23)*. Also, there were no significant associations between baseline serum vitamin E or dietary vitamin E or selenium—independent of vitamin E supplementation—and incidence of prostate cancer in the group as a whole *(22)*. Further clinical trials are needed to confirm the promising results for selenium and vitamin E found in these studies.

5. FUTURE DIRECTIONS IN PREVENTION RESEARCH

5.1. Large, Population-Based Phase III Prevention Trials

There is increasing evidence to justify a new large, population-based, Phase III primary prostate cancer chemoprevention trial. The Southwest Oncology Group (SWOG) is starting the intergroup SELECT trial, which will involve more than 32,000 men (white men over age 55 and African-American men over age 50 with normal PSA values) and randomize subjects in a 2×2 factorial design to daily supplements of vitamin E (400 IU) and/or selenium (200 mcg) and/or placebos for vitamin E and selenium. The trial is projected to last about 12 yr, including 7 yr of intervention and follow-up, with a primary endpoint of biopsy-proven prostate cancer based on clinical management practices and not on mandatory guidelines for exit biopsies as required in PCPT. Either a positive or a negative result will have profound implications for public-health prevention policy, as millions of health-conscious American men already use these dietary supplements.

Recent experience with β-carotene and lung cancer chemoprevention trials—in which the results showed an increase and not the expected decrease in lung cancer—illustrates the importance of prospectively testing the two-sided hypothesis that antioxidant micronutrients bring about the presumed beneficial effects and do not cause harm or have unanticipated negative clinical sequelae.

To further complement the large SELECT trial, the DCP plans to sponsor several short-term Phase II trials with selenium and/or vitamin E and/or lycopene to determine the biologic effects on markers of oxidative stress in high-risk cohorts, such as subjects with elevated PSA and negative biopsy. These short-term studies should foster improved ancillary studies for translational research in the large SELECT trial.

5.2. New Imaging Technologies, Functional Genomics, and Mathematical Modeling

Future prospects for translational science in chemoprevention research are extremely promising, thanks to the advances in biomedical engineering (CAIA), molecular genetics (DNA chip microarrays), proteomics (two-dimensional gels), and noninvasive medical imaging (magnetic resonance imaging [MRI]/magnetic resonance spectroscopy [MRS]). These new technologies will have a major impact on study design and cohort selection, biologic specimen sample processing, and the ability to categorize, stratify, and validate new intermediate endpoint markers with functional relevance.

Important advances are being made in histomorphometry (nuclear morphometry) using sophisticated computer algorithms combined with integrated workstations that consist of a microscope, camera, and personal computer. Histopathologic-derived parameters defined by CAIA represent an extension of the pathologist in quantitating the nuclear features of the precancer/cancer phenotype. Bartels and others (*3–5,56*) have now described malignancy-associated changes (MACs) in normal-appearing secretory epithelia of prostatic acini and ducts in prostates that harbor HGPIN and coexisting adenocarcinoma. These results suggest that the ability to detect and quantify MACs will improve the diagnostic accuracy, precision, and predictive value of sextant biopsies of the prostate and may allow for enhanced monitoring of biologic responses to chemopreventive agents.

The rapid emergence of new DNA microchip technology using cDNA probes and oligonucleotide arrays of expressed genes is revolutionizing the molecular assessment of multiplex gene expression. The NCI, through its Cancer Genome Anatomy Project (CGAP), is a major driving force in this research area (*2*). The overall aim of CGAP is to develop a user-friendly computer database that contains a complete catalog of all the genes expressed in cancer cells (tumor gene index). Expression libraries and databases of prostate specific expressed genes and sequences now exist that reflect the biologic continuum from normal to HGPIN to invasive prostate cancer *(50)*.

Chemoprevention applications of CGAP and DNA microchips include assessment of the patterns of differential gene expression in normal, premalignant, and cancer cells for risk stratification and histologic classification, as well as for monitoring the ability of chemopreventive agents to modulate gene expression *(14)*. This should lead to the development of panels of gene/protein expression arrays for assessing biologic response and predicting the reduction of cancer risk and cancer incidence. Combining the new DNA chip technology with techniques such as laser-capture microdissection, CAIA, and proteomics for acquiring homogeneous populations of cells should further enhance sensitivity, specificity, and predictive value.

Advances in noninvasive functional imaging will have a major impact on early diagnosis, identification of high-risk cohorts, biomarker development, and endpoint assessment for prostate cancer prevention strategies. One of the most promising methods under development involves use of MRI/MRS analyses of metabolite profiles. Recent studies suggest that MRI/MRS using choline-to-citrate ratios can improve early detection and the ability to monitor antitumor responses in early prostate cancer *(31)*. In the future, it may be possible to image and thus quantitate changes in HGPIN lesions. With the future promising more focal therapy—including gene-based intraprostatic strategies—techniques such as MRI/MRS lend themselves to better cohort selection and early detection of biologic response.

To further improve the throughput of new agent evaluation in Phase II, a critical decision point in agent development, Chronin et al. have developed a Bayesian sequential monitoring schema for interim analysis with as few as 30 subjects. The method (stopping rule) is conditioned on the choice of prior treatment effect (modulation of the biomarker) to stop quickly for ineffective agents but more slowly for active agents. Simulation of 50,000 Phase II chemoprevention trials using treatment effect sizes obtained from previous trials suggest that the Bayesian approach is comparable in accuracy, but more flexible and simple to interpret than well-known group sequential methods *(12)*. In essence, application of the new technologies for endpoint assessment such as CAIA, gene chip expression arrays, and MRI/MRS, combined with Bayesian methods, should further enhance the evaluation of new agents for biologic activity and proof-of-principle determination.

5.3. Translation of Chemoprevention Research for Public Health Benefit

The ultimate goal of chemoprevention research, whether directed at prostate cancer or cancers at other sites, is to either identify or develop safe, effective agents that can easily be administered to the general population to prevent clinical disease. However, having such agents as part of our arsenal does not automatically ensure their widespread use for public health approaches to cancer prevention, particularly in individuals who appear to be healthy. It will probably be necessary to convince both the healthcare community and the general population of the practical value of a chemopreventive approach to carcinogenesis in its early stages before clinical symptoms are manifested, similar to the use of calcium supplements to reduce risk for osteoporosis and the use of cholesterol-reducing medication to help prevent cardiovascular disease. We must remember that even men who are the "picture of health" are at risk for prostate cancer—some more than others, as a result of genetic susceptibilities and exposure to various environmental risk factors, including lifestyle choices. Developing methods that will enable clinicians to readily identify and stratify individuals at increased risk for prostate cancer is of critical importance, if we are to optimize the potential public health benefits of a chemopreventive approach to reducing the burden of this disease.

ACKNOWLEDGEMENTS

The authors gratefully acknowledge the excellent technical expertise and advice of Wael Sakr, M.D., and Charles Boone, M.D., in the preparation of Fig. 1.

REFERENCES

1. Ahlbom, A., P. Lichtenstein, H. Malmstrom, M. Feychting, K. Hemminki, and N. L. Pedersen. 1997. Cancer in twins: genetic and nongenetic familial risk factors. *J. Natl. Cancer Inst.* **89:** 287–293.
2. Anonymous. 1997. A catalog of cancer genes at the click of a mouse. *Science* **276:** 1023–1024.
3. Bacus, J. W. and J. V. Bacus. 1994. Quality control in image cytometry, DNA ploidy. *J. Cell. Biochem.* **19:** 153–164.
4. Bartels, P. A. 1992. Computer-generated diagnoses and usage analysis: an overview. *Cancer* **69:** 1636–1638.
5. Boone, C. W., J. W. Bacus, V. E. Steele, and G. J. Kelloff. 1997. Properties of intra-epithelial neoplasia relevant to cancer chemoprevention and to the development of surrogate endpoints for clinical trials. *Proc. Soc. Exp. Biol. Med.* **216:** 151–165.
6. Bostwick, D. G. 1995. High-grade prostatic intraepithelial neoplasia. *Cancer* **75:** 1823–1826.
7. Boyle, P., P. Maisonneuve, and P. Napalkov. 1995. Geographical and temporal patterns of incidence and mortality from prostate cancer. *Urology* **46:** 47–55.
8. Byar, D. and S. Piantadosi. 1985. Factorial designs for randomized clinical trials. *Cancer Treat. Rep.* **69:** 1055–1063.
9. Chan, J. M., M. J. Stampfer, and E. L. Giovannucci. 1998. What causes prostate cancer? A brief summary of the epidemiology. *Semin. Cancer Biol.* **8:** 263–273.
10. Clark, L. C., B. Dalkin, A. Krongrad, G. F. Combs, Jr., B. W. Turnbull, E. H. Slate, et al. 1998. Decreased incidence of prostate cancer with selenium supplementation: results of a double-blind cancer prevention trial. *Br. J. Urol.* **81:** 730–734.
11. Cote, R. J., E. C. Skinner, C. E. Salem, S. Mertes, F. Z. Stanczyk, B. Henderson, et al. 1998. The effect of finasteride on the prostate gland in men with elevated serum prostate-specific antigen levels. *Br. J. Cancer* **78:** 413–418.
12. Cronin, R. A., L. S. Freedman, R. Lieberman, A. L. Weiss, S. W. Beenken, and G. J. Kelloff. 1999. Bayesian monitoring of Phase II trials in cancer chemoprevention. *J. Clin. Epidemiol.* **52:** 705–711.
13. Cussenot, O., A. Valeri, P. Berthon, G. Fournier, and P. Mangin. 1998. Hereditary prostate cancer and other genetic predispositions to prostate cancer. *Urol. Int.* **60:** 30–34.
14. Duggan, D. J., M. Bittner, Y. Chen, and P. Meltzer. 1999. Expression profiling using cDNA microarrays. *Nat. Genet.* **21(Suppl.):** 10–14.
15. Feigl, P., B. Blumenstein, I. Thompson, J. Crowley, M. Wolf, B. S. Kramer, et al. 1995. Design of the Prostate Cancer Prevention Trial (PCPT). *Control. Clin. Trials* **16:** 150–163.
16. Fukutome, K., M. Watanabe, T. Shiraishi, M. Murata, H. Uemura, Y. Kubota, et al. 1999. N-acetyltransferase 1 genetic polymorphism influences the risk of prostate cancer development. *Cancer Lett.* **136:** 83–87.

17. Gann, P. H., J. Ma, E. Giovannucci, W. Willett, F. M. Sacks, C. H. Hennekens, and M. J. Stampfer. 1999. Lower prostate cancer risk in men with elevated plasma lycopene levels: results of a prospective analysis. *Cancer Res.* **59:** 1225–1230.

18. Giovannucci, E. 1998. Dietary influences of 1,25(OH)^2 vitamin D in relation to prostate cancer: a hypothesis. *Cancer Causes Control* **9:** 567–582.

19. Giovannucci, E. 1999. Tomatoes, tomato-based products, lycopene, and cancer: review of the epidemiologic literature. *J. Natl. Cancer Inst.* **91:** 317–331.

20. Giovannucci, E., E. B. Rimm, A. Wolk, A. Ascherio, M. J. Stampfer, G. Colditz, et al. 1998. Calcium and fructose intake in relation to risk of prostate cancer. *Cancer Res.* **58:** 442–447.

21. Haenszel, W. and M. Kurihara. 1968. Studies of Japanese migrants: I. Mortality from cancer and other diseases among Japanese in the United States. *J. Natl. Cancer Inst.* **40:** 43–68.

22. Hartman, T. J., D. Albanes, P. Pietinen, A. M. Hartman, M. Rautalahti, J. Tangrea, et al. 1998. The association between baseline vitamin E, selenium, and prostate cancer in the Alpha-Tocopherol, Beta-Carotene Cancer Prevention Study. *Cancer Epidemiol. Biomark. Prev.* **7:** 335–340.

23. Heinonen, O. P., D. Albanes, J. Virtamo, P. R. Taylor, J. K. Huttunen, A. Hartman, et al. 1998. Prostate cancer and supplementation with α-tocopherol and β-carotene: Incidence and mortality in a controlled trial. *J. Natl. Cancer Inst.* **90:** 440–446.

24. Ingles, S. A., R. K. Ross, M. C. Yu, R. A. Irvine, G. La Pera, R. W. Haile, et al. 1997. Association of prostate cancer risk with genetic polymorphisms in vitamin D receptor and androgen receptor. *J. Natl. Cancer Inst.* **89:** 166–170.

25. Ingles, S. A., G. A. Coetzee, R. K. Ross, B. E. Henderson, L. N. Kolonel, L. Crocitto, et al. 1998. Association of prostate cancer with vitamin D receptor haplotypes in African-Americans. *Cancer Res.* **58:** 1620–1623.

26. Jacobsen, B. K., S. F. Knutsen, and G. E. Fraser. 1998. Does high soy milk intake reduce prostate cancer incidence? The Adventist Health Study (United States). *Cancer Causes Control* **9:** 553–557.

27. Keetch, D. W., W. J. Catalona, and D. S. Smith. 1994. Serial prostate biopsies in men with persistently elevated serum prostate-specific antigen values. *J. Urol.* **151:** 1571–1574.

28. Kelloff, G. J., R. Lieberman, M. K. Brawer, E. D. Crawford, F. Labrie, and G. J. Miller. 1999. Strategies for chemoprevention of prostate cancer. *Prostate Cancer and Prostate Diseases* **2:** 27–33.

29. Kelloff, G. J., R. Lieberman, V. E. Steele, C. W. Boone, R. A. Lubet, L. Kopelovitch, et al. 1999. Chemoprevention of prostate cancer: concepts and strategies. *Eur. Urol.* **35:** 342–350.

30. Kolonel, L. N., A. M. Y. Nomura, and R. V. Cooney. 1999. Dietary fat and prostate cancer: current status (review). *J. Natl. Cancer Inst.* **91:** 414–428.

31. Kurhanewicz, J., D. B. Vigneron, H. Hricak, P. Narayan, P. Carroll, and S. Nelson. 1996. Three-dimensional H-1 MR spectroscopic imaging of the *in situ* human prostate with high (0.24-0.7-cm3) spatial resolution. *Radiology* **198:** 795–805.

32. Lee, M. M., R.-T. Wang, A. W. Hsing, F.-L. Gu, T. Wang, and M. Spitz. 1998. Case-control study of diet and prostate cancer in China. *Cancer Causes Control* **9:** 545–552.

33. Lieberman, R., J. A. Crowell, E. T. Hawk, C. W. Boone, C. C. Sigman, and G. J. Kelloff. 1998. Development of new cancer chemopreventive agents: role of pharmacokinetic/pharmacodynamic and intermediate endpoint biomarker monitoring. *Clin. Chem.* **44:** 420–427.

34. Lieberman, R., J. Thompson, H. Akaza, P. Greenwald, and W. Fair. 1999. Progress in new chemopreventive agent development for prostate cancer prevention: modulators of promotion and progression. *Prostate Cancer and Prostate Diseases* (in press).

35. McCormick, D. L., K. V. N. Rao, M. C. Bosland, V. E. Steele, R. A. Lubet, and G. J. Kelloff. 1995. Inhibition of rat prostatic carcinogenesis by dietary dehydroepiandrosterone but not by N-(4-hydroxy-phenyl)-all-*trans*-retinamide. *Proc. Am. Assoc. Cancer Res.* **36:** 126.

36. McCormick, D. L., K. V. N. Rao, L. Dooley, V. E. Steele, R. A. Lubet, G. Kelloff, et al. 1998. Influence of *N*-methyl-*N*-nitrosourea, testosterone, and *N*-(4-hydroxyphenyl)-all-*trans*-retinamide on prostate cancer induction in Wistar-Unilever rats. *Cancer Res.* **58:** 3282–3288.

37. McCormick, D. L., K. V. N. Rao, V. E. Steele, R. A. Lubet, G. J. Kelloff, and M. C. Bosland. 1999. Chemoprevention of rat prostate carcinogenesis by 9-*cis*-retinoic acid. *Cancer Res.* **59:** 521–524.

38. Messing, E. M., R. R. Love, K. D. Tutsch, A. K. Verma, J. Douglas, M. Pomplun, et al. 1999. Low-dose difluoromethylornithine and polyamine levels in human prostate tissue. *J. Natl. Cancer Inst.* **91:** 1416–1417.

39. Muir, C. S., J. Nectoux, and J. Staszewski. 1991. The epidemiology of prostatic cancer: geographical distribution and time-trends. *Acta. Oncol.* **30:** 133–140.

40. Parkin, D. M., P. Pisani, and J. Ferlay. 1999. Estimates of the worldwide incidence of 25 major cancers in 1990. *Int. J. Cancer* **80:** 827–841.

41. Pound, C. R., A. W. Partin, M. A. Eisenberger, D. W. Chan, J. D. Pearson, and P. Walsh. C. 1999. Natural history of progression after PSA elevation following radical prostatectomy. *JAMA* **281:** 1591–1597.

42. Prentice, R. 1989. Surrogate endpoints in clinical trials: definitive operational criteria. *Stat. Med.* **8:** 431–442.

43. Rao, K. V. N., D. L. McCormick, M. C. Bosland, V. E. Steele, R. A. Lubet, and G. J. Kelloff. 1996. Chemopreventive efficacy evaluation of liarozole fumarate, difluoromethylornithine, and oltipraz in the rat prostate. *Proc. Am. Assoc. Cancer Res.* **37:** 273.

44. Rao, K. V. N., M. C. Bosland, R. A. Lubet, V. E. Steele, G. J. Kelloff, and D. L. McCormick. 1997. Inhibition of rat prostate carcinogenesis by delayed administration of dehydroepiandrosterone. *Proc. Am. Assoc. Cancer Res.* **38:** 580.

45. Rebbeck, T. R., A. H. Walker, J. M. Jaffe, D. L. White, A. J. Wein, and S. B. Malkowicz. 1999. Glutathione *S*-transferase-μ (*GSTM1*) and -θ (*GSTM1*) genotypes in the etiology of prostate cancer. *Cancer Epidemiol. Biomark. Prev.* **8:** 283–287.

46. Ries, L. A. G., C. L. Kosary, B. F. Hankey, B. A. Miller, L. Clegg, and B. K. Edwards. 1999. SEER Cancer Statistics Review, 1973–1996. National Cancer Institute, Bethesda, MD.

47. Roberts, R. O., E. J. Bergstralh, S. K. Katusic, M. M. Lieber, and S. J. Jacobsen. 1999. Decline in prostate cancer mortality from 1980 to 1997, and an update in incidence trends in Olmsted County, Minnesota. *J. Urol.* **16:** 529–533.

48. Sakr, W. A., G. P. Haas, B. F. Cassin, J. E. Pontes, and J. D. Crissman. 1993. The frequency of carcinoma and intraepithelial neoplasia of the prostate in young male patients. *J. Urol.* **150:** 379–385.

49. Shimizu, H., R. K. Ross, L. Bernstein, R. Yatani, B. E. Henderson, and T. M. Mack. 1991. Cancers of the prostate and breast among Japanese and white immigrants in Los Angeles County. *Br. J. Cancer* **63:** 963–966.

50. Strausberg, R., C. A. Dahl, and R. D. Klausner. 1997. New opportunities for uncovering the molecular basis of cancer. *Nat. Genetics* **15:** 415–416.

51. Strom, S. S., Y. Yamamura, C. M. Duphorne, M. R. Spitz, R. J. Babaian, P. Pillow, et al. 1999. Phytoestrogen intake and prostate cancer: a case-control study using a new database. *Nutr. Cancer* **33:** 20–25.

52. Taylor, J. A., A. Hirvonen, M. Watson, G. Pittman, J. L. Mohler, and D. A. Bell. 1996. Association of prostate cancer with vitamin D receptor gene polymorphism. *Cancer Res.* **56:** 4108–4110.

53. Thompson, I. M., C. A. Coltman, O. W. Brawley, and A. Ryan. 1995. Chemoprevention of prostate cancer. *Semin. Urol.* **13:** 122–129.

54. Urban, D., R. Myers, U. Manne, H. Weiss, J. Mohler, D. Perkins, et al. 1999. Evaluation of biomarker modulation by fenretinide in prostate cancer patients. *Eur. Urol.* **35:** 429–438.

55. van der Meijden, A. P. M. 1999. Practical aspects of clinical trials on chemoprevention of prostate cancer. *Eur. Urol.* **35:** 515–518.

56. Veltrie, R. W., M. C. Miller, A. W. Partin, D. S. Coffey, and J. I. Epstein. 1996. Ability to predict biochemical progression using Gleason score and a computer-generated quantitative nuclear grade derived from cancer cell nuclei. *Urology* **48:** 685–691.

57. Yip, I., W. Aronson, and D. Heber. 1996. Nutritional approaches to the prevention of prostate cancer progression, in *Dietary Fats, Lipids, Hormones, and Tumorigenesis* (Heber, D. and D. Kritchevsky, eds.), Plenum Press, NY, pp. 173–181.

58. Yoshizawa, K., W. C. Willett, S. J. Morris, M. J. Stampfer, D. Spiegelman, E. Rimm, et al. 1998. Study of prediagnostic selenium level in toenails and the risk of advanced prostate cancer. *J. Natl. Cancer Inst.* **90:** 1219–1224.

59. Yu, H., R. E. Harris, Y.-T. Gao, R. Gao, and E. L. Wynder. 1991. Comparative epidemiology of cancers of the colon, rectum, prostate and breast in Shanghai, China, versus the United States. *Int. J. Epidemiol.* **20:** 76–81.

INDEX